MUNRO'S
Statistical Methods
for Health Care Research

SIXTH EDITION

Stacey Plichta Kellar, ScD, CPH
Professor
CUNY School of Public Health at Hunter College
New York, New York

Elizabeth A. Kelvin, PhD, MPH
Assistant Professor
CUNY School of Public Health at Hunter College
New York, New York

 Wolters Kluwer | Lippincott Williams & Wilkins
Health
Philadelphia · Baltimore · New York · London
Buenos Aires · Hong Kong · Sydney · Tokyo

Acquisitions Editor: Hilarie Surrena
Product Manager: Eric Van Osten
Editorial Assistant: Jacalyn Clay
Design Coordinator: Joan Wendt
Illustration Coordinator: Brett MacNaughton
Manufacturing Coordinator: Karin Duffield
Prepress Vendor: SPi Global

6th edition

Library of Congress Cataloging-in-Publication Data
Kellar, Stacey Plichta, 1965-
  Munro's statistical methods for health care research / Stacey Plichta Kellar, Elizabeth A. Kelvin. — 6th ed.
    p. ; cm.
  Statistical methods for health care research
  Rev. ed. of: Statistical methods for health care research / Barbara Hazard Munro. 5th ed. c2005.
  Includes bibliographical references and index.
  ISBN 978-1-4511-8794-6
  1. Nursing—Research—Statistical methods. 2. Medical care—Research—Statistical methods. I. Kelvin, Elizabeth A. II. Munro, Barbara Hazard. Statistical methods for health care research. III. Title. IV. Title: Statistical methods for health care research.
  [DNLM: 1. Health Services Research—methods. 2. Statistics as Topic. WA 950]

RT81.5.M86 2012
610.72'7—dc23
                                                                                              2011027645

Care has been taken to confirm the accuracy of the information presented and to describe generally accepted practices. However, the authors, editors, and publisher are not responsible for errors or omissions or for any consequences from application of the information in this book and make no warranty, expressed or implied, with respect to the currency, completeness, or accuracy of the contents of the publication. Application of this information in a particular situation remains the professional responsibility of the practitioner; the clinical treatments described and recommended may not be considered absolute and universal recommendations.

The authors, editors, and publisher have exerted every effort to ensure that drug selection and dosage set forth in this text are in accordance with the current recommendations and practice at the time of publication. However, in view of ongoing research, changes in government regulations, and the constant flow of information relating to drug therapy and drug reactions, the reader is urged to check the package insert for each drug for any change in indications and dosage and for added warnings and precautions. This is particularly important when the recommended agent is a new or infrequently employed drug.

Some drugs and medical devices presented in this publication have Food and Drug Administration (FDA) clearance for limited use in restricted research settings. It is the responsibility of the health care provider to ascertain the FDA status of each drug or device planned for use in his or her clinical practice.

Contributors

Jane K. Dixon, PhD
Professor
Yale University School of Nursing
New Haven, Connecticut

Anne E. Norris, PhD, RN, FAAN
Professor
College of Nursing
University of Central Florida
Orlando, Florida

Laurel S. Garzon Shepherd, PhD, PNP
Graduate Program Director
School of Nursing
Old Dominion University
Norfolk, Virginia

Emily Greene, MPH
Doctoral Student
Epidemiology Department
Columbia University
New York, New York

 This text makes extensive use of screen-shot reprints. The authors wish to thank SPPS, Inc., an IBM Company, for its permission to reprint screen-shots of SPSS procedures. All screenshot reprints are Courtesy of International Business Machines Corporation, © SPSS, Inc. SPSS was acquired by IBM in October, 2009. Screenshots appear on pages: 49–52, 101–102, 114–116, 135–136, 140–141, 164–166, 174–175, 193–195, 201–202, 226–227, 236–237, 252–255, 273–275, 277, 300–302, 307–309, 330–331, 385–387.

Reviewers

Diana Avans, PhD
Associate Professor, Lead Chair Natural
Sciences and Mathematics
Vanguard University of Southern California
Costa Mesa, California

Jo Azzarello, PhD, RN
Associate Professor
University of Oklahoma College of Nursing
Oklahoma City, Oklahoma

Wendy P. Blakely, PhD, RN
Associate Professor
Capital University
Columbus, Ohio

Joan Rosen Bloch, PhD, CRNP
Assistant Professor, Division of Graduate
Nursing, Doctor of Nursing Practice
Department
Drexel University
Philadelphia, Pennsylvania

Cecilia Borden, EdD, MSN, RN
Assistant Professor
Thomas Jefferson University: Jefferson School
of Nursing
Philadelphia, Pennsylvania

We are honored to be able to write this latest edition of Munro's Statistical Methods for Health Care Research. This book, now in its sixth edition, has been used by a generation of students in the health care professions. We tried our best to keep to the spirit of Munro by keeping this book user-friendly and accessible to students. We based this book on the organizational framework that Dr. Barbara Hazard Munro developed. In each chapter, you will find sections on the research question, examples from the literature, types of data required, assumptions, details of the specific technique under discussion, and a fully worked out example of how to compute the statistic using SPSS. For the simpler techniques, we have added a fully worked out example of how to compute the statistic by hand. We also updated the software to IBM SPSS 18, which is the latest version of SPSS at the time that this book went to press. The one substantive change that we made in this addition is that we discuss the nonparametric techniques in the same chapter as their parametric analogues, rather than in a stand-alone chapter. For example, we discuss the Mann-Whitney U-test in the same chapter as the independent *t* test. We also felt that the Chi-square test was important enough to merit a chapter of its own.

Text Organization

This book is organized into three sections: Section 1 focuses on obtaining and understanding your data, Section 2 focuses on analyzing the data (largely with bivariate statistics), and Section 3 focuses on model building and presenting your data. Section 1 is an expanded version of the original Section 1; it includes chapters on designing studies, organizing and displaying data, using univariate descriptive statistics, and understanding probability and hypothesis testing. Section 2 includes the first seven chapters of the original Section 2; it includes chapters on specific statistical techniques such as *t* tests, correlations, analysis of variance (ANOVA) models, and the Chi-square. Section 3 includes the chapters in Munro that addressed model building (logistic regression, linear regression, factor analysis, path analysis, and structural equation modeling). We also added a chapter on how to present your data in a poster, professional talk, or journal article.

Acknowledgments

We would like to thank both the users of the previous editions of this book and the reviewers of this newest edition who provided much useful feedback. We also want to thank our students and colleagues at both the City University of New York (CUNY) School of Public Health in Manhattan and at Old Dominion University in Norfolk, Virginia, who have taught us both much about teaching statistics. In particular, we want to thank our graduate students, Emily Greene, Linda McDowell, and Jessica Steier, who provided invaluable assistance in the production of this book. In addition, we would like to thank our editors, Eric Van Osten and Hilarie Surrena as well as the rest of the staff at LWW, who have been with us from the start of this project and are an unending source of support. Finally, Stacey Plichta Kellar would like to express her appreciation for the patience and support of her husband, Bill, and her daughters, Jesse and Samantha, and Elizabeth A. Kelvin would like to thank her parents, Phyllis and Norman, and sister, Jane, for their patience during this project.

Contents

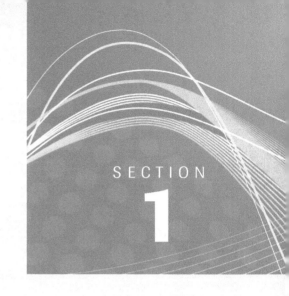

Obtaining and Understanding Data

Using Research and Statistics in Health Care

OBJECTIVES

After studying this chapter, you should be able to:

1. Understand the role of research in developing knowledge for use in evidence-based practice guidelines.
2. Discuss several ways that research can help policymakers.
3. Describe the differences between descriptive and inferential statistics.
4. Compose a study plan for the collection and analysis of data.

HISTORICAL NOTE

Nurses were at the forefront of the movement to use statistics to improve health care. For example, Florence Nightingale (1820–1910) used data from British army files to show how most of the deaths in the British army during the Crimean War (1853–1856) were not caused by direct combat, but rather by illnesses contracted off the field of battle or as a result of unattended wounds. Her statistical analyses convinced the British government to maintain field hospitals and supply nursing care to soldiers. Nightingale passed her passion for statistics on to her namesake, Florence Nightingale David, the eldest daughter of her closest friends. Florence Nightingale David (1909–1993) became a statistician and worked under Karl Pearson. She produced the first edition of Tables of the Correlation Coefficient in 1938. During World War II (1939–1945), she used statistical models to help England prepare for German bombing raids. David later left England for the United States and founded the Statistics Department at the University of California, Riverside in 1970 (Salsburg, 2001).

UNDERSTANDING THE ROLE OF EMPIRICAL RESEARCH

Nurses, allied health personnel, and public health professionals need a solid understanding of how information gained through observation, experience, or experimentation (e.g., empirical knowledge), is generated because evidence-based practice has become the standard by which clinical and public health guidelines are produced (Andrews and Redmond, 2004; McNaughton et al., 2004; Polit and Beck, 2008; Stevens, 2001). The widespread use of clinical guidelines since the 1980s has led to significant improvements in the outcomes of health care (Ahlqvist, Bogren, Hagman, et al. 2006; Brooks, 2004; Penney and Foy, 2007). These guidelines depend on a systematic review of the research evidence (Stevens, 2001), which, in turn, requires a sound understanding of statistics and research methods (Klardie, Johnson, McNaughton, & Meyers, 2004; Meyers, Johnson, Klardie, & McNaughton, 2004). The Cochrane Collaboration produces the largest collection of clinical guidelines (Cochrane Collaboration, 2010). This international nonprofit organization was founded in 1993 to develop and disseminate systematic reviews of health care interventions. In the United States, the U.S. Preventive Services Task Force (U.S. Preventive Services Task Force, 2007) has assumed primary responsibility for developing evidence-based guidelines for health care.

An example of an evidence-based clinical guideline concerns the use of bed rest for back pain (Hagen, Jamtvedt, Hilde, Winnem, 2005). Through a systematic review of the literature, Hagen and coworkers concluded that for people with acute low back pain, bed rest is less effective than staying active. They also concluded that for patients with sciatica, there is little or no difference in outcomes among those who stay active and those who rest in bed. Advances in clinical and public health depend on practitioners such as Hagen and coworkers who

develop guidelines based on empirical research (McCormack, 2003). Taking a leading role in research, however, demands an understanding of how to conduct empirical research, including competency in statistics.

Research can also help policymakers to identify health care problems that may lend themselves to policy solutions. For example, the ongoing nursing shortage is predicted to last for 10 years or more because of a number of demographic, environmental, and professional factors (Auerbach, Buerhaus, & Staiger, 2007). Health care organizations have responded to this shortage by encouraging the immigration of foreign nurses and calling for more graduates from nursing schools (Brush, Sochalski, & Berger, 2004). It appears, however, that some health care organizations are less concerned with the educational level of nurses and more concerned with simply having more nurses of any educational background (e.g., ADN, diploma, BSN).

The question suggested by this solution to the nursing shortage—whether the level of education of nurses in a given hospital affects patient outcomes—was studied by a team of nurse, medical, and sociologic researchers, and the results were published in the *Journal of the American Medical Society* (Aiken, Clarke, Cheung, et al., 2003). The findings of this study indicate that a 10% increase in the proportion of hospital nurses with baccalaureate degrees is associated with a 5% decline in mortality after common surgical procedures. The researchers used advanced statistical models to account for many factors, other than the nurses' education, that might explain the variation in hospital death rates. In addition to the educational preparation of these nurses, the study also took into account how ill patients were on admission, the size of the hospital, the technological capacity of the hospital, whether or not it was a teaching facility, the board certification of the attending surgeons, and patient-to-nurse staffing ratios. Even after statistically controlling for all of these factors, there was a clear positive effect of nurse education level on quality of care. These findings determined that the level of nursing education is critical and that increasing the number of nurses without concern for educational level has serious implications for critically ill patients.

TYPES OF RESEARCH STUDIES AND STATISTICS

Research studies serve many different purposes. Polit and Beck (2008) described the four main purposes of empirical research: description, exploration, explanation, and prediction and control (considered one category). In general, research studies use two different categories of statistics to analyze the data collected: descriptive and inferential. *Descriptive statistics* are simply numerical or graphical summaries of data, and may include charts, graphs, and simple summary statistics such as means and standard deviations to describe characteristics of a population sample. *Inferential statistics* are statistical techniques (e.g., chi-square test, the *t* test, the one-way ANOVA) that allow conclusions to be drawn about the relationships found among different variables in a population sample.

Descriptive Studies and Descriptive Statistics

Studies whose primary purpose is descriptive and explorative simply describe situations and events. These studies use descriptive questions such as: "What is the marital status of people in the United States?" and "What is the average length of stay in the hospital after being admitted for an asthma attack?". Descriptive statistics are typically used to analyze data in order to answer these types of questions (see Chapter 2 for more information about descriptive statistics). Table 1-1 illustrates the use of descriptive statistics to answer the question about the marital status of women in the United States by using data from the 2006-2008 American

Table 1-1	MARITAL STATUS OF U.S. WOMEN AGE 15 YEARS AND OLDER	
Status		**Percent**
Currently married		50.2
Never married		30.8
Divorced		10.6
Separated		2.2
Widowed		6.3

Source: U.S. Census Bureau. (2010). *2006-2008 American Community Survey 3-year estimates. S1201 Marital status*. Retrieved from http://factfinder.census.gov/servlet/STTable?_bm=y&-geo-id=01000US&-qr_name=ACS_2008_3YR_G00_S1201&-ds_name=ACS_2008_3YR_G00

Community Survey (U.S. Census Bureau, 2010). As shown in Table 1-1, the survey found that approximately 50.2% of women were currently married, 30.8% had never married, 10.6% were divorced, 2.2% were separated, and 6.3% were widowed (U.S. Census Bureau, 2010)

Explanatory Studies and Inferential Statistics

Studies that have the primary purpose of elucidating the relationships among variables are considered explanatory studies. Data for such studies are often collected through observational studies, those in which the researcher just collects information about the study participants' current, past or future status regarding the variables of interest without intervening in any way to change their status. The questions answered with these types of statistics are usually more complex than those answered by descriptive statistics. Their questions and lines of inquiry are often based on established theories from the research literature.

Explanatory studies depend on inferential questions such as: "Are women who are sedentary during the third trimester of pregnancy more or less likely to have a cesarean operation than women who exercise regularly during the third trimester?" or

"Do people with health insurance have a longer or shorter hospital stay after being admitted for an asthma attack than people without health insurance?". Explanatory studies do not necessarily attempt to establish causality but often attempt to understand how variables are related to each other. For example, a question might be: "Does length of hospital stay for an asthma attack differ depending on health insurance status?". Inferential statistics are used to examine how one variable is related to other variables; in other words, the relationship among variables (see Chapters 5 to 12 for more information about inferential statistics).

An example of an explanatory study is one conducted by Ludwig-Beymer and Gerc (2002), who examined the relationship between exercise behavior and receiving the flu vaccine in a sample of 999 health care workers. Table 1-2 shows the data from this study in a cross-tabulation table. A cross-tabulation table, sometimes referred to as a cross-tab, is a way to display the relationship between two variables. Table 1-2 shows that 48.1% of the health care workers who exercised regularly received the influenza vaccine compared with 52.4% of those who did not exercise regularly. Even though these numbers are not identical (48.1% versus 52.4%), a statistical test of probability (the chi-square test)

indicates that they are not statistically different, meaning that the two groups did not differ in their likelihood of obtaining the influenza vaccine more than one might expect just due to random chance, and therefore the small difference we see can probably just be attributable to chance rather than to exercise habits (see Chapter 12 for more information about chi-square analysis).

Prediction and Control Studies and Inferential Statistics

Prediction and control studies seek to determine which variables are predictive of other variables and to determine causality (e.g., one event causes another to happen). Data for prediction and control studies are typically collected using quasi-experimental or experimental study designs in which researchers introduce an intervention (e.g., change one of the variables being examined) as these types of studies are thought to have better validity, making causal inference more solid than with purely observational study designs. True experimental designs include random selection and random assignment of study participants to either the intervention group or to one or more control groups that do not receive the intervention. Quasi-experimental

Table 1-2	**RELATIONSHIP OF REGULAR EXERCISE TO OBTAINING A FLU VACCINATION IN 999 HEALTH CARE WORKERS**		
	RECEIVED FLU VACCINATION		
	n (%)	n (%)	Row Totals
Regular Exercise	Yes	No	Number in each gender group
Yes	235 (48.1)	254 (51.9)	489
No	267 (52.4)	243 (47.6)	510
Column totals (number in each vaccination group)	502	497	999

Note: Chi-square $p \leq .18$ (not statistically significant).
Source: Data from Ludwig-Beymer P, & Gerc SC. (2002). An influenza prevention campaign: the employee perspective. *Journal of Nursing Care Quality, 16*(3), 1–12.

designs are similar to experimental designs except that they lack one or more of the following: random assignment to the intervention or control group or, in some cases, a true control group (Polit & Beck, 2008).

Randomized control trials (RCTs) are considered experimental designs because study participants are randomly assigned to an intervention group or a control group and followed forward in time to determine if the intervention impacts on a specific health outcome. However, randomized control trials generally do not select study participants randomly from the population. Instead they have strict eligibility criteria that those interested in participating in the study must meet before they are allowed to participate. Anyone not meeting these eligibility criteria is excluded from the study. This departure from the random selection of study participants from the general population may limit the external validity of the study; in other words, the study results may not be generalizable to the general population.

In health-related research, quasi-experimental designs are often used, but their validity may not be much better than that of observational studies; therefore, experimental studies are considered the gold standard for causal inference. As with explanatory studies, prediction and control studies use inferential statistics to analyze the data and answer research questions about the relationship among variables.

TEN STEPS TO BUILDING A STUDY PLAN

All studies, no matter what the purpose, need to be well-planned. For example, in studies in which many variables are measured, it is easy to lose track of the initial purpose of the study and to generate "results" that appear to be useful. These results, however, are meaningless unless they exist in the context of an organized line of inquiry. Box 1-1 lists some of the common mistakes researchers make when embarking on research projects. These mistakes are often made when there is no study plan or when the plan is insufficiently detailed. Papers resulting from studies that have inadequate study plans often lack focus and clarity. Although several well-known methods for writing a study plan are available, they all follow the same basic principles.

A study plan is a written presentation of how the researcher is going to obtain and analyze the numerical data needed to answer the research questions. A good study plan keeps the analysis focused and relevant. It serves as the basis

---

BOX 1-1 COMMON MISTAKES IN RESEARCH

1. Undertaking a research project without reviewing the existing literature on the subject
2. Collecting data without a well-defined plan, hoping to make sense of it afterward
3. Defining terms in general or ambiguous language
4. Failing to base research on a sound theoretical foundation
5. Failing to make explicit and clear the underlying assumptions
6. Failing to recognize the limitations of the approach
7. Failing to anticipate rival hypotheses that would account for findings and that challenge interpretations and conclusions

Source: Courtesy of Dr. Brenda Nichols, Dean of the College of Arts and Sciences, Lamar University, Beaumont, Texas.

for the introduction and methods section of research papers after the data have been collected and analyzed. A study plan can also serve as the basis for the first sections of a dissertation or thesis. In addition, most grants require study plans similar to the one presented here.

The outline that a study plan should follow is summarized in Box 1-2 and described on this and the following pages. The method presented here is fairly standard, and similar ones can be found in guides to planning research (Ogden and Goldberg, 2002; Wood, 2006). A study plan begins with a statement of the research question(s) that the study is trying to answer (i.e., the purpose of the study) and a short description of the significance or importance of the question(s). The statement of purpose is the guiding force behind the entire research project, and the study should flow from it. A study plan also needs a theoretical or conceptual framework on which research questions and hypotheses are based. This framework presents a structured way of thinking about the interrelationships of the variables. Research questions are either very specific or broadly conceptual. The hypotheses, however, must be very specific because they provide the guide for the analysis of the data. The study plan should define key terms and variables, provide a description of the research design, and describe the sample and

how it was obtained. The plan should also state the statistical techniques that will be used to test each hypothesis. A good study plan lists any major assumptions and limitations of the study being described. And finally, a good study plan contains a brief description of how the findings obtained from the study will be disseminated.

Statement of the Purpose of the study and Its Significance

A study plan starts with a clear explanation of the purpose of the study and the significance of the problem to be studied. This explanation should include the reasons why the study is important and how the study fits into the existing body of research. This section orients researchers and interested readers to the study.

The statement of the problem should be no more than two or three sentences, and should clearly articulate what the study is seeking to accomplish. The rationale for the study should include a brief overview of the epidemiology of the problem being addressed. It should also include a discussion of the monetary and nonmonetary costs of the problem to society, to the health care system, and to people who have the problem. It should also provide a review of other studies in the literature that have examined similar issues. The rationale should then

---

BOX 1-2   TEN-STEP STUDY PLAN

1. Statement of the purpose of the study and its significance
2. Theoretical or conceptual framework
3. Research questions to be answered by the study
4. List of hypotheses to be tested
5. Definitions of key terms and variables
6. Description of the research study design
7. Description of the sample and how it was obtained
8. Description of the statistical analysis
9. Statement of assumptions, limitations, and delimitations
10. Dissemination plan

explain the weaknesses in the literature (e.g., what is not well documented, what is not known at all) and how the current study will add to the existing knowledge base. An example of a statement of the purpose of the study follows:

- *The purpose of the study of maintaining physical behavior is to examine the development of exercise habits over a 12-week period and to test the ability of the theory of planned behavior to predict actual participation in physical activity (Armitage, 2005).*

Theoretical or Conceptual Framework

All studies need to have an underlying framework that organizes the analysis by stating how all of the variables are expected to relate to one another. In writing a thesis or dissertation, this is accomplished by using (and testing) a theoretical model from the research literature. Theses and dissertations typically test and draw conclusions about the validity of theories that already exist in the literature. Even beyond the thesis and dissertation stage, models are vital. Models can keep the analyses organized and coherent. They provide a logical framework that connects the variables to each other and that helps to establish the relative importance of each variable in predicting the outcome. For example, when testing an intervention, the logical model being tested is that the intervention will affect health status or health behavior variables. Other factors, such as age and gender, are also expected to affect health status. A good model provides a framework that outlines the expected relationships among the different variables.

Numerous theories are used in health research. Some of these theories are disease specific, but many are general enough to be applied to numerous diseases. The two models discussed here are examples of theories that can facilitate empirical work: Andersen's model of health care use and the theory of planned behavior.

Andersen's Model of Health Care Use

Andersen's model of health care use postulates that the use of health services is a function of the perceived need for care, predisposing factors (e.g., cultural factors), and factors that enable patients to obtain care (e.g., knowledge, insurance) (Andersen, 1995). For example, in using Andersen's model to study condom use among adolescents, having easy access to condoms is viewed as an "enabling factor." The effect of easy access to condoms on condom use would be examined in the context of other factors discussed in the model, such as predisposing factors (e.g., age, gender) and need factors (e.g., adolescents' perceived need for contraception and/or disease protection).

Theory of Planned Behavior

A theory often used in the research of individual health behavior and behavioral intentions is the theory of planned behavior (Ajzen, 1991). According to this theory, the performance of any behavior depends on behavioral intention. Behavioral intention is viewed as being dependent on behavioral beliefs (e.g., attitude towards the behavior), normative beliefs, and control beliefs. Normative beliefs are beliefs about the expectations of others, and control beliefs are beliefs about the factors that may help or hinder the performance of the behavior. The framework for the study of physical activity discussed earlier by Armitage (2005) is based on this theory. That study found that behavioral beliefs, normative beliefs, and control beliefs all contribute to physical activity behavior.

Research Questions to Be Answered by the Study

Research questions should stem directly from the statement of the purpose of the study and the theoretical framework on which it is based. It is also important to ground research questions in the existing literature. This is where the significance section can be useful. Research questions should be clear about the relationships that are expected. Additionally, the research questions must relate directly to the data that will be collected by the researcher. For example, it does not make sense to have a research question that asks about the relationship of drinking to exercise behavior if data about alcohol use are not collected. Research questions asked in Armitage (2005) are listed below.

Descriptive Questions

- What is the level of intention to engage in physical activity among a group of adults who recently joined a fitness facility?
- What is the actual level of physical activity among a group of adults that recently joined a fitness facility?

Inferential Questions

- Does attitude toward exercise affect participation in physical activity?
- Does the extent to which participants perceive themselves as able to exercise (perceived behavioral control) affect participation in physical activity?
- Do subjective norms affect participation in physical activity?
- Does intention to exercise predict physical activity?

List of Hypotheses to Be Tested

A hypothesis is a tentative prediction or description of the relationship between two or more variables. The purpose of a hypothesis is to translate research questions into predictions of expected outcomes. The hypotheses, therefore, must stem directly from the research questions and be grounded in the theoretical framework

that is chosen. A hypothesis states the expected relationship between the variables. This relationship can be either an association in which no causal effect is presumed or a causal relationship in which one variable (the independent variable) is expected to cause changes in the other variable (the dependent variable). However, it is more common to express hypotheses in terms of association than causation as association requires fewer assumptions.

In some cases, the hypotheses stated are directional, that is, they are specific statements of the direction of the relationship between two variables. The hypothesized direction of the relationship can be either positive or direct (e.g., one variable increases the likelihood of the other variable), or they can be negative or inverse (e.g., one variable decreases the likelihood of the other variable). Directional hypotheses are considered to be one-sided as you are only testing whether or not one variable influences the other variable in one direction (e.g., one side) rather than in either possible direction (e.g., both sides). Sometimes, the hypothesis being tested is non-directional, and only states that the value of one variable is related to, or dependent on, the value of the other variable without stating the direction of the relationship. This non-directional hypothesis is called a two-sided hypothesis as it tests both the probability of a direct and of an inverse relationship. When conducting a one-sided test, the "direction of the relationship" should be based on the chosen theory and findings from previous research. If there are no previous findings, it is permissible to base hypotheses on expert opinion or a sound rationale.

In a research plan, the hypotheses serve as the guide for data analysis. There should be a specific hypothesis for each relationship that is being tested. In a dissertation, it is not unusual, for example, to have numerous hypotheses that are being tested. Of course, many of these can be grouped under headings (e.g., sociodemographic characteristics, physical activity). New researchers should be especially careful to write down each relationship that they plan to test to stay organized and focused. Hypotheses tested by Armitage (2005) include the following:

- Those who perceive themselves as being able to exercise will be more likely to engage in physical activity than those who do not.
- Those who perceive subjective norms that are supportive of exercise are more likely to exercise.
- Those with a positive behavioral intention to exercise are more likely to do so than those without a positive behavioral intention to exercise.

Definitions of Key Terms and Variables

In a research plan, it is important to clearly define key terms and variables. Terms are best defined when they first appear so that readers do not initially make assumptions about definitions only to discover later that different definitions apply. It is especially important to define terms that readers outside the field of study may not understand as intended. And finally, it is important to include units of measure in the definitions.

The variables used in a study must stem directly from the hypotheses. Specifically, variables should measure most, if not all, of the constructs discussed in the conceptual or theoretical model. Furthermore, it should be clearly indicated which variables are independent and which are dependent. Independent variables are those that are manipulated (i.e., by the intervention) or that may affect the outcome. Variables such as age, income, preexisting health conditions, and taking a medication are usually considered independent variables. Dependent variables are the outcomes of interest, in other words those variables that are expected to change in response to the characteristics, exposures or interventions being studied,

such as health status, use of healthcare services, and costs of inpatient stay. Some examples of variables used by Armitage (2005) include the following:

- Self-reported physical activity is defined as the participants' self-report of how many times they participated in physical activity in the past 3 months (rated on a 7-point scale that ranged from never to frequently).
- Perceived behavioral control is defined by averaging responses for four Likert scale items (responses ranged from 1 to 7; higher scores indicate greater levels of perceived behavioral control). The scale items were:
  1. To what extent do you see yourself as being capable of participating in physical activity? (incapable–capable)
  2. How confident are you that you will be able to participate in regular physical activity? (not very confident–very confident)
  3. I believe I have the ability to participate in regular physical activity. (definitely do not–definitely do)
  4. How much personal control do you feel you have over participating in regular physical activity? (no control–complete control).

Description of the Research Study Design

Every study plan must include a description of how the data will be collected (i.e., the design of the study). If secondary data (i.e., existing data) are used, it is likely that the data collection process is described in detail elsewhere, in which case a summary of how the data were collected is provided with a reference to the original source. When collecting original data, however, the study plan must describe in detail exactly how this will be accomplished.

For more detailed information, standard reference texts can be helpful (Babbie, 2007; Cook and Campbell, 1979; Polit and Beck, 2008).

Research design is the art and science of conducting studies that maximize reliability and validity of the findings and minimize bias or error. The research design also ensures that the relationship between the dependent and independent variables can be stated with as much certainty as possible. In addition, the type of research design may determine which types of statistical analysis can be used to examine the data. Each statistical technique makes assumptions about the data, and a good study plan maximizes the extent to which the data meet these assumptions. Details of these assumptions are explained later in the text when statistical techniques are discussed. The choice of design depends on several factors, including the type of problem, research setting, and available resources. Research designs commonly used in health care services research include observational studies, quasi-experimental studies, and experimental studies.

Observational Study Designs

Observational studies are those in which a phenomenon is simply observed and no intervention is instituted. They are appropriate when the purpose of the study is descriptive, when the hypotheses are exploratory, or when it is not possible to manipulate the exposure being studied, for example when the exposure is potentially harmful and therefore cannot ethically be assigned to study participants in an experimental study. The three main types of observational studies are cross-sectional studies, case-control studies, and longitudinal studies (also referred to as "cohort studies").

Cross-sectional studies involve the collection of data on the study participants' current outcome status and exposure status at one point in time. The study participants (the sample) can be selected randomly from the population or the research can use intact groups or convenience samples (e.g., members of a community center). Cross-sectional studies provide only indirect evidence about time order, in other words which variables occurred first. Because of this inability to determine time order, causal statements cannot be made from analyses of cross-sectional data. We cannot know that the presumed cause preceded the presumed outcome from a cross-sectional study.

Case-control studies involve the collection of data about the study participants' current outcome status (e.g., whether or not they have the health outcome being studied) and past exposure status. Although case-control studies provide some evidence that the presumed cause preceded the outcome, due to possible mis-recall of past exposures, most researchers avoid making causal statements from case-controls studies, and instead phrase their conclusions in terms of association rather than causation.

Longitudinal studies (i.e., prospective or cohort studies) are designed to collect data at more than one point in time, following study participants forward in time to identify future outcomes. Because longitudinal studies clearly determine that the presumed cause (the exposure) came before the presumed outcome, they are thought to provide stronger evidence for causation than cross-sectional or case control studies. However, even with longitudinal studies there may be alternate explanations for the associations found and therefore as with other observational study designs, conclusions are usually phrased in terms of association rather than causation.

Quasi-Experimental and Experimental Study Designs

Quasi-experimental and experimental study designs differ from observational study designs in that the researcher is an active agent in the experimental work. Both types of designs are prospective (follow participants forward in time) and involve measurements taken during at least two separate points in time, usually a pretest, or baseline, and a posttest measurement. Both types of designs involve a treatment or some type of intervention applied to some of the participants and a comparison group that does not receive the intervention (i.e., control group). These two groups are then compared in terms of the outcome of interest during the study follow-up. Any differences in the outcome between the two groups may be attributed to the treatment. Controlled experiments also involve the random selection of subjects from the population of interest and the assignment of the intervention being studied in a random fashion. In other words, each study participant has an equal chance of receiving the study treatment.

Quasi-experimental designs lack random selection and/or random assignment of the study intervention. Experimental designs differ from quasi-experimental designs primarily in the amount of control that the experimenter has over external sources of bias and random error, both of which might call into question the validity and reliability of the results. Evidence from experimental studies is considered to be stronger than evidence from both quasi-experimental studies and observational studies. A brief discussion of a study design based on Armitage's research (2005) follows:

- *This is an observational, longitudinal study of adult customers of a newly opened fitness center. All new members were invited to participate in the study. Those agreeing to participate completed a self-administered questionnaire at baseline and an identical questionnaire 3 months later.*

Description of the Sample and How It Was Obtained

The mechanism by which participants are selected to be in a study is a critical part of the research design and is such a complicated topic that it deserves its own section in the study plan. In general, studies attempt to find participants who represent all members of the population of interest because it is generally impossible to gather data from the entire population. For example, researchers interested in obtaining information about women with gestational diabetes may only be able to gather data from the clinic that serves such women. *Sampling* is the process of selecting a portion of the population to represent the entire population. A major consideration in assessing a sample is to make sure it represents the population being studied. It is important to state exactly what the target population is, that is, the group to which the researchers want to generalize the study results. Even with the use of an existing dataset, the study plan should contain an explanation of how people were chosen to be in the study. It should also contain a brief description of the sociodemographic characteristics of the sample.

Sampling can be either random (i.e., probability of being selected is known) or nonrandom (i.e., probability of selection unknown). In nonrandom sampling, convenience or subjective judgment is used to decide who is chosen for the sample. One disadvantage is that it is difficult to determine whether the sample includes members from all relevant segments of the population. Types of nonrandom samples include convenience sampling, snowball sampling, quota sampling, and systematic sampling. Random sampling is the selection of a group of subjects from a population so that each individual is chosen entirely by chance. In equal random sampling, each person in the population has the same probability of being chosen to be in the sample. This is also known as "self-weighted" sampling. Other more complicated random-sampling procedures in which samples are drawn randomly from within population subgroups are sometimes used in studies, particularly in some national surveys. The data from these studies must be analyzed with specialized software that accounts for the differences in the probability of each person's being selected into the study. Using a random sample of the population reduces the chances of bias in the study and increases the external validity, or generalizability of the study results. A short description of sampling from Armitage's research (2005), which employed a convenience sample, follows:

- All study participants were recruited from a single, newly opened fitness facility in the south of England.
- The final sample consisted of 94 new adult customers.
- Customers were 56% male, and the average age was 37.57 years (range, 18–65 years).

Description of the Statistical Analysis

Statistical analysis of the data occurs in four stages. First, the data must be entered into a database on the computer. Second, the data must be "cleaned." Third, descriptive statistics are used to describe the sample in terms of demographic characteristics. Descriptive statistics are also used to examine and describe the dependent and independent variables. Fourth, each hypothesis is listed with the inferential test that will be used to test it. The actual choice of test depends on the study design used to collect the data, the sample size, the measurement scale of the variables in the hypothesis, and the distribution of those variables. The tests chosen initially in the study plan may change as more information about the nature of the variables is obtained.

Data Entry

The very first step before any data analysis can occur involves entering the data into a database. There are a number of database software options which vary in terms of their ease of use. Some software options, such as Excel and SPSS, allow the user to enter data into a spreadsheet,

an interface in which rows represent study participants and columns represent variables. Appendix A contains detailed guidance on how to set up a data entry spreadsheet in SPSS.

Cleaning the Data

Once the data has been entered into a database, cleaning the data involves making certain that all of the variables have valid and usable values. This step is completed by running frequencies on every variable (see Chapter 2) and examining those frequencies carefully for invalid values, unusual values, large amounts of missing data, and adequate variability. For example, if the variable gender has a value of 0 for men and a value of 1 for women, any cases that listed a value of 3 for gender would have to be examined and explained. The frequency distribution of each variable is then checked for unusually large or small values to be sure that they were accurately entered into the database. For example, if a participant's weight is listed as 890 lb, it should be checked to see if it is not actually 89 lb because of a data entry error. In some cases, the paper copies from which the data were entered can be checked for accuracy. In other cases, especially if the study is based on secondary data, the data cannot be checked. All invalid and out-of-range values must then be defined as "system missing" so they will not be included in the final data analysis.

The next step in cleaning data is to check the variables with missing data. If too many participants are missing values for a given variable, the variable may not be usable. Additionally, the variables must be examined for adequate variability within each variable. If almost everyone answers the same way to a specific variable (e.g., if 99% of the group is female), then that variable cannot be used during the analysis because there are no male participants in your study to which you can compare the female participants.

Describing the Sample

The second step in data analysis is to describe the sample characteristics using descriptive statistics. It is common practice to create tables that display sample sociodemographic characteristics, such as age, gender, ethnicity, and education level. These descriptions help readers understand the study population. The overall values and distribution of the key independent and dependent variables are also described (see Chapter 2 for details).

Inferential Statistics Used to Test Each Hypothesis

The third step in data analysis is to list the inferential statistics that will be used to test the hypotheses. The hypotheses, including the independent and dependent variables in each hypothesis, should be clearly stated. The exact test performed to assess each hypothesis depends on the study design, sample size, distribution of the variables (i.e., normal vs. nonnormal), measurement scale of the variables in the hypothesis (nominal, ordinal, interval, ratio), and type of comparisons to be made. In general, nonparametric statistics, which do not require that the variables meet specific assumptions about distribution, are used for small sample sizes and for variables that are not normally distributed, while parametric statistics, which do require that certain distribution assumptions are met, are used for analyses of large sample sizes and with normally distributed variables. These techniques are described in Chapters 5–12. Some study plans may include multivariate statistical analyses to control for confounding variables and to eliminate rival hypotheses. These are discussed in Chapters 13–17.

Statement of Assumptions, Limitations, and Delimitations

Every study has assumptions, limitations, and delimitations, all of which must be stated explicitly. *Assumptions* are statements that are taken to be true even though the direct evidence of the truth is either absent or not well documented. For example, in the exercise study, it is assumed that participants were honest about their level of physical activity. *Limitations* are weaknesses or handicaps that potentially limit the validity of the results. For example, a limitation of the physical activity study is that it uses an intact group (i.e., clients of a single fitness facility) rather than a random sample of clients from several facilities. This may limit the ability of the study to be generalized to others in the population. Note that common limitations in "real-life" outcomes research are often small sample sizes (i.e., samples with fewer than 100 participants), poor response rates (e.g., many of those who were invited to participate in the study declined), poor follow-up rates, lack of random selection, lack of random assignment, and lack of diversity in the sample. *Delimitations* are boundaries in which the study was deliberately confined (e.g., the physical activity study focuses on adults only and did not include adolescents and children).

Dissemination Plan

A study is not truly complete until the knowledge gleaned from the work is disseminated for use. Arguably, the most important part of a research project is sharing the knowledge obtained from the project. Information can be shared in many different forms. First and foremost, the results of the study should be shared with the sites at which the study was conducted to help the sites improve their clinical practice. The results can also be more widely publicized throughout the local area through grand rounds, regional conferences, and newsletters.

A higher level of dissemination occurs when the paper is presented in peer-reviewed arenas (see Chapter 18). These forums include statewide conferences, national conferences, and peer-reviewed publications in professional journals.

Statewide conferences (e.g., annual meeting of the Virginia Public Health Association) typically provide space in which researchers can present their results in a poster format. National conferences (e.g., annual meeting of the American Public Health Association) typically provide opportunities to present research as posters, oral presentations on panels, and roundtables. Publishing in a peer-reviewed journal, however, provides the best way to widely disperse the results of a study. Most peer-reviewed journals are indexed in one or more electronic databases (e.g., Medline, Pubmed, or CINALH). These databases are commonly available at university libraries and on the Internet. Indexing in these databases makes the research available to millions of researchers and policymakers around the world.

CHAPTER REVIEW

Critical Thinking Concept Review

1. Find a peer-reviewed research article and do the following:
   a. Write the problem statement.
   b. Name the theoretical model used or briefly describe the overall conceptual model.
   c. Write out the main research questions. What is the rationale for the question?
   d. List the main hypotheses that the study is testing.
   e. Define the dependent variable and the main independent variables.
   f. Briefly describe the research design.
   g. Describe the sample (e.g., size, sociodemographic characteristics) and how it was obtained.
   h. List the statistics used to test the hypotheses.
   i. Identify the main assumptions and limitations.

2. Describe three studies that were critical to the practice of nursing, an allied health profession or public health practice in the United States.

3. Choose a topic in which you are interested and find (or conceptualize) a dataset related to that topic. State a research problem that can be answered by that dataset and write a 10-step study plan that will allow you to analyze your data.

Computational Problems

I. **Create a Database in SPSS**
   - Open SPSS
   - Go to VARIABLE VIEW (lower left hand corner of the screen)
   - In the field under the column labeled NAME, type the name of your variable (try to keep the name short, such as "ID" or "gender". Variable names must start with a letter)
   - Click on the field under TYPE and select the data type (i.e., date, number, string, which means text). Also you can define the number of digits (width and number of decimal points) that can be entered for that variable. Remember that usually we use numeric codes to stand for nominal data (i.e., 0 for male and 1 for female)

- Under LABEL, type the label for the variable (e.g., "participant ID number")
- Under VALUES you can assign labels to coded categorical data (i.e., 0 = male and 1 = female). Click on the field under VALUES and you will see a box appear. Click on the box. In the pop-up, type the numeric code (i.e., 0) in the VALUE space and the label (i.e., male) in the VALUE LABEL box, then click on ADD. You may add more values in the same fashion. When finished, click on OK.
- Repeat the process for the rest of your variables.

II. Data Entry
  - Click on DATA VIEW and enter the data in the table below, coding gender as "0" for male and "1" for female (e.g., enter "1" for females and "0" for males rather than typing in the word)

ID	Gender (0 = male, 1 = female)	Weight (lbs/kg)	Height (inches/cm)
1	1	150/68.0	65/165.1
2	0	187/84.8	68/172.7
3	0	135/61.2	58/147.3
4	1	167/75.75	64/162.6
5	1	240/108.8	69/175.3
6	1	206/93.4	65/165.1
7	0	128/58.0	64/162.6
8	0	188/85.3	66/167.6
9	0	190/86.2	69/175.3
10	1	134/60.8	67/170.2
11	1	162/73.5	68/172.7
12	0	118/53.5	60/152.4
13	0	212/96.2	64/162.6
14	0	137/62.2	62/157.5
15	0	170/77.1	63/160.0

Organizing, Displaying, and Describing Data

OBJECTIVES

After studying this chapter, you should be able to:

1. Discuss the nature, purpose, and types of statistics available for analyzing data.
2. Recognize and define mathematical symbols commonly used in statistics.
3. Correctly identify the measurement scale of a variable.
4. Explain the relationship between the measurement scale of a variable and the correct statistic to use.
5. Discuss the fundamental principles of data handling.
6. Construct and interpret frequency tables, bar charts, histograms, stem-and-leaf plots, frequency polygons, and cumulative frequency polygons.
7. Describe variables using appropriate measures of central tendency, dispersion, shape, and skewness.
8. Explain the use of percentiles.

THE NATURE OF STATISTICS

Statistics is a branch of applied mathematics that deals with the collection, organization, and interpretation of data by using well-defined procedures. Researchers use various techniques to gather these data, which become the observations used in statistical analyses. Thus, the raw materials of research are data, gathered from a sample that has been selected from a population.

Applying statistics to these data permits the researcher to draw conclusions and to understand more about the sample from which the data were obtained.

Statistics, as a field, uses its own language, including special symbols that represent formulas and other mathematical expressions and specialized terms that describe different types of variables. This chapter introduces and defines some of these specialized terms and symbols.

Symbols and formulas for descriptive statistics vary depending on whether one is describing a sample or a population. A *population* includes all members of a defined group; a *sample* is a subset of a population. Characteristics of populations are called *parameters*; characteristics of samples are called *sample statistics*. To distinguish between them, different sets of symbols are used. Usually, lowercase Greek letters are used to denote parameters, and Roman letters are used to denote statistics. Some of the more commonly used symbols can be found in Table 2-1.

This chapter also introduces descriptive statistics. These are the type of statistics that we use to describe variables by summarizing their values into more understandable terms without losing or distorting too much of the information. Frequency tables, bar charts, histograms, percentages, and measures of central tendency and dispersion are the most common statistics used to describe sample characteristics.

VARIABLES AND THEIR MEASUREMENT

Data are the raw materials of research and provide the numbers upon which we perform statistics. The most common way a researcher acquires data is by designing a study that will allow the collection of information (e.g., data) that will answer a specific research question.

Table 2-1	MATHEMATICAL SYMBOLS IN STATISTICS
Symbol	**Meaning**
Mathematical Functions	
+	Plus
−	Minus
×	Multiply
/	Divide
Σx_i	Sum of the numbers in the variable x; add up all the values of the variable x
Σx_i^2	Sum of the squared x's; square each value of the variable x and then add up all the squared values
$(\Sigma x_i)^2$	Sum of the x's, squared; add up all the values of the variable x and then square the total
<	Less than
≤	Less than or equal to
>	Greater than
≥	Greater than or equal to
=	Equal to
|x|	The absolute value of x
$p(A)$	Probability of event A happening (marginal probability)

(Continued)

Table 2-1	MATHEMATICAL SYMBOLS IN STATISTICS *(Continued)*
Symbol	**Meaning**
Mathematical Functions	
$p(A|B)$	Probability of event A happening if B happens (conditional probability)
$p(A \cap B)$	Probability of both event A and event B happening (intersection of A and B)
$p(A \cup B)$	Probability of event A happening or event B happening (union of A and B)
Statistical Symbols	
α	Alpha: the significance level set for the study
p	The *p*-value of the computed statistic
H_0	The null hypothesis
H_A	The alternative hypothesis
α error	Type I error in hypothesis testing
β error	Type II error in hypothesis testing
N	Population size
n	Sample size
f	Frequency
p_i, p_{95}	Percentile rank at the *i*th percentile, 95th percentile
μ	Mu, the population mean
$\bar{x}$	x-bar, the sample mean
σ^2	Sigma squared, the population variance
σ	Sigma, the population standard deviation
s^2	Sample variance
s	Sample standard deviation
CI	Confidence interval
df	Degrees of freedom
χ^2	Chi-square
ρ	Population correlation coefficient
r	Sample correlation coefficient

The researcher then attempts to answer the question by examining the data collected on the characteristics of interest in the study; in health research, this is usually about people or events. Sometimes researchers collect their own data, and sometimes they use data that may be available from other studies or government sources. Once collected, the data must be organized, examined, and interpreted using well-defined procedures.

Almost all quantitative studies involve data that are entered into a computer-based statistical spreadsheet or database for subsequent data analysis. The logistics and time required to collect data, enter it into a statistical spreadsheet or database, and prepare it for data analysis are often greatly underestimated and poorly understood. Davidson (1996) recommends taking control of the structure and flow of one's data from the beginning. It is hoped that this will help eliminate faulty data leading to faulty conclusions. Appendix A contains an overview of how a good computer database can be created in SPSS (the process is similar for other programs such as SAS and STATA) and how one's data can be initially cleaned so that it is suitable for analysis.

What Is a Variable?

In research, the specific characteristics or parameters of interest are commonly called variables. *A variable* is any characteristic that can and does assume different values for the different people, objects, or events being studied. We measure the value of the variable for each participant in our study, and then record these measurements in a spreadsheet or database to form a data set. This set of observed measurements collected from study participants allows us to describe the variables. For example, demographic variables describe the basic characteristics of human populations or study samples such as age, gender, ethnicity, marital status, number of children, education level, employment status, and income. Each observation within these variables is assigned a number using different rules: age is measured in years, gender is identified as male or female (can be coded "0" and "1"), income is measured in dollars earned per year, and so on.

It is important to note that for a characteristic to be considered a variable, it is critical that everyone in a given sample does not have the same value for the characteristic. For example, gender, which can assume two values (male and female), is not a variable when studying a sample of pregnant women. Because everyone in such a study is female, gender does not vary and is therefore a constant and not considered a variable.

Measurement Scale

Measurement, in the broadest sense, is the assignment of numerals to objects or events according to a set of rules (Stevens, 1946; Vogt, 2005). In measuring variables, four basic types of measurement are used: categorization, rank ordering, interval ordering, and numerical scoring. Each of these types of measurement corresponds to one of four measurement scales: nominal (categorization), ordinal (rank ordering), interval (interval ordering), and ratio (numerical scoring) (Babbie, 2007; Polit & Beck, 2008; Stevens, 1946). When analyzing data, the first task is to be aware of the type of measurement scale for each of the variables, because this knowledge helps in choosing the correct statistics to describe and display the data and examine the relationships among variables.

The scales can be thought of as occurring in ascending order, with the nominal scale being the lowest and ratio being the highest. This is because a variable measured on a higher scale can usually be converted into a lower scale but not vice versa. For example, weight measured on the ratio scale (e.g., pounds) can be converted into a categorical indicator for obese or not obese. However, if weight was originally collected as a categorical variable (obese vs. not obese), it cannot be reclassified into the ratio scale (pounds).

Nominal Scales

In the nominal scale, the numbers are simply used as codes representing categories or characteristics, and there is no order to the categories. Sometimes nominal variables are called categorical or qualitative. This type of scale allows the researcher to assign numeric values to categories of characteristics of people, objects, or events. These numeric values are usually assigned to the categories as codes for computer storage, but the choice of numerals for these codes is absolutely arbitrary, and the order of the numerals does not represent any kind of meaningful ordering in the categories. Examples of nominal variables are gender, ethnicity, religion, marital status, region of residence, adhering to an appointment. Note that the numbers could just as easily be assigned differently. In the example here, the males could have been assigned "1" and females assigned "0" without changing the nature of the variable.

Examples of Nominal-Level Variables	Values
Gender	0 = Male
	1 = Female
Ethnicity	1 = African-American
	2 = Caucasian
	3 = Hispanic
	4 = Other

Ordinal Scales

Ordinal scale variables are measured with numbers representing categories that can be placed in a meaningful numerical order (e.g., from lowest to highest) but for which there is no information regarding the specific size of the interval between the different values, and there is no "true zero." In this case, the characteristics are placed in categories that are ordered in some meaningful way (i.e., the assignment of numerals is not arbitrary). For example, it is possible to rank military personnel from lowest to highest (e.g., private, corporal, sergeant, lieutenant), but it is impossible to say anything about how much greater a corporal is than a private. It is also impossible to say whether the interval between a corporal and a private is the same as the interval between a sergeant and a lieutenant. Note than an ordinal variable can have the number "0" as one of its possible codes, but it will still not be a "true zero." For example, the value of "0" can be assigned to

the rank of private, a "1" to the rank of corporal, and so on. However, we could also assign the number "10" to the rank of private and the number "20" to the rank of corporal without changing the meaning of the variable so long as the higher ranks are assigned higher numbers.

All subjective rating scales are considered ordinal, including satisfaction scales, ratings of pain or discomfort, symptom checklists to evaluate psychological states such as depression, and so on. Variables based on the Likert scale are also considered ordinal. Likert-scale variables typically use the following format: "Please rate your level of agreement with the following statements on a scale of 1 to 5, where '1' is 'strongly disagree' and '5' is 'strongly agree'." Other ranges of response categories ('strongly like' to 'strongly dislike', 'very satisfied' to 'very dissatisfied') can also be used (Likert, Roslow, & Murphy, 1934). Likert scales were originally developed by Rensis Likert as part of his doctoral dissertation at Columbia University in the 1930s. Today, Likert scales are commonly used in many studies of health care quality and outcomes. Note that variables that are computed by adding a number of ordinal variables together are also considered ordinal (e.g., creating a scale by adding the responses to a number of questions, each of which elicits responses via a Likert scale).

Examples of Ordinal-Level Variables	Values
Health status	1 = Excellent
	2 = Good
	3 = Fair
	4 = Poor
	5 = Very poor
Pain intensity	0 = No pain
	1 = Minor/little pain
	2 = Moderate pain
	3 = Severe pain

Interval Scales

Interval-scale variables are measured with numbers that can be placed in meaningful numerical order and have meaningful intervals between values because the units of measure are in equal intervals. Because the units are in equal intervals, it is possible to add and subtract across an interval scale. However, interval scales do not have a "true zero," and ratios of scores cannot be meaningfully calculated. An interval scale provides information about the rank ordering of values and the magnitude of the difference between different values on the scale. Interval variables may be *continuous* (i.e., in theory, they may take on any numerical value within the variable's range) or they may be discrete (i.e., they may take on only a finite number of values between two points).

A good example of an interval scale is the PHQ-2 (Kroenke, Spitzer, & Williams, 2003), a validated screening tool for depression. The PHQ-2 asks the respondent over how many days in the previous 2-week period he or she had (a) been feeling down/depressed/hopeless and (b) felt little pleasure or interest in doing things. Each question is scored on a 4-point scale ranging from "none at all" (0) to "nearly every day" (3). The scores for each question are summed with a maximum number of 6 points possible. People whose composite scores are greater than or equal to 3 are screened as depressed. It is impossible to say that people who score 6 are twice as depressed as people who score a 3. Other examples of interval scales include most standardized educational tests, including the SAT exam, the GRE, the MCAT, and the LSAT.

Ratio Scales

Ratio-scale variables are measured with numbers that can be placed in a meaningful numerical order, have equal intervals between the numbers, and have the presence of a "true zero" point that is not arbitrary but is determined by nature. Most biomedical variables (e.g., weight, height, blood pressure, and pulse rate) are ratio variables. They all have a true zero, representing the absence of the phenomenon being measured, and the measurement of the variable needs to be anchored at 0 to be accurate. For example, if a patient's weight is 172 lb, it is assumed that the scale was balanced at "0" and not at "–5" before the patient stepped on it to be weighed. Ratio variables may be *continuous* (i.e., in theory, they may take on any numerical value within the variable's range) or they may be discrete (i.e., they take on only a finite number of values between two points).

With ratio scales, all mathematical operations (addition, subtraction, multiplication, and division) are possible. Thus, one can say that a 200-lb man is twice as heavy as a 100-lb man. Other examples of ratio-scale variables include age, income, and number of children. The distinction between interval and ratio variables is interesting, but for the purposes of this text, these two types of variables are handled the same way in analyzing data when the assumptions underlying the statistical test are met.

Measurement Scale Considerations

Researchers need to be very clear about the measurement scale of their study variables, particularly when it comes to classifying variables as ordinal, interval, or ratio (Burns & Grove, 2001). When measuring variables derived from psychosocial scales, psychological inventories, or tests of knowledge, there may be differences of opinion as to the variable's level of measurement. Many of these scales have arbitrary 0 points as determined by the test developer, and they have no accepted unit of measurement comparable to any standard measurement such as inches and feet. Technically, these variables are ordinal in nature, but in practice, researchers often think of them as interval- or ratio-level scales. This has been a controversial issue in the research literature for years. Gardner (1975) reviewed the early literature on this conflict, and Knapp (1990) has commented on more recent literature. In his original article on measurement (1946) and in a later article (1968), Stevens noted that treating ordinal scales as interval or ratio scales may violate a technical canon, but in many instances, the outcome had demonstrable use. More recently, Knapp (1990, 1993) and Wang, Yu, Wang, and Huang (1999) pointed out that such considerations as measurement perspective, the number of categories that make up an ordinal scale, the concept of *meaningfulness*, and the relevancy of measurement scales to permissible statistics may be important in deciding whether to treat a variable as ordinal or interval.

It is usually best to gather data at the highest level of measurement for research variables because this permits the researcher to perform more mathematical operations and gain greater precision in measurement. However, interval or ratio variables can be converted to ordinal or nominal variables. For example, diastolic blood pressure, as measured by a sphygmomanometer, is a ratio variable. However, for research purposes, blood pressure recorded as a ratio variable can easily be converted to a nominal variable indicating the pressure is either controlled or uncontrolled. By collecting blood pressure as a ratio variable, the researcher can choose to examine it as either a ratio or nominal variable and may decide to do both to answer different questions. But when no physiological basis for converting higher-order variables into lower-order variables exists, converting interval or ratio variables to lower-level nominal or ordinal variables can be unwise because it results in a loss of information. Cohen (1983) detailed the amount of degradation of measurement as a consequence of dichotomization and urged researchers to use all of the original measurement information.

USING DESCRIPTIVE STATISTICS AND VISUAL DISPLAYS

Descriptive statistics are used to describe and summarize data. This allows us to combine a group of individual measures into one or more summaries that make(s) them more meaningful. It is much easier to grasp the essence of a variable by looking at a graph or a chart, as opposed to simply scanning a spreadsheet with the raw data (the individual measurements). The three common ways of presenting and organizing data to describe a variable are frequency distributions, graphical displays, and descriptive statistics. The goal of presenting data in this manner is to help in understanding four things about each variable: its central tendency, dispersion, shape, and outliers.

Descriptive statistics help us to understand the central tendency, dispersion, and shape of the data that measure a variable. Measures of central tendency are the values that best represent the middle of a distribution; they provide information about the values that are most typical. The mean, median, and mode are all measures of central tendency. The measures of dispersion describe the extent to which the values of the variable are spread out around the measure of central tendency. The standard deviation (SD), interquartile range (IQR), and range are all measures of dispersion. Measures of skewness (asymmetry) and kurtosis (how peaked or flat the distribution is) can help us to quantify the shape of a distribution and the extent to which it deviates from a normal bell-shaped curve (more on this later in this chapter).

Graphical displays can help us to understand the shape of the distribution, to view outliers, and to visualize its central tendency and dispersion. This shape explains how the values of the variable are distributed (symmetrically or asymmetrically) around the measure of central tendency. For example, data that are normally distributed will have a characteristic "bell-shaped" curve. Outliers are those values that do not fit the pattern of the rest of the data; they are data points that are either much larger or much smaller than the rest of the values, and they stand out because they are unusual. The shape of the distribution is typically determined visually by using graphical methods such as histograms or stem-and-leaf plots.

RESEARCH QUESTION

Descriptive studies are those that simply seek to describe phenomena, without necessarily making statements about association or causation. In health-related research, these studies often seek to describe the health conditions in different sectors of society. The following studies provide examples of the use of descriptive statistics in practice. The first is a study of chronic conditions in the elderly, and the second is a study of the natural progression of heart disease. Overall, the use of descriptive statistics in these two studies allows readers to better understand the population on which the studies were focused. The descriptive statistics also serve to inform readers about the health conditions studied in each population.

Are There Ethnic Disparities in the Rates of Chronic Conditions in the Elderly?

A report from the Center on an Aging Society at Georgetown University used descriptive statistics to examine the rates of chronic conditions in patients by age and ethnicity (Center on an Aging Society, 2004). Because the increasingly diverse society in the United States challenges health care professionals to provide culturally competent care, it is important that providers understand how membership in different cultural groups (e.g., age, ethnicity, and religion) can affect health. In this study, the rates of chronic conditions were found to be higher among older African-Americans (77%) and Latinos (68%) than among Whites (64%) or Asian-Americans (42%). In addition, this report found that racial and ethnic minority elderly were less likely to have a primary care physician and health insurance. These data about elderly Americans can help to provide guidance to health sciences researchers, health care providers, policymakers, and educators who seek to address the disparities in health and access to health care in the United States.

How Does Cardiovascular Disease Progress in an Asymptomatic Population?

Another example of the use of descriptive statistics can be found in a paper based on the Pittsburgh Health Heart Project. This project followed a group of asymptomatic, community-dwelling adults for 3 years to examine the progression of subclinical cardiovascular disease (Stewart, Janicki, & Kamarck, 2006). The authors used descriptive statistics to describe the population at baseline and again at follow-up. At baseline, about half (50.9%) of the participants were women, and 13% were nonwhite; the average age was 60.1 years (SD, 4.6 years). Information about baseline risk factors was also provided: at baseline, 9.7% of the participants smoked, the average body mass index (BMI) was 27.5 kg/m^2 (SD, 4.6), and the average systolic blood pressure was 121.8 mm Hg (SD, 9.6). At the 3-year follow-up, the average systolic blood pressure was 118.9 mm Hg (SD, 9.1) and the average BMI had increased by 0.2 kg/m^2 (SD, 1.7) (Stewart et al., 2006). Data from a 3-year follow-up were compared with the original data so that the researchers could understand how the risk factors change over time.

USING VISUAL DISPLAYS TO DESCRIBE DATA

A summary of the data can be presented in a frequency table or in a chart. Frequency distribution tables offer two main advantages: They condense data into a form that can make them easier to understand (Morgan, Reichert, & Harrison, 2002), and they show many details in summary fashion. However, they do not provide a "picture" of the patterns in the data. Charts are very effective in giving the reader a picture of the differences and patterns in a set of data, but they do not provide the same level of detail as a frequency table (Wallgren et al., 1996). Providing both frequency tables and charts to the reader can help them to have a fuller understanding of the data from your study.

Frequency Distribution Tables

Frequency distribution tables provide a way of organizing data by using a table format. They allow readers to grasp the basic characteristics of the distribution of the variable quickly. When the data are organized into a table format, it is much easier for readers to glean information about the central tendency, dispersion, and outliers of the variable of interest. When the data are not organized, it is much harder to do so. For example, Table 2-2 presents the body weight (in pounds) of 39 diabetic women using data from the Behavioral Risk Factor Surveillance System (BRFSS) survey (Centers for Disease Control and Prevention, 2000). These data are an ordered array—they are rank ordered but not otherwise organized. From this table alone, it is not immediately obvious where the middle of the distribution lies, what the shape of the distribution is, or how many of the values are outliers.

A frequency distribution table shows the possible values of the variable grouped into class intervals (a set of defined range limits in which the data are grouped), the raw and relative frequencies of these intervals (i.e., numeric count and percentage within range), and the cumulative frequency (i.e., cumulative percentage up to the indicated range).

The frequency distribution shown in Table 2-3 was created from the data given in Table 2-2. Table 2-3 demonstrates how much easier it is to glean information from the data by using this format. The typical values of the variable (body weight), its dispersion, and the outliers are all

Table 2-2	RAW BODY WEIGHT DATA		
Person (No.)	Position	Weight (lb/kg)	Squared Weight
1	1	101/45.8	10,201/2097.6
2	2	115/52.2	13,225/2724.8
3	3	125/56.7	15,625/3214.9
4	4	126/57.2	15,876/3271.8
5	5	130/59.0	16,900/3481.0
6	6	135/61.2	18,225/3745.4
7	7	144/65.3	20,736/4264.1
8	8	145/65.8	21,025/4329.6
9	9	145/65.8	21,025/4329.6
10	10	147/66.7	21,609/4448.9
11	11	151/68.5	22,801/4692.3
12	12	161/73.0	25,921/5329.0
13	13	161/73.0	25,921/5329.0
14	14	165/74.8	27,225/5595.0
15	15	167/75.8	27,889/5745.6
16	16	177/80.3	31,329/6448.1
17	17	178/80.7	31,684/6512.5

(Continued)

| Table 2-2 | RAW BODY WEIGHT DATA *(Continued)* | | |
Person (No.)	Position	Weight (lb/kg)	Squared Weight
18	18	180/81.6	32,400/6658.6
19	19	180/81.6	32,400/6658.6
20	20	185/83.9	34,225/7039.2
21	21	185/83.9	34,225/7039.2
22	22	185/83.9	34,225/7039.2
23	23	185/83.9	34,225/7039.2
24	24	190/86.2	36,100/7430.4
25	25	190/86.2	36,100/7430.4
26	26	195/88.5	38,025/7832.3
27	27	195/88.5	38,025/7832.3
28	28	197/89.4	38,809/7992.4
29	29	200/90.7	40,000/8226.5
30	30	202/91.6	40,804/8390.6
31	31	208/94.3	43,264/8892.5
32	32	209/94.8	43,681/8987.1
33	33	220/99.8	48,400/9960.0
34	34	230/104.3	52,900/10878.5
35	35	235/106.6	55,225/11363.6
36	36	240/108.9	57,600/11859.2
37	37	240/108.9	57,600/11859.2
38	38	265/120.2	70,225/14448.0
39	39	319/144.7	101,761/20938.1
Sum	39	$\Sigma x = 7108$	$\Sigma x^2 = 1,367,436$

immediately obvious. For example, the majority of the women weigh between 180 and 199 lb (81.6–90.3 kg), but a fairly even number of women weigh either more or less than this. In addition, at least one outlier is obvious—the woman who weighs between 300 and 319 lb (136.0–144.7 kg).

Only limited frequency tables can be created for nominal-level variables. If the variable of interest is nominal, such as marital status, a table that shows the raw and relative frequency of each response category could be created. Table 2-4 is an example of a frequency table

created to describe the marital status of the 39 study participants from the BRFSS. There are no class intervals, and cumulative frequencies are not meaningful and therefore are not included. For example, from Table 2-4, a cumulative frequency might tell us that 71.7% of the sample is currently married or single, which is not particularly useful; therefore, cumulative frequencies are not included in Table 2-4. However, even with nominal variables, the categories should be listed in some natural order if one exists and then the frequencies indicated for each category.

Table 2-3	FREQUENCY DISTRIBUTION OF BODY WEIGHT		
Weight Range (Intervals of 20 lb [with kg conversions])	Raw Frequency (No.)	Relative Frequency (% of Total Sample)	Cumulative Frequency (Cumulative %)
100–119 (45.4–54.0)	2	5.1	5.1
120–139 (54.4–63.0)	4	10.3	15.4
140–159 (63.5–72.1)	5	12.8	28.2
160–179 (72.6–81.2)	6	15.4	43.6
180–199 (81.6–90.3)	11	28.2	71.9
200–219 (90.7–99.3)	4	10.3	82.1
220–239 (99.8–108.4)	3	7.7	89.7
240–259 (108.9–117.5)	2	5.1	94.9
260–279 (117.9–126.6)	1	2.6	97.4
280–299 (127.0–135.6)	0	0.0	97.4
300–319 (136.0–144.7)	1	2.6	100
Total	39	100.0	

Creating Frequency Distribution Tables

The five steps to creating a frequency distribution table for interval and ratio variables (some steps will not apply to nominal or ordinal variables) are as follows:

1. Create an ordered array of the data.
2. Determine which class intervals will be used.
3. Sort the data into the class intervals to obtain the raw frequencies of each class interval.
4. Compute the relative frequency of each class interval.
5. Compute the cumulative relative frequency of values along the class intervals.

Ordered Arrays

Most data will not come to us in an organized fashion. The first step in creating a frequency distribution table is to create an ordered array. This simply means taking the data points and putting them in order from the least value to the greatest value, as we did with the weight data from the diabetic women (Table 2-2).

Class Intervals

Class intervals group numeric data into categories. These categories should be of equal length and mutually exclusive and exhaustive, meaning that each data point should fit into only one class interval (i.e., class intervals should not overlap) and that there should be enough class intervals to account for all the data. The choice

Table 2-4	MARITAL STATUS	
Status	Raw Frequency	Relative Frequency
Married	21	53.8
Single	7	17.9
Divorced or separated	11	28.2
Total	39	100.0

of the width and number of intervals largely depends on the variable of interest. In general, the class intervals should be meaningful to the variable; interval widths of 5 to 10 units often work well but may depend on the expected range of the variable. It is unusual to use fewer than 5 or more than 15 class intervals, although again, the exact number used will depend on the variable that the class interval represents.

Authorities differ in their recommendations for the number of classes. Glass and Hopkins (1996) suggest there should be at least 10 times as many observations as classes until there are between 20 and 30 intervals. Freedman, Pisani, Purves, and Adhikari (1991) suggest 10 to 15 classes; Ott and Mendenhall (1990) suggest 5 to 20 classes; and Freund (1988) suggests 6 to 15 classes. Thus, it is up to the researcher to determine the number of intervals in a frequency distribution of a variable.

Usually, the clustering that best depicts the important features of the distribution of scores for the intended audience should be the major consideration. Too few or too many classes will obscure important features of a frequency distribution. Some detail is lost by grouping the values, but information is gained about clustering and the shape of the distribution.

The class intervals used in the above example (see Table 2-3) have a width of 20 lb each, making a total of 11 class intervals. These intervals are exhaustive and mutually exclusive. There are enough intervals to encompass all the data points (exhaustive), and the intervals do not overlap at all (mutually exclusive). The first class interval is 100 to 119 lb (45.4 to 54.0 kg), the second one is 120 to 139 lb (54.4 to 63.0 kg), and so on.

Raw Frequencies

The remaining columns in the frequency table provide summary information. The second column in the frequency table is the raw frequency column. This is the actual number of cases that fall into a given interval. For example, 11 of the study participants weigh between 180 and 199 lb, and so the number 11 is placed in the raw frequency column next to the class interval 180 to 199. The total at the bottom of the raw frequency column is the total number in the sample (i.e., 39).

Relative Frequencies

The third column in the frequency table is the relative frequency column. In this column, the percentage of cases that fall into each class interval is computed. For example, the relative frequency of the class interval 180 to 199 is 11 of 39, or 28.2%, of the total sample. The total at the bottom of the relative frequency column is 100, representing the sum of the relative frequencies (e.g., 100% of the cases).

Cumulative Relative Frequencies

The fourth column in the frequency table is the cumulative relative frequency. In this column, the percentage of the sample with values from the lowest value up to and including the value of the upper limit of the class interval is computed. For example, the cumulative relative frequency of the class interval 200 to 219 is 82%, because 82% of the sample weighs 219 lb or less. The cumulative relative frequency column is useful when computing percentiles, and we discuss this later in this chapter.

Summarizing Nominal or Ordinal Variables

Many of the above considerations will also apply to categorical variables (nominal and ordinal). However, with categorical variables, you will not have class intervals. Instead, you will place the name of each category in the first column. If there is any natural ordering or grouping of categories, the categories should be organized taking that ordering into account. The second column is where the raw frequency is reported, followed by the relative frequency and, if meaningful, the cumulative relative frequency.

Putting It All Together: Constructing Tables for Research Reports

The specific content of a table will vary depending on the variables that you are summarizing and/or the hypothesis that you are testing. It is wise to use a table only to highlight major facts. Most of the tables examined by researchers while analyzing their data do not need to be published in a journal. If a finding can be described well in words, then a table is unnecessary. Too many tables can overwhelm the rest of a research report (Burns & Grove, 2001).

The table should be as self-explanatory as possible. The patterns and exceptions in a table should be obvious at a glance once the reader has been told what they are (Ehrenberg, 1977). With this goal in mind, the title should state the variable, when and where the data were collected (if pertinent), and the size of the sample. Headings within the table should be brief and clear. Find out the required format for tables in the research report. If the report is being submitted to a particular journal, examine tables in recent past issues. Follow the advice about table format for publication in a manual of style, such as the *Publication Manual of the American Psychological Association* (APA, 2010). Morgan et al. (2002) offer several principles that should guide table construction (Box 2-1).

An Overview of Charts/Graphical Displays of Data

Although there are many different kinds of graphical displays of data (generally referred to as charts), most are based on several basic types that are built with lines, areas, and text. These include bar charts, histograms, stem-and-leaf plots, pie charts, scatter plots, line charts, flow charts, and box plots. Charts can quickly reveal facts about data that might be gleaned from a table only after careful study. They are often the most effective way to describe, explore, and summarize a set of numbers (Tufte, 1983). Charts, the visual representations of frequency distributions, provide a global, bird's-eye view of the data and help the reader gain insight. Box 2-2 contains some general questions from Wallgren et al. (1996) to keep in mind when constructing charts.

BOX 2-1   GUIDELINES FOR MAKING FREQUENCY TABLES

1. Don't try to do too much in a table. Model tables after published exemplars of similar research to find the right balance for how much a table should contain.
2. Use white space effectively so as to make the layout of the table pleasing to the eye, and to aid in comprehension and clarity.
3. Make sure that tables and text refer to each other; however, not everything displayed in a table needs to be mentioned in the text.
4. Use some aspect of the data to order and group rows and columns. This could be size (largest to smallest), chronology (first to last), or to show similarity or invite comparison.
5. If appropriate, frame the table with summary statistics in rows and columns to provide a standard of comparison. Remember that, when making a table, values are compared down columns more easily than across rows.
6. It is useful to round numbers in a table to one or two decimal places because they are more easily understood when the number of digits is reduced.

> **BOX 2-2   GENERAL SUGGESTIONS FOR CONSTRUCTING CHARTS**
>
> - **Is the chart easy to read?** Simplicity is the hallmark of a good chart. What you want to display in a chart should be quickly and clearly evident. Keep in mind the target audience for whom you are constructing the chart. Keep grid lines and tick marks to a minimum. Avoid odd lettering and ornate patterns (Schmid, 1983).
> - **Is the chart in the right place?** Locate the chart close to the place in the text where the topic is discussed. Make sure that the chart is well positioned on the page.
> - **Does the chart benefit from being in color (if color is used)?** Color should have a purpose; it should not be used solely for decorative reasons.
> - **Have you tried the chart out on anybody?** Try the chart out on someone whom you consider to correspond to the target group before you make the final diagram. Ask that person questions about the chart to gain information on how the person perceives the chart.

An important description of a variable includes the shape and symmetry of the distribution of its values. Charts can be used to help describe this characteristic. Distributions can have various symmetrical and asymmetrical (i.e., right-skewed, left-skewed) patterns (Fig. 2-1). Symmetrical distributions have a well-defined centerline or median, with an equal number of data points to the left and right of this centerline. The normal distribution is an important symmetrical, bell-shaped distribution.

Not all symmetrical distributions qualify as normal distributions; for example, a bimodal distribution (two peaks) might be symmetrical but would not be normal (see Chapter 3 and Chapter 4 for a discussion on the normal distribution and its importance in statistics). The triangular and rectangular distributions shown in Figure 2-1 are both symmetrical, but they do not have the characteristic bell-shaped curve of a normal distribution. For most statistics used in health sciences research, the type of distribution (i.e., normal or other) determines which statistics can be used to analyze the data.

In general, the idea of skewness refers to the extent to which the data are not symmetrical about the centerline. Right-skewed data, sometimes called positively skewed data, have a pronounced tail trailing off to the right-hand side of the graph (toward the higher numbers). This occurs when relatively few cases have very high values. Distributions of income are often right skewed. Left-skewed data, also called negatively skewed data, have a pronounced tail trailing off to the left-hand side (toward the lower numbers). This occurs when relatively few cases have very low values. Two measures of skewness are discussed in detail later in this chapter.

Kurtosis is also a characteristic of data shapes; specifically, it refers to the steepness, or peakedness, of the mound or mode. A distribution with a wide, flat mound with thick tails on each side is called platykurtic, whereas a distribution with a tall peak and long skinny tails on each side is called leptokurtic. A distribution with medium kurtosis (i.e., somewhere between platykurtic and leptokurtic) is referred to as mesokurtic. A normal distribution is an example of a mesokurtic distribution.

Creating Histograms

A histogram is a graphical display used to show the shape of the distribution of variables that are of interval and ratio measurement scale.

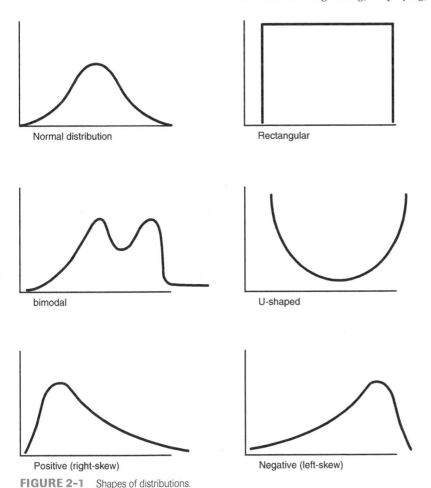

FIGURE 2-1   Shapes of distributions.

In some cases, histograms can also be used for ordinal data that are continuous and have a wide range of values. Histograms are essentially visual depictions of frequency distributions. They consist of an *x*-axis, on which the class intervals are listed, and a *y*-axis, on which the raw or relative frequencies are graphed. Figure 2-2 shows a histogram of the weight data from the 39 diabetic women mentioned earlier. It was created from the frequency distribution given in Table 2-3.

Creating a histogram from a frequency distribution table is easy. First, the values of the class intervals (from smallest to largest) are placed on the *x*-axis. The class intervals must be mutually exclusive, exhaustive, and of equal width. Second, the raw (or relative) frequency is placed on the *y*-axis. The length of the *y*-axis should be roughly two-thirds to three-fourths that of the *x*-axis so that the histogram looks proportional (Schmid, 1983). Third, it is important that the bars of the histogram touch. Finally, the choice of the correct number of class intervals is as much art as science, as shown in the two histograms in Figure 2-3: one uses five class intervals, and the other uses 20. If there are too few bars,

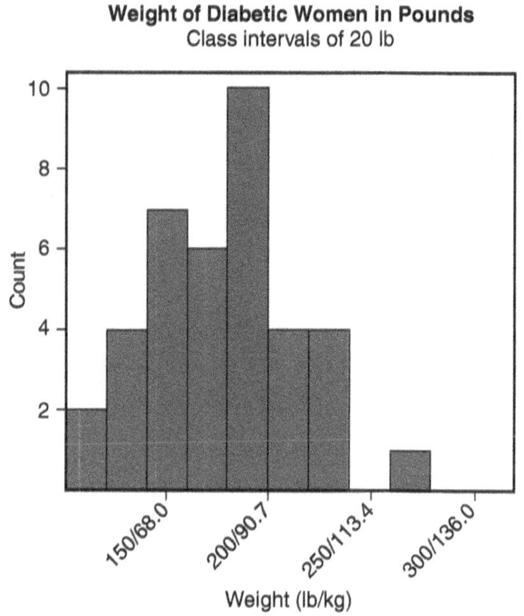

Weight of Diabetic Women in Pounds
Class intervals of 20 lb

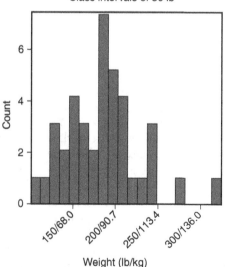

FIGURE 2-2   Histogram of the variable "weight" for diabetic women, from SPSS.

Frequency Polygons

The frequency polygon, a chart for interval or ratio variables, is equivalent to the histogram but appears smoother. For any set of data, the histogram and the frequency polygon will both have equivalent total areas of 100%. A frequency polygon provides a rough estimate of the shape of the distribution. It is constructed by using a histogram. First, a dot is placed in the middle of each class interval bar on the histogram. Second, the dots are connected in order using straight lines. Third, the histogram is erased, leaving a rough estimate of the shape of the data distribution. When comparing different frequency distributions, it is sometimes easier to use a frequency polygon than a histogram. Figure 2-4 presents a frequency polygon based on the histogram in Figure 2-2.

Stem-and-Leaf Displays

Stem-and-leaf displays, also known as *stemplots*, are alternative ways of graphing data (Cleveland, 1988). They are similar to histograms in that they provide information regarding the range

information is lost, and if there are too many bars, the histogram looks cluttered; either too few or too many bars makes it impossible to get a good picture of the distribution of the data.

Weight of Diabetic Women in Pounds
Class intervals of 50 lb

Weight of Diabetic Women in Pounds
Class intervals of 50 lb

FIGURE 2-3   Two different versions of the weight histogram.

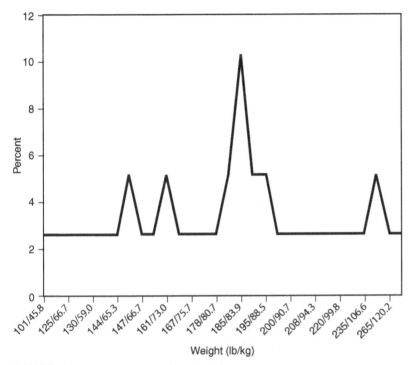

FIGURE 2-4   Frequency polygon of body weight.

of values, center of the data, and shape of the data. One advantage of stem-and-leaf plots is that they preserve the individual values of the variable. Stem-and-leaf plots can also be easily constructed by hand, without the need for a computer or complex statistical software. They are best used with small data sets (less than or equal to 100 cases) because constructing them with large data sets is cumbersome.

The data and stem-and-leaf plot for the variable "age of onset of diabetes" from the BRFSS are presented in Table 2-5. The age range for diabetes onset in this sample was 5 to 52 years. The "stem" of the stem-and-leaf plot consists of one or more of the initial digits of measurement. In this example, the "stem" is the first digit, or the number filling the tens position, of the "age of onset" variable, which ranges from 0 for those who are 5 years old to 5 for those in their 50s. The "leaf" consists of the remaining digit, the digit in the "ones" position. For example, for

the person who is 25 years old, the "stem" is 2, and the "leaf" is 5. The stems form an ordered column, or vertical axis, with the numbers in ascending order such that the smallest stem is at the top and the largest is at the bottom. Stems are separated from the leaves by a vertical line, followed by the leaf value of each participant.

One strength of the stem-and-leaf plot is that each participant is recorded. When using variables that have decimal places (e.g., age 32.5 years), the decimal is often dropped to make the display easier to read. In the BRFSS example, three people in the study had an age of onset of 45 years, and so three leaves with a value of 5 were put on stem 4 (representing 40). From the stem-and-leaf plot in Table 2-6, it is clear that most of the women were diagnosed with diabetes while in their 40s. The earliest age of onset was 5 years, and the latest age of onset was 52 years. The shape of the plot shows that the data are skewed toward a later age of onset.

Table 2-5	STEM-AND-LEAF PLOT FOR AGE OF ONSET OF DIABETES

Raw Data: Age of Onset of Diabetes

Age of Onset (Years)	Frequency
5	1
7	1
11	1
12	1
14	1
19	1
20	1
23	3
25	1
29	1
32	1
33	1
34	1
35	1
36	2
37	1
38	2
39	1
41	2
42	2
43	1
44	2
45	3
46	1
47	1
48	1
50	1
51	2
52	1

Table 2-6	STEM-AND-LEAF PLOT FOR AGE OF ONSET OF DIABETES

Stem	Leaf
0	5 7
1	1 2 4 9
2	0 3 3 3 5 9
3	2 3 4 5 6 6 7 8 8 9
4	1 1 2 2 3 4 4 5 5 5 6 7 8
5	0 1 1 2

Note. Raw data appear in chart below.

that value lies. For example, the 50th percentile, represented by p_{50}, is the value of the variable at which 50% of the data are below and 50% are above. In Box 2-3, we can see that a weight of 185 lb is at the 50th percentile because half the values lie below that value and half lie above it. The 50th percentile is also called the *median*.

One way of obtaining percentile ranks is from a graph called an ogive, which is a graphical representation of the cumulative frequency distribution from the frequency distribution table. An ogive of the weight data from the diabetic women is shown in Figure 2-5. As is evident in this figure, the 25th percentile is 147 lb (66.7 kg), and the 75th percentile is 202 lb (91.6 kg). This means that 50% of the women weigh between 147 and 202 lb (66.7 and 91.6 kg). Percentile ranks are particularly useful when individual scores are compared with a standardized distribution.

Percentile Rank, Cumulative Frequencies, and Ogives

The percentile rank of a value of a variable shows the position in the distribution where

Bar Charts

A bar chart, the simplest form of chart, is used for nominal or ordinal data. When constructing such charts, the category labels are usually listed horizontally in some systematic order, and then vertical bars are drawn to represent the frequency or percentage in each category. A space separates each bar to emphasize the nominal or ordinal nature of the variable. The spacing

BOX 2-3   CONSTRUCTING PIE CHARTS

When constructing a pie chart, Wallgren et al. (1996) recommend the following:
- Use the pie chart to provide overviews: Readers find it difficult to get precise measurements from a circle.
- Place the different sectors in the same order as would be found in the bar chart, beginning either in an ascending or a descending order, if applicable. Retain the order between the variables.
- Use the percentages corresponding to each category rather than the absolute frequency of each category.
- Read the pie chart by beginning at the 12 o'clock position and proceeding clockwise.
- Use no more than six sectors in a given pie chart; clarity is lost with more than six sectors.
- Use a low-key shading pattern that does not detract from the meaning of the pie chart.
- Make sure that the sum of the pie chart sectors equals 100%.

and the width of the bars are at the researcher's discretion, but once chosen, all the spacing and widths should be equal. Figure 2-6 shows a bar chart of the variable "marital status." From this bar chart, it is easy to see that the majority of study participants are married and that about half as many are separated or divorced.

Pie Chart

The pie chart, an alternative to the bar chart, is simply a circle that has been partitioned into percentage distributions of qualitative variables. Simple to construct, the pie chart has a total area of 100%, with 1% equivalent to 3.6° of the

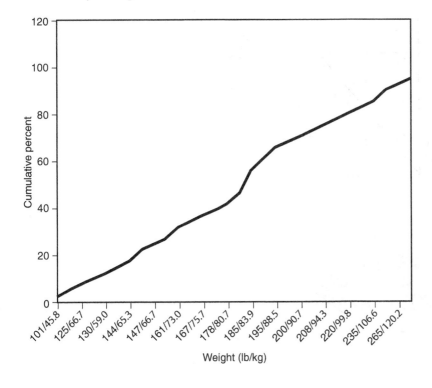

FIGURE 2-5 Ogive of the body weight.

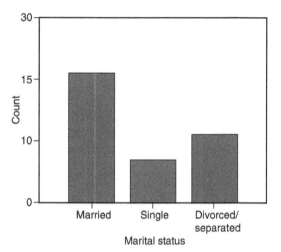

FIGURE 2-6 A bar chart showing the marital status of women in the study.

circle. The percentages depicted in each slice of the pie chart must add up to 100% (the total pie).

In the 2007 to 2008 National Health and Nutrition Examination Survey (NHANES) administration, a subset of participants was asked to gauge personal health status by answering the following question: "Would you say your general health is ..." with one of five answers (or don't know/refuse to answer)—excellent, very good, good, fair, or poor. The pie chart in Figure 2-7 summarizes the self-reported health status of the NHANES participants. Some tips for constructing pie charts from Wallgren et al. (1996) can be found in Box 2-3.

DESCRIBING DATA WITH SIMPLE STATISTICS

Graphical displays are useful, but it is also important to use descriptive statistics to describe each variable. The four characteristics that can be described with descriptive statistics are central tendency, dispersion, skewness, and kurtosis. The different measures of central tendency reveal the "typical" value of the variable, and the measures of dispersion reveal the "spread"

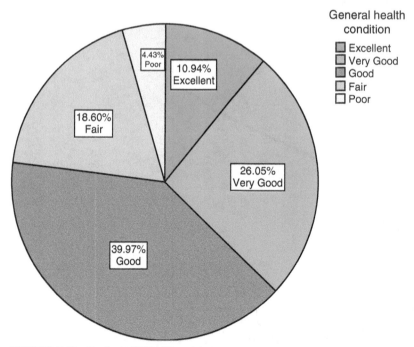

FIGURE 2-7 Pie chart of NHANES participants.

of the data. In addition, measures of skewness and kurtosis can help the reader to understand the shape of the distribution. When presenting a measure of central tendency, it is important to present the correct measure of dispersion at the same time because neither measurement is meaningful in isolation. Although less commonly done, it is also useful to say something about the extent to which the data deviate from the normal distribution with measures of skewness and kurtosis. For example, imagine that a personal health education program is conducted for two groups. The participants' average age is 25 years. Although both groups have a mean age of 25 years, the first group has a range (i.e., dispersion) of 5 to 65 years of age, and the second group has a range of 18 to 29 years of age. Clearly, the content of the program will look quite different for the two groups. The content of the program might also change if the data were skewed so that most of the group was older or younger than the mean might make it appear.

Measures of Central Tendency

The three measures of central tendency—the *mode*, *median*, and *mean*—each provide a single number about which the other observations tend to cluster. The choice of which measure of central tendency to use depends on the measurement scale and the distribution of the variable. In many cases, it is appropriate to present more than one of these measures of central tendency at the same time.

Mode

The mode is simply the most frequently occurring value. It is possible for a distribution to have multiple modes. If all of the scores in a distribution are different, then there is no mode. The mode is an appropriate measure of central tendency for variables at all levels of measurement: nominal, ordinal, interval, and ratio. When describing a nominal variable, the modal category would be reported. The mode is the only measure that we can use for nominal variables. In the example of body weight (see Table 2-2), the mode is 185 lb (83.9 kg) because that is the value that occurs most frequently (four times). A useful measure of dispersion to report with the mode is the range. If the variable is nominal, all the possible values of the variable are listed to represent the range.

Median

The median is the value that is in the middle of the distribution; it is also called the 50th percentile, and it is sometimes represented as "p_{50}." The median is the point or value below which 50% of the distribution falls. The median is an appropriate measure of central tendency for ordinal, interval, and ratio-level variables. One way to find the median value is to rank order the data and find the value that is in the exact middle of the distribution. In the example of the 39 diabetic women, the median value is the value in the 20th position because 19 of the values lie below this position and 19 lie above it (see Table 2-2). Thus, the median weight of this sample is 185 lb (83.9 kg). If the median of a distribution with an even number of values must be computed, the two values in the middle of the distribution are averaged. For example, when computing the median for the variable BMI (the higher the BMI, the more overweight the person is) in Table 2-7, there are only 38 values

Table 2-7	RELATIONSHIP OF REGULAR EXERCISE TO OBTAINING A FLU VACCINATION IN 999 HEALTH CARE WORKERS	
Person (No.)	**Position**	**Body Mass Index**
1	1	18.47
2	2	19.13
3	3	20.52
4	4	21.63
5	5	22.14
6	6	23.04

(Continued)

Table 2-7	RELATIONSHIP OF REGULAR EXERCISE TO OBTAINING A FLU VACCINATION IN 999 HEALTH CARE WORKERS (Continued)	
Person (No.)	Position	Body Mass Index
7	7	25.51
8	8	26.52
9	9	26.63
10	10	26.88
11	11	27.63
12	12	28.13
13	13	28.32
14	14	28.52
15	15	28.53
16	16	28.57
17	17	29.05
18	18	29.58
19	19	29.75
20	20	29.95
21	21	30.89
22	22	31.47
23	23	31.61
24	24	31.75
25	25	31.75
26	26	33.28
27	27	33.47
28	28	33.61
29	29	33.63
30	30	34.61
31	31	34.95
32	32	35.51
33	33	35.87
34	34	36.49
35	35	36.80
36	36	37.59
37	37	38.27
38	38	44.09

(one person did not answer the height question). The median BMI is the average of the value at the 19th and 20th positions; these are 29.75 and 29.95, respectively, and so the median BMI is

$$\frac{29.75 + 29.95}{2} = 29.85$$

The most common measures of dispersion for the median are the range and the IQR. The median is a robust measure (e.g., one or two extreme values will not change it greatly) and is a good measure of central tendency to use when the data are skewed or have a few extreme values.

Mean

The mean is the arithmetic average of the distribution and the measure of central tendency with which most people are familiar. The mean is most appropriately used to describe ratio- and interval-level data, but in some cases, it may also be used to describe ordinal data. To calculate the mean, you add up the values of each observation in the data set and then divide by the number of observations. In the example of weight, the mean weight of the sample is

$$\frac{7108}{39} = 182.26 \text{ lb}$$

The formula used to compute a mean is

$$\bar{x} = \frac{\sum x_i}{n} \qquad (2\text{-}1)$$

Note that x-bar ($\bar{x}$) stands for the mean, $\sum x_i$ stands for the sum of all of the values of x from the first to the last (or ith) value, and n stands for the number of data points. The most common measure of spread reported with a mean is the SD.

The mean has some interesting properties. It is the fulcrum, or true center, of the distribution, meaning that it is the point that is the shortest total distance (sum of the distance from each value) from all other points in the distribution. This is illustrated in Table 2-8. This table presents five numbers chosen at random (4, 4, 10, 5, 7). In this distribution, the $\sum x_i = 30$, $n = 5$, the mean is 6, the median is 5, and the mode is 4. If the mean is subtracted from each value in the distribution, the result is a quantity called the "deviation from the mean" of each point. The sum of these deviations always equals 0. As illustrated in Table 2-8, however, the sum of the deviations from the mode or median does not equal 0 except when the mode or median is equal to the mean. The concepts of "deviation from the mean," "squared deviation from the mean," and "sums of squared deviation from the mean (or sums of squares, for short)" are used throughout this text when we discuss computing various inferential statistics.

Another property of the mean is that when repeatedly drawing random samples from the same population, the means will vary less among themselves and less from the true population mean than will other measures of central tendency. However, the mean is sensitive to outliers and skewness (e.g., a few extreme values or a nonnormal distribution can drastically change the value of the mean).

Choosing the Correct Measure of Central Tendency

The question of which measure of central tendency to use commonly arises in cases in which the variable is from the interval or ratio measurement scale. The mean is the most commonly used measure of central tendency. One of the advantages of using the mean is that it is unique, meaning there is just one in any given data set and its calculation uses every single value in the distribution. However, the mean is also a *sensitive* measure, meaning that a single very large (or very small) value can dramatically change the mean. If a distribution is not symmetrical, the mean will not truly reflect the center of the distribution.

The median is a more *robust* measure of central tendency because a few outliers or a skewed distribution will not affect its value very much. If a distribution has large outliers or is skewed, the median may provide a better measure of a "typical" observation because it will be closer to the center of the data set. As shown in Figure 2-8, with data that are skewed to the right, the mean is larger than the median, and with data that are skewed to the left, the mean is smaller than the median.

The main use of the mode is for calling attention to a distribution in which the values cluster at one or more places. It can also be used for making rough estimates. In addition, the mode is the only measure of central tendency available for nominal data.

When a distribution is normal, meaning that it has only one mode and is symmetrical, the mean, median, and mode will have, or very

Table 2-8	DEMONSTRATION OF SHORTEST DISTANCE FROM MEASURES OF CENTRAL TENDENCY			
Values	Values of x	$x =$ Mean	$x =$ Median	$x =$ Mode
1	4	$4 - 6 = -2$	$4 - 5 = -1$	$4 - 4 = 0$
2	4	$4 - 6 = -2$	$4 - 5 = -1$	$4 - 4 = 0$
3	5	$5 - 6 = -1$	$5 - 5 = 0$	$5 - 4 = 1$
4	7	$7 - 6 = 1$	$7 - 5 = 2$	$7 - 4 = 3$
5	10	$10 - 6 = 4$	$10 - 5 = 5$	$10 - 4 = 6$
Sum	30	0	5	10

Note. Mean value = 4 + 4 + 5 + 7 + 10/5 = 6; median value = 5, and modal value = 4.

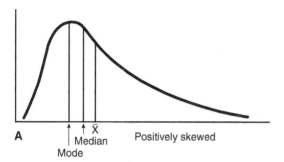

A   Median   Positively skewed
   Mode

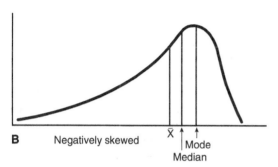

B   Negatively skewed   Mode
                          Median

FIGURE 2-8   Depiction of the mean and median of skewed distributions.

nearly have, the same value. In a skewed, or nonsymmetrical, distribution such as those in Figure 2-8, the mode is the value under the high point of the distribution, the mean is pulled to the right or the left by the extreme values in the tail of the distribution, and the median usually falls in between. Thus, if the mean is greater than the median, then the distribution is *positively skewed*, with the mean being dragged to the right by a few high scores. If the mean is less than the median, then the distribution is *negatively skewed*, with the mean being pulled to the left by a small number of low scores. Weisberg (1992) points out that it is not always necessary to select only a single measure of central tendency because these statistics provide different information. Sometimes it is useful to examine multiple aspects of a distribution.

Measures of Dispersion

The dispersion of a variable refers to the spread of scores or variation in the data set. When describing a variable, it is important to describe both a measure of central tendency and a measure of dispersion. Reporting only an average without an accompanying measure of variability, or dispersion, is a good way to misrepresent a set of data. A common story in statistics classes tells of the woman who had her head in an oven and her feet in a bucket of ice water. When asked how she felt, the reply was: "On the average, I feel fine." Researchers tend to focus on measures of central tendency and neglect how the data are scattered, but variability is at least equally important (Tulman & Jacobsen, 1989). Two data sets can have the same average but very different variabilities. If scores in a distribution are similar, they are *homogeneous* (having low variability); if scores are not similar, they are *heterogeneous* (having high variability).

The five most commonly used measures of dispersion are the *range, IQR, variance, SD,* and *coefficient of variation*. Again, which measure of dispersion to use depends on the measurement scale of the variable. It is often useful to present more than one measure of dispersion because they each contain different, albeit related, information about the dispersion of the data.

Range

The range is the simplest measure of variability. It is defined as the difference between the highest and the lowest value in a data set. In the example of body weight (see Table 2-2), the range is 319 to 101 lb (144.7 to 45.8 kg), or 218 lb (98.9 kg). Typically, though, the range is reported as the lowest and the highest number (e.g., the weight ranged from 101 to 319 lb [45.8 to 144.7 kg]). The range is appropriate for ordinal-, interval-, and ratio-level variables. Note that the range can be unstable because it is based on the two most extreme values in the data set. For example, if the heaviest person in the data set weighed 721 lb (327.0 kg), the range would be from 721 to 101 (327.0 to 48.5 kg), or 620 lb (281.2 kg), even though all but one of the data points was at 319 lb (144.7 kg) or lower.

Interquartile Range

The IQR is the middle 50% of the data, that is, the 75th to 25th percentile. It is typically reported when a median value is used for the measure of central tendency. In the example of body weight, the IQR is from 147 to 202 lb (66.7 to 91.6 kg) (an IQR of 55 lb). This is typically reported as "50% of the women weighed between 147 and 202 lb." The IQR is appropriate for ordinal-, interval-, and ratio-level variables.

Standard Deviation and Variance

The SD is the square root of the variance, and it shows the average absolute distance of each point from the mean. It is typically reported as

a measure of dispersion when the mean is presented as the measure of central tendency. The larger the number, the more widely scattered about the mean are the individual values of the variable. The SD is obtained by first computing the variance (the sum of the squared deviations about the mean) and then taking the square root of the variance. The sample variance is represented by the symbol s^2, and the sample SD is represented by the symbol s. The two formulas to compute the sample variance are the *basic formula* and the *shortcut formula*. The basic formula is useful in understanding exactly what the SD is, as you will actually calculate the distance from the mean of each point, square the distance, and then sum it up. The shortcut formula is easier computationally, particularly with larger data sets.

Table 2-9 shows how to compute the **sum of the squared deviations from the mean**:

$$\left(\sum (x_i - \bar{x})^2 \right) \qquad (2\text{-}2)$$

Table 2-9	STEP-BY-STEP COMPUTING: THE SQUARED DEVIATION FROM THE MEAN OF BODY WEIGHT		
Person (No.)	Weight (x) (lb [kg])	Deviation from the Mean ($x - 182.26$)	Squared Deviation from the Mean ($x - 182.26$)^2
1	101 (45.8)	–81.26	6,603.19
2	115 (52.2)	–67.26	4,523.91
3	125 (56.7)	–57.26	3,278.71
4	126 (57.2)	–56.26	3,165.19
5	130 (59.0)	–52.26	2,731.11
6	135 (61.2)	–47.26	2,233.51
7	144 (65.3)	–38.26	1,463.83
8	145 (65.8)	–37.26	1,388.31
9	145 (65.8)	–37.26	1,388.31
10	147 (66.7)	–35.26	1,243.27
11	151 (68.5)	–31.26	977.19
12	161 (73.0)	–21.26	451.99
13	161 (73.0)	–21.26	451.99

(Continued)

Table 2-9	STEP-BY-STEP COMPUTING: THE SQUARED DEVIATION FROM THE MEAN OF BODY WEIGHT *(Continued)*		
Person (No.)	Weight (x) (lb [kg])	Deviation from the Mean ($x - 182.26$)	Squared Deviation from the Mean ($x - 182.26)^2$
14	165 (74.8)	–17.26	297.91
15	167 (75.7)	–15.26	232.87
16	177 (80.3)	–5.26	27.67
17	178 (80.7)	–4.26	18.15
18	180 (81.6)	–2.26	5.11
19	180 (81.6)	–2.26	5.11
20	185 (83.9)	2.74	7.51
21	185 (83.9)	2.74	7.51
22	185 (83.9)	2.74	7.51
23	185 (83.9)	2.74	7.51
24	190 (86.2)	7.74	59.91
25	190 (86.2)	7.74	59.91
26	195 (88.5)	12.74	162.31
27	195 (88.5)	12.74	162.31
28	197 (89.4)	14.74	217.27
29	200 (90.7)	17.74	314.71
30	202 (91.6)	19.74	389.67
31	208 (94.3)	25.74	662.55
32	209 (94.8)	26.74	715.03
33	220 (99.8)	37.74	1,424.31
34	230 (104.3)	47.74	2,279.11
35	235 (106.6)	52.74	2,781.51
36	240 (108.9)	57.74	3,333.91
37	240 (108.9)	57.74	3,333.91
38	265 (120.2)	82.74	6,845.91
39	319 (144.7)	136.74	18,697.83
Sum	$\sum x_i = 7,108$	$\sum x_i - \bar{x} = 0$	$\sum (x_i - \bar{x})^2 = 71,957.44$

The mean value is subtracted from each participant's observed value for the variable. The sum of the mean deviations about the mean is 0 (since there will be an equal value of positive and negative mean deviations), and so the sum of the squared deviations about the mean is used instead. This is often referred to as the "sum of squares about the mean," or, in shorthand, the "sums of squares."

The **basic formula for the sample variance** is

$$S^2 = \frac{\sum (x_i - \bar{x})^2}{n - 1} \qquad (2\text{-}3)$$

The **shortcut formula for sample variance** is

$$S^2 = \frac{\sum x_i^2 - \frac{\left(\sum x_i\right)^2}{n}}{n - 1} \qquad (2\text{-}4)$$

In the basic formula (Equation 2-3), the sample variance is computed by squaring each deviation from the mean, adding them, and dividing the sum by $n - 1$ (one less than the sample size). It may seem odd to divide by $n - 1$ rather than n, but it is a mathematical necessity when using sample data rather than population data and involves a theoretical consideration called *degrees of freedom*. Dividing by $n - 1$ gives an unbiased estimator of the sample variance and SD by correcting for the fact that only certain members of the population are measured. Sophisticated mathematical analyses have proved that if the sum of the squared deviations from the mean were simply divided by the sample size and not $n - 1$, the variance estimate would be too small. This consideration assumes more importance with small samples.

Box 2-4 shows how to compute the sample variance and the sample SD using both the basic and the shortcut formulas. To use the shortcut

---

BOX 2-4   COMPUTING THE VARIANCE AND STANDARD DEVIATION OF BODY WEIGHT

Using the basic formula

$$s^2 = \frac{\sum (x_i - \bar{x})^2}{n - 1}$$, do the following:

Step 1: Compute the sum of the squared deviations about the mean (see Table 2-9).

$$\sum (x_i - \bar{x})^2 = 71,957.44$$

Step 2: Divide by the sample size $n - 1$.
$71957.44/(39 - 1) = 71957.44/38 = 1893.62$
The sample variance, $s^2 = 1893.62$. The sample standard deviation (SD), $s = (1893.62)^{1/2} = 43.52$.

Using the **shortcut formula**

$$s^2 = \frac{\sum x_i^2 - \frac{\left(\sum x_i\right)^2}{n}}{n - 1}$$, do the following:

Step 1: Compute

$$\sum x_i^2$$

by squaring each value of the variable and summing them up (see Table 2-9).

$$\sum x_i^2 = 1,367,436$$

(Continued)

BOX 2-4   COMPUTING THE VARIANCE AND STANDARD DEVIATION OF BODY WEIGHT *(Continued)*

Step 2: Compute

$$\left(\sum x_i\right)^2$$

by summing up the values of the variable (Table 2-9) then squaring the total:

$$\left(\sum x_i\right)^2 = (7108)^2 = 50,523,664$$

Step 3: Plug these two values into the formula, remembering that $n =$ the number of participants in the study:

$$s^2 = \frac{\left(\sum x_i^2 - \frac{\left(\sum x_i\right)^2}{n}\right)}{n-1} = \frac{1,367,436 - \frac{50,523,664}{39}}{39-1}$$

$$= (1,367,436 - 1,295,478.56)/38$$
$$= 71,957.44/38$$
$$= 1,893.62$$

The sample variance, $s^2 = 1,893.62$. The sample SD, $s = (1,893.62)^{1/2} = 43.52$.

Computing the Coefficient of Variation:

$$cv = \frac{s}{\|\overline{x}\|} \times 100$$

Step 1: Compute the SD: s = 43.52.
Step 2: Divide the SD by the absolute value of the mean:
cv = (43.52 lb/182.26 lb) × 100 = 23.88%
The coefficient of variation is 23.88%.

formula, only two values need to be computed: the sum of the squared values of the variable and the sum of the values of the variable. These values are then plugged into the shortcut formula. Table 2-2 shows how to compute these two values for body weight, and Box 2-4 shows how to use these two values to compute the SD.

The variance and SD, like the mean, are sensitive to extreme values. For example, in Table 2-2, the SD of weight is 43.52, but if the weight of the heaviest individual is changed from 319 to 400 lb (144.7 to 181.4 kg), SD changes to 51.43, a large

inflation from the original SD. Therefore, the SD serves best for distributions that are symmetrical and have a single peak. In general, if it is appropriate to calculate the mean, then it is appropriate to calculate the SD.

The SD has a straightforward interpretation if the distribution is bell-shaped or normal. (The normal curve is discussed in detail in the next chapter.) If the distribution is perfectly normal, 68% of the values will be within 1 SD of the mean, 95% of the values will be within 2 SD of the mean, and more than 99% of the data will be within 3 SD of the mean. For example, consider the basic statistics for the approximately bell-shaped distribution of the weight of 39 individuals. The mean weight is 182.26 lb (82.67 kg), and the SD is 43.52. To determine the range of individuals falling ±1 SD from the mean, you subtract the SD from the mean to determine the lower limit (182.26 − 43.52 = 138.74) and add the SD to the mean to determine the upper limit (182.26 + 43.52 = 225.78). Twenty-seven of the 39 individuals, approximately 69%, had weights that fell within 1 SD of the mean weight (between 138.74 and 225.78). This suggests that the distribution of weight is very close to a normal distribution. Even if the distribution is not perfectly symmetrical, however, this percentage holds fairly well. Chebyshev's theorem maintains that even in oddly shaped distributions, at least 75% of the data will fall within 2 SD of the mean (Freund, 1988).

The SD is useful for examining the spread of data for a single variable or among variables measured in the same units, such as pounds. However, to compare the variation of two different variables, such as body weight and blood glucose level, the SD cannot be used because they are measured in different units. Instead, a unitless measure of dispersion called the *coefficient of variation* is used.

Coefficient of Variation

The coefficient of variation is used when comparing the variation of two or more different variables that are measured in different units. It is defined as the ratio of the SD to the absolute value of the mean and is expressed as a percentage. The coefficient of variation is a unitless measure that depicts the size of the SD relative to its mean. The coefficient of variation for body weight is 23.88%. The computation of this is also shown in Box 2-1.

The formula for the coefficient of variation is

$$cv = \frac{s}{\|\bar{x}\|} \times 100 \qquad (2\text{-}5)$$

Population Mean, Variance, and Standard Deviation

When working with population data, different symbols for the mean, variance, and SD are used. A slightly different formula is used to compute the variance and SD of an entire population. A population consists of the entire group that will be described. In nursing and allied health, it is rare to have these types of data. Population data for health care providers provide an indication of the impact of a specific health issue such as infection rates of syphilis or rates of preterm births within a specified region. Each state collects these types of data, which may be used as population health indicators. Examples of nationwide data can be found on the Centers for Disease Control and Prevention's (CDC's) Web site (www.cdc.gov). For population-based data, the symbol for the *population mean* is μ, and the following symbols and formulas are used:
The formula for the population mean is

$$\mu = \frac{\sum x_i}{n} \qquad (2\text{-}6)$$

The basic formula for the population variance is

$$\sigma^2 = \frac{\sum (x_i - \mu)^2}{n} \qquad (2\text{-}7)$$

The shortcut formula for population variance is

$$\sigma^2 = \frac{\sum x_i^2 - \dfrac{\left(\sum x_i\right)^2}{n}}{n} \qquad (2\text{-}8)$$

The population SD is the square root of the population variance:

$$\sqrt{\sigma^2} \qquad (2\text{-}9)$$

Measures of Skewness or Symmetry

In addition to central tendency and variability, *symmetry* is an important characteristic of a distribution. A *normal distribution* is *symmetrical* and bell-shaped, having only one mode. When a variable's distribution is asymmetrical, it is skewed. A skewed variable is one whose mean is not in the center of the distribution, and when the variable is skewed, the mean and the median are different. If there is positive skewness, there is a pileup of cases to the left and the right tail of the distribution is too long. Negative skewness results in a pileup of cases to the right and a too-long left tail (Tabachnick & Fidel, 2001). For a positively skewed variable, the mean will be greater than the median, whereas for a negatively skewed variable, the mean will be less than the median.

Two sets of data can have the same mean and SD but different skewness. Two measures of symmetry are considered here: Pearson's measure and Fisher's measure. Although rarely mentioned in research reports, these statistics are very useful in determining the degree of symmetry of a variable's distribution. Researchers routinely compute them using statistics produced when running frequency distributions and descriptive statistics on study variables.

Pearson's Skewness Coefficient

The Pearson's Skewness Coefficient is easily calculated and is useful for quick estimates of symmetry. It is defined as

$$\text{Skewness} = \frac{\bar{x} - \text{Median}}{s}$$

For a perfectly symmetrical distribution, the mean will equal the median, and the skewness coefficient will be 0. As shown in Figure 2-8, if the distribution is positively skewed, the mean will be more than the median, and the coefficient will be positive. If the coefficient is negative, the distribution is negatively skewed, and the mean will be less than the median. In general, skewness values will fall between –1 and +1 SD units. Values falling outside this range indicate a substantially skewed distribution (Hair et al., 2009).

Hildebrand (1986) states that skewness values above 0.2 or below –0.2 indicate severe skewness.

For the weight data of Table 2-2, the Pearson skewness coefficient is (182.26 – 185.00)/43.52 = –0.06. The resulting value of –0.06 is close to 0. Using Hildebrand's guideline, the value of –0.06 indicates minor, not severe, skewness.

Fisher's Measure of Skewness

The formula for Fisher's skewness statistic, found in Hildebrand (1986), is based on deviations from the mean to the third power. A symmetrical curve will result in a value of 0. If the skewness value is positive, then the curve is skewed to the right, and vice versa for a distribution skewed to the left. For the weight data in Table 2-2, Fisher's skewness measure is 0.727. The measure of skewness can be interpreted in terms of the normal curve. (This concept is explained further in the next chapter.) A z-score is calculated by dividing the measure of skewness by the standard error for skewness (0.727/0.378 = 1.92). Values above +1.96 or below –1.96 are significant at the 0.05 level because 95% of the scores in a normal distribution fall between +1.96 and –1.96 SD from the mean. Our value of 1.92 is less than 1.96, indicating that this distribution is not significantly skewed. Because this statistic is based on deviations to the third power, it is very sensitive to extreme values.

MEASURES OF KURTOSIS OR PEAKEDNESS

Fisher's Measure of Kurtosis

This statistic, indicating whether a distribution has the right bell shape for a normal curve, measures whether the bell shape is too flat or too peaked. Fisher's measure, based on deviations from the mean to the fourth power, can also be found in Hildebrand (1986). However, the calculation is tedious and is ordinarily done by a computer program. A curve with the correct bell shape will result in a value of 0. If the kurtosis value is a large positive number, the distribution is too peaked to be normal (*leptokurtic*). If the kurtosis value is negative, the curve is too flat to be normal (*platykurtic*). For the weight data in Table 2-2, the kurtosis statistic is given as 1.40, a value close to 0, indicating that the shape of the bell for this distribution can be called normal. Dividing this value by the standard error for kurtosis (1.40/0.741 = 1.89), our distribution is not significantly kurtosed; that is, the value is not beyond ±1.96 SD. Because this statistic is based on deviations to the fourth power, it is very sensitive to extreme values. If a distribution is markedly skewed, there is no particular need to examine kurtosis because the distribution is not normal.

OBTAINING FREQUENCY TABLES, DESCRIPTIVE STATISTICS, AND HISTOGRAMS IN SPSS

The method for obtaining frequencies, descriptive statistics, and histograms in SPSS is shown in Box 2-5, and the output is shown in Box 2-6. In step 1, the data are entered into the SPSS data window. Of note, there are two variables: "Caseid" and "Weight." Caseid is simply the unique identifier of each woman in the data set, and Weight is the woman's self-reported weight in pounds. After the data are entered, the menu system is used to obtain a frequency distribution, descriptive statistics, and a histogram.

For step 2, from the menu bar, "Analyze ... Descriptive Statistics ... Frequencies" are selected successively. For step 3, the variable "Weight" is selected and moved over to the "Variables" slot, making sure that the "Display Frequency Tables" box is checked to obtain a frequency distribution. Clicking on the "Statistics" button to obtain descriptive statistics continues the process. After the popup box appears for step 4, the statistics that will be computed are selected. In this example, the mean, median, mode, quartiles, SD, and minimum and maximum values will be computed. "Sum" gives the Σx_i, allowing the work to be checked. In step 5, a histogram is chosen by

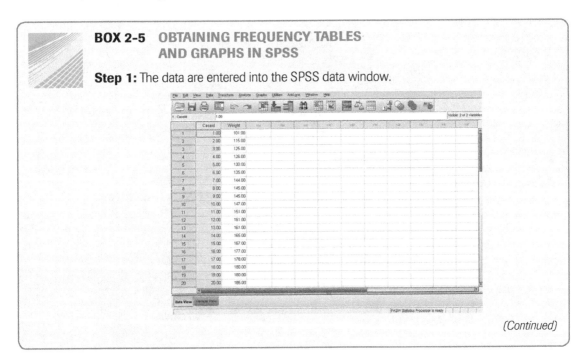

BOX 2-5   OBTAINING FREQUENCY TABLES AND GRAPHS IN SPSS

Step 1: The data are entered into the SPSS data window.

(Continued)

**BOX 2-5 OBTAINING FREQUENCY TABLES AND GRAPHS
IN SPSS** *(Continued)*

Step 2: The menu bar is used to click on "Analyze" and then to select "Descriptive Statistics" and "Frequencies."

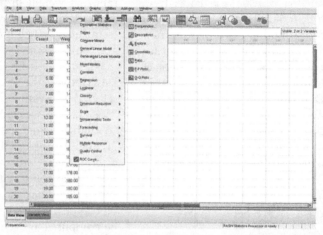

Step 3: In the "Frequencies" popup box, the variable "Weight" is moved over to the slot labeled "Variable(s)." The "Display Frequency Tables" box is checked.

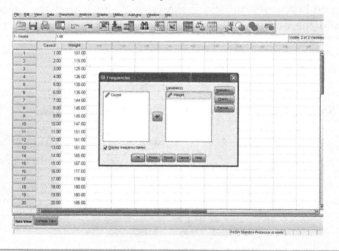

**BOX 2-5   OBTAINING FREQUENCY TABLES AND GRAPHS
IN SPSS** *(Continued)*

Step 4: Click on the "Statistics" button. In the "Statistics" popup box, the "Quartiles" box is checked under "Percentile Values," and the "Mean," "Median," "Mode," and "Sum" boxes are checked under "Central Tendency," as shown. Also check the boxes for "Std deviation," "S.E. Mean," "Minimum," "Maximum," and "Variance" under "Dispersion." The "Continue" button is then clicked.

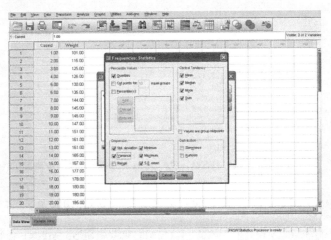

Step 5: In the "Frequencies" popup box, the "Charts" button is clicked.

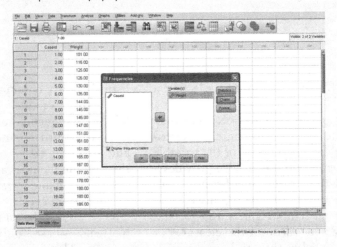

(Continued)

BOX 2-5   OBTAINING FREQUENCY TABLES AND GRAPHS IN SPSS (Continued)

Step 6: In the "Frequencies: Charts" popup box, "Histograms" is checked, and the "Continue" button is clicked.

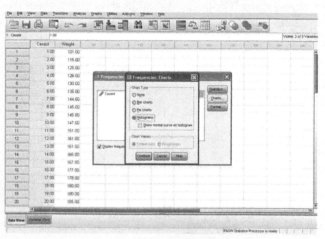

Step 7: When the "OK" button is clicked, the output appears in the output window (see Box 2-6).
Alternatively, when the "Paste" button is clicked, SPSS syntax is generated, which, when run, will generate the output in the output window.

clicking the "Charts" button and selecting a histogram.

The SPSS output lists the statistics that were requested in the first box and an exact distribution of each and every value of the variable "Weight" in the second box. It also provides a histogram. All three measures of central tendency are in the first box: the mean weight is 182.26 lb, the median weight is 185 lb, and the mode is 185 lb. Also, all the measures of dispersion are found in the first box: the SD is 43.52 lb, and the range is 218 lb (with a minimum weight of 101 lb and a maximum weight of 319 lb).

The frequency distribution provided by SPSS is in the second box (see Box 2-6). This listing has five columns. The first column lists the actual weights. The second column is labeled "Frequency" and lists the raw frequencies. The third column is labeled "Percent" and lists the relative frequencies. However, this column includes any missing values in the computation and *should not* be used to report relative frequencies. The fourth column is labeled "Valid Percent" and lists the relative frequencies based *only* on valid values of the variable. This column is used to report relative frequencies. Note that because there are no missing values in this data set, the "Percent" and "Valid Percent" are the same. That would not be the case if some participants were missing information about their weight. The last

BOX 2-6 SPSS OUTPUT FROM THE FREQUENCIES COMMAND FREQUENCIES

Statistics

Weight

N	Valid	39
	Missing	0
Mean		182.2564 (82.671)
Standard error of mean		6.96809
Median		185.0000 (83.9145)
Mode		185.00 (83.91)
Standard deviation		43.51571
Variance		1,893.617
Minimum		101.00 (45.81)
Maximum		319.00 (144.70)
Sum		7,108.00
Percentiles	25	147.0000 (66.6780)
	50	185.0000 (83.9145)
	75	202.0000 (91.6256)

Weight

		Frequency	Percent	Valid Percent	Cumulative Percent
Valid	101.00 (45.81)	1	2.6	2.6	2.6
	115.00 (52.16)	1	2.6	2.6	5.1
	125.00 (56.70)	1	2.6	2.6	7.7
	126.00 (57.15)	1	2.6	2.6	10.3
	130.00 (58.97)	1	2.6	2.6	12.8
	135.00 (61.23)	1	2.6	2.6	15.4
	144.00 (65.32)	1	2.6	2.6	17.9
	145.00 (65.77)	2	5.1	5.1	23.1
	147.00 (66.68)	1	2.6	2.6	25.6
	151.00 (68.49)	1	2.6	2.6	28.2
	161.00 (73.03)	2	5.1	5.1	33.3

(Continued)

BOX 2-6   SPSS OUTPUT FROM THE FREQUENCIES COMMAND FREQUENCIES (Continued)

	Frequency	Percent	Valid Percent	Cumulative Percent
165.00 (74.84)	1	2.6	2.6	35.9
167.00 (75.75)	1	2.6	2.6	38.5
177.00 (80.29)	1	2.6	2.6	41.0
180.00 (81.65)	2	5.1	5.1	48.7
185.00 (83.91)	4	10.3	10.3	59.0
190.00 (86.18)	2	5.1	5.1	64.1
195.00 (88.45)	2	5.1	5.1	69.2
197.00 (89.36)	1	2.6	2.6	71.8
200.00 (90.72)	1	2.6	2.6	74.4
202.00 (91.63)	1	2.6	2.6	76.9
208.00 (94.35)	1	2.6	2.6	79.5
209.00 (94.80)	1	2.6	2.6	82.1
220.00 (99.79)	1	2.6	2.6	84.6
230.00 (104.33)	1	2.6	2.6	87.2
235.00 (106.59)	1	2.6	2.6	89.7
240.00 (108.86)	2	5.1	5.1	94.9
265.00 (120.20)	1	2.6	2.6	97.4
319.00 (144.70)	1	2.6	2.6	100.0
Total	39	100.0	100.0	

column is labeled "Cumulative Percent" and lists the cumulative frequency distribution. For example, 10.3% of the sample weighs exactly 185 lb (83.9 kg) (valid percent), and overall, 59.0% of the sample weighs 185 lb or less (cumulative percent). In SPSS, the frequency table is not automatically put into class intervals. To create a frequency table with even class intervals such as the one in Table 2-3, a version of the variable "Weight" that was grouped into class intervals would have to be created.

Putting It All Together
The results would be reported as follows: the mean weight of the women was 182.26 lb (82.67 kg), ranging from 101 to 319 lb (45.8 to 144.7 kg). The SD was 43.52 lb, and the coefficient of variation was 23.88%. The Fisher's measure of skewness of the distribution was 0.727 (SD = 0.378) and the Fisher's measure of kurtosis was 1.401 (SD = 0.741).

CHAPTER REVIEW

Multiple-Choice Concept Review

1. The equation Σx_i^2 is best known as the
   a. sum of all the squared values of the variable x in the data set.
   b. product of all the values of the variable x in the data set.
   c. square of the sum of all the values of the variable x in the data set.
   d. sum of all the values of the variable x in the data set.

2. The equation $(\Sigma x_i)^2$ is best known as the
   a. sum of all the squared values of the variable x in the data set.
   b. product of all the values of the variable x in the data set.
   c. square of the sum of all the values of the variable x in the data set.
   d. sum of all the values of the variable x in the data set.

3. A nominal level of measurement is used when the values of a variable have which of the following properties?
   a. They can be placed in meaningful order, but there is no information about the size of the interval between each value.
   b. They can be placed in meaningful order, have meaningful intervals, and have a true zero.
   c. They can be placed in meaningful order and have meaningful intervals between the times, but there is no true zero.
   d. They simply represent categories.

4. Class intervals should be
   a. of equal length.
   b. mutually exclusive.
   c. overlapping intervals.
   d. a and b only.

5. Symmetrical distributions are best described by which of the following statements?
   a. They have an equal number of data points that appear to the left and to the right of the center.
   b. They are normally distributed.
   c. They have a U-shaped distribution.
   d. They have small standard deviations.

6. Skewness refers to the
   a. shape of the top of the curve.
   b. extent to which data are not symmetrical about the center.
   c. presence of outliers.
   d. sample.

7. Which of the following statements best describes a stem-and-leaf display?
   a. It shows the range of values of the variable.
   b. It shows the shape of the distribution of the variable.
   c. It preserves the individual values of the variable.
   d. All of the above are correct.

8. Standard deviation is best described by which of the following statements?
   a. It can be used to compare variation between two or more variables.
   b. It is the average distance of each point from the mean.
   c. It is the variance squared.
   d. Both a and b are correct.

9. Descriptive statistics have which of the following properties?
   a. They are numerical or graphical summaries of data.
   b. They are used to examine relationships between variables in a data set.
   c. They are used to see how well sample data can be generalized to the population.
   d. All of these.

10. Inferential statistics have which of the following properties?
    a. They are numerical or graphical summaries of data.
    b. They are used to examine relationships between variables in a data set.
    c. They are used to see how well sample data can be generalized to the population.
    d. Both b and c are correct.

Choosing the Correct Measurement Scale

For each of the following variables (1 to 20) listed below, select the correct measurement scale (a to d).
   a. Nominal
   b. Ordinal
   c. Interval
   d. Ratio

1. Gender

2. Temperature in Celsius

3. Weight in pounds

4. Weight in kilograms

5. Age in years

6. Age in categories (0 to 6 months, 7 to 12 months, 13+ months)

7. Blood type

8. Ethnic identity

9. Number of years spent in school

10. Highest educational degree obtained

11. Satisfaction with nursing care received (on a scale of 1 to 10)

12. Religion

13. IQ score

14. Smoking status (nonsmoker vs. smoker)

15. Birth order

16. Reaction time in seconds

17. Marital status

18. Number of children

19. Score on a satisfaction scale that sums Likert items

20. Annual income in dollars

Computational Problems

1. For each of the following two data sets, do the following by hand and in SPSS:
   a. Create a frequency distribution.
   b. Create a histogram.
   c. Create a stem-and-leaf plot (by hand only).
   d. Compute the measures of central tendency (i.e., mean, median, and mode) and dispersion (i.e., range, interquartile range, and standard deviation).

Data set 1: Number of Hospitals in 25 Selected Counties in Yunnan, China

8	12	60	79	48
53	18	54	25	36
13	16	23	30	30
49	14	22	44	35
13	20	38	24	28

Data set 2: Blood Cholesterol (in mg/dL) Levels of 32 Participants at a Community Health Fair

180	185	200	198
211	203	199	195
210	190	210	200
180	197	188	198
187	240	189	178
185	220	188	200
188	259	195	221
200	196	194	196

2. From the data in the table below, determine the following:
   a. What percentage of this group is married?
   b. What is the mean age and standard deviation of age?
   c. How many participants are older than 30 years?
   d. What percentage of this group is older than 30 years?
   e. What percentage of this group is male?
   f. What are the mean and standard deviation of years of work experience?
   g. What percentage of this group has a BS degree?

Data set: Selected Demographic Information for 17 Health Care Students Who Attend a State University

ID No.	Gender	Age (Years)	Marital Status	Years Worked	Degree
101	M	27	Married	6	BS
102	F	51	Married	29	MS
103	F	41	Married	19	MS
104	F	26	Married	4	BS
105	F	27	Single	4	BS
106	F	47	Divorced	25	MS
107	F	49	Divorced	20	MS
108	F	42	Married	19	MS
109	F	37	Married	17	BS
110	F	50	Married	28	BS
111	F	39	Single	7	MS
112	M	42	Married	10	MS
113	F	27	Married	5	BS
114	F	49	Divorced	30	BS
115	M	33	Married	11	BS
116	F	30	Married	11	BS
117	F	43	Single	20	MS

3. For the following data set, do the following by hand and in SPSS:
   a. For each group, do the following:
      - Construct the stem-and-leaf plot (by hand only).
      - Construct the histogram.
      - Construct the frequency distribution.
      - Compute the mean, median, mode, standard deviation, and interquartile range.
   b. What does a comparison of the two groups suggest?

Data set: Age (in Years) of 140 Inpatients in Two Departments of One Hospital

Department A

37	37	52	49	48	40	60
37	37	52	54	43	40	54
37	37	52	38	33	40	53
18	37	40	41	45	39	52
57	38	40	34	42	41	46
58	38	40	64	26	41	43
78	33	40	64	40	41	35
18	43	40	53	40	41	35
19	43	41	58	40	31	35
19	43	51	56	35	31	35

Department B

19	84	39	56	78	31	35
19	48	46	56	74	36	25
19	65	35	55	68	79	40
18	65	36	53	66	37	40
20	65	41	53	59	25	31
28	65	41	53	45	18	36
28	43	44	52	52	34	37
47	47	29	47	44	41	31
63	52	30	42	46	41	57
45	52	30	48	40	41	37

4. For the following data set, do the following by hand and in SPSS:
   a. For each group, do the following:
   - Construct the stem-and-leaf plot (by hand only).
   - Construct the histogram.
   - Construct the frequency distribution.
   - Compute the mean, median, mode, standard deviation, and interquartile range.
   b. What does a comparison of the two groups suggest?

Data set: Measured Weight (in Pounds [kg]) of 48 Employees of Two Groups in a Health Care Department					
Group A					
155 (70.3)	160 (72.6)	155 (70.3)	200 (90.7)	125 (56.7)	130 (59.0)
240 (108.9)	118 (53.5)	200 (90.7)	180 (81.6)	130 (59.0)	270 (122.5)
145 (65.8)	180 (81.6)	220 (99.8)	150 (68.0)	154 (69.9)	132 (59.9)
201 (91.2)	100 (45.4)	162 (73.5)	150 (68.0)	228 (103.4)	130 (59.0)
Group B					
182 (82.6)	180 (81.6)	245 (111.1)	203 (92.1)	200 (90.7)	181 (82.1)
192 (87.1)	260 (117.9)	145 (65.8)	165 (74.8)	245 (111.1)	165 (74.8)
225 (102.1)	243 (110.2)	185 (83.9)	200 (90.7)	160 (72.6)	210 (95.3)
115 (52.2)	212 (96.2)	198 (89.8)	145 (65.8)	225 (102.1)	280 (127.0)

Data set Exercises

1. Access the data set called MUNRO04.SAV, which contains data collected using the survey form available on thePoint. Either bring it into SPSS or convert it into a file for SAS or whatever software you are using. Print the dictionary, which contains a list of the variables, formats, and labels. In most versions of SPSS for Windows, this is done by clicking on Utilities, and then on File Info. Once the file is in the output screen, it can be printed from the File menu.

2. Compare the file information with the survey form on thePoint. Note that the variable names have been selected to reflect each variable, making it easy to recognize them when working with the file. Variable labels and value labels have been added to enhance the output. Look for any discrepancies between the survey form and the file information.

3. Produce charts/graphs. Many options are available for producing charts in statistical software programs. They may be produced within specific techniques and in separate graphics sections. We will confine ourselves to requesting graphics that are available with the specific techniques. The following can be requested as part of the output from frequencies in most software programs. Within the frequencies program, request a bar graph for GENDER, a histogram for SATCURWT, and a histogram with a polygon (normal curve) for SATCURWT.

Key Principles Underlying Statistical Inference: Probability and the Normal Distribution

OBJECTIVES

After studying this chapter, you should be able to:

1. Explain the importance of probability theory for statistical inference.

2. Define the characteristics of a probability measure, and explain the difference between a theoretical probability distribution and an empirical probability distribution (*a priori* vs. *a posteriori*).

3. Compute marginal, joint, and conditional probabilities from a cross-tabulation table and correctly interpret their meaning.

4. Define and derive sensitivity, specificity, predictive value, and efficiency from a cross-tabulation table.

5. Identify and describe the characteristics of a normal distribution.

6. Use a standard normal distribution to obtain *z*-scores and percentiles.

7. Explain the importance of the central limit theorem.

FUNDAMENTAL CONCEPTS IN RESEARCH

One of the main objectives of research is to draw meaningful conclusions about a population, based on data collected from a sample of that population. Sometimes researchers focus on what a sample can tell us about a whole population, sometimes they focus on how a sample compares with the whole population, and at other times they make comparisons between different groups. Researchers may also compare measurements on the same group that are taken over time (e.g., to test how a weight-loss program is performing). In all these cases, researchers use statistical inference as their tool for obtaining information from a sample of data about the population from which the sample is drawn. Statistical inference uses probability to help the researchers to assess the meaning of their findings. A particularly important probability distribution for statistical inference in health-related research is the normal (or Gaussian) distribution. This chapter focuses on the fundamental concepts of probability and the normal distribution, both of which are crucial to understanding the statistical techniques contained in the subsequent chapters of this book.

Estimating Population Probabilities Using Research

One example of using statistical inference to draw conclusions about a population from a sample comes to us from a recent population-based study of an urban area using the New York City Health and Nutrition Examination Survey (NYCHANES). In this study, the authors found that the prevalence of diabetes (diagnosed and undiagnosed combined) among adults aged 20 and above was 12.5%. (Thorpe et al., 2009) Population-based studies have also been used to estimate the baseline prevalence of an exposure or disease. For example, in order to determine the efficacy of the human papillomavirus (HPV) vaccine, the baseline population prevalence for HPV must be determined. Using biological samples collected as part of the 2003 to 2004 NHANES cycle, it was estimated that the overall prevalence of HPV was 28.6% among women aged 14 to 59 years (Dunne et al., 2007).

PROBABILITY: THE MATHEMATICS THAT UNDERLIES STATISTICS

An understanding of probability is critical to an understanding of statistical inference. Competency in probability is needed to comprehend statistical

significance (e.g., interpreting p-values), read cross-tabulation tables, and understand frequency distributions, all of which are used in health care research extensively (see Chapters 2 and 10). In particular, correctly reading cross-tabulation tables (commonly referred to as "cross-tabs") is a critical skill for researchers and for clinicians and administrators who need to understand the research literature. Using cross-tabs requires an understanding of joint, conditional, and marginal probabilities. Thus, after a brief discussion of definitions and concepts necessary to an understanding of probability, we will illustrate the principles of probability with examples from cross-tabulation tables.

Defining Probability

The general concept of objective probability can be categorized under two areas: *a priori* (theoretical or classical) probability and *a posteriori* (empirical or relative frequency) probability (Daniel, 2008; Mood, Graybill, & Boes, 1974). In theoretical probability, the distribution of events can be inferred without collecting data. For example, we can compute the probability of getting "heads or tails" on a coin flip without actually flipping the coin. In empirical probability, data must be collected by some process, and the probability that each event will occur must be estimated from the data. In health care research, empirical probability is used when reporting characteristics of a sample (e.g., 35% of the sample was female) and classical probability (e.g., theoretical probability distributions) is used when making statistical inferences about the data.

Probability provides a numerical measure of uncertainty by giving a precise measurement of the likelihood that an event will occur. An event can be as simple as a single outcome (e.g., one card is picked out of a deck of cards) or it can be composed of a set of outcomes (e.g., five cards are picked out of a deck of cards). It can be an event from which results are inferred (e.g., a coin flip) or an event for which data need to be collected (e.g., percentage of premature births in a hospital). Events that are uncertain are those that may or may not occur. For example, there is a small chance that a lottery ticket will be a winner (i.e., the "event"), but there is a much larger chance that it will not be a winner. People who purchase lottery tickets are essentially willing to pay for the uncertainty (the probability) of winning.

Several definitions, notations, and formulas—all of which are used throughout this chapter—are useful for an understanding of probability (Table 3-1). It is particularly critical to understand two of these ideas, sample space and probability distribution, when using statistics. Simply put, *sample space* is the set of all possible outcomes of a study. For example, if a coin is flipped, the sample space has two possible outcomes: heads and tails; if a six-sided die is rolled, the sample space has six possible outcomes. Similarly, the sample space for gender has two outcomes: female and male.

A *probability distribution* is the set of probabilities associated with each possible outcome in the sample space. The probability distribution of a variable can be expressed as a table, graph, or formula; the key is that it specifies all the possible values of a random variable

and the respective probabilities (Daniel, 2008). The probability distributions computed in Chapter 2 are examples of empirical probability distributions. The probability distributions used in inferential statistics (e.g., normal distribution, binomial distribution, chi-square distribution, and Student's *t* distribution) are examples of theoretical probability distributions.

Probability theory is based on the three axioms stated by Kolmogorov (1956). These axioms are illustrated by examples in the next section:

1. The probability that each event will occur must be greater than or equal to 0 and less than or equal to 1.
2. The sum of the probabilities of all the mutually exclusive outcomes of the sample space is equal to 1. Mutually exclusive outcomes are those that cannot occur at the same time (e.g., on any given flip, a coin can be either heads or tails but not both).
3. The probability that either of two mutually exclusive events, *A* or *B*, will occur is the sum of the probabilities of their individual probabilities.

Table 3-1	PROBABILITY SYMBOLS AND DEFINITIONS
Symbol or Term	**Meaning**
Sample space	The set of all possible outcomes of a study
Probability distribution	The set of probabilities associated with each event in the sample space
$p(A)$	The marginal probability that event A will occur
$p(\overline{A})$	The probability that event A will not occur
$p(A|B)$	The conditional probability that event A will occur if event B occurs
$p(A \cap B)$	The joint probability that both events A and B will occur; also called the intersection of A and B
$p(A \cup B)$	The probability that event A will happen and/or event B will happen; also called the union of A and B
Addition rule	$p(A \cup B) = p(A) + p(B) - p(A \cap B)$
Multiplication rule	$p(A \cap B) = p(A) \times p(A|B)$
Independence of events A and B	If $p(A) = p(A|B)$, then A and B are independent

In this section, we illustrate the different types of probability using a cross-tabulation table from a study of emergency department (ED) services for sexual assault victims in Virginia (Table 3-2) (Plichta, Vandecar-Burdin, Odor, Reams, & Zhang, 2007). This study examined the question: Does having a forensic nurse trained to assist victims of sexual violence on staff in an ED affect the probability that a hospital will have a relationship with a rape crisis center? Some experts thought that having a forensic nurse on staff might actually reduce the chance that an ED would have a connection with a rape crisis center. The two variables of interest here are "forensic nurse on staff" (yes/no) and "relationship with rape crisis center" (yes/no). A total of 53 EDs provided appropriate responses to these two questions, and it turned out that 33 EDs had a forensic nurse on staff and 41 EDs had a relationship with a rape crisis center.

Marginal Probability

The marginal probability is simply the number of times the event occurred divided by the total number of times that it could have occurred. When using relative frequency probability, the probability of an event is the number of times the event occurred divided by

the total number of trials. This is expressed mathematically as

$$p(A) = \frac{\#Times\_A\_occurs}{N} \qquad (3\text{-}1)$$

where N is the total number of trials. In health care research, the number of trials (N) is typically the number of subjects in the study. "Subjects" may refer to individual human beings, individual institutions (e.g., EDs), or even individual laboratory samples.

First, the simple probability, also called the marginal probability, of each of the two variables is computed. The probability that the ED will have a forensic nurse on staff is

$$p(A) = \frac{33}{53} = .6226$$

In other words, 62.26% of the EDs have a forensic nurse on staff. The probability of not having a forensic nurse on staff, $p(\text{not } A)$, is

$$p(\bar{A}) = \frac{20}{53} = .3774$$

Because having a nurse on staff and not having a nurse on staff are mutually exclusive and exhaustive events, their probabilities add up to 1 (.6626 + .3774 = 1.0). Similarly, the probability that the ED will have a relationship with a rape crisis center is

$$p(B) = \frac{41}{53} = .7736$$

Table 3-2	**CROSS-TABULATION TABLE: FORENSIC NURSE ON EMERGENCY DEPARTMENT STAFF BY EMERGENCY DEPARTMENT LINKAGE TO A RAPE CRISIS CENTER**		
	RAPE CRISIS CENTER LINKAGE		
Forensic Nurse on EMERGENCY DEPARTMENT Staff	No	Yes	Total
No	8	12	20
Yes	4	29	33
Total	12	41	53

In other words, 77.36% of the hospitals have such a relationship, and the probability that the ED will not have a relationship with a rape crisis center is

$$p(\bar{B})=\frac{12}{53}=.2264$$

Conditional Probability

Conditional probability is the probability that one event will occur *given that* another event has occurred. In mathematical notation, conditional probability is written as $p(B|A)$, the probability of event B occurring *given that* event A has occurred. In practice, using conditional probabilities means that only a subset of the data is being studied. It is very important to use the correct denominator when computing conditional probability.

Conditional probabilities are often compared in cross-tabulation tables. For example, in the ED study, the research question is: Does having a forensic nurse on staff affect the probability that the ED will have a relationship with the local rape crisis center? To answer this question, we need to compare two conditional probabilities: (a) *given that* the ED does not have a forensic nurse on staff, what is the probability that the ED will have a relationship with a rape crisis center and (b) *given that* the ED does have a forensic nurse on staff, what is the probability that the ED will have a relationship with a rape crisis center?

The correct denominator for the first probability is 20 because 20 EDs reported no forensic nurse on staff, and the correct denominator for the second probability is 33 because 33 EDs reported that they do have a forensic nurse on staff. The conditional probabilities are computed as follows:

p(relationship with rape crisis center|no forensic nurse)

$$=p(B\,|\,\bar{A})=\frac{12}{20}=.6000$$

p(relationship with rape crisis center|forensic nurse)

$$=p(B\,|\,A)=\frac{29}{33}=.8788$$

In other words, 60% of the EDs without a forensic nurse on staff have a relationship with a rape crisis center compared with 87.88% of EDs with a forensic nurse on staff. Although it certainly looks like the presence of a forensic nurse increases the chances of having such a relationship, inferential statistics (in this case, a chi-square test, discussed in Chapter 10) must be used to see whether this difference was statistically significant or simply attributable to chance.

Joint Probability

Joint probability is the cooccurrence of two or more events. The key to understanding joint probability is to know that the words "both" and "and" are usually involved. For example, if the research question asked about the probability of an ED in our sample having *both* a forensic nurse on staff *and* a relationship with a rape crisis center, a joint probability would be computed.

In mathematical notation, this probability is written as:

$$p(A\cap B) \qquad (3\text{-}2)$$

In this example, the probability would be computed as

p(forensic nurse on staff $\cap$ relationship with rape crisis center)

$$p(A\cap B)=\frac{29}{53}=.547$$

In other words, 54.7% of the EDs have *both* a forensic nurse on staff *and* a relationship with a local rape crisis center. In this case, the denominator is the entire sample and the numerator is the number of EDs with both conditions.

Addition Rule

The addition rule is used to compute the probability that either one of two events will occur; this means that one, the other, or both will occur. Usually, the term *and/or* indicates this type of probability. For example, if one wanted to know how many hospitals had a forensic nurse on staff *and/or* a relationship with a rape crisis center, the addition rule would be used. The general rule is expressed mathematically as shown in Equation 3-3:

$$P(A \cup B) = p(A) + P(B) - p(A \cap B) \quad (3\text{-}3)$$

The reason that the joint probability is subtracted is that if the events A and B are nonmutually exclusive (e.g., they have some overlap), the probability of the overlap is added twice. In the example above, the two marginal probabilities and the joint probability of these two outcomes are used to compute the probability of the event of either occurring:

$$p(A) = p(\text{forensic\_nurse\_on\_staff}) = \frac{33}{53}$$

$$p(B) = p(\text{relationship\_with\_rape\_crisis\_}$$
$$\text{center}) = \frac{41}{53}$$

$$p(A \cap B) = p(\text{forensic\_nurse} \mid \text{rape\_crisis\_}$$
$$\text{center}) = \frac{29}{53}$$

Thus,

$$p(A \cap B) = \frac{33}{53} + \frac{41}{53} - \frac{29}{53} = \frac{45}{53} = .849$$

In other words, 84.9% of the EDs have a forensic nurse on staff *and/or* a relationship with a rape crisis center.

Another version of the addition rule is useful when computing the probability that either of two mutually exclusive events will occur. When two events are mutually exclusive, they never occur together, and thus, their joint probability

is 0. Therefore, the addition rule for mutually exclusive events is reduced to

$$p(A \cup B) = p(A) + p(B) \quad (3\text{-}4)$$

since $p(A \cap B) = 0$

Multiplication Rule

The multiplication rule in probability allows certain types of probabilities to be computed from other probabilities. This is particularly useful when only the probabilities that the events will occur, not the raw data, are available. These probabilities can be used to compute joint probabilities. The general multiplication rule is

$$p(A \cap B) = p(A) \times p(B \mid A) \quad (3\text{-}5)$$

For example, if only marginal and conditional probabilities from the ED study were available, the joint probability could be computed as shown in Equation 3-5 using the marginal and conditional probabilities as such:

$$p(A) = p(\text{forensic\_nurse\_on\_staff}) = \frac{33}{53} = .6226$$

$$p(B \mid A) = p(\text{relationship with rape crisis center}$$
$$\text{and forensic nurse on staff}) = \frac{29}{33} = .8788$$

$$p(A \cap B) = .6226 \times .8788 = .5471$$

This is the same result achieved when joint probability was computed directly from the table:

$$\frac{29}{53} = .5471$$

Independent Events

Two events are independent when the occurrence of either one does not change the probability that the other will occur. In mathematical terms, this is defined by saying that events

A and B are independent if $p(A|B) = p(A)$. In this case, the multiplication rule reduces to

$$p(A \cap B) = p(A) \times p(B) \qquad (3\text{-}6)$$

It is important to understand that independent events are not mutually exclusive events; they can and do cooccur. Mutually exclusive events are not independent insofar as the occurrence of one depends on the other one's *not* occurring.

An example of two independent events is rolling a 3 on a die and flipping a tail on a coin. Rolling a 3 does not affect the probability of flipping the tail. If events are independent, then the joint probability that both will occur is simply the product of the probabilities that each will occur. This is written as

$$p(A \cap B) = p(A) \times p(B) \qquad (3\text{-}7)$$

which means the

$$p(A \text{ and } B) = p(A) \times p(B) \qquad (3\text{-}8)$$

For example, the probability of rolling a 3 on a die is .17, and the probability of flipping a tail on a coin is .5. Then the probability of both rolling a 3 on a die and flipping a tail on the coin is

$$.17 \times .05 = .085$$

Sensitivity, Specificity, Predictive Value, and Efficiency

Cross-tabulation tables can also provide us with information on the quality of diagnostic tests. Clinicians routinely order tests to screen patients for the presence or absence of disease. There are four possible outcomes to diagnosing and testing a particular patient: True Positive (TP), where the screening test result correctly identifies someone who has the disease as having the disease (i.e., both diagnosis and screening test result are positive for the disease); True Negative (TN), where the screening test result correctly identifies someone who does not have the disease as not having the disease (i.e., both diagnosis and screening test are negative); False Positive (FP), where the screening test result incorrectly

identifies someone who does not have the disease as having the disease (i.e., diagnosis is negative and the screening test result is positive for the disease); and False Negative (FN), where the screening test result incorrectly classifies someone as not having the disease when, in fact, that person does have the disease (i.e., the diagnosis is positive for the disease and the screening test result is negative for it) (Kraemer, 1992). Essex-Sorlie (1995) notes that a type I error resembles an *FP outcome*, occurring when a screening test result incorrectly indicates disease presence. A type II error is comparable to an *FN outcome*, indicating a screening test result incorrectly points to disease absence. The following 2 × 2 table is often used as a way to depict the relationship between the various outcomes.

	DIAGNOSIS	
Screening	Condition Present	Condition Absent
Test Result Positive	True Positive (TP)	False Positive (FP)
Test Result Negative	False Negative (FN)	True Negative (TN)

The terms used to define the clinical performance of a screening test result are sensitivity, specificity, positive predictive value, negative predictive value, and efficiency. Test *sensitivity* (Sn) is defined as the probability that the test result is positive when given to a group of patients who have the disease. It is determined by the formula

$$Sn = (TP/[TP + FN]) \times 100 \qquad (3\text{-}9)$$

and is expressed as the percentage of those with the disease who are correctly identified as having the disease. In other words, sensitivity can be viewed as **1 − the false negative rate**, expressed as a percentage.

For example, Harvey, Roth, Yarnold, Durham, and Green (1992) undertook a study to assess the use of plasma D-dimer levels for diagnosing deep venous thrombosis (DVT) in

105 patients hospitalized for stroke rehabilitation. Plasma samples were drawn from patients within 24 hours of a venous ultrasound screening for DVT. Of the 105 patients in the study, 14 had DVTs identified by ultrasound. The optimal cutoff for predicting DVT was a D-dimer level of greater than 1,591 ng/ml. Test results showed the following:

	Positive Ultrasound	Negative Ultrasound
D-Dimer > 1,591 ng/ml	13 (TP)	19 (FP)
D-Dimer ≤ 1,591 ng/ml	1 (FN)	72 (TN)
	14 (TP + FN)	91 (FP + TN)

Using the above formula, Sn = (TP/[TP + FN]) × 100 = 13/14 × 100 = 93, the sensitivity for the D-dimer test for diagnosing DVTs is 93%. The larger the sensitivity, the more it is likely to confirm the disease. The D-dimer's test for diagnosing the presence of DVT is accurate 93% of the time.

The *specificity* (Sp) of a screening test is defined as the probability that the test will be negative among patients who do not have the disease. Its formula is

$$Sp = (TN/[TN + FP]) \times 100 \qquad (3\text{-}10)$$

and can be understood as 1 – the FP rate, expressed as a percentage.

In the same example, the specificity for the D-dimer test was 79% (Sp = (72/[72 + 19]) × 100 = 72/91 × 100 = 79). A large Sp means that a negative screening test result can rule out the disease. The D-dimer's specificity of 79% indicates that the test is fairly good in ruling out the presence of DVTs in rehabilitation stroke patients. Seventy-nine percent of those who do not have DVTs are correctly identified as not having DVTs on the D-dimer screening test.

The *positive predictive value* (PPV) of a test is the probability that a patient who tested positive for the disease actually has the disease. The formula for PPV is:

$$PPV = (TP/[TP + FP]) \times 100 \qquad (3\text{-}11)$$

Again using the D-dimer test for predicting DVT, its PPV is calculated as PPV = (13/[13 + 19]) × 100 = 13/32 × 100 = 40.6 or 41%. This means that only 41 out of every 100 people who test positive for DVTs on the D-dimer screening test actually have DVTs, and 59 out of 100 of those who test positive do not actually have DVTs (they are false-positives).

The *negative predictive value* (NPV) of a test is the probability that a patient who tested negative for a disease really does not have the disease. It is calculated as

$$NPV = (TN/[TN + FN]) \times 100 \qquad (3\text{-}12)$$

Using this formula in the above D-dimer test example, NPV = (72/[72 + 1]) × 100 = 72/73 × 100 = 98.6 or 99%. This value indicates that 99 out of 100 patients who screen negative for DVTs on the D-dimer test truly do not have DVTs. Thus, the D-dimer test is outstanding at ruling out DVTs in rehabilitation stroke patients who test negative for their presence.

The *efficiency* (EFF) of a test is the probability that the test result and the diagnosis agree (Kraemer, 1992) and is calculated as

$$EFF = ([TP + TN]/[TP + TN + FP + FN]) \times 100 \qquad (3\text{-}13)$$

In the D-dimer test example, EFF = ([13 + 72]/[13 + 72 + 19 + 1]) × 100 = 85/105 × 100 = 80.9. Thus, the efficiency of the D-dimer test in diagnosing rehabilitation stroke patients with DVTs is almost 81%.

NORMAL DISTRIBUTION

The Normal distribution, also referred to as the Gaussian distribution, is one of the most important theoretical distributions in statistics. It is a theoretically perfect frequency polygon in which the mean, median, and mode all coincide in the center, and it takes the form of a symmetrical bell-shaped curve (Fig. 3-1). It is a continuous frequency distribution that is expressed by the following formula:

$$f(x) = 1 \frac{1}{\sqrt{2\pi\sigma^2}} \times e^{\frac{-(x-\mu)^2}{2\sigma^2}} \qquad (3\text{-}14)$$

where μ is the overall mean of the distribution and σ^2 is the variance. Although knowing the actual formula is not important when using a normal distribution, it is helpful to see the formula to understand that a normal distribution is a theoretical distribution where the shape is determined by two key parameters: the population mean (shown as μ) and the population standard deviation (SD) (shown as σ). The usefulness of this is that for phenomena that are normally distributed, if we know the mean and SD of a population, we can infer the distribution of the variable for the entire population without collecting any data.

In practice, this distribution is among the most important distributions in statistics for three reasons (Vaughan, 1998). First, although most distributions are not exactly normal, many biological and population-level variables (such as height and weight) tend to have approximately normal distributions. Second, many inferential statistics assume that the populations are distributed normally. Third, the normal curve is a probability distribution and is used to answer questions about the likelihood of getting various particular outcomes when sampling from a population. For example, when we discuss hypothesis testing, we will talk about the probability

(or the likelihood) that a given difference or relationship could have occurred by chance alone. Understanding the normal curve prepares you for understanding the concepts underlying hypothesis testing.

Useful Characteristics of the Normal Distribution

A normal distribution is displayed in Figure 3-1. It possesses several key properties: (a) it is bell shaped; (b) the mean, median, and mode are equal; (c) it is symmetrical about the mean; and (d) the total area under the curve above the x-axis is equal to 1.

The baseline of the normal curve is measured off in SD units. These are indicated by the Greek letter for SD, σ, in Figure 3-1. A score that is 1 SD above the mean is symbolized by $+1\alpha$, and -1α indicates a score that is 1 SD below the mean. For example, the Graduate Record Exam verbal test has a mean of 500 and an SD of 100. Thus, 1 SD above the mean ($+1\alpha$) is determined by adding the SD to the mean (500 + 100 = 600), and 1 SD below the mean (-1α) is found by subtracting the SD from the mean (500 – 100 = 400). A score that is 2 SD above the mean is 500 + 100 + 100 = 700; a score that is 2 SD below the mean is 500 – (100 + 100) = 300.

These properties have a very useful result: The percentage of the data that lies between the mean and a given SD is a known quantity. Specifically, 68% of the data in a normal distribution lie within ±1 SD from the mean, 95% of

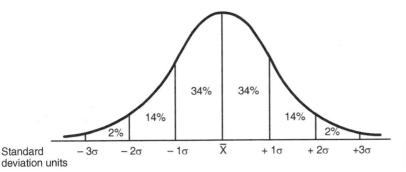

Standard deviation units

FIGURE 3-1   Normal distribution with Standard deviation units.

the data lie within ±2 SD from the mean, and 99.7% of the data lie within ±3 SD from the mean. Many distributions are nonnormal in practice. When the distribution is shaped so that the mean is larger than the median or mode, the distribution is said to be positively skewed. Similarly, when the distribution is shaped so that the mean is smaller than the median or mode, it is said to be negatively skewed (Fig. 3-2).

STANDARD NORMAL DISTRIBUTION AND UNDERSTANDING Z-SCORES

The *standard normal distribution* is a particularly useful form of the normal distribution in which the mean is 0 and the SD is 1. Data points in any normally distributed data set can be converted to a standard normal distribution by transforming the data points into z-score test results. The z-score shows how many SD a given

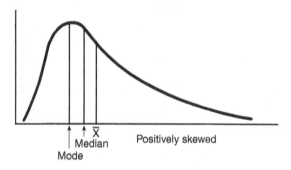

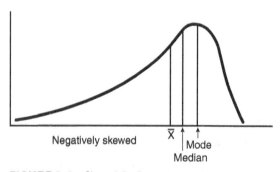

FIGURE 3-2   Skewed distributions.

score is above or below the mean of the distribution. These z-scores are very useful because they follow a known probability distribution, and this allows for the computation of percentile ranks and the assessment of the extent to which a given data point is different from the rest of a data set.

Understanding and Using z-Scores

A z-score measures the number of SDs that an actual value lies from the mean; it can be positive or negative. A data point with a positive z-score has a value that is above (to the right of) the mean, and a negative z-score indicates that the value is below (to the left of) the mean. Knowing the probability that someone will score below, at, or above the mean on a test can be very useful. In health care, the criteria that typically define laboratory test results (e.g., glucose, thyroid, and electrolytes) as abnormal are based on the standard normal distribution, with scores that occur less than 95% of the time. In particular, those with a z-score of ±2 or greater (representing very large and very small values) are defined as abnormal (Seaborg, 2007).

Using Z-Scores to Compute Percentile Ranks

Percentiles allow us to describe a given score in relation to other scores in a distribution. A *percentile* tells us the relative position of a given score and allows us to compare scores on tests that have different means and SDs. A percentile rank is calculated as

$$\frac{\text{Number of scores at or below a given score}}{\text{Total number of scores}} \times 100$$

$$(3\text{-}15)$$

Suppose you received a score of 90 on a test given to a class of 50 people. Of your classmates, 40 had scores lower than 90. Your percentile rank would be

$$(40/50) \times 100 = 80$$

You achieved a higher score than 80% of the people who took the test, which also means that almost 20% did as well or better than you.

To compute the percentile rank of a single value (data point) of a variable from a normal distribution, a z-score is first computed, and then that z-score is located in a z-table to obtain the percentile rank. The equation to calculate z-scores is

$$z = \frac{x - \mu}{\sigma} \qquad (3\text{-}16)$$

where x is the value of the data point, μ is the mean, and σ is the SD.

For example, the ages of the 62 young women who participated in a program run by an adolescent health clinic are listed in Table 3-3. The ages range from 10 to 22 years and are roughly normally distributed. The average age is 16 years, with an SD of 2.94. To find out what percentage of the girls are 14 years of age or younger, the percentile rank of 14 is found by computing the z-score of 14 using Equation 3-16:

$$z = \frac{14 - 16}{2.94} = -0.6802$$

After this value is computed, we take the absolute value ($|-0.6802| = 0.6802$), and look up this z-score in the z-table, which is also called the "Table of the Area under the Normal Curve" (see Appendix B). By looking up the first digit and first decimal place in the column labeled "z," the value 0.6 can be found in the column. Then, across the top of the table, the hundredth decimal place can be found; in this case, .08. The number that is located at the intersection of the row and column (25.17) is the percentage of the area *under the curve between the z-score of 0.68 and the mean (recall that the mean in the standard normal distribution is 0)*. A positive z-score is above the mean, whereas a negative z-score falls below the mean.

The z-score table provides the z-scores for the positive side of the distribution, but

Table 3-3	AGES OF PARTICIPANTS IN A PROGRAM FOR ADOLESCENT GIRLS	
	Age (Years)	
10	20	18
11	11	19
12	12	12
13	13	13
14	14	14
15	15	15
15	15	15
15	15	15
16	16	16
16	16	16
17	17	17
17	17	17
18	18	18
18	18	13
19	19	14
19	10	15
20	20	15
21	21	16
22	22	16
17	18	
20	11	

because the distribution is symmetrical, we can look up the absolute value of a negative z-score on the table. So, we can calculate the percentage of girls who are 14 years old or younger as $50 - 25.17 = 24.83$. In other words, according to the computed percentile rank, 24.83% of the girls were 14 years old or younger. Looking at the other side of the distribution, $50 + 25.17 = 75.17\%$ of the girls were older than 14 years. Some commonly computed percentile ranks are the 25th percentile, 50th percentile (also known as the median), and 75th percentile.

However, do not assume that converting variable raw scores to z-scores will result in a normal distribution: A distribution of z-scores has exactly the same distribution as the original distribution. When the data are not exactly normally distributed, the percentile rank that is computed using z-scores differs somewhat from the one computed using the data. Obviously, if the distribution of the data is very nonnormal, then z-scores provide a poor estimate of the percentile ranks.

CENTRAL LIMIT THEOREM

The central limit theorem allows confidence intervals to be computed around the population mean from a single sample mean (Mood et al., 1974). In general, the central limit theorem states that when a number of different samples are drawn from the same population, the distribution of the sample means tends to be normally distributed. If you draw a sample from a population and calculate its mean, how close have you come to knowing the mean of the population? Statisticians have provided us with formulas that allow us to determine just how close the mean of our sample is to the mean of the population.

When many samples are drawn from a population, the means of these samples tend to be normally distributed; that is, when they are charted along a baseline, they tend to form the normal curve. The larger the number of samples, the more the distribution approximates the normal curve. Also, if the average of the means of the samples is calculated (the mean of the means), this average (or mean) is very close to the actual mean of the population. Again, the larger the number of samples, the closer this overall mean is to the population mean.

It also states that the SD of the distribution of the sample means (i.e., the standard error of the mean used in constructing confidence intervals) can be computed using this equation:

$$se_{\overline{X}} = \frac{s}{\sqrt{n}} \qquad (3\text{-}17)$$

The larger the sample size, the smaller the standard error (and thus the more accurate the measure). In general, the approximation to normality of the sampling distribution of the mean becomes better as the sample size increases. A sample size of 30 or greater has been found to be sufficient for the central limit theorem to apply (Vaughan, 1998).

CHAPTER REVIEW

Multiple-Choice Concept Review

1. The $p(A)$ is most accurately defined as the
   a. joint probability of event A.
   b. marginal probability of event A.
   c. proof of event A.
   d. marginal probability that event A will not occur.

2. The $p(\overline{B})$ is most accurately defined as the
   a. joint probability of event B.
   b. marginal probability of event B.
   c. proof of event B.
   d. marginal probability that event B will not occur.

3. The $p(B \mid A)$ is most accurately defined as the
   a. joint probability that events A and B will occur.
   b. addition rule.
   c. conditional probability that event B will occur.
   d. multiplication rule.

4. The $P(A \cup B) = P(A) + P(B) - p(A \cap B)$ describes the
   a. joint probability that events A and B will occur.
   b. addition rule.
   c. conditional probability that event B will occur.
   d. multiplication rule.

5. If the $p(A \mid B) = p(A)$, then
   a. two events are independent.
   b. two events are mutually exclusive.
   c. $p(A) = p(B)$.
   d. none of the above apply.

6. A normal distribution is characterized by
   a. a bell shape.
   b. a mean, median, and mode that are equal.
   c. a total area under the curve above the x-axis that is 1.
   d. all of the above.

7. A z-score can give information about
   a. the mean of a distribution.
   b. the standard deviation (SD) of a distribution.
   c. the percentile rank of a data point.
   d. none of the above.

8. A z-score of 0 corresponds to the
   a. mean.
   b. SD.
   c. interquartile range.
   d. 75th percentile.

9. The 50th percentile is always the
   a. mean.
   b. median.
   c. SD.
   d. a and b.

10. A sample population curve is more likely to look like the population curve when
    a. the bell shape is wide.
    b. the sample size is small.
    c. the sample size is greater than 30.
    d. none of the above.

Conceptual Questions

1. In a positively skewed distribution, the "tail" extends toward the _____ (right/ left) or toward _____ (higher/lower) scores of the distribution.

2. When raw scores are converted to standard scores, the resulting distribution has a mean equal to _____ and a standard deviation equal to _____.

Computational Problems

1. Consider the following cross-tabulation table from a 12-week study of diet and exercise. Compute all of the marginal, joint, and conditional probabilities.

	Achievement of Goal Weight		
Weight Loss Strategy	Achieved Goal Weight	Did Not Achieve Goal Weight	Total
Diet alone	20	80	100
Diet and exercise	60	40	100
Total	80	120	200

2. Consider the following cross-tabulation table from a national study of women's health. It seeks to examine the relationship between education level and smoking. Compute all of the marginal, joint, and conditional probabilities.

	Smoking Status		
Education Level	Does Not Smoke (n)	Smokes (n)	Total
Less than high school diploma	250	75	325
High school diploma or GED	620	235	855
2-year college degree (AA/AS)	554	154	708
4-year college degree (BA/BS)	369	72	441
Postgraduate degree (MA/MS/PhD/MD/JD)	167	23	190
Total	1,960	559	2,519

3. A standardized exam is known to be normally distributed with a mean score of 82 and a standard deviation of 6.58 in the examination. A study group of four students obtains scores of A) 78, B) 82, C) 88, D) 95. For each score, compute the corresponding z-score and find its percentile rank. Round the z-scores to the nearest hundredth place.

4. Scores on a particular test are normally distributed with a mean of 70 and an SD of 15. Between what two scores would you expect
   a. 68% of the scores to fall between: _____ and _____?

    b. 96% of the scores to fall between: _____ and _____?

5. Scores on a different test are normally distributed with a mean of 70 and an SD of 5. The following four scores were drawn from that distribution: 58, 65, 73, and 82.

    a. Transform the raw scores to z-scores.

    b. Calculate the percentile for each score.

6. At your hospital, there were 1,500 deliveries last year; 364 of the women had cesarean operations. What is the probability of having a cesarean operation at your hospital?

7. You are reading a review paper discussing the use of serum ferritin as a diagnostic test for iron deficiency anemia, with the results summarized as follows:

		Anemia Present	Anemia Absent	Total
Serum ferritin	+ (Positive)	731	270	1,001
Test result	– (Negative)	78	1,500	1,578
	Total	809	1,770	2,579

    a. Calculate the sensitivity (Sn), specificity (Sp), positive predictive value (PPV), negative predictive value (NPV), and efficiency (EFF).

    b. Describe the clinical performance of the serum ferritin test as a diagnostic tool.

Hypothesis Testing with Inferential Statistics

OBJECTIVES

After studying this chapter, you should be able to:

1. Write a testable hypothesis and explain the difference between the null and alternative hypotheses.

2. Define statistical significance and explain the meaning of a *p*-value.

3. Discriminate between type I and type II errors.

4. Recognize the importance of statistical power in conducting analyses.

5. Interpret the rejection region for one- and two-tailed tests and assess the significance of a statistical test.

6. Compare a sample mean with a population mean using a one-sample *z*-test.

RESEARCH QUESTION

Statistical inference helps us to answer two types of questions: questions about parameter estimation (e.g., describing a sample or population in terms of its characteristics) and questions about hypothesis testing (e.g., testing statements of relationships between two or more variables). *Parameter estimation* takes two forms: point estimation and interval estimation. When an estimate of the population parameter is given as a single number, it is called a *point estimate*. The sample mean, median, variance, and standard deviation would all be considered point estimates. In contrast, *interval estimation* of a parameter involves more than one point; it consists of a range of values within which the population parameter is thought to be. A common type of interval estimation is the construction of a confidence interval (CI) and the upper and lower limits of the range of values, called confidence limits. Both point and CI estimates are types of statistical estimates that let us *infer* the true value of an unknown population parameter using information from a *random sample* of that population. Hypothesis testing involves first constructing a hypothesis about the relationship of two or more variables and then testing that hypothesis with the appropriate statistical test. The following studies provide examples of parameter estimation and hypothesis testing.

Parameter Estimation: What Is the STI Prevalence Rate among Women Aged 14 to 19 in the United States?

The National Health and Nutrition Examination Survey (NHANES), conducted by the Centers for Disease Control and Prevention (CDC), is a program of studies designed to assess the health and nutritional status of adults and children in the United States. The survey is unique in that it combines interviews and physical examinations (http://www.cdc.gov/nchs/nhanes.htm). In the 2003 to 2004 NHANES, women aged 14 to 19 years were asked to provide biological samples (urine, sera, and self-collected vaginal swabs) for testing to estimate the prevalence of sexually transmitted infections (STIs) in this group. The study found that 24.1% (95% CI: 18.4% to 30.9%) of women aged 14 to 19 years had at least one STI. The most common STIs were human papillomavirus (HPV), which infected an estimated 18.3% (95% CI: 13.5% to 24.8%) of these women, and chlamydia, which infected 3.9% (95% CI: 2.2% to 6.9%) of the women (Forhan, 2009).

Hypothesis Testing: Is the Oral Health of Children Admitted to a PICU Significantly Different from that of Children in the General Population?

An example of hypothesis testing and group comparisons can be found in a study on the oral health of children admitted to a pediatric intensive care unit (PICU) in England (Franklin, Senior, James, & Roberts, 2000). The purpose of this study was to assess the oral health care needs of hospitalized children and to determine whether these needs were being met while the children were in the hospital. In this study, the main question was: Is the oral health of children in the PICU different from the oral health of other children in England? We can state this question as a hypothesis that can be tested with inferential statistics as such: "the oral health of children in the PICU will not be different from that of the general population of children in England." The researchers tested this hypothesis by comparing data on the presence of oral caries (cavities) from the group of children in the PICU with data from the entire population of children in England. The authors reported that the number of dental caries among children in the PICU was not statistically significantly different than the number of dental caries reported among children of the same age in the general population (Franklin et al., 2000).

FORMULATING HYPOTHESES

Hypothesis testing is a key feature of health services research. If we have a good theoretical or conceptual model, an underlying theoretical structure, a representative sample, and an appropriate research design, then we can develop and test hypotheses. We use statistics to test whether the data support our hypotheses. Even if the data support a hypothesis, we do not claim to prove that our hypothesis is absolutely true. Since one study does not provide irrefutable evidence, it is always possible that some error has distorted the findings.

Hypotheses provide a way for researchers to articulate the expected relationships between variables. They must stem directly from the research questions and should be grounded in theory or on a strong conceptual model. The expected relationship can be either an association (i.e., no causal effect presumed) or a causal relationship (i.e., in which the independent variable is said to cause changes in the dependent variable). A testable hypothesis identifies the groups that are being compared, the variables on which they are being compared, and the expected relationships.

There are two types of hypotheses: null and alternative. The *null hypothesis* proposes that there is no difference or relationship between the variables of interest. Often written as H_0, the null hypothesis is the foundation of the statistical test. When you statistically test a hypothesis, you assume that H_0 correctly describes the state of affairs between the two variables of interest. If a significant difference or relationship is found, the null hypothesis is rejected; if no difference or relationship is found, H_0 is accepted.

The alternative hypothesis is also known as the acting hypothesis or the research hypothesis, represented by H_r or H_a (Agresti & Finlay, 1997). The alternative hypothesis is expressed in one of two ways: directional or nondirectional. A *directional hypothesis* states that there will be a relationship between two variables and gives the expected direction of that relationship. A *nondirectional hypothesis* simply states that there will be a statistically significant relationship between two variables, but the direction is not stated. For example, the first main hypothesis from the study of oral health in the PICU (Franklin et al., 2000) can be stated in three ways:

- **Null hypothesis (H_0):** The oral health of children in the PICU will not differ from that of children in the general population.
- **Nondirectional alternative hypothesis (H_A):** The oral health of children in the PICU will be significantly different from the oral health of children in the general population.
- **Directional alternative hypothesis (H_A):** The oral health of children in the PICU will be significantly worse than the oral health of children in the general population.

TESTING HYPOTHESES

Hypothesis testing is the classical approach to assessing the statistical significance of findings (Hubberty, 1993). Hypotheses are tested by using the appropriate inferential statistic and interpreting the results. In each of the hypotheses about the PICU, the word "significantly" is used; this refers to the statistical significance of the results of the test of the hypothesis. In the broadest sense, the value of a computed statistic is considered significant when it is much different from what is expected by chance alone.

Current convention is to state hypotheses in their alternative forms. This makes sense because it gives readers (and researchers) a clear idea of why the study is being conducted and what relationships are expected. Technically, though, inferential statistics only test the null hypothesis. Practically, this means that after performing the correct statistical test, a decision is made about the null hypothesis. The decision can be one of two: to either reject or to accept the null hypothesis. Rejecting the null hypothesis means that researchers believe that the variables are significantly associated with each other. Accepting the null hypothesis means that researchers believe that the variables are not significantly associated. The criteria that are used to either reject or to accept the null hypothesis are based on the α-level that is set in advance of the study and the p-value of the computed statistic. Some texts discuss this in terms of rejecting the null hypothesis or failing to reject the null hypothesis.

Statistical Significance

The p-value (e.g., probability value) of any statistical test represents the probability that the results were obtained by chance alone. It represents the precise chance of getting that result, and it is derived from the value of the computed test statistic. The actual p-value of a statistical test is computed from the data and is not known until the test is completed.

The specific level of the p-value that is defined as "statistically significant" is called the alpha-level (α-level). *This value is defined by the researcher before any statistical tests are conducted.* Common α-levels used are .10, .05, and .01. An α-level of .10 means that for a result to be significant, it cannot occur more than 10% of the time by chance. Similarly, an α-level of .05 means that the result cannot occur more than 5% of the time by chance, and an α-level of .01 means that it cannot occur more than 1% of the time by chance.

For example, in the study of emergency departments, which we discussed in Chapter 3 (Plichta, Vandecar-Burdin, Odor, Reams, & Zhang, 2007), we examined the association between having a forensic nurse on staff at an emergency department and that emergency department having a relationship with a rape crisis center. Note that the hypothesis has two parts: the null and the alternative. Written out, it looks like this:

H_0: There will be no statistically significant association between an emergency department having a forensic nurse on staff and having a relationship with a rape crisis center.

H_A: There will be a statistically significant association between an emergency department having a forensic nurse on staff and having a relationship with a rape crisis center.

In advance, we set an α-level of .05. We tested the cross-tabulation (Table 4-1) with a chi-square statistic and found that the associated p-value of the chi-square statistic was .019. Since this was less than the preset α-level of .05, we rejected the null hypothesis and reported the result—that emergency departments with a forensic nurse were more likely to have a relationship with a rape crisis center—as statistically significant.

Types of Errors

The two potential mistakes are to either reject the null hypothesis when it is true (a type I error) or to accept the null hypothesis when it is false (a type II error). There is, of course, no way to know whether a type I or type II error has been committed in any given study. This is why it is important not to rely on just one study but to have a large body of evidence from many studies before conclusions about a phenomenon can be drawn. Drawing the wrong conclusion is called an *error of inference*.

Table 4-2 shows the four possible things that can happen when we make a decision about a hypothesis. If H_0 is true and we accept that hypothesis, we have responded correctly. The incorrect response would be to reject a true null hypothesis (type I error). If H_0 is false and we reject it, we have responded correctly. The incorrect response would be to accept a false null hypothesis (type II error).

Type I Errors

A type I error is made when a null hypothesis is rejected when it is true. You can think of this as saying a finding is significant, when it is really

Table 4-1	RELATIONSHIP OF FORENSIC NURSE ON STAFF TO RELATIONSHIOP WITH RAPE CRISIS CENTER FOR HOSPITALS IN VIRGINIA		
	Relationship with Rape Crisis Center	No Relationship with Rape Crisis Center	Totals
Forensic nurse on staff	29	4	33
No forensic nurse on staff	12	8	20
Totals	41	12	53

Table 4-2	TYPES OF ERRORS	
	Null Hypothesis (H_0)	
Decision	True	False
Accept H_0	OK	Type II
Reject H_0	Type I	OK

not. The probability of making a type I error is defined by the α-level of the study. Given an α-level of .10, it is known that 10% of the time, a type I error will be made and the null hypothesis rejected when it is actually true. For example, in the study of forensic nurses and emergency departments (Plichta et al., 2007), we found that those hospitals with forensic nurses were more likely to have a relationship with a rape crisis center than those hospitals without forensic nurses. However, we may have obtained a sample of hospitals that were biased (e.g., if those with a relationship were more likely to respond to our study than were other hospitals). If, in reality, there was no difference in the presence of a relationship with a rape crisis center by type of nurse, we would have committed a type I error. In terms of the screening tests discussed in the previous chapter, a type I error is similar to a false positive on a screening test—the test screens a patient as having a disease (alternate hypothesis) when, in reality, he or she does not (null hypothesis).

Type II Errors

A type II error is made when a null hypothesis is not rejected when it is false. In terms of the screening tests discussed in the previous chapter, a type II error is similar to a false negative on a screening test—the test screens a patient as not having a disease (null hypothesis) when, in reality, he or she does (alternate hypothesis). We can think of this as missing a significant finding. The probability of making a type II error is referred to as β (beta).

Given a β-level of .20, it is known that 20% of the time, a null hypothesis will be accepted when a relationship between the variables actually exists. The probability of making a type II error decreases as the power of a study increases.

The Relationship between Type I and Type II Errors

The probability of making a type I error can be *decreased* by setting a more stringent significance level. In other words, you could set the α-level at .01 instead of .05; then there is only 1 chance in 100 (1%) that the result termed significant could occur by chance alone. If you do that, however, you will make it more difficult to find a significant result; that is, you will decrease the *power* of the test and increase the risk of a type II error.

If the data showed no significant results, the researcher would accept the null hypothesis. If there were significant differences, a type II error would have been made. To avoid a type II error, you could make the level of significance less extreme. There is a greater chance of finding significant results if you are willing to risk 10 chances in 100 that you are wrong ($p = .10$) than there is if you are willing to risk only 5 chances in 100 ($p = .05$). Other ways to decrease the likelihood of a type II error are to increase the sample size and decrease sources of extraneous variation.

Power of a Study

The power of a statistical test is its ability to detect statistically significant differences; it is defined as $1 - \beta$. Failure to consider *statistical power* when results appear to be nonsignificant prevents an accurate interpretation of the results. Researchers conducting a study with low power have a high probability of committing a type II error, that is, of saying no statistical differences exist between groups when differences actually do exist. For example, a study with low power might wrongly conclude that an experimental medication was ineffective; thus, the medication, which actually is effective, would not be produced. Unfortunately, many studies ignore issues of power. For example, a substantial number of studies have been found to be underpowered in recent reviews of orthopedic research (Freedman, 2001; Lochner, Bhandari, & Tornetta, 2001), psychogeriatrics (Chibnall, 2003) systemic lupus erythematosus (Ginzler & Moldovan, 2004), and occupational therapy (Ottenbacher & Maas, 1999). The importance of making sure that a study is sufficiently powered to detect statistically significant results cannot be overstated (Burns, 2000; Cohen, 1992; Devane, Begley, & Clark, 2004; Polit & Beck, 2008).

The specific equation needed to compute the power of a statistical analysis depends on the type of comparison being made (e.g., comparing two means or comparing three means or comparing proportions) (Cohen, 1988). The actual computation of power is beyond the scope of this text; however, interested readers can learn more by consulting the Cohen text (1988) for the exact method of computing power. Other writers provide health care–focused explanations of how to compute power and how to decide on an appropriate sample size for a study (Burns, 2000; Devane et al., 2004; Polit & Beck, 2008). Several computer programs, including SPSS SamplePower and nQuery, estimate power and necessary sample sizes (nQuery, 2007; SPSS SamplePower, 2007).

The two most common power analyses are used to compute either the power of a study or to compute the necessary sample size for a desired level of power (usually set at greater than or equal to .80). All statistical power analyses use the relationships among the four quantities used in statistical inference, namely, the α-level, power $(1 - \beta)$, sample size (n), and population effect size (γ) (Cohen, 1988, 1992). The key to understanding power analysis is in knowing that any one of these can be computed from the other three.

The first three quantities are fairly straightforward. The α-level is set by the researcher before the start of the study. Typical α-levels are .10, .05, and .01. As noted previously, the probability of making a type II error is β, and the power is $1 - \beta$. The level of power that is conventionally sought is .80; higher levels of power are even more desirable but may pose unrealistic sample-size requirements (Cohen, 1988). The sample size (n) is simply the number needed in the study. If two or more groups are being compared, the sample size referred to here is the size of each group.

The population effect size is represented by γ and is somewhat more complicated to explain. In short, the effect size represents the magnitude of the relationship between the variables. The metric on which effect size is measured differs based on the type of comparison. For example, when comparing two means, the effect size is the difference in means divided by the standard deviation, and when comparing correlations, the effect size is represented as the correlation coefficient (r). Table 4-3 presents a list of common statistical tests, the index on which the effect size is based for that test, and a suggested interpretation of the magnitude of the effect size (Cohen, 1992). The actual effect size that is chosen for the power analysis is fairly subjective. It should be based on both what would be regarded as clinically and substantively meaningful and on what previous studies in the same subject area have found.

A number of strategies are available to increase the power of studies (Burns, 2000). Power always increases with sample size, and so the first strategy is to increase the size of the study sample as much as possible. The second strategy is to use smaller effect sizes. The choice of effect size is subjective, and a range of reasonable effect sizes can be tested. The third way to increase the power of a study is to increase the α-level. Of course, increasing the α-level leads to an increased risk of a type I error, but these are the types of tradeoffs that need to be considered before a study is conducted.

Table 4-3	**POWER AND EFFECT SIZES**				
			Effect Size		
Test	Population Effect Size Index	Small	Medium	Large
1. m_A vs. m_B for independent means	$d = \dfrac{m_A - m_B}{B}$	.20	.50	.80
2. Significance of product–moment r	r	.10	.30	.50
3. r_A vs. r_B for independent r's	$q = z_A - z_B$ (where z = Fisher's z)	.10	.30	.50
4. $p = .5$ and the sign test	$g = p - .50$	.05	.15	.25
5. p_A vs. p_B for independent proportions	$h = \varnothing_A - \varnothing_B$ (where $\varnothing$ = arcsine transformation)	.20	.50	.80
6. Chi-square for goodness of fit and consistency	$w = \sqrt{\sum_{[m]}^{\kappa} \dfrac{(P_{ti} - P_{oi})^2}{P_{oi}}}$	.10	.30	.50
7. One-way analysis of variance	$f = \dfrac{O_m}{B}$	.10	.25	.40
8. Multiple and multiple partial correlation	$f^2 = \dfrac{R^2}{1 - R^2}$	.02	.15	.35

Source: Reprinted with permission from Cohen, J. (1992). The power primer. *Psychological Bulletin, 112*(3), 155–159. Can be obtained from Plichta, Stacey, Garzon, Laurel (2009) *Statistics for Nursing and Allied Health*, Philidelphia, PA, Lippincott Williams & Wilkins.

A SIX-STEP PROCESS FOR TESTING HYPOTHESES

In empirical research, hypotheses are tested using inferential statistics (e.g., t test, chi-square, ANOVA). In this chapter, we present a six-step process for testing hypotheses with inferential statistics. Variations on this general procedure are widely used and can be found in a number of texts (Daniel, 2008; Kuzma & Bohnenblust, 2005). The application of these specific steps for each inferential technique is covered in Chapters 5 to 17. The general procedure is as follows:

1. State the hypothesis (both null and alternative versions).
2. Define the significance level (i.e., the α-level) for the study, choose the appropriate test statistic, determine the critical region, and state the rejection rule.
3. Make sure that the data meet the necessary assumptions to compute the test statistic.
4. Compute the parameters that are being compared by the test statistic (e.g., means and proportions).
5. Compute the test statistic, and obtain the p-value of the computed statistic.
6. Determine whether the result is statistically significant and clearly state a conclusion.

Using the Six-Step Process to Conduct a One-Sample z-Test

We will introduce the first statistic that this book covers—the one-sample z-test—and use it to illustrate the use of the six-step process. The one-sample z-test is used to compare the mean value of a variable obtained from a sample with the population mean of that variable to see whether the sampled value is statistically significantly different from the population value.

As an example, we will use data to answer the question "Do women who attend a local church-based health fair have significantly higher BMI measures than women in the general U.S. population?" Our data come from a sample of women attending a health fair at a community church that has an active health ministry. Because obesity is increasingly a threat to the health of the US population, particularly among low-income African-Americans (Truong & Sturm, 2005), the researchers wanted to know how the BMIs of the women in the sample compared with those of US women in general. Note that a BMI of 25 to 29.99 indicates being overweight and a BMI of 30.00 or higher indicates obesity (WHO, 2000).

Keep in mind that because these data are not perfect and represent only a sample of the entire population, it cannot be definitively stated that the null hypothesis is true or false. At best, it can be stated that the null hypothesis should be rejected or not rejected (Polit & Beck, 2008).

Step 1: State the Null and Alternative Hypotheses

- H_0: The BMIs of the women attending the church health fair will not be significantly different from those of the US population.
- H_A (nondirectional): The BMIs of the women attending the church health fair will be significantly different from those of the US population.

Step 2: Define the Significance Level (α-Level), Choose the Appropriate Test Statistic, Determine the Rejection Region, and State the Rejection Rule

α-Level: The α-level for this study is .05. This means that if the value of the computed test statistic occurs by chance 5% of the time or less,

the null hypothesis will be rejected. The conclusion will then be that the BMIs of the women attending the health fair are significantly different from those of the general population.

Choose the appropriate test statistic: Each of the test statistics available to researchers has a different purpose, and each makes certain assumptions about the data. If the test statistic is used when the assumptions are not met, there is a threat to the statistical validity of the conclusions. We will use the one-sample z-test to test our hypothesis about BMI.

The one-sample z-test is used to assess whether a sample mean is significantly different from a population mean. It assumes that the data from the sample are normally distributed and that both the population mean (μ) and the population standard deviation (σ) are known. If the population standard deviation is not known, the one-sample t test is an alternative test that can be used.

Determine the critical region and state the rejection rule: As stated earlier, the value of a statistic is considered significant when its computed value is much different from what would be expected by chance alone. The α-level is how "by chance alone" is defined. In this case, it is .05, meaning that the null hypothesis will be rejected if the computed value of the statistic is so extreme that it is different from 95% of the values and that the null hypothesis will be accepted if the computed value falls within the 95% range. To reject the null hypothesis, the computed value of the statistic needs to exceed the critical value for the one-sample z-test.

The range of values in which the null hypothesis is rejected is called the "critical region," and the cutoff values of the z-test at which the null hypothesis is rejected are called the "critical values." A nondirectional hypothesis simply tests whether the mean is significantly different from the population mean (e.g., it can be much smaller or much larger). In this case, a two-tailed z-test should be used to test the hypothesis because it is important to know whether the computed value of the statistic falls within the middle 95%, in which case the null hypothesis would not be rejected, or whether it falls in the extreme (outer) 5% of z-scores (i.e., the top 2.5% or bottom 2.5%), in which case the null hypothesis would be rejected. Figure 4-1 provides a graphic example of this for a two-tailed z-test. For an α-level of .05 and a two-tailed test, the critical values are +1.96 and –1.96. Differences in means with computed z-scores at or above +1.96 and at or below –1.96 are considered statistically significant.

A one-tailed test is technically meant to be used with directional hypotheses. In this case, whether the sample mean is significantly greater than (or less than) the population mean is being tested. If the hypothesis stated that the mean BMI of the sample is greater than that of the US population, it would be important to know whether the computed z-score falls within the range of the lower 95% of values. If the computed z-score fell within the lower 95%, the null hypothesis would not be rejected. If the computed z-score fell in the top 5% of values, the null hypothesis would be rejected. Figure 4-2 provides a graphic example of this. For an α-level of .05 and a positive one-tailed test, the critical

value for the upper tail is +1.65. If the z-score for a mean difference (one-tailed) is above +1.65, the sample mean is considered to be significantly greater than the population mean. If testing the hypothesis that the mean BMI of the sample is significantly lower than that of the U.S. population, then the critical value for the lower region, –1.65, would be used and the null hypothesis would be rejected for the computed values of z that fell into the lower rejection region.

Standard use of two-tailed tests: The current standard is to use a two-tailed test in all research even when testing directional hypotheses (Chow, 2000; Dubey, 1991; Moye & Tita, 2002; Polit & Beck, 2008). This standard was set by the US Food and Drug Administration, which generally opposes the use of one-tailed tests (Chow, 2000). The controversy in the health services literature about which test to use dates back to the 1950s (Hick, 1952). However, using a two-tailed test for both directional and nondirectional hypotheses is the standard practice in almost all peer-reviewed health journals and most US National Institutes of Health–sponsored research. Therefore, the two-tailed test is used throughout this text. It is also important to note

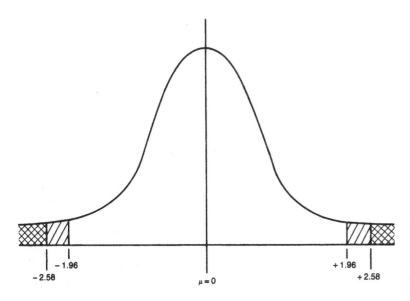

FIGURE 4-1   Critical region for a two-tailed z-test (α = .05).

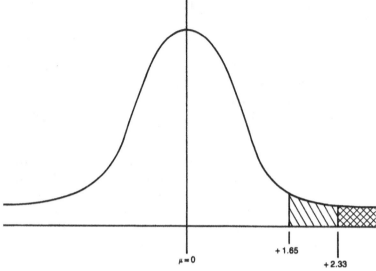

FIGURE 4-2   Critical region for a one-tailed z-test ($\alpha = .05$).

that most statistical software packages (including SPSS) return two-tailed values as the default measure. If a one-tailed test is needed, it needs to be specified before the program is run, and the researcher should clearly state in the methods section that a one-tailed test is being employed.

Step 3: Make Sure That the Data Meet the Necessary Assumptions to Compute the Statistic

The BMI data are normally distributed in the 48 women. The mean and population standard deviation of BMI in the United States is known; in 1999 to 2000, the mean BMI for US women was 27.9, with a standard deviation of 5.4 (Okusun, Chandra, & Boev, 2004). The two assumptions of the one-sample z-test have been met, and so the test can proceed.

Step 4: Compute and State the Parameters That are Being Compared by the Test Statistic

The mean BMI of the 48 women in the sample was 29.2, with a standard deviation of 3.4.

Step 5: Compute the Test Statistic and Obtain Its p-Value

The formula for the z-test is

$$z = \frac{\bar{X} - \mu}{\sigma / \sqrt{n}}$$

The z-test for this example is computed using this equation:

$$z = \frac{29.2 - 27.9}{5.4 / \sqrt{48}} = \frac{1.3}{5.4 / 6.928} = \frac{1.3}{.7794} = 1.67$$

Therefore, the computed value of the z-test (the z-score) is 1.67. This value does not exceed the critical value of 1.96, and so it does not fall into the rejection region.

The exact p-value for this computed statistic can be obtained from the z-table (Appendix B). The first two digits are looked up first, and the first decimal is placed in the column labeled z; in this case, the value is 1.6. Then, going across the top of the table, the hundredth decimal place is found (in this case, .07). The number that is located at the intersection of the row and column is the area under the curve at and below the z-value; in this case, the value is .9525. Therefore, the approximate p-value for a one-tailed test is 1 − .9525, or .0475. The exact p-value for a two-tailed test is 2 × .0475, or .095. The interesting thing about this result is that it would have been identified as statistically significant if a one-tailed z-test had been chosen.

Step 6: Determine Statistical Significance and Clearly State a Conclusion

The computed z-statistic did not fall into the critical region; for it to do so, it would have had to have an absolute value of 1.96 or greater. Because the computed value of the z-statistic did not exceed the critical value, the null hypothesis is accepted. Another way to view this is to look at the p-value of the test. Because the specific p-value of .095 is greater than the α-level (.05) for this study, the null hypothesis (H_0) is accepted. Overall, we conclude that the mean BMI of the women who attended the church fair is not significantly different from that of the general population.

COMPUTING THE CONFIDENCE INTERVAL AROUND A MEAN

Most studies are conducted using only a sample of data from the population of interest. The assumption made is that the results obtained from the sample are a valid representation of the whole population. However, an estimate of a mean made from sample data does not provide the exact value of the true mean of the population. One way to assess how good an estimate is when obtained from the sample is to compute confidence intervals (CIs) around the estimate of the mean.

For example, let us consider data from a program for adolescent girls. This program had 62 participants from a midsize city in the northeastern United States. The mean age of the participants was 16.0 years, with a standard deviation of 2.94 years. However, there are many more adolescents in that city who

could have participated; these 62 participants represent the larger population of all adolescent girls who could have enrolled in the program. Then, it would be reasonable to ask the following question: How good an estimate is the mean age that was computed from the data of the true mean age of all adolescent girls who could have participated? One way to answer this question is to construct a confidence interval (CI) around the mean.

Constructing a Confidence Interval

The question of how good an estimate is the sample mean ($\bar{x}$) of the population mean (μ) can be answered by constructing a CI around the sample mean. In broad terms, a CI gives the range of values of a sample statistic that is actually likely to contain the true population value (Vogt, 2005). CIs are typically constructed as either 95% or 99% CIs. A 95% CI is interpreted as follows: If the study were repeated over and over again, drawing different random samples of the same size from the same population, 95% of the time, the population mean (μ) would fall within the 95% CI. Of course, that means that 5% of the time, the population mean (μ) does not fall within the 95% CI, meaning that we will be wrong 5% of the time.

In order to compute a CI, we need to know the reliability factor and the standard error of the mean. The reliability coefficient is obtained from the z-table. The specific reliability coefficient used depends on the level of CI you want to construct. For example, the reliability coefficient for a 95% CI is 1.96, and the reliability coefficient for a 99% CI is 2.58. These reliability coefficients are based on z-scores. A z-score of 1.96 is equivalent to a percentile rank of 2.5%, and a z-score of +1.96 is equivalent to a z-score of 97.5%. Thus, the area under the normal curve *between* these two values is 95%. In other words, the boundaries for the 95% CI are ±1.96 standard errors of the estimate of the mean. Similarly, a z-score of -2.58 is equivalent to a percentile rank of 0.5%, and a z-score of $+2.58$ is equivalent to a percentile rank of 99.5%. The area under the normal curve *between* these two values is 99%.

The standard error of the mean is computed as

$$se_{\bar{X}} = \frac{s}{\sqrt{n}}$$

where s is the sample standard deviation and n is the sample size.

The equation for **computing a 95% CI around the mean is**

$$95\%\,CI = \bar{x} \pm (1.96 \times se_{\bar{x}})$$

The equation for **computing a 99% CI is**

$$99\%\,CI = \bar{x} \pm (2.58 \times se_{\bar{x}})$$

The **95% CI around the value of the mean for** the age of the adolescent girls is computed as follows:

Standard error:

$$se_x = \frac{s}{\sqrt{n}} = \frac{2.94}{\sqrt{62}} = 0.3734$$

A **95% CI around the mean** is computed as

$$
\begin{aligned}
95\%\,CI &= \bar{x} \pm (1.96 \times se_{\bar{x}}) \\
&= 16.0 \pm (1.96 \times .3734) \\
&= 16.0 \pm .7319 \\
95\%\,CI &= (15.27,\ 16.73)
\end{aligned}
$$

Thus, researchers can state that they are 95% confident that the true mean age of girls who could have participated in the program is between 15.27 and 16.73 years.

A **99% CI** is computed as

$$
\begin{aligned}
99\%\,CI &= \bar{x} \pm (2.58 * se_{\bar{x}}) \\
&= 16.0 \pm (2.58 * .3734) \\
&= 16.0 \pm .9634 \\
99\%\,CI &= (15.04,\ 16.96)
\end{aligned}
$$

Thus, researchers can state that they are 99% confident that the true mean age of girls who could participate in the program is between 15.04 and 16.96 years.

SUMMARY

Topics covered in this chapter provide the foundation to testing hypotheses with the statistical techniques covered in the subsequent chapters of this book. Researchers must understand the trade-offs required between type I and type II errors and the statistical power of the study in order to set useful α-levels. Researchers then need to follow the process dictated by these choices, compute the statistical results, and provide results with a stated CI.

CHAPTER REVIEW

Multiple-Choice Concept Review

1. The null hypothesis states
   a. the expected direction of the relationship between the variables.
   b. that no relationship will be found.
   c. that a relationship will be found, but it will not state the direction.
   d. none of the above.

2. The α-level is defined by
   a. the probability of making a type I error.
   b. the probability of making a type II error.
   c. the researcher at the start of a study.
   d. a and c only.

3. The one-sample t test is used to compare a sample mean to a population mean when
   a. the population mean is known.
   b. the population standard deviation (SD) is not known.
   c. the sample size is at least 30.
   d. all of the above occur.

4. Power is defined by
   a. the α-level.
   b. the sample size.
   c. the effect size (γ).
   d. all of the above.

5. A type I error occurs when the
   a. null hypothesis is accepted when it is false.
   b. null hypothesis is rejected when it is true.
   c. sample size is too small.
   d. effect size (γ) is not defined in advance.

6. A type II error occurs when the
   a. null hypothesis is accepted when it is false.
   b. null hypothesis is rejected when it is true.
   c. sample size is too small.
   d. effect size (γ) is not defined in advance.

7. Power can be increased by doing which of the following?
   a. Increasing the α-level.
   b. Increasing the sample size.
   c. Increasing the effect size (γ).
   d. All of the above.

8. A researcher conducts a small study and finds that no statistically significant relationship exists between smoking and lung cancer. This is most likely
   a. a type I error.
   b. a type II error.
   c. both a and b.
   d. none of the above.

9. Which of the following is more likely to contain the "true" population value of the mean?
   a. A 90% confidence interval (CI).
   b. A 95% CI.
   c. A 99% CI.
   d. All of the above.

10. If a statistical test is significant, it means that
    a. it has important clinical applications.
    b. the study had acceptable power.
    c. the null hypothesis was rejected.
    d. all of the above are true.

Critical Thinking Concept Review

1. Read the article by Baibergenova, A., Kudyakov, R., Zdeb, M., and Carpenter, D. (2003) titled "Low Birth Weight and Residential Proximity to PCB-contaminated Waste Sites," which can be found in *Environmental Health Perspectives*, *111* (i10), 1352–1358. Write the five hypotheses that this study is testing. Write both the null and alternative hypotheses for each one.
2. Choose a research article from your field. Write the five hypotheses that this study is testing. Write both the null and alternative hypotheses for each one.
3. Imagine that you are going to conduct a study. Write the purpose of the study, research questions, and main hypotheses. Write both the null and alternative hypotheses for each one.

Computational Problems

1. Compute z-tests and find the one-tailed and two-tailed p-value for each of the following situations. Then, write up the results of the analysis in a single sentence. Use α less than or equal to .05 as your definition of statistical significance.
    a. The mean BMI for US men is 26.8, with a standard deviation of 4.6. You have data from a sample of 25 men with type II diabetes, who are attending a diabetes health promotion program. The mean BMI of the sample is 31.3.
    b. The mean age for US citizens is 45.2 years, with a standard deviation of 17.5 years. The 36 men in the sample have a mean age of 47 years.
    c. The average adult in the United States travels 40 miles each day (mostly by car), with a standard deviation of 8.2 miles. You have data from a group of 49 urban women who travel 38.2 miles each day.
2. You have measured 120 subjects on a particular scale. The mean is 75, and the SD is 6.
    a. What is the standard error of the mean?
    b. Set up the 95% CI for the mean.
    c. Set up the 99% CI for the mean.

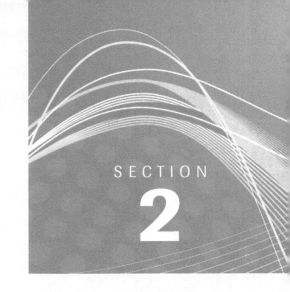

Analyzing the Data

The Independent *t* Test and the Mann-Whitney *U*-Test: Measuring the Differences Between the Means of Two Unrelated Groups

OBJECTIVES

After studying this chapter, you should be able to:

1. Determine when to use the independent samples *t* test or the Mann-Whitney *U*-test.

2. Discuss how the mean difference, group variability, and sample size are related to the statistical significance of the *t*-statistic.

3. Discuss how the results of the homogeneity of variance test are related to choice of *t* test formula (pooled variances or separate variances).

4. Hand compute an independent samples *t*-statistic and a Mann-Whitney *U*-test and determine whether the computed statistic is statistically significant.

5. Use SPSS to obtain an independent samples *t*-statistic and a Mann-Whitney *U*-test statistic.

6. Correctly interpret SPSS output from an independent samples *t* test and a Mann-Whitney *U*-test.

OVERVIEW OF THE INDEPENDENT SAMPLES *t* TEST AND THE MANN-WHITNEY *U*-TEST

Many research projects are designed to test the differences between two groups. In this and subsequent chapters, we will refer to the variable that defines the groups as the "grouping variable" and the other variable as the "characteristic of interest." Note that the grouping variable is usually the independent variable (i.e., the exposure or hypothesized cause), and the characteristic of interest is usually the dependent variable (i.e., the outcome). For example, if we were to study the relationship of gender to height, we would need two variables. The grouping variable would be "gender," and it would have two categories: (1) male and (2) female. The characteristic of interest would be height, and we could measure it in centimeters. In addition, we would not expect men's heights to in any way influence women's heights, making these two groups (men and women) unrelated to, or independent of, each other (two independent samples).

If we want to compare the distribution of a numerical variable for two different groups, we can use the independent samples *t* test (compare the mean for each group) or the Mann-Whitney *U*-test (compares the distribution of values for each group). These two tests perform similar functions, but they are used under different conditions. The *independent samples t test* is a parametric test, meaning that the variable must meet certain assumptions regarding its distribution for the test to be valid, which allows the comparison of the *means* of the two groups. The Mann-Whitney *U*-test is a nonparametric test that is similar to the independent samples *t* test, but it compares the *overall distribution of values* of the two groups. Both tests essentially provide the same information, whether the two groups differ significantly on the distribution of the characteristic of interest. The Mann-Whitney *U*-test has fewer assumptions and thus can be used more freely, but it is not as sensitive as the independent *t* test, meaning that it is not as likely to detect differences between groups.

The *t* test was developed by an Englishman, William Sealy Gosset (1876 to 1937), who published under the pseudonym "Student." He originally developed the independent *t* test for the Guinness brewery for quality control in beer brewing. To do this, Gosset needed to develop a way to analyze small data samples. The modern version of Student's *t*-distribution was derived by R.A. Fisher (1890 to 1962) in 1925 (O'Connor & Robertson, 2003). The Mann-Whitney *U*-test was developed by an economist,

Henry B. Mann, and a graduate student, D. Ransom Whitney, at Ohio State University in 1947 (Salsburg, 2001). It was one of the first nonparametric tests (i.e., a test that does not depend on data having a specific underlying distribution). It was initially used in economics to compare average wages across different years but has since become quite useful in health sciences research.

RESEARCH QUESTION

When we compare two groups on a particular characteristic, we are asking whether the groups are different. Statistically, we are asking whether the difference we find greater is greater than that which could occur by chance alone. The null hypothesis for the *t* test and the Mann-Whitney *U*-test states that any differences that occur between the two groups is due to random error and not because the samples are drawn from two different populations. In short, the null hypothesis states that there is no true difference between the two groups. When we use the *t* test or the Mann-Whitney *U*-test to interpret the significance of the difference between groups, we are asking the statistical question: "What is the probability of getting a difference of this magnitude in groups this size if we were comparing random samples drawn from the same population?" In other words: "What is the probability of getting a difference this large by chance alone?" The following are two examples of questions that these two tests can help to answer.

Do Sleeping Problems Affect the Health-Related Quality of Life of Elderly Patients With Chronic Heart Failure?

This study looking at sleeping problems in the elderly provides a good example of the use of the independent *t* test. It is an observational cross-sectional study of 223 elderly patients with chronic heart failure (Brostrom, Stromberg, Daahlstrom, and Fridlund, 2004). The study tested the hypothesis that patients with chronic heart failure who reported sleeping difficulties would have lower average health-related quality of life scores than those who experienced no sleeping difficulties. The grouping variable is "sleeping difficulty," and it has two categories: (1) has sleeping difficulty or (2) does not have sleeping difficulty. The outcome variable of interest is "health-related quality of life," the scores for which are obtained from the Minnesota Living with Heart Failure Questionnaire. This is an ordinal-level variable in which higher scores indicate a worse quality of life.

In this study, the grouping variable (sleeping difficulty) is the independent variable and health-related quality-of-life score is the dependent variable. The researchers used the independent samples *t* test to test their hypothesis and concluded that the average quality-of-life score among chronic heart failure patients who had sleeping difficulties was significantly lower than that of patients without sleeping difficulties.

Does Oral Misoprostol Lead to a Faster Delivery Than a Placebo?

A double-blind, randomized trial (i.e., a true experimental study) involved 156 pregnant women whose labor was induced to see whether oral misoprostol acted as a cervical priming agent and promoted labor (Beigi, Kabiri, & Zarrinkoub, 2003). The first hypothesis tested was that the women who took oral misoprostol would deliver their babies more quickly than the women who took a placebo. The grouping variable is the "type of drug," misoprostol or placebo, and the outcome variable is "time from ingestion of the drug to delivery of the infant" (in hours). In this case, the grouping variable is the independent variable and the outcome variable is the dependent variable. The researchers used the Mann-Whitney *U*-test and concluded that women who took oral misoprostol had significantly shorter delivery times than the women who took a placebo.

THE INDEPENDENT SAMPLES *t* TEST: TYPE OF DATA REQUIRED

Researchers must choose between the independent samples *t* test and the Mann-Whitney *U*-test to answer questions such as the ones presented here. The independent samples *t* test is a parametric test in which the following assumptions must be met if the test is to be valid:

- The grouping variable (usually the independent variable) must be dichotomous (i.e., it must have only two categories and these categories must be mutually exclusive).
- The two categories must be independent of each other (e.g., the values of one group do not influence the values of the other group).
- The variable measuring the characteristic of interest (usually the dependent variable) must be normally distributed and continuous.

Some people have criticized the use of the term continuous rather than specifying the level of measurement of the variable (ordinal, interval, ratio). However, even when data are measured at the ordinal level, they may be appropriate for use in parametric analyses if they approximate the data required to meet the assumptions of a given analysis. Nunnally and Bernstein (1994) consider any measure that can assume 11 or more levels as continuous and state that, under some circumstances, even fewer measures with fewer than 11 levels can be treated as continuous. Scales with fewer items are considered discrete. For ease of expression, we use the term continuous to describe scale scores.

Note that if the independent samples *t* test is used when one or more of its assumptions are not met, its internal validity (i.e., statistical conclusions) may be threatened because the computed *p*-value may not be correct. However, the *t* test can be used with confidence when one or more of its assumptions are somewhat violated, particularly if the sample size is large

> **BOX 5-1   CHOOSING BETWEEN THE INDEPENDENT *t* TEST AND THE MANN-WHITNEY *U*-TEST**
>
> **The independent *t* test can be used when**
>
> - The grouping variable is dichotomous.
> - The variable measuring the characteristic of interest is normally distributed and continuous.
> - The measures of each value of the variable, which measures the characteristic of interest, constitute an independent random sample.
>
> **The Mann-Whitney U-test can be used when**
>
> - The grouping variable is dichotomous.
> - The measures of each value of the variable, which measure the characteristic of interest, constitute an independent random sample.
> - The measurement scale of the variable, which measures the characteristic of interest, is at least ordinal.
> - The total sample size is at least 8.

(i.e., ≥30 cases), the data are not badly skewed, and there is a fairly large range of values across the ordinal or ratio variable (Box 5-1). If you are not sure that the assumptions of the independent samples *t* test are met, the Mann-Whitney *U*-test (covered later in this chapter) is a good alternative.

Finally, it is important to note that there are two versions of the independent samples *t* test, pooled and separate. When the two groups being compared have equal variances (e.g., homogeneity of variance), the *t* test formula for pooled samples is used; when the two groups have variances that are significantly different (e.g., heterogeneity of variance), the *t* test formula for separate samples is used (Daniel, 2008; Kuzma & Bohnenblust, 2001).

COMPUTING THE INDEPENDENT SAMPLES *t* TEST

Pooled Variances Formula

The computational procedure that we introduced in this chapter for the independent *t* test is illustrated here using data to answer the following typical research question: Do men lose weight faster than women? One way to answer this question is to design a longitudinal, observational study using an existing group of dieters. People who are all at least 20% overweight are invited into the study, and their average weight loss after 3 months on a diet is examined. The grouping variable is "gender," and it has two categories, male and female, and so it is *dichotomous*. The outcome variable of interest is the "pounds of weight lost in the past 3 months" (a ratio-level variable). In this case, the grouping variable is the independent variable. The computational method for the independent samples *t* test that is used when the variances are equal is presented in this example. The hand computation for cases with different variances is more complicated and is not presented here; however, the use of the independent samples *t* test for separate variances using SPSS is covered.

First, a local dieting support group is approached, and 32 members, all of whom are at least 20% overweight and agreed to participate in the study, are randomly selected. The participants—17 male dieters and 15 female dieters—are followed over a 3-month period to see how much weight they lose. The data are shown in Table 5-1, and the distribution of the variable "weight" is shown in the stem-and-leaf plots in Table 5-2. The step-by-step hand computational process is shown in Box 5-2, and the procedure for computing the *t* test using SPSS is shown in Box 5-3. The SPSS output from this procedure is shown in Table 5-3. In order to help you understand how the independent samples *t* test is computed, we show the computation by hand. However, when actually conducting research, SPSS or another statistical package will most likely be used to perform the computations.

Step 1: State the Null and Alternative Hypotheses

- H_0: There will be no difference in the mean weight loss of men versus women.
- H_A: Male dieters will achieve a significantly higher weight loss than female dieters.

Step 2: Define the Significance Level (α-Level), Determine the Degrees of Freedom, and Find the Critical Value for the Computed Independent Samples *t* Test Statistic

To say that a statistically significant difference exists in the means of the two groups, the computed value of the independent samples

Table 5-1	THREE-MONTH WEIGHT LOSS FOR FEMALE AND MALE DIETERS							
Person No.	Gender	Weight Loss (*X*)	$(x_i - \overline{x})^2$	Person No.	Gender	Weight Loss (*X*)	$(x_i - \overline{x})^2$
1	F	3	83.357	16	M	9	91.968
2	F	5	50.837	17	M	9	91.968
3	F	6	37.577	18	M	13	31.248
4	F	8	17.057	19	M	13	31.248
5	F	8	17.057	20	M	14	21.068
6	F	10	4.537	21	M	15	12.888
7	F	12	0.017	22	M	17	2.528
8	F	13	0.757	23	M	19	0.168
9	F	13	0.757	24	M	19	0.168
10	F	13	0.757	25	M	19	0.168
11	F	16	14.977	26	M	19	0.168
12	F	16	14.977	27	M	21	5.808
13	F	18	34.457	28	M	23	19.448
14	F	20	61.937	29	M	24	29.268
15	F	21	78.677	30	M	25	41.088
				31	M	27	70.728
				32	M	30	130.188
Sum	–	182	417.734	–	–	316	580.118

Table 5-2	STEM-AND-LEAF PLOTS FOR WEIGHT-LOSS DATA

Overall and by Gender

(Stem Width: 10.00; Each Leaf: 1 case)

Total Group

Frequency	Stem-and-Leaf Plot
1.00	0.3
6.00	0.568899
8.00	1.02333334
9.00	1.566789999
5.00	1.566789999
2.00	2.57
1.00	3.0

Women Only

Frequency	Stem-and-Leaf Plot
1.00	0.3
4.00	0.5688
5.00	1.02333
3.00	1.668
2.00	2.01

Men Only

Frequency	Stem-and-Leaf Plot
2.00	0.99
3.00	1.334
6.00	1.579999
3.00	2.134
2.00	2.57
1.00	3.0

t-statistic must exceed the critical value. The computed value is the t test statistic that is computed by hand (see Box 5-2) or using SPSS (see Box 5-3), and the critical value of the t test is obtained from the table of critical values for the t-statistic, given the degrees of freedom and α-level (see Appendix C). The critical values are what define the rejection region that is discussed in Chapter 4. The critical value of the t-statistic is the threshold to which the computed value of the t test is compared to determine whether the null hypothesis is rejected.

For two-tailed tests, the null hypothesis is rejected when the computed value is either greater than the critical value at the positive end of the tail or less than (more negative) the value at the negative end of the tail. Although directional hypotheses (such as the one here) should technically be tested using a one-tailed test, the current practice is to use a two-tailed test for these as well. Note that the default for SPSS is a two-tailed test for most procedures, including the independent samples t test. Using SPSS, an exact p-value of the computed t test statistic is automatically computed, and so it is not necessary to find the critical value at which we would reject the null hypothesis.

However, when computing an independent t test by hand, it is necessary to find the critical value in a t-table to determine statistical significance. In this example, an α-level of .05 and a two-tailed test are used. The degrees of freedom are computed for a t test by subtracting 2 from the total sample size ($n - 2$). Because there are 32 people in the analysis, the degrees of freedom are $n - 2$, which equals 30. The critical value is found by looking in the t test table (see Appendix C). The critical value is 2.042, which can be found by looking at the column labeled "two-tailed test, $\alpha = .05$" and the row "degrees of freedom = 30."

Step 3: Make Sure That the Data Meet All the Necessary Assumptions

The data (see Table 5-1) are reviewed and appear to meet all the necessary assumptions. The grouping variable is dichotomous (i.e., gender has two categories). The men and women in this study constitute an independent random sample because they were drawn at random from a weight-loss group and are not related

(Text continues on page 104)

BOX 5-2 **STEP-BY-STEP COMPUTING: THE INDEPENDENT *t* TEST STATISTIC**

Step 1: State the null and alternative hypothesis.

- **H₀:** There will be no difference in the means of the two groups.
- **Hₐ:** Male dieters will achieve a significantly different amount of weight loss than female dieters.

Step 2: Define the significance level (a-level), determine the degrees of freedom, and find the critical value.

- The α-level is .05.
- The total degrees of freedom are 30 $(n-2)$.
- The critical value for the *t*-statistic is 2.0423.

Step 3: Make sure that the data meet all the necessary assumptions.

- The grouping variable is dichotomous.
- Data points are independent of one another.
- Data are normally distributed (see Table 5-2).
- Weight loss is a ratio variable.

Step 4: Compute the mean, standard deviation, and variance for weight loss by gender.

Gender	Mean Weight Loss (lb)	Standard Deviation	Variance
Women	12.13	5.46	29.81
Men	18.59	6.02	36.26
Overall	15.56	6.55	42.90

Computations for Step 4

The mean for the weight loss among women is

$$\frac{\sum X_1}{n_1} = \frac{182}{15} = 12.13 \, \text{lb}$$

The variance for weight loss among women is

$$s^2 = \frac{\sum X_i^2 - \frac{(\sum X)^2}{n}}{n-1} = \frac{2626 - \frac{182^2}{15}}{15-1} = 29.84$$

The standard deviation for weight loss among women is

$$\sqrt{29.84} = 5.463$$

The mean for weight loss among men is

$$\frac{\sum X_2}{n_2} = \frac{316}{17} = 18.59 \, \text{lb}$$

The variance for weight loss among men is

$$s^2 = \frac{6454 - \frac{316^2}{17}}{17-1} = 36.26$$

(Continued)

BOX 5-2   STEP-BY-STEP COMPUTING: THE INDEPENDENT
_t_ TEST STATISTIC (Continued)

The standard deviation for weight loss among men is

$$\sqrt{36.26} = 6.02$$

Step 5: Test for homogeneity of variance

The critical value for the _f_-statistic is 2.44.
The computed value is

$$\frac{36.26}{29.84} = 1.22$$

Because the computed _f_-statistic does not exceed the critical value, it can be concluded that there is homogeneity of variance and that the independent _t_ test for pooled samples can be used.

The formula for the computed _t_-statistic (pooled samples) is

$$t = \frac{\bar{X}_1 - \bar{X}_2}{\sqrt{\left(\dfrac{\sum(X_{1i} - \bar{X}_1)^2 + \sum(X_{2i} - \bar{X}_2)^2}{n_1 + n_2 - 2}\right)\left(\dfrac{1}{n_1} + \dfrac{1}{n_2}\right)}}$$

The computed _t_-statistic using the above formula is

$$t = \frac{12.13 - 18.59}{\sqrt{\left(\dfrac{417.734 + 580.118}{15 + 17 - 2}\right)\left(\dfrac{1}{15} + \dfrac{1}{17}\right)}}$$

$$t = \frac{-6.46}{\sqrt{(33.262)(0.067 + 0.059)}} = \frac{-6.46}{\sqrt{4.191}} = -3.156$$

The 95% confidence interval (CI) about the mean difference is

$$95\% \, CI = (\bar{X}_1 - \bar{X}_2) \pm t_{df,\alpha}(SE_{pooled})$$

Standard error of the mean difference when you have homogeneity of variance is.

$$SE_{pooled} = \sqrt{\left(\dfrac{\sum(X_{1i} - \bar{X}_1^2) + \sum(X_{2i} - \bar{X}_2)^2}{n_1 + n_2 - 2}\right)\left(\dfrac{1}{n_1} + \dfrac{1}{n_2}\right)}$$

The critical value is $t_{30,\,0.05}$ = 2.042. To compute the 95% CI for the dieting example
SE_{pooled} = 2.047.
Critical value: 2.042

$$95\% \, CI = (\bar{X}_1 - \bar{X}_2) \pm t_{df,\alpha}(SE_{pooled})$$
$$95\% \, CI = 18.59 - 12.13 \pm 2.042(2.047)$$
$$95\% \, CI = 6.46 \pm 4.180$$
$$= (2.28, 10.64)$$

Step 6: Determine the statistical significance and state a conclusion.

Because the absolute value of the computed _t_-statistic is 3.16, which is greater than the critical value of 2.042, the null hypothesis can be rejected. It can be concluded that, in this sample, the male dieters had a statistically significant greater weight loss than female dieters over a 3-month period.

BOX 5-3   OBTAINING AN INDEPENDENT *t* TEST USING SPSS

Step 1: The data must be entered into an SPSS data set. Note that you must assign numeric codes to represent gender (1 = female and 2 = male).

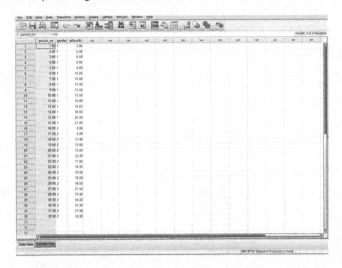

Step 2: The menu system is used to click on "Analyze" and then to select "Compare Means" and "Independent-Samples *t* test."

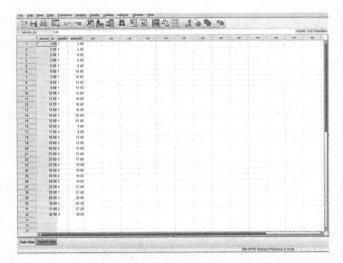

Step 3: When the "Independent- Samples *t* test" popup box appears, "wtlosslb" is selected and moved over to the slot labeled "Test Variables." The variable, "gender," is

(Continued)

BOX 5-3 **OBTAINING AN INDEPENDENT *t* TEST USING SPSS** *(Continued)*

selected and moved over to the slot labeled "Grouping Variable." The "Define Groups" button is clicked. A 1 is put in the slot labeled "group 1," and a 2 is put in the slot labeled "group 2." These are the two values of the grouping variable "gender." When the button labeled "OK" is clicked, the output appears in the output window (see Table 5-3).

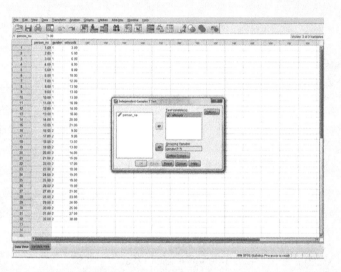

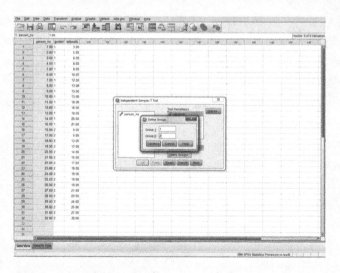

Table 5-3   SPSS OUTPUT

Group Statistics

Wtlosslb	Gender	N	Mean	Standard Deviation	Standard Error Mean
	1	15	12.1333	5.46243	1.41039
	2	17	18.5882	6.02141	1.46041

Independent Samples Test

	Levene's Test for Equality of Variances		*t* test for Equality of Means					95% Confidence Interval of the Difference	
	F	Significance	*t*	Degrees of Freedom	Significance (two-tailed)	Mean Difference	Standard Error Difference	Lower	Upper
wtlosslb Equal variances assumed	.078	.782	-3.159	30	.004	-6.45490	2.04304	-10.62735	-2.28246
Equal variances not assumed			-3.179	29.969	.003	-6.45490	2.03027	-10.60144	-2.30836

to one another (independent). The total sample size is greater than 30 ($n = 32$). Weight loss is approximately normally distributed (see the stem-and-leaf plots in Table 5-2) and is of a ratio measurement scale. Because all the assumptions are met, the independent samples t test can be used. If one or more of these assumptions were violated, the Mann-Whitney U-test would have been used instead. These decisions are made on a case-by-case basis and depend on how many assumptions are violated and how severe the violations are.

Step 4: Compute the Mean, Standard Deviation, and Variance of Each Group

Because the means of two groups are compared, the first pieces of information that are necessary are the values of those means and the size of the difference between the two values. In this example, the mean weight loss achieved by the male dieters was 18.59 lb (8.43 kg) with a standard deviation of 6.02, and the mean weight loss achieved by the female dieters was 12.13 lb (5.50 kg) with a standard deviation of 5.46. Overall, the men lost an average of 6.46 lb (2.93 kg) more than the women. The details of these computations are found in Step 4 in Box 5-2.

Step 5: Compute the Test Statistic

The t test can help determine whether this average difference is statistically significant or whether it is just due to chance. An independent samples t test statistic is then computed and compared with the critical value for a two-tailed t test at $\alpha = .05$ and 30 degrees of freedom. If the average difference is not statistically significant (i.e., the computed t-statistic is smaller than the critical value), the null hypothesis is not rejected. This means that, based on the collected data, there is no real difference in weight loss between the two groups and that any observed differences are the result of random error.

Choose the Correct Independent Samples *t Test* to Use

There are two ways to compute the independent samples t test. The first way is used when the variances of the two groups are equal, and the other is used when the variances of the two groups are significantly different. The correct test is chosen by examining the variances of the two groups being compared. When the variances of the two groups are the same, the *independent samples t test formula for pooled samples* is used; when the variances are different, the *independent samples t test formula for separate samples* is used. The computational method used when the variances are equal is presented in this text. The hand computation for groups with different variances is more complicated and is not presented here. However, discussions about how to compute both in SPSS and how to choose between the two versions of the independent samples t test when reading an SPSS output are presented.

There are a number of tests that can be used to ascertain whether the variances are equal. One of the simpler tests is the Hartley test, also known as the F_{max} test. For this test, an f-statistic is computed by dividing the larger variance (maximum variance) by the smaller variance (minimum variance). Then the critical value of the f-statistic is located in the f-table (see Appendix F) under the appropriate degrees of freedom ($n - 1$) for each group and the chosen significance level. If the computed f-statistic exceeds the critical value, there is heterogeneity of variance. If the computed f-statistic does not exceed the critical value, then there is homogeneity of variance. If there is homogeneity of variance, the independent t test for pooled variances is used. If there is heterogeneity of variance, the independent t test for separate variances is used. The F_{max} test is relatively easy to calculate, but it assumes that the distribution of the variable in both populations is normal and is very sensitive to departures from this assumption. A somewhat less sensitive test is Levene's test of homogeneity of variance, which is the test used by SPSS. For this example, however, we will use the F_{max} test.

In the example, the critical value of the *f*-statistic is found in the *f*-table for $p < .05$ by looking at numerator degrees of freedom = 16 and denominator degrees of freedom = 14; the critical value is 2.44. Then, the *f*-statistic is computed by dividing the larger variance (i.e., that of the male dieters) by the smaller variance (i.e., that of the female dieters). It is important to remember that variance is the square of the standard deviation. Therefore, the computed *f*-statistic is

$$\frac{6.02^2}{5.46^2} = \frac{36.24}{29.81} = 1.22$$

Because the computed *f*-statistic of 1.22 is less than the critical value of 2.44, it can be concluded that the two variances are not significantly different from one another, and so there is homogeneity of variance. Therefore, the independent samples *t* test for pooled variance is chosen. If there was no homogeneity of variance, the alternative independent samples *t* test for different variances formula would be used, which can be obtained from SPSS.

Compute the t-Statistic Using the Formula for Pooled Variances

The formula for the independent samples *t*-statistic is

$$t = \frac{\bar{x}_1 - \bar{x}_2}{SE_{pooled}}$$

$$SE_{pooled} = \sqrt{s^2_{pooled}\left(\frac{1}{n_1} + \frac{1}{n_2}\right)}$$

$$S^2_{pooled} = \frac{(n_1 - 1)s^2_1 + (n_2 - 1)s^2_2}{n_1 + n_2 - 2} \qquad (5\text{-}1)$$

$$s^2 = \frac{1}{n-1}\sum(x_i - \bar{x})^2$$

$$t = \frac{\bar{x}_1 - \bar{x}_2}{\sqrt{\left(\dfrac{\sum(x_{1i} - \bar{x}_1)^2 + \sum(x_{2i} - \bar{x}_2)^2}{n_1 + n_2 - 2}\right)\left(\dfrac{1}{n_1} + \dfrac{1}{n_2}\right)}}$$

The independent *t*-statistic is computed using Equation 5-1:

$$t = \frac{12.13 - 18.59}{\sqrt{\left(\dfrac{417.734 + 580.118}{15 + 17 - 2}\right)\left(\dfrac{1}{15} + \dfrac{1}{17}\right)}}$$

$$t = \frac{-6.46}{\sqrt{(33.262)(0.067 + 0.059)}} = \frac{-6.46}{\sqrt{4.191}} = -3.156$$

independent $t = -3.156$

The detailed steps for computing this formula are shown in Step 5 in Box 5-2.

Compute the 95% Confidence Interval around the Difference between the Means

When the two variances are equal, computing the 95% confidence interval around the difference between the means is straightforward. Computing the confidence interval when there is no homogeneity of variance is somewhat more complicated and beyond the scope of this text. Most statistical packages, including SPSS, compute the confidence intervals for us.

To compute a confidence interval about the difference between the means when the two group variances are equal, the pooled standard error must be computed (SE_{pooled}). This is given by the bottom half of the equation for computing the independent *t* test, which has already been computed to be 2.047. It is then necessary to determine the critical value for the two-tailed independent *t* test at .05 and the appropriate degrees of freedom ($n_1 + n_2 - 2 = 17 + 15 - 2 = 30$, in this example). If a 90% or 99% confidence interval was computed, the critical value for the two-tailed test would be .10 or .01, respectively. In this case, the critical value is 2.042 for two-tailed test at $\alpha = .05$. After these two quantities have been computed, the upper and lower bounds of the 95% confidence interval are computed with the following formula:

$$95\% \, CI = (\bar{x}_1 - \bar{x}_2) \pm t_{df, \alpha}(SE_{pooled}) \qquad (5\text{-}2)$$

The 95% confidence interval for the dieting example is computed using equation 5-2.

This means that 95% of the estimates of differences in weight loss between men and women, which are computed from a sample size of 32, will lie between 2.28 and 10.64 lb (1.03 and 4.83 kg).

Step 6: Determine the Statistical Significance and State a Conclusion

The computed independent t test is statistically significant if the *absolute value* of the t-statistic calculated in Step 6 is larger than the critical value of the t-statistic determined in Step 5. In other words, if the computed statistic falls into the rejection region, the difference is statistically significant, and the means are significantly different from one another. In this example, the absolute value of the computed t-statistic (3.156) is greater than the critical value of 2.042 ($|-3.156|$ > 2.46). This indicates that the actual p-value is well below .05. Another way to ascertain statistical significance is to use the 95% confidence interval around the mean difference: 95% confidence intervals that do not cross 0 (e.g., either positive or negative difference in the means) are statistically significant differences. Because our 95% confidence interval ranged from 2.28 to 10.64, it does not cross 0, and therefore, the difference in weight loss by gender is statistically significant at the α = .05 level.

Step-by-Step Procedure for Using SPSS to Compute the Independent Samples *t* Test

It is fairly easy to compute an independent samples t test using SPSS. Box 5-3 illustrates the process with images from the SPSS program. First, the data must be entered into the data editor. There should be three variables: the person ID, gender (1 = female; 2 = male), and weight loss (in pounds). After the data have been entered, the menu system is used to obtain the independent t test statistic. The SPSS output (see Table 5-3) provides the mean and standard deviation of each group as well as an independent t test to see whether any differences found in weight loss are statistically significant.

The SPSS output has two parts. The first part of the output provides the means and standard deviations of the two groups. The second part of the output provides four pieces of information: (1) whether or not there is homogeneity of variance, (2) the value of the computed t-statistic for both pooled variances and separate variances, (3) the actual p-value of the computed t-statistic, and (4) the 95% confidence interval around the mean differences.

The box labeled "Group Statistics" is examined first. This is where the mean weight loss and standard deviations are found for each group. Note that the women (group 1) had a mean weight loss of 12.13 lb (5.50 kg) (standard deviation, 5.462), and the men had a mean weight loss of 18.59 lb (8.43 kg) (standard deviation, 6.021). This box also provides the standard error of each mean.

Second, from the table labeled "Independent Samples Test," *Levene's test for equality of variances* needs to be examined. This test helps researchers choose the proper independent t test when the equality of variances is assumed (e.g., homogeneity of variance) or when equal variances are not assumed (e.g., heterogeneity of variance). Because the actual p-value of this test is .782 (and greater than the α-level of .05), it can be determined that the variances of the two groups are not significantly different and that there is homogeneity of variance. Therefore, the row labeled "Equal variances assumed" is examined to obtain the correct independent samples t test value. The computed value of the independent t-statistic (equal variances assumed) is listed as −3.159, with 30 degrees of freedom and a p-value of .004. Because the actual p-value of this statistic is lower than the α-level of .05, it can be concluded that male dieters have a significantly greater weight loss over a 3-month period than do female dieters.

Note that Levene's test is a more sophisticated way to test for homogeneity of variance than the *f*-test that is used when computing this by hand.

Third, the section of the output labeled "95% Confidence Interval of the Difference" is examined. A 95% confidence interval is obtained from the row labeled "Equal variances assumed." The confidence intervals are –10.627 (the lower bound) and –2.282 (the upper bound). This is the confidence interval around the female minus male means, which is a negative number because males lost more weight than females. Note that above we calculated the confidence interval around the male minus female mean, which is a positive difference, and this is why our confidence interval was positive 2.28 to 10.64.

Putting It All Together

After the mean weight loss for each group, the independent *t* test, and the confidence interval have been computed, conclusions can be stated. It is important to state both the magnitude and the direction of the difference (i.e., men lost 6.46 lb more than women) and whether the difference was statistically significant. This is done so that readers can judge both the statistical significance and the clinical significance of the findings.

In this study, it was concluded that the dieters lost an average of 15.56 lb (7.06 kg) (standard deviation, 6.55) over a 3-month period, with men losing an average of 18.59 lb (8.43 kg) (standard deviation, 6.02) and women losing an average of 12.13 lb (5.50 kg) (standard deviation, 5.46). Furthermore, it was concluded that men lost significantly more weight than women (6.46 lb [2.93 kg] more) by the independent *t* test at the $\alpha = .05$ level and that researchers were 95% sure that the true weight loss difference between men and women after 3 months lies somewhere between 2.28 and 10.64 lb (1.03 and 4.83 kg).

CONCEPTUAL UNDERSTANDING OF THE INDEPENDENT SAMPLES *t* TEST

In the study of the relationship of weight loss to gender among dieters, a sample of 32 dieters (17 men and 15 women) from the entire population of dieters was used. Inferences were made about the population of all dieters based on the results from the sample to answer the question "Do men lose a different amount of weight over a 3-month period than women?" In the sample, there was an average difference of 6.46 lb (2.93 kg). If the study was conducted repeatedly, using a different group of 32 men and women ($n = 32$) who were randomly selected, it is unlikely that the exact difference of 6.46 lb would occur in each study. There would be some random error, and the estimate of the two means would be somewhat different every time a different random sample was selected.

The collection of these estimates of the difference of two normally distributed variables with the population variance unknown is in itself a variable that is assumed to follow the *t*-distribution. Therefore, by transforming any given estimate of the mean difference (e.g., 6.46 lb [2.93 kg]) into a *t*-statistic, a *t*-table can be consulted (see Appendix C) to find out what the probability is of getting a *t*-statistic as large as or larger than the one computed. It is this assumption of an underlying theoretical probability distribution as opposed to using an empirical distribution that allows the computation of the appropriate *p*-value for the estimate of the mean difference.

What is really being tested with the independent samples *t* test is the null hypothesis that the difference between the two means is essentially equal to 0 (i.e., men and women do not differ in the amount of weight they lose). By using the independent samples *t* test, it is possible to answer the question "What is the probability of getting a difference of a given magnitude between two means from normally distributed samples?" The *t*-table lists the probabilities for the family of *t*-distributions (each degree of freedom has a slightly different set of probabilities associated with it and a slightly different graph; see Appendix C). The *t*-distribution for this example is shown in Figure 5-1, which looks similar to the normal distribution (i.e., equal mean, median, and mode; symmetrical about the mean; bell shaped). In general, this similarity increases with sample size, and for degrees of freedom over 200, the *t*-distribution is indistinguishable from the normal curve. Two things of interest should be noted: (a) the value of the independent *t* test is larger (and thus more likely to be statistically significant) when the difference between the two means is larger, and (b) the value of the independent *t* test is larger when the variance within each group is smaller (see Fig. 5-1).

The *t*-distributions are detailed in Appendix C. The shape of the distributions varies depending on the size of the samples drawn from the populations. Unlike the *z*-distributions, which are based on the normal curve and estimate the theoretical population parameters, the *t*-distributions are based on sample size and vary according to the degrees of freedom. Theoretically, when an infinite number of samples of equal size are drawn from a

normally distributed population, the mean of the sampling distribution will equal the mean of the population. If the sample sizes were large enough, the shape of the sampling distribution would approximate the normal curve.

To answer research questions through the use of the *t* test, we compare the difference we obtained between our means with the sampling distribution of such differences. In general, the larger the difference between our two means, the more likely it is that the *t* test will be significant. However, two other factors are taken into account: the variability and the sample size. An increase in variability leads to an increase in error, and an increase in sample size leads to a decrease in error.

Given the same mean difference, groups with less variability will be more likely to be significantly different than groups with wide variability. This is because in groups with more variability, the error term will be larger. If the groups have scores that vary widely, there is likely to be considerable overlap between the two groups; thus, it will be difficult to ascertain whether a difference exists. Groups with less variability will have distributions more clearly distinct from each other; that is, there will be less overlap between their respective distributions. With more variability (thus, larger error), we need a larger difference to be reasonably "sure" that a real difference exists.

The estimate of the mean difference in weight loss between men and women is based on one

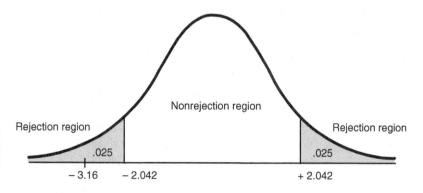

FIGURE 5-1 Rejection and acceptance regions using the independent *t* test for *p* < .05 and degrees of freedom = 30.

study of 32 people. It is, therefore, a "point" estimate; after all, if the study was conducted again (with a different random sample of 32 dieters), the exact same estimate of the difference in weight loss would not be obtained. A reasonable question to ask is "How good an estimate is it?" In addition to ascertaining whether the weight loss is different between men and women, the *t*-distribution can also help to compute a confidence interval around the estimate of the mean difference in weight loss. The confidence interval can help researchers understand how good the point estimate of the difference in weight loss is between men and women.

In general, confidence intervals provide a measure of how well the true value of the parameter is estimated. They are usually computed as 95% confidence intervals, although confidence intervals of 90% and 99% are also common. The interval has two parts: a lower bound (the lowest estimate of the difference that is likely to be obtained if the experiment is repeated again and again) and an upper bound (the highest estimate of the difference that is likely to be obtained if the experiment is repeated again and again). A narrow interval, in which there is little difference between the lower and the upper bound, indicates a better and more precise estimate than does a wide interval. Researchers can say that they are 95% sure that the "true" population value of the difference in weight loss will fall somewhere between the lower and upper bounds.

SAMPLE SIZE CONSIDERATIONS AND POWER OF THE *t* TEST

How many subjects do you need for a *t* test? Cohen (1987) provides tables for determining sample size based on power and effect size determinations, or a computerized program can be used. To enter the tables, we must first decide whether we will be conducting a one- or two-tailed test and what our α or probability level will be. If there is sufficient theoretical rationale and we can hypothesize that one group will

score significantly higher than the other, we will be using a one-tailed test. If we simply want to answer a question such as "Is there a difference between the two groups on the outcome measure?" then we will use a two-tailed test. When planning a study, the sample size is set based on the planned analysis that will require the highest number of subjects. If you were going to run three *t* tests and one would be two tailed, you would base your sample on that, because it requires more subjects than the one-tailed tests.

The power of the test of the null hypothesis is "the probability that it will lead to the rejection of the null hypothesis" (Cohen, 1987, p. 4) when the null hypothesis is false (in other words). A power of .80 means, therefore, that there is an 80% chance of rejecting a false null hypothesis. The higher the desired power, the more the subjects required. Cohen (1987) suggests that for the behavioral scientist, a power of .80 is reasonable, given no other basis for selecting the desired level.

The effect size should be based on previous work, if it exists, rather than simply picking a "moderate" effect from the Cohen (1987) tables. The effect size for the *t* test is simply the difference between the means of the two groups divided by the standard deviation for the measure. Cohen's moderate effect size is set at .50, which means half of a standard deviation unit. As an example, the graduate record examinations (GRE) have a mean of 500 and a standard deviation of 100. Half of a standard deviation unit on that measure would be 50 (100/2). Thus, a moderate effect would be a difference of 50 points on the GRE between two groups.

In a test of the model of transitional nursing care (Brooten et al., 1995), the LaMonica-Oberst Patient Satisfaction Scale was used. A 17-point difference was found between the experimental and control groups. The standard deviation of the scale was 24. If we were going to use that scale again in a similar experiment, what would our expected effect size be? Divide the difference between the means of 17 by the standard deviation of 24 (17/24), which gives an effect size of .71.

Table 5-4 gives a section of Cohen's tables. The top section has the table for a two-tailed test (a_2) at the .05 level (or a one-tailed test at the .025 level). Given an effect size of .70 (numbers across the top of the table) and a power of .80 (numbers down the left side of the table), we would need 33 subjects in each of our groups. If we had used the moderate effect (defined by Cohen as .50),

Table 5-4	POWER TABLES FOR t-TEST (N TO DETECT D BY t TEST)										

$a_2 = .05\ (a_1 = .025)$

Power	.10	.20	.30	.40	.50	.60	.70	.80	1.00	1.20	1.40
.25	332	84	38	22	14	10	8	6	5	4	3
.50	769	193	86	49	32	22	17	13	9	7	5
.60	981	246	110	62	40	28	21	16	11	8	6
2/3	1144	287	128	73	47	33	24	19	12	9	7
.70	1235	310	138	78	50	35	26	20	13	10	7
.75	1389	348	155	88	57	40	29	23	15	11	8
.80	1571	393	175	99	64	45	33	26	17	12	9
.85	1797	450	201	113	73	51	38	29	19	14	10
.90	2102	526	234	132	85	59	44	34	22	16	12
.95	2600	651	290	163	105	73	54	42	27	19	14
.99	3675	920	409	231	148	103	76	58	38	27	20

$$a_1 = .05\ (a_2 = .10)$$
$$d$$

Power	.10	.20	.30	.40	.50	.60	.70	.80	1.00	1.20	1.40
.25	189	48	21	12	8	6	5	4	3	2	2
.50	542	136	61	35	22	16	12	9	6	5	4
.60	721	181	81	46	30	21	15	12	8	6	5
2/3	862	216	96	55	35	25	18	14	9	7	5
.70	942	236	105	60	38	27	20	15	10	7	6
.75	1076	270	120	68	44	31	23	18	11	8	6
.80	1237	310	138	78	50	35	26	20	13	9	7
.85	1438	360	160	91	58	41	30	23	15	11	8
.90	1713	429	191	108	69	48	36	27	18	13	10
.95	2165	542	241	136	87	61	45	35	22	16	12
.99	3155	789	351	198	127	88	65	50	32	23	17

From Cohen, J. (1987). *Statistical power analysis for the behavior sciences* (Rev. ed.). Hillsdale, NJ: Lawrence Erlbaum Assoc. pp. 54–55.

we would need 64 subjects in each of our groups at the same power level. The larger effect size indicates a larger difference between the mean scores and can be detected by fewer subjects.

Now look at the lower section, which includes a one-tailed test at the .05 level ($a_1 = .05$). Given an effect size of .70 and a power of .80, we would need 26 subjects per group. Thus, we can see that a one-tailed test is more powerful; that is, we need fewer subjects to detect a significant difference.

To summarize, for sample size with the *t* test, you must determine

- One-tailed versus two-tailed test
- Alpha level
- Effect size
- Power

You must also estimate how many subjects will be "lost" during data collection and oversample to be sure of having the appropriate numbers for analysis.

MANN-WHITNEY *U*-TEST

The Mann-Whitney *U*-test is a nonparametric test used to determine whether a relationship exists between two groups when one variable is dichotomous and the other variable is at least ordinal. It can be used in situations in which the assumptions for the independent *t* test are not met (e.g., small sample sizes, nonnormally distributed data, ordinal data). The Mann-Whitney *U*-test tests the null hypothesis, which states that the distribution of the two groups is equal. It is analogous to the parametric independent *t* test, which tests whether the means of the two groups are equal.

STEP-BY-STEP PROCEDURE FOR COMPUTING THE MANN-WHITNEY *U*-TEST

To illustrate the computational procedure for the Mann-Whitney *U*-test, data are used from a research question in physical therapy: Is there a difference in the level of pain relief among patients with rib fractures who use painkilling drugs and those who use transcutaneous nerve stimulation (TENS)? A small study that involved 30 people with rib fractures was conducted in an orthopedic office. Usable data were collected from 23 of the patients (response rate, 76.7%). The grouping variable is "type of pain control used," and it has two categories—drugs or TENS. The outcome variable of interest is "level of pain" as rated by the patient on a scale from 0 to 20, where 0 is no pain relief and 20 is complete pain relief. In this case, the grouping variable is the independent variable, and the level of pain relief variable is the dependent variable. There are 11 people in the TENS group and 12 people in the painkilling drug group. The data are shown in Table 5-5, and a summary of the ranking process is shown in Table 5-6. The procedure for computing the Mann-Whitney *U*-test using SPSS is shown in Box 5-4, and the SPSS output is shown in Table 5-7.

Step 1: State the Null and Alternative Hypotheses

- H_0: There will be no difference in pain relief scores between patients who use painkilling drugs and patients who use TENS.
- H_A: Patients who use TENS will experience a different distribution of pain relief scores than patients who use painkilling drugs.

Step 2: Define the α-Level, Determine the Degrees of Freedom, and Find the Critical Value for the Computed Mann-Whitney *U*-Statistic

To say that the two groups are significantly different from one another when using the Mann-Whitney *U*-test, the computed value of the *U*-statistic must be smaller than the critical value. In this example, an α-level of .05 and a two-sided test are used. There are 11 people

Table 5-5	DATA FROM THE TENS STUDY SELF-RATED PAIN-RELIEF SCORES				
Person Number	Group (1 = TENS)	Self-Rated Pain Relief	Person Number	Group (2 = Painkillers)	Self-Rated Pain Relief
1	1	17	12	2	13
2	1	12	13	2	10
3	1	16	14	2	4
4	1	14	15	2	5
5	1	16	16	2	7
6	1	16	17	2	6
7	1	14	18	2	6
8	1	16	19	2	9
9	1	15	20	2	4
10	1	14	21	2	11
11	1	17	22	2	3
			23	2	16

in the TENS group (group n) and 12 people in the painkilling drug group (group m). The critical value is obtained from Appendix D. The critical value can be obtained by looking at the intersection of $n = 11$ and $m = 12$ for .05 (two-tailed test). In this case, the critical value is 34.

Step 3: Make Sure That the Data Meet All the Necessary Assumptions

The data appear to meet all the assumptions. The grouping variable, "type of pain relief," is dichotomous, and the other variable, "self-rated pain relief," in which high scores mean more pain relief, is ordinal. The measurements constitute an independent random sample, and the total sample size is at least 8.

Step 4: Compute the Median and Interquartile Range for Each Group

It is useful to calculate some descriptive statistics for the sample. Because the median is more robust than the mean—being less impacted by

outliers—when using a nonparametric test, it is common to report the median and the interquartile range for the two groups being compared. The first pieces of information that are needed are the values of those medians and the size of the difference between them. In this example, the median pain relief achieved by the group is 13, and the interquartile range is 10 (16 – 6). The median value for pain relief in the TENS group is 16 (interquartile range, 2), and the median value for pain relief in the painkiller group is 6.5 (interquartile range, 7). Overall, the TENS group seems to have experienced much more pain relief than the painkiller group. A Mann-Whitney U-test is computed and compared with the critical value of the U-statistic at $p \leq .05$ to see whether this difference is truly statistically significant.

Step 5: Compute the Mann-Whitney U-Test Statistic

First, all of the data points in both groups are ranked according to the size of the number, beginning with the smallest, keeping track of

(Text continues on page 116)

Table 5-6	RANKING THE DATA		
Group	Actual Score	Position (*N*)	Rank of Score
2	3	1	1
2	4	2	2.5 (tied for ranks 2 and 3)
			2 + 3/2 = 2.5
2	4	3	2.5 (tied for ranks 2 and 3)
2	5	4	4
2	6	5	5.5 (tied for ranks 5 and 6)
2	6	6	5.5 (tied for ranks 5 and 6)
2	7	7	7
2	9	8	8
2	10	9	9
2	11	10	10
1	12	11	11
2	13	12	12
1	14	13	14 (tied for ranks 13, 14, and 15)
			(13 + 14 + 15)/3 = 14
1	14	14	14 (tied for ranks 13, 14, and 15)
1	14	15	14 (tied for ranks 13, 14, and 15)
1	15	16	16
2	16	17	19 (tied for ranks 17, 18, 19, 20, and 21)
			(17 + 18 + 19 + 20 + 21)/5 = 19
1	16	18	19 (tied for ranks 17, 18, 19, 20, and 21)
1	16	19	19 (tied for ranks 17, 18, 19, 20, and 21)
1	16	20	19 (tied for ranks 17, 18, 19, 20, and 21)
1	16	21	19 (tied for ranks 17, 18, 19, 20, and 21)
1	17	22	22.5 (tied for ranks 22 and 23)
1	17	23	22.5 (tied for ranks 22 and 23)

Note. All scores are listed from lowest to highest within the specific group (1 or 2). All position numbers (1 – *n* or 1 – 23) are listed; there are as many position numbers as there are people in the study. When the ranks are computed, tied scores are averaged.

Table 5-7	SPSS OUTPUT

Hypothesis Test Summary			
Null Hypothesis	Test	Significance	Decision
1 The distribution of PainScore is the same across categories of group.	Independent samples Mann-Whitney *U*-test	.000	Reject the null hypothesis

Asymptomatic significances are displayed. The significant level is .05.

BOX 5-4 COMPUTING THE MANN-WHITNEY *U*-STATISTIC USING SPSS

Step 1: The data are entered into an SPSS data set.

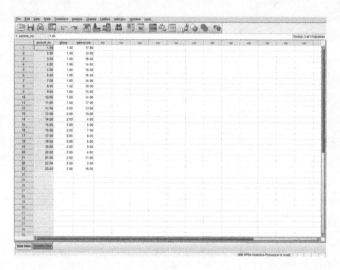

Step 2: The menu system is used to click on "Analyze" and then to select "Nonparametric Tests" and "Independent Samples."

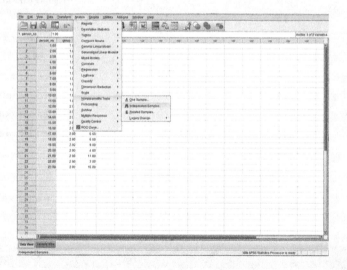

Step 3: When the "Nonparametric tests: two of more independent samples" popup box appears, click on "Fields." Move Painscore into the "TestFields" box; the variable group is

(Continued)

BOX 5-4 **COMPUTING THE MANN-WHITNEY *U*-STATISTIC USING SPSS** *(Continued)*

then selected and moved over to the slot labeled "Groups." Note that the group must be identified as a nominal variable and Painscore as a scale variable in your data (in the "Data View" window, the variable group should have "Nominal" listed and Painscore should have "Scale" indicated under "Measure").

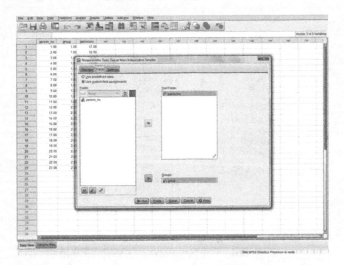

Click on "Settings" in the popup box. Select "Customize tests," then "Mann-Whitney *U* (2 samples)." When "Run" is clicked, the results appear in the output window (see Table 5-6).

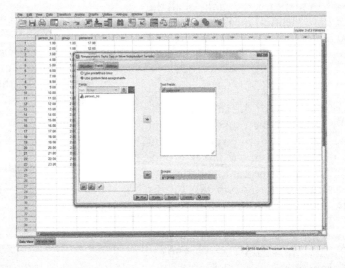

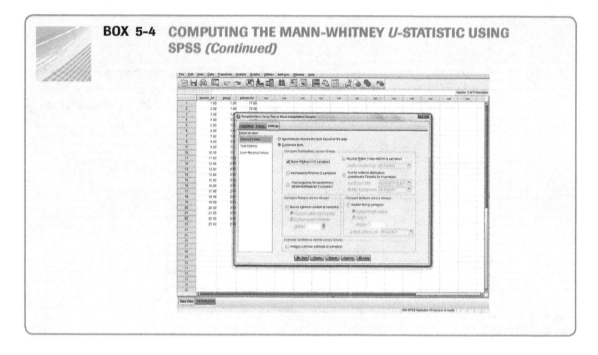

BOX 5-4   COMPUTING THE MANN-WHITNEY *U*-STATISTIC USING SPSS *(Continued)*

which numbers are in which group. Table 5-6 shows how to do this in detail. The smallest number gets a rank of 1, the second smallest a rank of 2, and so on. Where there are two or more measures with the same value, they are "tied for rank." In that case, the ranks of all the positions that have identical measures are averaged. For example, if two data points are tied for fifth place, the rank 5.5 is assigned:

$$5.5 = \frac{5+6}{2}$$

R_n, the sum of the ranks of the smaller group, is obtained by summing the ranks of the data points in the smaller group (group n), and R_m, the sum of the ranks of the larger group, is obtained by summing the ranks of the data points in the larger group (group m). In this example, the sum of ranks is computed as follows:

TENS (group n): R_n = 11 + 14 + 14 + 14 + 16 + 19 + 19 + 19 + 19 + 22.5 + 22.5 = 190

Painkiller (group m): R_m = 1 + 2.5 + 2.5 + 4 + 5.5 + 5.5 + 7 + 8 + 9 + 10 + 12 + 19 = 86.

After the sum of ranks has been obtained, the Mann-Whitney *U*-test statistic can be obtained. The basic formula for the Mann-Whitney *U*-test is

$$U = R_n - \frac{n(n+1)}{2} \qquad (5\text{-}3)$$

$$U' = n \times m - U \qquad (5\text{-}4)$$

where n is the size of the smaller sample, m is the size of the larger sample, and R_n is the sum of the ranks of the smaller sample.

In this example, the *U*-statistic is calculated by using Equation 5-3 as follows:

$$U = 190 - \frac{11(12)}{2} = 190 - 66 = 124$$
$$U = 124$$

U' is computed by using Equation 5-4 as follows:

$$U' = (11 \times 12) - 124 = 132 - 124 = 8$$
$$U' = 8$$

Step 6: Determine the Statistical Significance and State a Conclusion

When the number of measures in both groups is fewer than 20, whichever answer (*U* or *U*') is smaller is used, and this computed value is compared with the critical value in the Mann-Whitney *U* table discussed in Step 2. If the number of measures in either group is more than 20, the tables cannot be used. Instead, a *z*-score is computed, and the critical value is found in the *z*-table (Appendix B). This is done by using the equation

$$z = (t - mn/2)/(nm \, [n + m + 1]/12) \quad (5\text{-}5)$$

SPSS will compute this and give the exact *p*-value for the *U*-statistic.

In this example, $U = 124$ and $U' = 8$. The smaller of the two values, 8, is compared with the critical value of 34. Because the computed *U*-statistic of 8 is less than the critical value of 34, the statistic is well within the rejection region for $p < .05$, and the null hypothesis should be rejected. It can be concluded that, in the sample, the TENS group had significantly higher pain relief scores than the pain-killer group.

Step-by-Step Procedure for Using SPSS to Compute the Mann-Whitney *U*-Statistic

It is fairly easy to compute a Mann-Whitney *U*-test using SPSS (see Box 5-4). First, the data are entered into the data editor. There are three variables: the person ID, group (1 = TENS, 2 = painkillers), and pain-relief score. After the data are entered, the menu system can be used to obtain the Mann-Whitney *U*-test. The SPSS output (see Table 5-7) provides the *p*-value of the Mann-Whitney test (see Box 5-4).

The output is presented (see Table 5-7) and shows the *p*-value for the Mann-Whitney *U*-test. Because the actual *p*-value is listed as .000, which is well below the α-level of .05, it can be concluded that people who use TENS experience significantly greater subjective pain relief than people who use painkillers.

Conceptual Understanding of the Mann-Whitney *U*-Test

The Mann-Whitney *U*-test is based on the relative ranks of the measurements in each group. Ranking allows researchers to use the relative magnitude of the distribution of observations in each group. The data in the two groups are ordered, and each group is assigned a rank independent of the group from which it comes. If the two distributions are similar, the sum of the ranks is equal, and the value of *U* and *U'* is similar (and large). If one distribution is much larger than the other, one rank sum will also be much larger than the other, and a small (statistically significant) value of *U* is obtained.

Putting It All Together

After the median pain reduction for each group and the Mann-Whitney *U*-test have been computed, it is time to state the conclusion. In this study, people with rib fractures who use TENS units had a median pain relief score of 16.0, and people with rib fractures who use painkillers had a median pain relief score of 6.5. The Mann-Whitney *U*-test is significant with a $p < .05$. It can be concluded that people who use TENS experience significantly more pain relief than people who use painkillers.

| CHAPTER REVIEW |

Multiple-Choice Concept Review

1. The independent samples t test is best described as
   a. a type of Mann-Whitney U-test.
   b. a parametric test.
   c. a nonparametric test.
   d. none of the above.

2. The independent samples t test is used to determine differences in the means of
   a. two groups only.
   b. three groups only.
   c. four groups only.
   d. any number of groups.

3. If the variances of the two groups being compared are significantly different, which independent samples t test should be used?
   a. The independent samples t test for pooled variances
   b. The independent samples t test for separate variances
   c. Either test so long as the sample size is over 30 cases
   d. The Mann-Whitney U-test

4. Student's independent samples t test is best used when the measurement scale of the characteristic of interest is
   a. nominal.
   b. ordinal.
   c. interval or ratio.
   d. all of the above.

5. Student's independent samples t test is best used when
   a. the total sample size is at least 30.
   b. the grouping variable is dichotomous.
   c. the data are paired.
   d. a and b only.

6. Consider the following question: Do women make more visits to their primary care physician in a year than men? Which variable is the grouping variable?
   a. Gender
   b. Number of visits to the physician
   c. Both
   d. Neither

7. Consider the following question: Do people who exercise three times a week or more have lower systolic blood pressure than people who exercise less than three times a week? Which variable should be normally distributed?
   a. Frequency of exercise
   b. Systolic blood pressure
   c. Both
   d. Either one

8. Consider the following question: Do children who are immunized against chickenpox miss fewer days of school than children who are not immunized? Which is the grouping variable?
   a. Number of days of school missed
   b. Immunization status
   c. Either one
   d. Neither one

9. Consider the following question: Do people without health insurance spend more money a year on over-the-counter drugs than people who have some form of health insurance? How many levels (or possible values) does the variable "health insurance" have?
   a. One
   b. Two
   c. Three
   d. Can't tell

10. Consider the following question: Among people with chronic back pain, do those who have their back pain treated by a chiropractor miss fewer days of work than those who are treated by a primary care physician? Is it possible to use an independent *t* test if the variable "number of days missed" is recoded into three-category variables (none, less than 3, more than or equal to 3)?
    a. No
    b. Yes
    c. Only if at least 60 people are in the study
    d. Only if an independent random sample is available

11. The Mann-Whitney *U*-test is best described as
    a. a special type of independent *t* test.
    b. a parametric test.
    c. a nonparametric test.
    d. none of the above.

12. The Mann-Whitney *U*-test is used to determine differences in the distribution of a variable in
    a. two groups only.
    b. three groups only.
    c. four groups only.
    d. any number of groups.

13. If data are normally distributed in only one group, then which of the following tests can be used?
    a. Independent *t* test for pooled variances
    b. Independent *t* test for separate variances
    c. Either test as long as the sample size is over 30 cases
    d. Mann-Whitney *U*-test

14. The Mann-Whitney U-test is best used when the measurement scale of the characteristic of interest is
    a. nominal.
    b. ordinal.
    c. interval or ratio.
    d. b and c.

15. The Mann-Whitney U-test is best used when
    a. the total sample size is at least 8.
    b. the grouping variable is dichotomous.
    c. the data are paired.
    d. a and b only are true.

16. Consider the following question: Do people who eat after 8 PM sleep fewer hours than people who do not eat after 8 PM? Which variable is the grouping variable?
    a. Eating before or after 8 pm
    b. Number of hours of sleep
    c. Both
    d. Neither

17. Consider the following question: Do people who exercise at least three times a week have lower systolic blood pressure than people who exercise less than three times a week? Which of the following variables should be normally distributed to perform a Mann-Whitney U-test?
    a. Frequency of exercise
    b. Systolic blood pressure
    c. Both
    d. Neither, because a normal distribution is not an assumption

18. Consider the following question: Do children who are immunized against chickenpox miss fewer days of school than children who are not immunized? Which of the following variables should be dichotomous to perform a Mann-Whitney U-test?
    a. Number of days of school missed
    b. Immunization status
    c. Both
    d. Neither, because a normal distribution is not an assumption

19. Consider the following question: Is there a relationship between insurance status and the number of days absent from work? To use an independent t test, how many possible values should the variable "health insurance" have?
    a. One
    b. Two
    c. Three
    d. Can't tell from the information given

20. Consider the following question: Do people with chronic back pain who are treated by a chiropractor miss fewer days of work than people who are treated by a primary care physician? Can a Mann-Whitney *U*-test be used if the variable "number of days missed" is recoded into two-category variables (none, 1 or more)?
   a. No
   b. Yes
   c. Only if nonparametric data are available
   d. Only if an independent random sample is available

Critical Thinking Concept Review

1. Develop five hypotheses that could be tested with the independent *t* test or the Mann-Whitney *U*-test.

2. Find the critical value of the independent *t* test for each of the following *p*-values and sample sizes. In each case, assume you are conducting a two-tailed test.
   a. $p = .05$; sample size = 23 _____
   b. $p = .01$; sample size = 47 _____
   c. $p = .10$; sample size = 180 _____
   d. $p = .05$; sample size = 19 _____
   e. $p = .10$; sample size = 102 _____
   f. $p = .01$; sample size = 14 _____

3. Find the critical value of the Mann-Whitney *U*-test for each of the following *p*-values and sample sizes. Assume a two-tailed test.
   a. $p = .05$; $n = 10$; $m = 13$ _____
   b. $p = .01$; $n = 17$; $m = 5$ _____
   c. $p = .10$; $n = 20$; $m = 20$ _____
   d. $p = .05$; $n = 2$; $m = 9$ _____
   e. $p = .10$; $n = 8$; $m = 12$ _____
   f. $p = .01$; $n = 14$; $m = 7$ _____

Computational Problems

For each of the following five problems, state the most likely hypothesis and compute an independent *t* test for problems 1 to 4 to determine whether a statistically significant difference exists between the two groups in question. Use an α-level of .05 and a two-tailed test for questions 1 to 4. Compute a *t* test statistic only (no Mann-Whitney *U*) for problem 5, which may take a little extra thought. Perform the computations for problems 1 to 4 both by hand and using SPSS. Do problem 5 by hand only.

1. A study was conducted to examine the effect of an herbal formula for insomnia. A group of 13 volunteers was recruited and randomly assigned to take either the herbal formula or a placebo. The following table lists the hours of sleep that each person had on the night he or she took either the formula or placebo.

Group	Hours of Sleep	Group	Hours of Sleep
Placebo	3.8	Formula	4.6
Placebo	5.2	Formula	6.2
Placebo	6.7	Formula	3.9
Placebo	3.7	Formula	5.2
Placebo	4.3	Formula	5.4
Placebo	2.1	Formula	4.1
Placebo	5.0		

2. A study was conducted to see whether the type of child care (e.g., home with full-time caretaker, full-time day care) was related to aggressive behavior in 2-year-old children.

Group	Number of Aggressive Acts in a 4-Hour Period	Group	Number of Aggressive Acts in a 4-Hour Period
Home	5	Day care	1
Home	3	Day care	3
Home	4	Day care	4
Home	1	Day care	4
Home	2	Day care	2
Home	3	Day care	0
Home	2		

3. A study was conducted in a major urban area to examine the relationship between health insurance and the number of visits made to a physician's office in the past year.

Person Number	Insurance Type	Number of Visits	Person Number	Insurance Type	Number of Visits
1	None	0	31	Private	0
2	None	0	32	Private	0
3	None	0	33	Private	1
4	None	0	34	Private	1
5	None	0	35	Private	1
6	None	0	36	Private	1
7	None	1	37	Private	2
8	None	1	38	Private	2
9	None	1	39	Private	2
10	None	1	40	Private	2

(Continued)

Person Number	Insurance Type	Number of Visits	Person Number	Insurance Type	Number of Visits
11	None	1	41	Private	2
12	None	1	42	Private	2
13	None	1	43	Private	2
14	None	1	44	Private	2
15	None	1	45	Private	3
16	None	1	46	Private	3
17	None	2	47	Private	3
18	None	2	48	Private	3
19	None	2	49	Private	3
20	None	2	50	Private	3
21	None	2	51	Private	3
22	None	2	52	Private	3
23	None	3	53	Private	4
24	None	3	54	Private	4
25	None	3	55	Private	4
26	None	3	56	Private	4
27	None	4	57	Private	4
28	None	4	58	Private	5
29	None	5	59	Private	5
30	None	5	60	Private	6
			61	Private	6

4. Data from a study examining the relationship between poverty and depression are listed in the following table. A total of 67 people took part in this study. Note that a higher score indicates a higher level of depression.

Person Number	Poverty Level	Depression Score	Person Number	Poverty Level	Depression Score
1	Below poverty	12	32	Above poverty	10
2	Below poverty	12	33	Above poverty	9
3	Below poverty	11	34	Above poverty	8
4	Below poverty	11	35	Above poverty	8
5	Below poverty	11	36	Above poverty	8
6	Below poverty	11	37	Above poverty	7
7	Below poverty	9	38	Above poverty	7

Person Number	Poverty Level	Depression Score	Person Number	Poverty Level	Depression Score
8	Below poverty	9	39	Above poverty	7
9	Below poverty	8	40	Above poverty	6
10	Below poverty	8	41	Above poverty	6
11	Below poverty	7	42	Above poverty	6
12	Below poverty	7	43	Above poverty	5
13	Below poverty	7	44	Above poverty	5
14	Below poverty	7	45	Above poverty	5
15	Below poverty	7	46	Above poverty	5
16	Below poverty	6	47	Above poverty	5
17	Below poverty	6	48	Above poverty	5
18	Below poverty	6	49	Above poverty	5
19	Below poverty	6	50	Above poverty	5
20	Below poverty	6	51	Above poverty	5
21	Below poverty	6	52	Above poverty	5
22	Below poverty	5	53	Above poverty	5
23	Below poverty	4	54	Above poverty	5
24	Below poverty	4	55	Above poverty	4
25	Below poverty	4	56	Above poverty	4
26	Below poverty	3	57	Above poverty	4
27	Below poverty	3	58	Above poverty	3
28	Below poverty	2	59	Above poverty	3
29	Below poverty	2	60	Above poverty	3
30	Below poverty	0	61	Above poverty	3
31	Below poverty	0	62	Above poverty	3
			63	Above poverty	2
			64	Above poverty	2
			65	Above poverty	1
			66	Above poverty	1
			67	Above poverty	0

5. A study was conducted to examine the professional behavior of dental hygienists. Information was available on whether they read professional journal articles on a regular basis and the number of years that they had been in practice. The question of interest is "Have people who read journal articles in their field on a regular basis been in practice longer than people who do not regularly read journal articles?"

Group	Group Size	Mean Years in Practice	Standard Deviation
Does not read journal articles regularly	120	11.83	7.67
Reads articles regularly	107	15.71	8.84

The Paired t Test and the Wilcoxon Matched-Pairs Signed Rank Test: Comparing the Means/Medians of Two Related Groups

OBJECTIVES

After studying this chapter, you should be able to:

1. Determine when the paired t test and Wilcoxon matched-pairs signed rank test are appropriate to use and select the correct test.

2. Hand compute a paired t-statistic and a Wilcoxon matched-pairs signed rank statistic and determine whether they are statistically significant.

3. Use SPSS to compute a paired t test statistic and a Wilcoxon matched-pairs test.

4. Correctly interpret SPSS output from a paired t test and a Wilcoxon matched-pairs test.

5. Write up the results of the paired t test and the Wilcoxon matched-pairs test.

OVERVIEW OF THE PAIRED t TEST AND THE WILCOXON MATCHED-PAIRS SIGNED-RANK TEST

The pretest/posttest and matched-pairs designs are two common research designs used for health services research. In both designs, the data are "paired"; that is, the measurements of the same variable at two different points are compared. By "paired," we mean that the two observations are in some way connected and therefore are not independent of each other. The paired observations of the variable can be measured on the same person at two different points in time, or they can be measured at the same time on two different people who are "matched" on some condition (e.g., age, gender, and twins), where one of them experiences an intervention and the other serves as the control. Usually, but not always, this variable is the dependent variable.

The statistical analysis of paired data assumes that measures are likely to be correlated because they are taken from the same or very similar participants. To measure differences in the central tendency (e.g., mean and median) in such data, either the paired t test or the Wilcoxon matched-pairs signed rank test is used. For brevity, we will refer to the Wilcoxon matched-pairs signed rank test as simply the Wilcoxon matched-pairs test. The paired t test is a parametric test that allows a comparison of the means of the two correlated (paired) groups. However, the data must meet certain assumptions. This test uses the same family of t-distributions discussed in the previous chapter. The Wilcoxon matched-pairs test is a nonparametric test that is similar to the paired t test, but it compares the medians of the two correlated groups rather than the means and has fewer assumptions. Essentially, the same information is provided by both tests, whether the two groups differ significantly on the measure of central tendency of the characteristic of interest. The Wilcoxon matched-pairs test has fewer assumptions and can be used more often, but it is not as sensitive as the paired t test.

RESEARCH QUESTION

The research question being asked here is "Are the means or medians of two related groups different from one another?" Pretest/posttest designs are used in studies that examine the effect of an intervention on a study participant by comparing posttest values of the dependent variable after an intervention to the pretest values of that same variable before the intervention. For example, researchers may want to examine weight loss after some intervention by comparing the study participants' postintervention weight with their preintervention weight. In many of these cases, the participant is serving as his or her own control. Matched-pairs designs are used to examine the effect of an intervention in which each participant who receives the intervention is matched to a control who does not receive the intervention. Matched-pairs designs commonly use twins or siblings who share biologic or sociodemographic characteristics (e.g., age, gender, and ethnicity). For example, researchers may want to examine differences in how weight loss occurs in diet plans with and without exercise. A group of twins could be studied as matched pairs; one twin would be assigned to a diet-alone group and the other to a diet with exercise group. Then, the mean weight loss of the twin in the diet-alone group is compared with that of the twin in the diet with exercise group.

If the two groups being compared are matched or paired on some basis, the scores are likely to be similar. The differences between the two groups due to chance will not be as large as when they are drawn independently. In the paired t test and the Wilcoxon matched-pairs test, a correction is made to account for this.

When we compare two related groups on a particular characteristic, we are asking whether the two groups are different, controlling for the fact that they are already related (e.g., because they are drawn from the same people or from matched controls, we would expect them to be more similar than two unrelated groups). The statistical question asks how different the groups are; that is, is the difference greater than we would expect to find by chance alone. For the paired t test, the null hypothesis is that there is no difference in the mean between the two groups; for the Wilcoxon matched-pairs signed rank test, the null hypothesis is that there is no difference between the distributions. Conceptually, what we are asking is "What is the probability of getting a difference of this magnitude in the means/medians in two groups that are related to one another?" For the paired t test, the larger the test statistic, the lower its associated probability (p-value) will be. In other words, larger paired t test statistics mean that the differences in means are less likely to have occurred by chance. For the Wilcoxon matched-pairs signed rank test, the smaller the test statistics, the lower its associated probability (p-value) will be. In other words, smaller

Wilcoxon matched-pairs signed rank test statistic values mean that the difference in distributions is less likely to have occurred by chance.

The following studies provide examples of how the paired *t* test and the Wilcoxon matched-pairs test are used in practice. The first study discussed provides an example of a matched case–control study. The second two studies provide examples of pretest/posttest studies where the participants serve as their own control.

Does Breast-feeding Affect Bone Density?

One retrospective, matched, case control twin study collected data from the Bone Research Program in a twins database to examine whether breast-feeding affects bone density (Paton et al., 2002). This study examined bone density in 58 female twin pairs (a total of 116 people) in which one twin had breast-fed a child and the other had not. In this case control study, the measurements in the "case" were compared with the measurements in the "control." The researchers used the paired *t* test to compare bone density in the twin who had breast-fed and the twin who had not. The researchers found that there were no detectable differences in bone density of the spine, hip, and total body between twins. They concluded that breast-feeding does not affect bone density.

Does a Depression Education Program Change the Knowledge Base of Residents in Obstetrics and Gynecology?

A group of researchers tested a 5-hour educational intervention (one lecture and two workshops) for residents in obstetrics and gynecology at eight different hospitals (Learman et al., 2003). Each of the residents took a depression knowledge and self-efficacy test before the intervention and again 3 months after the intervention. The investigators found that the data were normally distributed and met the assumptions for a paired *t* test. The researchers found that self-efficacy in caring for depressed patients increased significantly ($p \leq .001$) but that knowledge did not, although it approached significance.

Does a Minimal-Contact Intervention Promote Walking Among Sedentary Women?

A study examined the effect of a 6-week minimum contact intervention on increasing walking among sedentary women (Dinger, Heesch, & McClary, 2005). The intervention consisted of an orientation session, use of a free pedometer, three commercial brochures about walking, and one e-mail a week for 6 weeks; the e-mails contained information about how to begin and maintain a physical activity program involving walking. This study used a one-group, pretest/posttest design in which participants served as their own controls. Outcome variables, including the number of minutes walked per week, were collected at baseline and again at the end of the 6 weeks. Because the walking data were not normally distributed, the researchers chose to use the Wilcoxon matched-pairs test to examine the pretest to posttest differences in minutes walked each week. At pretest, women reported walking a median of 55 minutes a week, and at posttest, they reported walking a median of 245 minutes a week; this was a statistically significant increase as tested by the Wilcoxon matched-pairs test ($p \leq .001$).

TYPES OF DATA REQUIRED

For both the paired *t* test and the Wilcoxon matched-pairs test, we need two measures of the same dependent variable taken on either the same person at two different points in time or on a participant and a matched control. For the paired *t* test, the dependent variable will ideally be of interval/ratio measurement scale. However, even data measured at the ordinal level can be appropriate for the paired *t* test if the data approximate the type of data needed.

In particular, if the dependent variable is ordinal, it can still be analyzed using a paired *t* test if the scale has 11 or more categories and the data are normally distributed (Nunnally & Bernstein, 1994). For the Wilcoxon matched-pairs test, the data need to be of at least an ordinal measurement scale. For both tests, the independent variable is categorical, either the intervention received (e.g., drug vs. placebo) or simply time (e.g., time 1 compared with time 2).

ASSUMPTIONS

The choices for comparing the means or medians of two correlated groups are the paired *t* test and the Wilcoxon matched-pairs test. The paired *t* test is a parametric test, but to use it, some assumptions must be met. Specifically, it is necessary to know the following: (a) that only two measurements (either pretest/posttest on the same person or the same measure taken on a participant and a matched control subject) are compared, (b) the total sample size, (c) whether the two measures of the variable are normally distributed, and (d) the measurement

scale of the variable measuring the characteristic of interest.

If the paired *t* test is used when one or more of its assumptions are not met, there is a threat to its internal validity (i.e., statistical conclusions) because the computed *p*-value may not be correct. However, the paired *t* test can be used with confidence, and there is a relatively low risk of error if just a few assumptions are violated (e.g., if the sample size is relatively large, the data are not too skewed, and there is a fairly large range of values).

The Wilcoxon matched-pairs test has fewer assumptions and can be used with ordinal-, interval-, or ratio-level data. It simply assumes that there are at least five paired measures to compare. For a summary of the differences between the two tests, see Box 6-1.

COMPUTING THE PAIRED *t* TEST

The paired *t* test is a parametric test used to determine whether a difference exists in the means of two correlated variables that are interval or ratio in measurement scale and normally

---

BOX 6-1 **CHOOSING BETWEEN THE PAIRED *t* TEST AND THE WILCOXON MATCHED-PAIRS TEST**

The paired *t* test can be used when

- There are two paired measurements of the characteristic of interest (i.e., either one pretest and one posttest measurement on the same person or one measurement on a participant and one measurement on a matched control).
- The two measures that are compared are normally distributed, or there are at least 30 pairs and a distribution that is not too badly skewed.
- The measurement scale is either interval or ratio (sometimes ordinal is acceptable as well).

The Wilcoxon matched-pairs test can be used when

- There are two paired measurements of the characteristic of interest (i.e., either one pretest and one posttest measurement on the same person or one measurement on a participant and one measurement on a matched control).
- The measurement scale of the characteristic is ordinal, interval, or ratio.
- The total sample size contains at least five pairs of measurements.

distributed. If the data are not exactly normally distributed, the paired *t* test can still be used if there are at least 30 pairs of measures. The paired *t* test scores the null hypothesis that the difference between the two-paired (correlated) means is not statistically different from 0.

Step-by-Step Procedure for Hand-Computing the Paired *t* Test

To illustrate the paired *t* test, we will use data from a study that asked the following research question: Does a multisession cardiovascular health education program for teenagers increase their knowledge about cardiovascular health? To answer this question, a group of teenagers is invited to participate in a health education program. At the beginning of the first session, a 20-item quiz about cardiovascular health (with scores 0 to 100) is given. At the end of the last session, the same quiz is administered. The posttest scores are compared with the pretest scores to see whether there was a significant change in knowledge about cardiovascular health. Note that because the pretest and posttest data come from the same person, the data points are correlated (not independent of one another), and so a statistical technique for matched pairs must be used. The pretest and posttest quiz scores are shown in Table 6-1, and the stem-and-leaf plots for these data are shown in Table 6-2. Computation of the paired *t* test for this example is illustrated in Boxes 6-2 and 6-3.

Step 1: State the Null and Alternative Hypotheses

- H_0: There will be no difference in mean pretest and posttest knowledge scores.
- H_A: Mean posttest knowledge score will be significantly different from the mean pretest knowledge score.

Step 2: Define the Significance Level (α-Level), Determine the Degrees of Freedom, and Find the Critical Value for the Computed *t* Test Statistic

To say that a statistically significant difference exists in the means of the two measures, the computed value of the paired *t*-statistic must exceed the critical value. The computed value is the numeric value of the paired *t*-statistic computed from the data. The critical value is the value of the paired *t* test that is obtained from the table of critical values for the *t* test (Appendix C). The critical value is the value at which the probability of obtaining that value or higher is at or below our predetermined α-level.

In this example, an α-level of .05 and a two-tailed test are used. The degrees of freedom for a *t* test are computed by subtracting 1 from the total number of pairs in the study. This example includes 31 pairs, and so the degrees of freedom are $n-1$, which equals 30. The critical value is found by looking in the *t* test table (see Appendix C) and finding the column labeled "Two-tailed test = .05" and the row "Degrees of freedom = 30." The critical value is 2.042.

Step 3: Make Sure That the Data Meet All the Necessary Assumptions

The data presented in Table 6-1 appear to meet all the assumptions. There are two measures of the dependent variable (pretest and posttest) for each of the 31 teenagers, the data are of ratio measurement scale (score on a 100-point quiz), and the scores are approximately normally distributed (see the stem-and-leaf plots in Table 6-2). Because all the assumptions are met, the paired *t* test is used. If one or more of these assumptions had been violated, the Wilcoxon matched-pairs test would be used instead. These decisions are made on a case-by-case basis and depend on the number and severity of the assumptions that are violated.

Table 6-1	PRETEST AND POSTTEST HEALTH QUIZ SCORES FOR 31 TEENAGE PARTICIPANTS IN A HEALTH EDUCATION PROGRAM			
		Knowledge Score		
Subject Number	After Program	Before Program	Difference in Scores (d)	Square of Difference (d^2)
1	73	48	25	625
2	78	56	22	484
3	67	58	9	81
4	74	60	14	196
5	72	61	11	121
6	73	61	12	144
7	65	62	3	9
8	79	63	16	256
9	77	64	13	169
10	80	66	14	196
11	78	66	12	144
12	79	66	13	169
13	70	67	3	9
14	74	67	7	49
15	86	68	18	324
16	83	70	13	169
17	86	71	15	225
18	80	72	8	64
19	80	72	8	64
20	70	72	−2	4
21	75	73	2	4
22	87	73	14	196
23	75	74	1	1
24	87	74	13	169
25	90	76	14	196
26	82	77	5	25
27	78	78	0	0
28	77	79	−2	4
29	83	81	2	4
30	83	84	−1	1
31	86	88	−2	4
Sum	2,427	2,147	280	4,106

Table 6-2	STEM-AND-LEAF PLOTS FOR PRETEST AND POSTTEST QUIZ SCORES	
Pretest	**Posttest**
Stem-and-Leaf Plot	Stem-and-Leaf Plot
4.8	6.57
5.68	7.0023344
6.666778	7.557788899
6.666778	8.0002333
7.012223344	8.66677
7.6789	9.0
8.14	
8.8	

Step 4: Compute the Mean and Standard Deviation of Each Group

Because the means of a variable measured at two points in time (pretest and posttest) are compared, the values of these means and the size of the difference between them must be obtained. In this example, the mean pretest quiz score was 69.26 (standard deviation, 8.61) and the mean posttest quiz score was 78.29 (standard deviation, 6.21). Overall, the posttest quiz scores were higher than the pretest scores by an average of 9.03 points.

Step 5: Compute the Paired t Test Statistic

The paired *t* test can help to determine whether this average difference is statistically significant or whether it is probably just due to chance. A paired *t* test statistic is computed and compared with the critical value for the *t*-statistic at $\alpha = .05$ and 30 degrees of freedom. If the average difference is not statistically significant, then no real difference exists in the two quiz scores, and any observed differences are the result of random error.

The formula for the paired *t* test statistic is

$$t = \frac{(\overline{x}_d - \mu_0)}{SE_{\overline{x}_d}}$$

$$\overline{x}_d = (\overline{x}_1 - \overline{x}_2)$$

$$SE_{\overline{x}_d} = \frac{s_d}{\sqrt{n_d}}$$

$$s = \sqrt{\frac{\sum d_i^2 - \frac{\left(\sum x_i\right)^2}{n_d}}{(n_d - 1)}}$$

where *d* represents the difference in pretest and posttest values, and μ_d is the mean difference under the null hypothesis, or 0. Thus,

$$t = \frac{\overline{x}_1 - \overline{x}_2 - 0}{\sqrt{\frac{\sum d_i^2 - \frac{\left(\sum x_i^2\right)}{n_d}}{n_d(n_d - 1)}}} \tag{6-1}$$

To use this formula, each posttest value is subtracted from its paired pretest value to get the difference, then the mean difference is computed, and the sum of the difference scores (Σd_i) and the sum of the squared difference scores (Σd_i^2) must be computed. Table 6-1 contains these numbers. $\Sigma d_i = -280$ and $\Sigma d_i^2 = 4,106$. After these values are plugged into the equation, the paired *t*-statistic can be computed using Equation 6-1 as follows:

$$t = \frac{69.26 - 78.29 - 0}{\sqrt{\frac{(4106) - \frac{(-280)^2}{31}}{31(30 - 1)}}}$$

$$= \frac{-9.03}{\sqrt{\frac{4106 - 2529.032}{930}}}$$

$$= -6.935$$

BOX 6-2 STEP-BY-STEP COMPUTING: THE PAIRED *t* TEST STATISTIC

Step 1: State the null and alternative hypotheses.
  H$_0$: There will be no difference in the means of the two groups.
  H$_A$: The mean knowledge score after participating in the program will be significantly different from the mean knowledge score before participating in the program.
Step 2: Define the significance level (α-level), determine the degrees of freedom, and find the critical value for the computed t-statistic.
  The α-level is .05.
  The total degrees of freedom equal the number of pairs minus 1 ($31 - 1 = 30$).
  The critical value for the *t*-statistic, two-tailed test $= t_{\alpha/df} = t_{.05/30} = 2.042$.
Step 3: Make sure that the data meet all the necessary assumptions.
  The measures of the dependent variables for the two means are correlated.
  The dependent variable, "knowledge," is a ratio variable.
  The dependent variable has a normal distribution.
Step 4: Compute the mean, standard deviation, and variance for each group.

Program	Mean Knowledge Score	Standard Deviation	Variance
Before	69.26 points	8.61	74.06
After	78.29 points	6.21	38.55

Step 5: Compute the paired *t*-statistic.

The paired *t*-statistic formula is

$$t = \frac{\bar{X}_1 - \bar{X}_2 - 0}{\sqrt{\dfrac{\sum d_i^2 - \dfrac{\left(\sum x_i\right)^2}{n_d}}{n_d(n_d - 1)}}}$$

Computations for Σd can be found in Table 6-1.
$\Sigma d = -25 - 22 - 9 - 14 - 11 - 12 - 3 - 16 - 13 - 14 - 12 - 13 - 3 - 7 - 18 - 13 - 15 - 8 - 8 + 2 - 2 - 14 - 1 - 13 - 14 - 5 - 0 + 2 - 2 + 1 + 2 = -280.$
Computations for Σd^2 can be found in Table 6-1.
$\Sigma d^2 = 625 + 484 + 81 + 196 + 121 + 144 + 9 + 256 + 169 + 196 + 144 + 169 + 9 + 49 + 324 + 169 + 225 + 64 + 64 + 4 + 4 + 196 + 1 + 169 + 196 + 25 + 0 + 4 + 4 + 1 + 4 = 4,106.$
Plug the values for Σd and Σd^2 into the paired *t*-statistic formula to get the following:

$$t = \frac{69.26 - 78.29 - 0}{\sqrt{\dfrac{(4106) - \dfrac{(-280)^2}{31}}{31(30 - 1)}}}$$

$$= \frac{-9.03}{\sqrt{\dfrac{4106 - 2529.032}{930}}}$$

$$= -6.935$$

Paired *t*-statistic $= -6.935$

BOX 6-2 STEP-BY-STEP COMPUTING: THE PAIRED t TEST STATISTIC *(Continued)*

Step 6: Determine the statistical significance and state a conclusion.

The critical value is 2.042. Because $|-6.935| = 6.935 > 2.042$, the two means are significantly different from one another.

Because the value of the absolute value of the computed paired t-statistic is 6.935, which is greater than the critical value of 2.042, it can be concluded that the knowledge score after taking the educational program was significantly higher than the knowledge score before taking the program.

BOX 6-3 COMPUTING THE PAIRED t TEST STATISTIC USING SPSS

Step1: The data are entered into an SPSS data set.

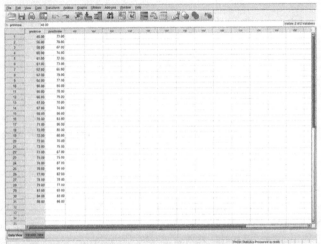

Step 2: The menu system is used to click on "Analyze" and then to select "Compare Means" and "Paired-Samples t Test."

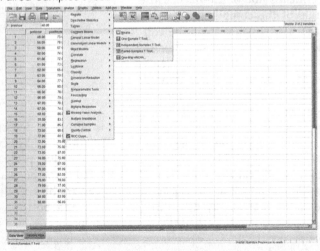

(Continued)

> **BOX 6-3** **COMPUTING THE PAIRED *t* TEST STATISTIC USING SPSS**
> *(Continued)*
>
> **Step 3:** In the "Paired-Samples *t* Test" popup box, "preknow" and "postknow" are selected and moved over to the slot labeled "Pair" under "Variable1" and "Variable2," respectively. When the button labeled "OK" is clicked, the results appear in the output window, which is shown in Table 6-3.
>
>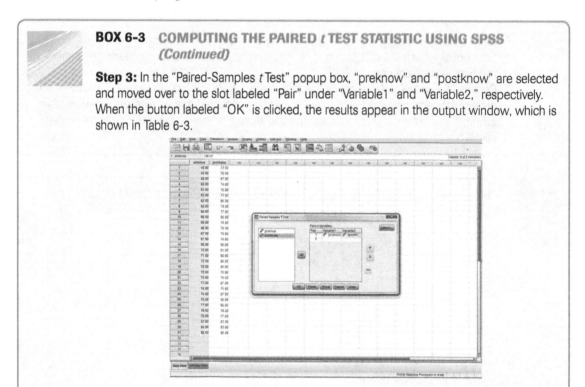

Step 6: Determine Statistical Significance and State a Conclusion

To determine statistical significance, the absolute value of the computed *t*-statistic is compared with the critical value of 2.042. Because the absolute value of the computed *t*-statistic is greater than the critical value, it can be concluded that the two means are significantly different from one another at $p \leq .05$ (two-tailed test). Because a two-tailed test is used, the computed *t* test is statistically significant if the absolute value of the computed paired *t*-statistic is larger than the critical value of the *t*-statistic determined by using the *t*-table; thus, the computed *t*-statistic of –6.935 is still considered statistically significant. In other words, if the computed statistic falls into the rejection region, the difference is statistically significant, and the paired means are significantly different from one another.

It can be concluded that the teenagers in this sample had significantly higher mean scores (an average gain of 9.02 points) on the quiz after going through the educational program. When stating these conclusions, it is important to state both the magnitude and the direction of the difference (9.02 points higher) as well as whether the difference was statistically significant.

Step-by-Step Procedure for Using SPSS to Compute the Paired *t* Test

It is fairly easy to compute a paired *t* test using SPSS. Box 6-3 illustrates the process with images from the SPSS program. First, the data must be entered into the data editor. There should be three variables: person ID number, pretest quiz score, and posttest quiz score. Note that the data for this test are set up somewhat differently than usual in that the data in each group (pretest and posttest) will have their own test score variables—so data for the pretest-only group's scores will be entered into one column in SPSS while the scores for the posttest will be entered into a separate column (usually we would have two different variables, one for test score and one for group—pretest vs. posttest). After the data are entered, the menu system is used by clicking on "Analyze" and selecting "Compare Means" and then "Paired-Samples *t* Test." While in the "Paired-Samples *t* Test" popup box, "preknow" and "postknow" are selected and moved over to the slot labeled "Pair" under "Variable1" and "Variable2," respectively. The button labeled "OK" is clicked next, and the results appear in the output window shown in Table 6-3.

After the paired *t* test has been run, the output must be examined (see Table 6-3).

The first portion of the output provides the means and standard deviations of the pretest and posttest values. The second portion of the output shows the correlation between the two means; note that they are indeed correlated ($p = .001$). The third portion of the output provides four useful pieces of information: (a) the average difference between the two values (paired differences mean = −9.032), (b) the 95% confidence interval around the difference (−11.692, −6.373), (c) the value of the computed *t*-statistic (−6.936), and (d) the actual *p*-value associated with the computed statistic ($p = .000$, or $p < .001$).

First, the output under "Paired Samples Statistics" must be examined to find the pretest and posttest means, as well as their standard deviations. Second, the output under "Paired Samples Test" must be examined to find the result of the *t* test. In this section, the average gain in points from pretest to posttest (9.032) is shown. Also, the 95% confidence interval of this estimate, which is 6.373 to 11.692 (the absolute values to make it a comparison of posttest–pretest is shown). This is the range of values one would expect to find 95% of the time if this study were repeated over and over again with different samples of 31 teenagers. It can be viewed as an estimate of where the "true" difference in points might lie.

Conceptual Understanding of the Paired *t* Test

The paired *t* test essentially asks the question: What is the probability of getting a difference of a given magnitude between two means from correlated, normally distributed samples? For example, in the study about the relationship of knowledge to program participation among teenagers, a sample of 31 teenagers from the entire population of teenagers was used. Two measures of knowledge must be taken from the same person to answer the question: Does knowledge change as a result of the intervention? Because these were multiple measures from the same person, the two variables are not independent of one another (i.e., the knowledge score at posttest of each person is likely to be related to what is known at pretest). Therefore, the independent *t* test cannot be used because the correlation between the two measures must be taken into account. This is done by obtaining the standard error of the difference score and computing a *t*-statistic that uses this standard error. (The distribution of the difference of two *t*-distributed variables will follow a student's *t*-distribution.) In this case, a 95% confidence interval around the mean difference was computed rather than around the means themselves.

COMPUTING THE WILCOXON MATCHED-PAIRS TEST

The Wilcoxon matched-pairs test is a nonparametric test used to determine whether a relationship exists between two correlated measures of the same variable in which the measurement scale of the variable is at least ordinal. It is analogous to the paired *t* test and can be used in situations in which the assumptions for the paired *t* test are not met (e.g., small sample sizes, nonnormally distributed data, and ordinal level of measurement). The Wilcoxon matched-pairs test tests the null hypothesis that the medians of the two correlated groups are equal.

| Table 6-3 | **SPSS OUTPUT FROM A PAIRED *t* TEST** |

Paired Samples Statistics

		Mean	N	Standard Deviation	Standard Error Mean
Pair 1	Preknow	69.26	31	8.606	1.546
	Postknow	78.29	31	6.209	1.115

Paired Samples Correlations

		N	Correlation	Significance
Pair 1	Preknow and Postknow	31	.562	.001

Paired Samples Test

Paired Differences

		Mean	Standard Deviation	Standard Error Mean	95% Confidence Interval of the Difference Lower	Upper	*t*	df	Significance (two-tailed)
Pair 1	Pretest–Posttest	–9.032	7.250	1.302	–11.692	–6.373	–6.936	30	.000

Putting It All Together

The educational intervention significantly increased the teenagers' knowledge about cardiovascular health. The students gained an average of 9.03 points (95% confidence interval, 6.37, 11.69) on a knowledge test after completing the program. This gain is statistically significant at $p \leq .05$ by the paired τ test (two-tailed).

Step-by-Step Procedure for Hand Computing the Wilcoxon Matched-Pairs Test

To illustrate the Wilcoxon matched-pairs test, the following research question is used: Does talk therapy combined with exercise alleviate depressive symptoms more than talk therapy alone? To answer this question, people who were newly diagnosed with mild depression were invited to participate in the study. Study participants were carefully matched on age, race, and gender. One person from each pair was assigned to the therapy-alone group, and the other was assigned to the therapy plus exercise group. Twelve weeks later, the depression levels of the two groups were compared to see which of the two groups had a lower number of depressive symptoms. Because the participants were matched, the two measures of depression (therapy vs. therapy plus exercise) were correlated, and a technique for matched data must be used.

In this study, there were 20 patients resulting in 10 pairs of participants. One person in each pair was assigned to the therapy-alone group, and the other person in each pair was assigned to the therapy plus exercise group. Sample data (with ranks) are shown in Table 6-4, and stem-and-leaf plots are shown in Table 6-5. The

BOX 6-4   STEP-BY-STEP COMPUTING: THE WILCOXON MATCHED-PAIRS TEST

Step 1: State the null and alternative hypotheses.

H_0: There will be no difference in the median depression score of the two groups.

H_A: The median depression score of the therapy and exercise group is different from that of the therapy-alone group.

Step 2: Define the significance level (α-level) and find the critical value for the computed Wilcoxon matched-pairs test.

The α-level is .05.

There are 10 pairs.

The critical value for a 10-pair sample is 8.

Step 3: Make sure that the data meet all the necessary assumptions.

The measures of the dependent variables are correlated.

The dependent variable (depression score) must be at least ordinal.

There must be at least five pairs.

Step 4: Compute the median and interquartile range for each group.

Program	Median Depression Score	Interquartile Range
Therapy only	28	(24.0, 32.5)
Therapy plus exercise	26.5	(17.25, 31.25)

Step 5: Compute the Wilcoxon matched-pairs statistic.

The Wilcoxon matched-pairs statistic is simply the smaller of two sums of ranks: the sum of the negative ranks $\Sigma R-$ and the sum of the positive ranks $\Sigma R+$.

Obtain the difference scores and rank them according to their absolute value (see Table 6-4).

Compute $\Sigma R- = 5.5 + 8.5 + 3 + 1.5 = 18.5$.

Compute $\Sigma R+ = 4 + 7 + 5.5 + 10 + 1.5 + 8.5 = 36.5$.

The smaller of these two ranks is the computed statistic; thus, $18.5 < 36.5$. The critical value is 8 and $18.5 > 8$.

Step 6: Determine the statistical significance and state a conclusion.

Because the computed statistic, 18.5, is greater than the critical value of 8, no significant difference exists. It can be concluded that no difference exists in the median depression score of the people in the therapy-alone group versus the therapy plus exercise group.

procedure for computing a Wilcoxon matched-pairs statistic is shown in Box 6-4, and the procedure for obtaining the Wilcoxon matched-pairs test using SPSS is shown in Box 6-5. The output from the Wilcoxon matched-pairs test is shown in Table 6-6.

Step 1: State the Null and Alternative Hypotheses

- H_0: There will be no difference in median depression score between participants in the therapy-alone group and participants in the therapy plus exercise group.

BOX 6-5   **COMPUTING THE WILCOXON MATCHED-PAIRS STATISTIC USING SPSS**

Step 1: Enter the data into the SPSS data set.

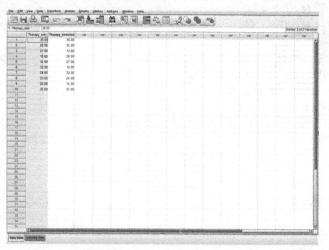

Step 2: The menu system is used to click on "Analyze," then select "nonparametric tests," and then "Related samples."

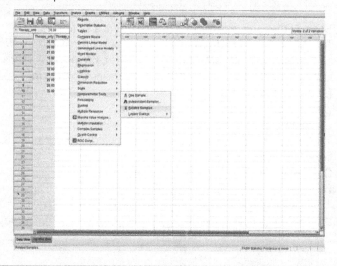

BOX 6-5   COMPUTING THE WILCOXON MATCHED-PAIRS STATISTIC USING SPSS *(Continued)*

Step 3: Then click on the "Fields" tab at the top of the popup box. Move both variables (group and groupex) into the "Test fields" box (note that the box variables must be defined as scale variables in the "Measure" box in variable view).

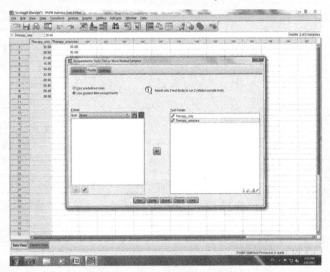

Step 4: Click on the "Settings" tab at the top of the popup box and select "Customize tests," then "Wilcoxon matched-pair signed-rank (2 samples)." Click on "Run," and the results will appear in the output window (see Table 6-6).

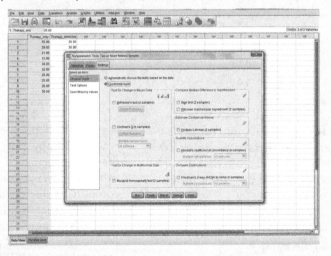

Table 6-4	POSTINTERVENTION DEPRESSION SCORES			
	Postintervention Depression Score (CES-D)		Rank of the Absolute	
Subject Number	Therapy Only	Therapy Plus Exercise	Difference Scores	Values of the Difference Scores
1	35	30	5	4.0
2	28	35	−7	5.5
3	21	12	9	7.0
4	15	26	−11	8.5
5	34	27	7	5.5
6	32	18	14	10.0
7	28	32	−4	3.0
8	25	24	1	1.5
9	26	15	11	8.5
10	30	31	−1	1.5
	Details of the Ranking Procedure			
Subject Number	Difference Scores	Rank of the Absolute Values of the Difference Scores		
10	−1	1.5		
8	1	1.5		
7	−4	3		
1	5	4		
2	−7	5.5		
5	7	5.5		
3	9	7		
4	−11	8.5		
9	11	8.5		
6	14	10		

- H_A: Median depression score for the participants in the therapy plus exercise group will be different from that of the participants in the therapy-alone group.

Step 2: Define the Significance Level (α-Level) and Find the Critical Value for the Wilcoxon Matched-Pairs Test

The significance level is defined by setting the α-level and finding the critical value for the computed Wilcoxon matched-pairs statistic. To

say that the depression level in participants who receive therapy plus exercise is different than that of participants who receive therapy only, using the Wilcoxon matched-pairs test, the computed value of the statistic must be smaller than the critical value.

In this example, an α-level of .05 is used. Because there are 10 pairs, the Wilcoxon signed rank table is used (see Appendix E) to find the critical value, which is under the column "$n = 10$." For $n = 10$ pairs, a computed signed rank score of 8 or lower is needed to have

Table 6-5	STEM-AND-LEAF PLOTS FOR DEPRESSION SCORES	
Frequency	**Stem-and-Leaf Plot**	
Therapy Only		
1.00	1.5	
2.00	2.15	
3.00	2.688	
3.00	3.024	
1.00	3.5	
Therapy Plus Exercise		
1.00	1.2	
2.00	1.58	
1.00	2.4	
2.00	2.67	
3.00	3.012	
1.00	3.5	

statistical significance at $\alpha = .05$. The Wilcoxon signed rank table gives exact *p*-values for each and every possible value of the statistic at different sample sizes (number of pairs) from 5 to 30.

Step 3: Make Sure That the Data Meet All the Necessary Assumptions

The data appear to meet all the assumptions for the Wilcoxon matched-pairs test. The measure of depression (Center for Epidemiologic Studies Depression Scale [CES-D] score) is ordinal. The measurements are paired, and the total sample size is over five pairs. Because the values are not

normally distributed (see Tables 6-4 and 6-5), the paired *t* test could not be used.

Step 4: Compute the Median and Interquartile Range for Each Group

Because two medians are compared, the values of these medians are needed. In this example, the median depression score of the participants in the therapy-only group is 28 (interquartile range, 24 to 32.5), and the median depression score of the participants in the therapy plus exercise group is 26.5 (interquartile range, 17.25 to 31.25).

Step 5: Compute the Wilcoxon Matched-Pairs Statistic

The Wilcoxon matched-pairs statistic is simply the smaller of the two sums of ranks: the sum of positive ranks and the sum of the negative ranks. The first step in computing the statistic is to compute the difference in scores between each pair (see Table 6-4). Then, the absolute value of the scores is ranked from smallest to largest using the same ranking procedure as used for the Mann-Whitney *U*-test described in Chapter 5. The two sums of ranks are computed separately. First, the ranks of all of the negative differences are added. Then, the ranks for all of the positive differences are added. The value of the computed statistic is whichever of these is smaller. In this case, the sum of the negative ranks is 18.5, and the sum of the positive ranks is 36.5. Therefore, 18.5 is taken as the value of the Wilcoxon matched-pairs test.

Table 6-6	SPSS OUTPUT FROM A WILCOXON MATCHED-PAIRS TEST			
Hypothesis Test Summary				
Null Hypothesis	**Test**	**Significance**	**Decision**	
1 The median of differences between CES-D therapy and CES-D therapy plus exercise equals 0.	Related-samples Wilcoxon signed ranks test	.358	Retain the null hypothesis	

Asymptomatic significances are displayed. The significant level is .05.

Step 6: Determine Statistical Significance and State a Conclusion

Because the test statistic of 18.5 is larger than the critical value of 10, it can be concluded that no significant difference exists in median depression scores between the therapy-only group and the matched group that received therapy plus exercise.

Step-by-Step Procedure for Using SPSS to Compute the Wilcoxon Matched-Pairs Test

After the data have been entered, the menu system is used to obtain the Wilcoxon matched-pair statistic, as shown in Box 6-5 and Table 6-6. The first step is to enter the data into the computer. The data for this test are set up somewhat differently than usual in that data in each group will have its own CES-D variable—so data for the therapy-only group's CES-D scores will be entered into one column in SPSS while the CES-D data for the therapy plus exercise group will be entered into a separate column. In this example, the two variables are (1) CES-D score for the therapy-only group and (2) the CES-D score for the therapy plus exercise group. Each matched pair's data (CES-D for therapy only and CES-D for therapy plus exercise) are entered on a separate row. In this case, the depression variable for the person in the pair who only had therapy is named "group," and the depression variable for the person in the pair who had therapy plus exercise is named "groupex." Second, the SPSS menu is used to generate the output,

as shown in Box 6-5 (see Table 6-6). The exact *p*-value for this sum of ranks is .358. Because the *p*-value is larger than .05, it can be concluded that no statistically significant difference exists in the median depression score between the two matched groups.

Conceptual Understanding of the Wilcoxon Matched-Pairs Test

The Wilcoxon matched-pairs test is based on the relative ranks of the difference scores between the matched pairs. The sums of the ranks of the negative differences and positive differences are obtained. If the size of the positive differences is similar to size of the negative differences, the sum of the ranks of the negative and positive differences should also be similar (and large enough not to be significant). If, for example, there are many more (or larger) positive differences than negative ones, the rank sum of the positive differences would be a large number, and the rank sum of the negative differences would be a much smaller and possibly significant number.

Putting It All Together

In this study, it can be concluded that no significant difference exists in median depression level between participants in therapy only and participants in therapy plus exercise.

CHAPTER REVIEW

Multiple-Choice Concept Review

1. The paired *t* test is
   a. a type of Wilcoxon matched-pairs test.
   b. a parametric test.
   c. a nonparametric test.
   d. described by both a and b.

2. The paired *t* test is used to determine whether the means of which of the following are different from one another?
   a. Two repeated measures
   b. Three repeated measures
   c. Measures from a case and a matched control
   d. Both a and c

3. The paired *t* test is best used when the measurement scale of the characteristic of interest is
   a. nominal.
   b. ordinal.
   c. interval or ratio.
   d. any of the above.

4. The Wilcoxon matched-pairs test is best used when the measurement scale of the characteristic of interest is
   a. nominal.
   b. ordinal.
   c. interval or ratio.
   d. b or c.

5. Which of the following statistical tests can be used if the data are paired but normally distributed in only one of the measures being compared?
   a. *t* test for pooled variances
   b. Paired *t* test
   c. Wilcoxon matched-pairs test
   d. Mann-Whitney *U*-test

6. Data are considered paired if
   a. two measures of the same variable are taken on the same person.
   b. measures of the same variable are taken on a case and a matched control.
   c. measures of the same variable are taken on a case group and an unmatched control group.
   d. both a and b are true.

7. Which of the following measures of central tendency are tested by the Wilcoxon matched-pairs test to determine whether two groups are significantly different?
   a. Means
   b. Medians
   c. Modes
   d. Interquartile ranges

8. The Wilcoxon matched-pairs test is most likely to be significant when
   a. the sums of the ranks of the negative and positive differences are about equal.
   b. the sum of the ranks of the negative differences is substantially greater than that of the positive differences.
   c. the sum of the ranks of the positive differences is substantially greater than that of the negative differences.
   d. both b and c are true.

9. When analyzing the mean or median differences of paired data, which of the following are considered most important?
   a. Magnitude of the difference
   b. Statistical significance of the difference
   c. Sample size
   d. Both a and b are equally important

10. The Wilcoxon matched-pairs test is best used when
   a. there are two matched groups to compare.
   b. there are three or more matched groups to compare.
   c. the data are normally distributed.
   d. the data are from an entire population rather than just a sample.

Choosing the Best Statistical Test

For each of the following scenarios (1 to 10), pick the most appropriate test (a to d) from the following choices:
   a. Independent t test
   b. Mann-Whitney U-test
   c. Paired t test
   d. Wilcoxon matched-pairs test

1. A total of 75 nursing students take a professional board preparation course, and 65 other nursing students study on their own. Which test could be used to reveal which group had the higher board scores, assuming the board scores were normally distributed?

2. Which test could be used to determine the difference in the average number of times in a month people exercise before and after a 3-hour exercise orientation program? There were 50 people in the sample, and the number of times people exercised was not normally distributed.

3. Which test would be most appropriate to answer the following research question: Do patients with a history of cocaine use have more gumline cavities than other patients? There were 15 people in the sample (7 with a history of cocaine use and 8 without), and the number of gumline cavities was not normally distributed.

4. Which test would be most appropriate to answer the following research question: Is there a difference in the number of outpatient medical visits a year between people who live in urban areas and those who live in rural areas? There were 22 people in the sample (half in each group), and the number of visits was normally distributed.

5. Which test would be most appropriate to answer the following research question: Is there a difference in the number of outpatient medical visits a year between military dependents and civilian dependents? There were 37 people in the sample, and the number of visits was left-skewed.

6. Which test would be most appropriate to answer the following research question: Is there a difference in the mean weight loss by women in two age groups

(18 to 44 years and 45 to 64 years) over a 3-month period? There were 87 women in the sample, and weight loss was normally distributed.

7. Which test would be most appropriate to answer the following research question: Are women who are treated at a public health department with a dual diagnosis of unplanned pregnancy and sexually transmitted disease (STD) younger than those who have an unplanned pregnancy but do not have an STD? There were 250 women in the study, and their ages were normally distributed.

8. Patients in a critical care unit, who are matched on age, receive either experimental oral care or control oral care. Which test would be most appropriate to answer the following research question: Does the type of oral care received by the patients have any effect on their length of stay in the critical care unit? There were 36 pairs of patients, and their length of stay was not normally distributed.

9. Which test would be most appropriate to answer the following research question: Is there any relationship between having children (having none compared with having one or more) and pay measured as an hourly wage? There were 1,021 people in the sample, and wages were left-skewed.

10. In a twin study of infant sucking behavior, one infant is shown pictures of faces, and the other is shown pictures of random geometric shapes. Which test would be most appropriate to answer the following research question: Do the infants who are shown the faces evidence more vigorous sucking behavior? There were 38 pairs of infants, and sucking frequency was normally distributed.

Critical Thinking Concept Review

1. Develop five hypotheses that could be tested with the paired *t* test or the Wilcoxon matched-pairs test.

2. Find the critical value of the Wilcoxon matched-pairs for each two-sided test of the following *p*-values and sample sizes.
   a. $p = .05$, 8 pairs _____
   b. $p = .01$, 8 pairs _____
   c. $p = .10$, 25 pairs _____
   d. $p = .05$, 9 pairs _____
   e. $p = .10$, 16 pairs _____

3. Briefly describe the difference between a study with a case and matched-control design and a study that has each person act as his or her own control.

Computational Problems

For each of the following four problems, state the most likely hypothesis and compute a paired *t* test to determine whether a statistically significant difference exists between the two groups in question. Use an α-level of .05 and a two-tailed test. For problems 1 to 3, perform the computations both by hand and by using SPSS. Note that questions 1 and 2 may not meet all the assumptions for a paired *t* test; they are included to start you off with problems that are easier to compute. Use SPSS only to compute problem 4.

Repeat the instructions for problems 1 to 4 but compute a Wilcoxon matched-pairs test instead. Perform the computations both by hand and by using SPSS for problems 1 to 3; use SPSS only to compute problem 4.

1. A hairstyle researcher wants to conduct a study to see whether blonds really do have more fun. She obtains a sample of 10 people. She has them rate how much fun they had in the past week on a 7-point Likert-item scale in which higher scores mean more fun. She then sends each of them home with a blond wig with instructions to wear the wig for an entire week. At the end of the week, the participants return to the hairstylist and again rate how much fun they had in the past week (on the same 7-point scale). Do blonds have more fun? Here are the data.

Subject Number	Brown Hair	Blond Hair
1	5	4
2	3	5
3	3	4
4	4	6
5	3	5
6	1	6
7	4	6
8	1	5
9	2	4
10	3	4

2. A food company wants to know which type of salad would be best received by its customers. It sets up an experiment in which 10 people are given two types of salads: type A and type B. Each salad is carefully weighed at exactly 15 oz. After 20 minutes, the remainder of the salad is weighed, and the amount of each type of salad remaining for each person is calculated. It is assumed that subjects would eat more of the type of salad they prefer. Which salad was preferred? Here are the data.

Subject Number	Salad A (Ounces Left)	Salad B (Ounces Left)
1	12	11
2	5	7
3	15	15
4	13	12
5	4	13
6	2	5
7	13	14
8	10	11
9	4	15
10	6	10

3. A study is conducted to see whether an educational intervention for nurse practitioner students increases their knowledge about domestic violence victims. Was the intervention successful? Here are the pretest and posttest knowledge scores for each student.

Person Number	Posttest Score	Pretest Score
1	2	3
2	4	3
3	4	4
4	5	4
5	6	5
6	5	5
7	6	5
8	6	6
9	5	6
10	6	6
11	7	6
12	8	7
13	7	7
14	3	7
15	7	8
16	8	8
17	9	9

4. A health educator wants to evaluate a smoking cessation program in terms of helping participants smoke less. A total of 35 male smokers participate in the study. The number of cigarettes they smoke daily is recorded before and after they participate in the smoking cessation program. Did the program work? Here are the data.

Participant Number	Number of Cigarettes Smoked Daily Before Participating in the Program	Number of Cigarettes Smoked Daily After Participating in the Program
1	12	10
2	11	6
3	13	8
4	13	8
5	10	6
6	20	9
7	10	7
8	17	12
9	11	6
10	14	8

(*Continued*)

Participant Number	Number of Cigarettes Smoked Daily Before Participating in the Program	Number of Cigarettes Smoked Daily After Participating in the Program
11	10	8
12	13	6
13	14	9
14	22	10
15	16	8
16	17	8
17	11	6
18	19	6
19	15	7
20	14	10
21	18	6
22	15	6
23	16	7
24	13	6
25	12	6
26	11	8
27	10	7
28	17	8
29	16	6
30	14	9
31	10	10
32	20	11
33	21	9
34	15	6
35	15	7

The One-Way ANOVA and the Kruskal-Wallis *H*-Test: Comparing the Means of Three or More Unrelated Groups

OBJECTIVES

After studying this chapter, you should be able to:

1. Determine when one-way ANOVA and the Kruskal-Wallis *H*-test are appropriate to use.
2. Choose between one-way ANOVA and the Kruskal-Wallis *H*-test.
3. Describe between-group, within-group, and total variance.
4. Hand compute a one-way ANOVA and a Kruskal-Wallis *H*-test and determine whether the results are statistically significant.
5. Use SPSS to compute a one-way ANOVA and a Kruskal-Wallis *H*-test and correctly interpret the output.
6. Explain the use of *post hoc* tests and *a priori* comparisons.
7. Report the results of one-way ANOVA in a summary table.

OVERVIEW OF THE ONE-WAY ANOVA AND THE KRUSKAL-WALLIS *H*-TEST

One-way analysis of variance (ANOVA) is used to compare the means of three or more groups, and the Kruskal-Wallis *H*-test (its nonparametric analogue) is used to compare the distribution of three or more groups. ANOVA models were developed by Sir Ronald A. Fisher (1890 to 1962), one of the grandfathers of experimental statistics, to further agricultural research. He worked as a statistician at Rothamsted Experimental Station in England, where he refined the science of experimental design (Fisher, 1925). The ANOVA models were later applied to many different types of research, including health services research.

It is fairly common for a health services or clinical research question to involve a comparison of several groups on a particular measure. In Chapter 5, we discussed the independent samples t test and the Mann-Whitney U-test as methods for examining the difference between two groups. When we have more than two groups and are interested in the differences among these groups, we are dealing with different combinations of means or distributions. If we choose to analyze the differences by independent samples t test analysis, we would need to do a number of independent samples t tests. Suppose we had four different groups—A, B, C, and D—that we wanted to compare a particular variable. If we were interested in the differences among the four groups, we would need to do an independent t test for each of the possible pairs that exist in the four groups. We would have A versus B, A versus C, A versus D, B versus C, B versus D, and C versus D. In all, we would have six separate comparisons, each requiring a separate analysis.

The problem with conducting such multiple-group comparisons relates to the underlying concept of statistical analysis. Each test is based on the probability that the null hypothesis is true. Therefore, each time we conduct a test, we are running the risk of a type I error. The probability level we set as the point at which we reject the null hypothesis is also the level of risk with which we are comfortable. If that level is .05, we are accepting the risk that 5 out of 100 times, our rejection of the null hypothesis will be in error. However, when we calculate multiple t tests on independent samples that are being measured on the same variable, the rate of error increases exponentially by the number of tests conducted. For example, with our four-group problem, the error rate increases to 18 out of 100 times, a substantial increase. The calculation of the rate of type I errors is determined by the following formula:

Probability of a type I error $= 1 - (1 - \alpha)^t$

where α is the level of significance for the tests and t is the number of test comparisons used. In our example, the calculation would give us

Probability of a type I error
$= 1 - (1 - 0.05)^4 = .18$

In order to avoid this increased probability of making a type I error, instead of using a series of individual comparisons (e.g., 6 t tests), we examine the differences among the groups through an analysis that considers the variation across all groups at once. This test is the ANOVA or its nonparametric analogue, the Kruskal-Wallis H-test (sometimes referred to as the Kruskal-Wallis ANOVA).

RESEARCH QUESTION

The research question that one-way ANOVA asks is "Are the means of the three or more independent groups significantly different from one another?" In particular, we are testing the null hypothesis that the means of the three or more groups are equivalent. "One-way" refers to the fact that the test has only one grouping variable, as compared with the "n-way" ANOVA (presented in Chapter 8), which can have multiple independent variables in the same model.

The Kruskal-Wallis H-test is a nonparametric test that is similar to a one-way ANOVA and can be used when the data do not meet the assumptions for a one-way ANOVA. It asks the question "Are the distributions of the three or more independent groups significantly different from one another?" In this case, we are testing the null hypothesis that the distribution of the three or more groups is equivalent. Typically, we report the median when using the Kruskal-Wallis ANOVA rather than reporting the mean. Note that the Kruskal-Wallis H-test is not as sensitive as a one-way ANOVA and thus less likely to detect significant differences between groups.

The following studies provide examples of how one-way ANOVA and the Kruskal-Wallis *H*-test are used in practice. The first study uses one-way ANOVA to examine the effect of school closures on respiratory disease rates in children. The second study uses the Kruskal-Wallis *H*-test to examine the effect of different educational programs on low-income women.

Should Elementary Schools Close During Flu Epidemics?

This is a question that researchers addressed when they examined the effect of school closure on the incidence of respiratory diseases among Israeli children (Heymann, Chodick, Reichman, Kokia, & Laufer, 2004). Schools were closed during the peak incidence of infectious disease to determine whether school closure could reduce the transmission of the disease. During three regularly scheduled 2-week periods of school closure affecting 186,094 children aged 6 to 12 years, data were collected on the occurrence of respiratory infections based on recorded diagnoses and symptoms, physician visits, and medication purchases.

Outcome rates of infectious diseases were compared using a one-way ANOVA. This was followed by a pairwise Tukey *post hoc* test, which compared the 14-day closure periods. During the closure periods, there were significant decreases in the rates of respiratory diseases, physician visits, and medication purchases. This study provided quantitative data to support school closure during influenza pandemics.

Which Educational Approach Is Most Likely to Increase Knowledge about HIV/AIDS Among Women Participating in the Women, Infants, and Children Program?

This question was examined in a study of 217 women who were assigned to one of three groups: a control group that received written material, a nurse-educated group, and a videotape-educated group. The grouping variable, "type of education," is nominal with three levels. The outcome variable, "knowledge score," is ratio. The study used a Kruskal-Wallis *H*-test and found that both the nurse-educated group and the videotape-educated group had significantly higher posttest knowledge scores than did the control group (Ashworth, DuRant, Gaillard, & Rountree, 1994).

TYPE OF DATA REQUIRED

With both one-way ANOVA and the Kruskal-Wallis *H*-test, the independent variable is at the nominal level. A one-way ANOVA means that there is only one independent variable (often called a factor or grouping variable). This is also true for the Kruskal-Wallis *H*-test. Gender would be an independent variable with two levels (male/female), whereas ethnicity might have varying levels, depending on how it was defined. For example, we could define ethnicity as a four-level variable (African-American, Hispanic, Caucasian, other.) The factor serves as the grouping variable, and it defines the groups whose distributions we are comparing. The dependent variable must be continuous (e.g., of an interval or ratio measurement scale); this is the variable whose mean or distribution we will compare for each of the groups. In the study of educational approaches to increase knowledge about HIV/AIDS (Ashworth et al., 1994), "type of education" is the grouping variable.

ASSUMPTIONS

ANOVA has been shown to be fairly robust. This means that even if the variables do not rigidly adhere to the assumptions required for the test, the results may still be close to the truth. The risk of error is lower if the sample size is large, the design is balanced (i.e., the groups are of roughly the same size), and the data are not badly skewed.

BOX 7-1 CHOOSING BETWEEN THE ONE-WAY ANOVA AND THE KRUSKAL-WALLIS *H*-TEST

The one-way ANOVA can be used when the following assumptions are met:
- The measures of the characteristic of interest constitute an independent random sample.
- The grouping variable has three or more categories.
- The variable measuring the characteristic of interest is normally distributed.
- The variable measuring the characteristic of interest is a continuous interval or ratio variable.
- There is homogeneity of variance among all of the groups.

The Kruskal-Wallis *H*-test can be used when the following assumptions are met:
- The measures of each value of the variable measuring the characteristic of interest constitute an independent random sample.
- The grouping variable has at least three groups.
- The measurement scale of the variable measuring the characteristic of interest is at least ordinal.

The assumptions for ANOVA are the same as those for the *t* test; that is, the characteristic of interest should be a continuous variable that is normally distributed, the groups (in this case, three or more) should be mutually exclusive and independent of each other, and the groups should have equal variances (homogeneity of variance requirement).

The Kruskal-Wallis *H*-test is a nonparametric test, meaning that it has fewer assumptions and can be used in those situations in which the one-way ANOVA cannot work because of violations of one or more assumptions. It simply assumes that there are three or more mutually exclusive, independent groups to compare on some characteristic. The characteristic can be an ordinal, integer, or ratio measurement; it need not be continuous nor does it have to be normally distributed. Box 7-1 displays the differences between the two tests.

(referred to as "*k*" groups) is present on a variable of a normally distributed interval or ratio measurement scale. The "*k*" categories or levels of the independent variable (the factor) define the different groups that are compared. Technically, unlimited levels of the factor are possible (as long as there are adequate numbers in each group), but it is unusual to see comparisons made between more than six groups at a time.

Students are often confused when we say that ANOVA tells us whether the means of groups differ significantly and then proceed to talk about analyzing variance. The *t* test was clearly a test of mean difference, because the difference between the two means was contained in the numerator of the *t* test formula. It is important to understand how analyzing the variability of groups on some measure can tell us whether their measures of central tendency (means) differ.

ONE-WAY ANOVA

The one-way ANOVA is a parametric test used to determine whether a statistically significant difference in the means of three or more groups

Using Variance to Compare Means

The one-way ANOVA is a little different from other tests of the mean in that it uses the ratio of two different types of variance to test a hypothesis about differences between the means. These two types of variance are the within-group variance and the between-group variance, which, when added together, represents the total variance within the sample (Fig. 7-1). The within-group variance is the spread of data within each group; this should be roughly equal for the groups because the one-way ANOVA assumes homogeneity of variance. The within-group variance is also referred to as the "error" or "residual" variance. The between-group variance is a measure of the distance between the means of the different groups.

In one-way ANOVA, the two variances are computed, and then an *f*-statistic is computed by obtaining a ratio of the between-group variance to the within-group variance. In general, the larger the between-group variance (relative to the within-group variance), the larger the *f*-statistic will be. The ratio of the two variances follows an *f*-distribution (see Appendix F). If the *f*-statistic is sufficiently large, it will be greater than the critical value and therefore statistically significant, and it will be possible to conclude that at least one of the group means is significantly different from the other group means.

With ANOVA, the variance of each group is measured separately; all the subjects are then lumped together, and the variance of the total group is computed. If the variance of the total group (total variation) is about the same as the average of the variances of the separate groups (within-group variation), the means of the separate groups are not different. This is because if total variation is the sum of within-group variation and between-group variation and if within-group variation and total variation are equal, there is no between-group variation. This should become clearer in the diagrams that follow. However, if the variance of the total group is much larger than the average variation within the separate groups, a significant mean difference exists between at least two of the groups. In that case, the within-group variation does not equal the total variation. The difference between them must equal the between-group variation.

To visualize the difference in the types of variation, consider three groups exposed to three

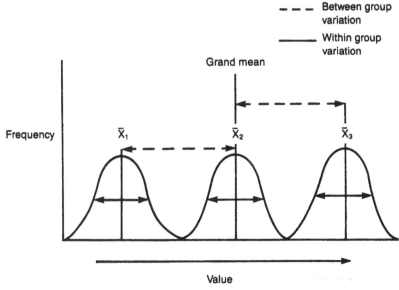

FIGURE 7-1   Between-group and within-group variation: The case of no overlap.

different experimental conditions. Suppose that the three conditions yielded such widely different scores that there was no overlap among the three groups in terms of the outcome measure (Fig. 7-1). We could then represent our three groups in terms of their relationship to each other and in terms of a total group. Each group would then have its own mean and its own distribution around its mean. At the same time, there would be a *grand mean*, which is a mean for all the groups combined. As shown in Figure 7-1, we can look at the variation within the groups and between the groups. The combination of the within-group and between-group variation equals the total variation.

The ANOVA test examines the variation and tests whether the between-group variation exceeds the within-group variation. When the between-group variance is greater (statistically greater) than the within-group variance, the means of the groups must be different. However, when the within-group variance is approximately the same as the between-group variance, the groups' means are not significantly different. This relationship between the difference among groups and the different types of variance is shown in Figure 7-2.

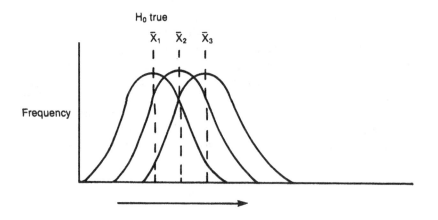

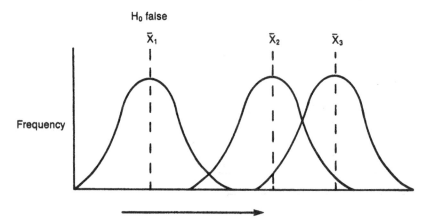

FIGURE 7-2   Relationship of variation to null hypothesis.

When the null hypothesis (H_0) is true (i.e., the means of all groups are equal), the groups overlap to a large extent, and the within-group variation exceeds the between-group variation. When the null hypothesis is false, the groups show little overlapping and the distance between groups is greater. In the lower portion of Figure 7-2, we see that group 1 overlaps very little with group 2 and not at all with group 3. Groups 2 and 3 do overlap. In that case, it may be that group 1 scored significantly lower than groups 2 and 3 and that groups 2 and 3 do not differ significantly from each other. Thus, the group variation and the deviation between group means determine the likelihood that the null hypothesis is true.

Figure 7-3 illustrates the fact that when the variation within a group or groups is great, the difference between the groups must be greater than when the distribution within groups is narrow in order to reject the null hypothesis. In the same way, when the group distributions are narrow (low within-group variance), relatively small between-group differences will be significant.

Note that one-way ANOVA can only reveal that at least one group mean is significantly different from the others; it cannot reveal which means are different. To find out which of the group means are significantly different from each other, a *post hoc* test must be performed.

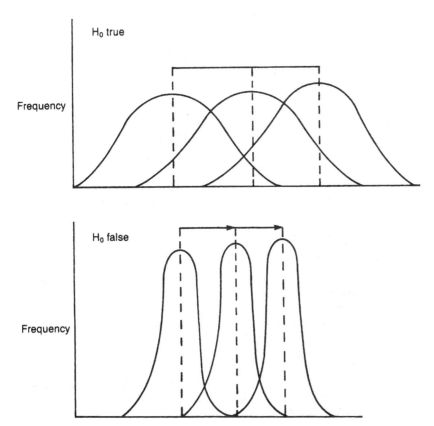

FIGURE 7-3 Effect of within-group variation on null hypothesis.

Post Hoc Tests in ANOVA

After a significant f-test for the one-way ANOVA has been obtained, the null hypothesis can be rejected, and it can be said that at least one of the group means is different from the others. However, more tests must be performed to determine which of the means are different. A series of t tests might be computed to compare all of the possible pairs of means. The problem with a series of t tests, however, is that it would lead to multiple comparisons and thus be likely to lead to a type I error.

A type of statistical test called a "*post hoc* test" decreases the likelihood of making a type I error. The *post hoc* test allows us to figure out which group(s) is different and is conducted only after a significant ANOVA test. Many *post hoc* tests are available to health sciences researchers (Fig. 7-4). The choice of a *post hoc* test depends largely on the type of data and the comparisons that are wanted, although the results are usually similar even with different types of *post hoc*

tests. An extended discussion of these tests is beyond the scope of this text; good overviews can be found in the SPSS *Base 15 User's Guide* (SPSS, 2006) in Toothaker (1993). A very useful decision flowchart from which *post hoc* tests can be chosen is presented in the text by Gaddis and Gaddis (1990).

The Bonferroni test is reported frequently. In the Bonferroni test, the desired α level is divided by the number of comparisons. For example, with an α of .05 and four comparisons, the significance level would have to be equal to or less than .05/4 = .0125 for the paired comparison to be significant. This is discussed further in the "Computing the One-Way Analysis of Variance" section.

THE ANOVA TABLE

The results of the calculations leading to the f-ratio for the ANOVA test are summarized in a table format that is standard for presenting

Bonferroni correction	The desired α level is divided by the number of comparisons.
Duncan test	This test is computed in the same way as the student Newman-Keuls, but the critical value is less stringent.
Least significant difference test	This test is equivalent to multiple t tests. The modification is that a pooled estimate of variance is used rather than variance common to groups being compared.
Scheffé test	A frequently used test. The formula is based on the usual formula for the calculation of a t test or f-ratio. The critical value used for determining whether the resulting f-statistic is significant is different.
Student Newman-Keuls	This test is similar to Tukey's honestly significant difference (HSD), but the critical values do not stay the same. They reflect the variables being compared.
Tukey's HSD	This is the most conservative comparison test and, as such, is the least powerful. The critical values for Tukey remain the same for each comparison, regardless of the total number of means to be compared.
Tukey's wholly significant difference	This test uses critical values that are the average of those used in Tukey's HSD and Student Newman-Keuls. It is therefore intermediate in conservatism between those two measures.

FIGURE 7-4 Commonly used *post hoc* tests for analysis of variance models.

ANOVA results. This presentation of the results is called the Summary of ANOVA table, or sometimes simply the ANOVA table (Table 7-1). This table displays all the elements necessary to compute the *f*-ratio between the within-group variance and the between-group variance. This computed *f*-ratio is compared with the critical value (obtained from a standard *f*-table, Appendix F) to see whether the one-way ANOVA is statistically significant.

The typical one-way ANOVA table has six columns and three rows. The first column lists the sources of variance, as described by the two rows (between-group variance and within-group variance). The next three columns contain the numbers that are needed to compute the two types of variance and obtain the *f*-ratio. These are the sums of squares, the degrees of freedom, and the mean square. The fifth column contains the actual value of the *f*-ratio, and the sixth column lists whether it is a statistically significant value. We will now go over how to compute each of these quantities using a real-life example.

Step-by-Step Procedure for Computing the One-Way ANOVA

The research question that will be used to illustrate the use of the one-way ANOVA is "Do people with private health insurance visit their physicians more frequently than people with no insurance or other types of insurance?" This question will be answered by using data from a study of 108 adult attendees of a community-based health fair. At entry to the health fair, each person was given a questionnaire that asked for information about his or her health status, use of health services, health insurance, and other information about seeking health care. The grouping variable of interest in this analysis, "type of insurance," has four categories: no insurance, Medicare, TRICARE (insurance for military dependents), and private insurance. The dependent variable, "number of physician visits in the past year," is of ratio measurement scale.

The data are shown in Table 7-2 together with computations that are used to obtain the one-way ANOVA. The distribution of the variable "number of visits to the physician" is shown in stem-and-leaf plots in Table 7-3. A summary of the computational process is shown in Box 7-2, and the procedure for computing a one-way ANOVA using SPSS (with a printout) is shown in Box 7-3. The text follows along with these tables.

Step 1: State the Null and Alternative Hypotheses

- H_0: None of the groups differ on the mean number of visits to the physician.
- H_A: At least one of the groups has a different mean number of physician visits than the other groups.

Table 7-1	**ONE-WAY ANOVA TABLE**				
Source of Variance	**Sum of Square (SS)**	**Degrees of Freedom (df)**	**Mean Square (MS)**	**f-Ratio**	**p-Value**
Between groups	SS_b	df_b	MS_b	MS_b/MS_w	Look in *f*-table
Within groups	SS_w	df_w	MS_w		
Total	SS_t				

df_b, degrees of freedom for the between-groups variance; df_w, degrees of freedom for the within-groups variance; MS_b, mean square between; MS_w, mean square within; SS_b, sum of squares between; SS_t, sums of squares total; SS_w, sum of squares within.

| Table 7-2 | NUMBER OF OUTPATIENT VISITS TO A PHYSICIAN IN THE PAST YEAR BY INSURANCE TYPE | | | | | | |

No Insurance		Private Insurance		Medicare		TRICARE	
X	X^2	X	X^2	X	X^2	X	X^2
0	0	1	1	1	1	1	1
0	0	1	1	2	4	1	1
1	1	2	4	2	4	2	4
1	1	2	4	2	4	2	4
1	1	2	4	2	4	2	4
1	1	3	9	3	9	3	9
1	1	3	9	3	9	3	9
2	4	3	9	3	9	3	9
2	4	3	9	3	9	3	9
2	4	4	16	4	16	4	16
2	4	4	16	4	16	4	16
2	4	4	16	4	16	4	16
2	4	4	16	4	16	4	16
2	4	4	16	4	16	4	16
2	4	5	25	4	16	5	25
3	9	5	25	4	16	5	25
3	9	5	25	5	25	5	25
3	9	5	25	5	25	5	25
3	9	5	25	5	25	5	25
3	9	5	25	5	25	6	36
3	9	6	36	6	36	6	36
3	9	6	36	6	36	6	36
3	9	6	36	6	36	7	49
4	16	6	36	7	49	8	64
4	16	7	49	7	49		
4	16	7	49	8	64		
4	16	8	64				
5	25	9	81				
5	25						
6	36						
$N = 30$		$N = 28$		$N = 26$		$N = 24$	
$\sum x = 77$		$\sum x = 125$		$\sum x = 109$		$\sum x = 98$	
$\sum x^2 = 259$		$\sum x^2 = 667$		$\sum x^2 = 535$		$\sum x^2 = 476$	

Table 7-3	STEM-AND-LEAF PLOT FOR THE NUMBER OF VISITS TO THE PHYSICIAN
Stem Width: 1	Each Leaf: 1 Case
Frequency	Stem-and-Leaf
2.00	0.00
10.00	1.0000000000
18.00	2.000000000000000000
20.00	3.00000000000000000000
21.00	4.000000000000000000000
17.00	5.00000000000000000
11.00	6.00000000000
5.00	7.00000
3.00	8.000
1.00	9.0

BOX 7-2 STEP-BY-STEP COMPUTING: THE ONE-WAY ANOVA

Step 1: State the null and alternative hypotheses.
- **H₀:** There is no difference in the means of the four groups.
- **Hₐ:** The mean number of doctor visits in at least one of the four is different from the mean number of visits in the other groups.

Step 2: Define the significance level (α-level), determine the degrees of freedom, and obtain the critical value for the *f*-test.
- α-level = .05.
- The degrees of freedom between groups (df_b) = $k - 1 = 4 - 1 = 3$.
- The degrees of freedom within groups (df_w) = total $n - k = 108 - 4 = 104$.
- The critical value from the *f*-table for $f_{3,104}$ at $\alpha = .05$ is 2.70. (Use the value at $f_{3,100}$, which is as close as you can get from the *f*-table.)

Step 3: Make sure that the data meet all the necessary assumptions.
- The measures constitute an independent random sample.
- The grouping variable, "type of insurance," has at least three levels.
- The dependent variable, "number of visits," is normally distributed.
- The measurement scale of the dependent variable is interval or ratio.
- There is homogeneity of variance (see computations below).

Test for homogeneity of variance
- The group with the largest variance is private insurance: $s^2 = 4.04$; df = 27.
- The group with the smallest variance is no insurance: $s^2 = 2.12$; df = 29.
- Computed *f*-test: 4.04/2.12 = 1.91.
- Critical value for $f_{27,29}$ at $\alpha = .05 = 1.901$.

(Continued)

BOX 7-2   STEP-BY-STEP COMPUTING: THE ONE-WAY ANOVA *(Continued)*

- Because the computed value is very close to the critical value, it can be concluded that the assumption of homogeneity of variance is not grossly violated. Because the one-way ANOVA is a robust technique and there is a large sample size with groups that are roughly equal in size, the one-way ANOVA can still be used.

Step 4: Compute the mean, standard deviation, and variance for each group.

Measure	No Insurance	Private Insurance	Medicare	TRICARE
Mean number of visits	2.57	4.46	4.19	4.08
Standard deviation	1.46	2.01	1.77	1.82
Variance	2.12	4.04	3.12	3.30

Computations for the means and variances:

Group	Mean	Variance	Standard Deviation
	$\bar{X} = \dfrac{\sum x_i}{n}$	$S^2 = \dfrac{\sum x_i^2 - [(\sum x)^2 / n]}{n-1}$	$s = \sqrt{s^2}$

No insurance:

$$\frac{77}{30} = 2.57 \qquad S^2 = \frac{259 - \dfrac{77^2}{30}}{30-1} = 2.12 \qquad s = \sqrt{2.12} = 1.45$$

Private insurance:

$$\frac{125}{28} = 4.46 \qquad S^2 = \frac{667 - \dfrac{125^2}{28}}{28-1} = 4.04 \qquad s = \sqrt{4.04} = 2.01$$

Medicare group:

$$\frac{109}{26} = 4.19 \qquad S^2 = \frac{535 - \dfrac{109^2}{26}}{26-1} = 3.12 \qquad s = \sqrt{3.12} = 1.77$$

TRICARE group:

$$\frac{98}{24} = 4.08 \qquad S^2 = \frac{476 - \dfrac{98^2}{24}}{24-1} = 3.30 \qquad s = \sqrt{3.30} = 1.82$$

BOX 7-2   STEP-BY-STEP COMPUTING: THE ONE-WAY ANOVA *(Continued)*

Step 5: Perform the computations necessary to complete the one-way ANOVA and perform post hoc tests if needed.
Sum of squares between (SS_b):

$$SS_b = \sum_{i=1}^{k} n_i (\overline{X}_i - \overline{X})^2$$

$$SS_b = 30(2.57 - 3.79)^2 + 28(4.46 - 3.79)^2 + 26(4.19 - 3.79)^2 + 24(4.08 - 3.79)^2$$
$$SS_b = 44.65 + 12.57 + 4.16 + 2.02 = 63.4$$

Sum of squares within (SS_w):

$$SS_w = \sum_{i=1}^{k} (n_i - 1)s_i^2$$

$$SS_w = (30 - 1)1.45^2 + (28 - 1)2.01^2 + (26 - 1)1.77^2 + (24 - 1)1.82^2$$
$$SS_w = 60.97 + 109.08 + 78.32 + 76.19 = 324.56$$

Sum of squares total (SS_t):
$SS_t = SS_b + SS_w = 63.4 + 324.56 = 387.96$
Calculate the mean squares and the *f*-ratio:
Mean square between groups (MS_b):

$$MS_b = \frac{SS_b}{df_b}$$
$$MS_b = \frac{63.4}{3}$$
$$MS_b = 21.13$$

Mean square within groups (MS_w):

$$MSw = \frac{SSw}{dfw}$$
$$MSw = \frac{324.56}{104}$$
$$MSw = 3.12$$

Compute the *f*-statistic and *post hoc* tests (*f*-ratio):

$$f = \frac{MS_b}{MS_w}$$
$$f = \frac{21.13}{3.12}$$
$$f = 6.772$$

(Continued)

BOX 7-2 STEP-BY-STEP COMPUTING: THE ONE-WAY ANOVA *(Continued)*

The critical value is 2.70. Because 6.772 is greater than 2.70, at least some of the means are significantly different from some of the other means.

ANOVA Table

Source of Variance	Sum of Squares	Degrees of Freedom	Mean Square	*f*-Ratio	*p*-Value
Between groups	63.4	3	21.13	6.772	<.05
Within groups	324.56	104	3.12		
Total	387.96				

Step 6: Determine statistical significance and state a conclusion.

The type of insurance is significantly associated with the number of outpatient visits made in a year ($p < .05$). Post hoc tests (from SPSS) revealed that people with no insurance made significantly fewer visits a year (2.57) than those with private insurance (4.46), Medicare (4.19), or TRICARE (4.08). No other differences were found between the groups. Note: Differneces in the hand-computations and the SPSS answers in this exercise are due to using rounded values of the means and standard deviations in this excercise (rounded to two decimal places).

BOX 7-3 OBTAINING ONE-WAY ANOVA USING SPSS

Step 1: The data are entered into an SPSS data set.

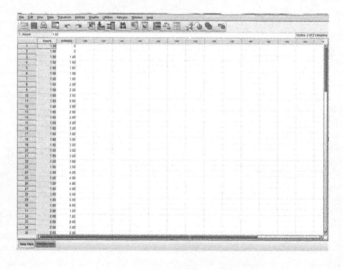

BOX 7-3   OBTAINING ONE-WAY ANOVA USING SPSS *(Continued)*

Step 2: The menu bar is used to click on "Analyze" and then to select "Compare Means" and "One-Way ANOVA."

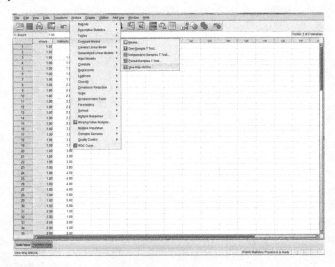

Step 3: When the "One-Way ANOVA" popup box appears, "mdvisits" is moved to the "Dependent List" and "insure" is moved to the "Factor" box.

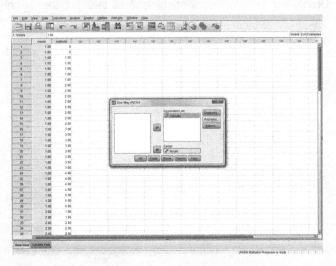

(Continued)

BOX 7-3 **OBTAINING ONE-WAY ANOVA USING SPSS** *(Continued)*

Step 4: Click on *"Post hoc."* When the "One-Way ANOVA: *Post-Hoc* Multiple Comparisons" box appears, the *post hoc* test "Bonferroni" is selected. In this case, the Bonferroni test is chosen. The "Continue" button is then clicked.

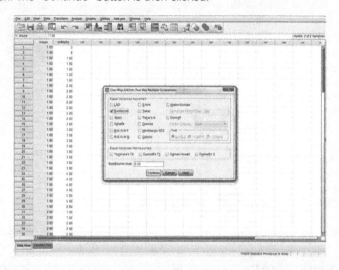

Step 5: Click on "Options." When the "One-Way ANOVA: Options" box appears, "Descriptive" and "Homogeneity of variance test" and then "Continue" are selected.

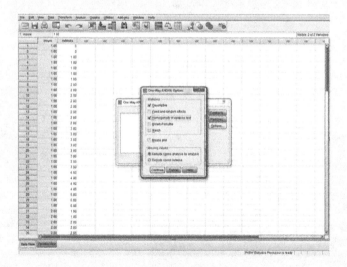

Step 6: When the "OK" button is clicked, the results appear in the output window.

Step 2: Define the Significance Level (α-Level), Determine the Degrees of Freedom, and Obtain the Critical Value for the f-Test

To be able to say that a statistically significant difference between the means exists, the computed value of the f-statistic must exceed the critical value for the α-level that is chosen. The computed value is the f-ratio that is computed from the data, and the critical value is the value of the f-ratio that is obtained from the table of critical values for the f-test (Appendix F). The critical value is the value at which the probability of obtaining that value or higher is at or below the predetermined α-level.

In this example, an α-level of .05 is used. The degrees of freedom must be determined for the between-groups variance (df_b) and for the within-groups variance (df_w). The degrees of freedom for the between-groups variance is the total number of groups (k) minus 1, and the degrees of freedom for the within-groups variance is the total number of observations (n) minus the total number of groups (k). The $df_b = (k - 1) = (4 - 1) = 3$ and the $df_w = (n - k) = (108 - 4) = 104$. The critical value for the f-ratio at the intersection of these degrees of freedom can be found in the f-table (Appendix F): df_b is the numerator and df_w is the denominator.

In the example, the degrees of freedom between groups (df_b) is 3 and the degrees of freedom within groups (df_w) is 104. We will use the coordinates of 3, 100 (since 104 is not in our table). We locate the between-groups df on the row across the top of the table, and we locate the within-groups df on the column on the left side of the table. With these points as coordinates, we locate two critical values for f. The top value (in light print for $\alpha = .05$) is 2.70. This is the value required to reject the null hypothesis at a probability level of .05. The value below (in bold print) is 3.98—the value required to reject the null hypothesis at the 0.01 level. Therefore, the computed f-statistic must exceed 2.70 in

order for us to reject the null hypothesis and to be able to say that the means are significantly different from each other at $p < .05$.

Step 3: Make Sure That the Data Meet All the Necessary Assumptions

The data, as shown in Table 7-2, meet all the necessary assumptions. The people in this study constitute an independent random sample because they were randomly selected from among attendees at a community health fair, and the individuals in the four groups are not related to each other (i.e., independent). The grouping variable, "type of insurance," has four levels: no insurance, Medicare, private insurance, and TRICARE. The total sample size is fairly large ($N = 108$), so that any minor deviations from normality and homogeneity should not substantively affect the results. The dependent variable, "number of visits to the physician," is approximately normally distributed (see the stem-and-leaf plots in Table 7-3) and is of a ratio measurement scale.

To test for homogeneity of variance between the groups, the Hartley test, also known as the F_{max} test, can be used. This F_{max} test is conducted by taking the variance of the group with the largest variance and dividing it by the variance of the group with the smallest variance. Then the computed value of the f-statistic is compared with the critical value obtained from the f-table (see Appendix F). If homogeneity of variance exists between the two groups with the most extreme values, then homogeneity will exist between all the other groups. When computing a one-way ANOVA using SPSS, Levene's test is used to test for homogeneity of variance (see Chapter 5 for details).

The data meet almost all the assumptions, and so a one-way ANOVA will be used. Although the assumption of homogeneity of variance is not quite met, this study has a large sample size, and the groups are nearly equal in size. Because a one-way ANOVA is robust under these conditions (meaning it will still give a correct answer even if the assumptions are somewhat violated), a one-way ANOVA is chosen. If one or more of these assumptions had been grossly violated, the Kruskal-Wallis *H*-test should be used instead. These decisions are made on a case-by-case basis and depend on how many assumptions are violated and how severe the violations are.

Step 4: Compute the Mean, Standard Deviation, and Variance for Each Group

The means are computed using the totals shown in Table 7-2. People with private insurance made the most visits to their physicians in the previous year (4.46; standard deviation, 2.01), followed by those with Medicare (4.19; standard deviation, 1.77) and TRICARE (4.08; standard deviation, 1.82), with the least number of visits being made by those with no insurance (2.57; standard deviation, 1.45). Although it appears that the "no insurance" group is different from the others, the one-way ANOVA must be performed, followed by post hoc tests, to confirm these impressions.

Step 5: Perform the Computations Necessary to Complete the One-Way Analysis of Variance Table

The first step in completing the one-way ANOVA table is to compute the sums of squares. Three sums of squares must be computed: the SS_t, SS_b, and SS_w. After they have been computed, they are written in the appropriate places in the ANOVA table. In this example, $SS_t = 388.1$, $SS_b = 63.89$, and $SS_w = 324.2$ (see Step 5 in Box 7-2 for computational details). The formulas for the different sums of squares are as follows:

$$SS_t = SS_b + SS_w$$

$$SS_b = \sum_{i=1}^{k} n_i (\overline{x}_i - \overline{x})^2$$

$$SS_w = \sum_{i=1}^{k} (n_i - 1) s_i^2$$

In these formulas, k represents the number of groups, n_i represents the sample size of group i, $\overline{x}_i$ represents the sample mean of group i, and $\overline{x}_i$ represents the grand mean (the mean of all observations in all the groups). The second step in completing the ANOVA table is to fill in the degrees of freedom obtained in Step 2, and then compute the mean squares and *f*-ratio and put them in the ANOVA table. The *f*-ratio is simply the ratio of the MS_b / MS_w, or 21.13/3.12. As shown in Table 7-3, this equals 6.772. The formulas are as follows:

$$MS_b = \frac{SS_b}{df_b}$$

$$MS_w = \frac{SS_w}{df_w}$$

$$f_{ratio} = \frac{MS_b}{MS_w}$$

The final step in completing the one-way ANOVA table is to compare the computed *f*-ratio (6.772) with the critical value obtained in Step 2 (2.70). If the computed *f*-ratio exceeds the critical value, as it does in this case, then at least one of the means is significantly different from the others.

Because there is a significant *f*-test, then it is known that at least one of the means is significantly different from the others. However, a post hoc test must be conducted to find out which of the means are really different. Computing a post hoc test by hand is beyond the scope of this text; however, we will discuss how to obtain post hoc tests using SPSS in the next section.

Step 6: Determine Statistical Significance and State a Conclusion

Because the one-way ANOVA is statistically significant, it can be concluded that the mean number of physician visits is significantly different for at least one type of insurance.

Step-by-Step Procedure for Using SPSS to Compute a One-Way ANOVA

It is fairly easy to compute a one-way ANOVA, using SPSS. Box 7-3 illustrates the process with images from the SPSS program. First, the data must be entered into the data spreadsheet (in data view). Two variables should be used: insurance (named: insure; coded: 1 = no insurance, 2 = private, 3 = Medicare, 4 = TRICARE or military dependent) and number of visits (named: mdvisits).

After the data have been entered, the menu system is used to obtain the one-way ANOVA by clicking on "Analyze" and then selecting "Compare Means" and then "One-Way ANOVA." When the "One-Way ANOVA" pop-up box appears, the variable "mdvisits" is moved to the "Dependent List," and the group variable "insure" is moved to the "Factor" box. Then, the button labeled "*Post-Hoc*" is clicked. In the "One-Way ANOVA: *Post-Hoc*" popup box, the test that is wanted is selected (in this case, a Bonferroni *post hoc* test). The significance level is set at .05.

The "Continue" button is clicked next, and then the "Options" button is clicked. In the "Options" pop-up box, "Descriptive" and "Homogeneity of variance test" are selected. Then the "Continue" button and the "OK" button are clicked (or click on "Paste" and then run the syntax). The results appear in the output window. The SPSS output (see Table 7-4) provides the mean and standard deviation of each group as well as the one-way ANOVA.

The first portion of the SPSS output is labeled "Descriptives." This is where the mean and standard deviation of each group can be found. This portion also contains the 95% confidence intervals for the mean of each group, as well as the minimum and maximum values. Note that the group means are identical to those computed by hand and discussed earlier.

The second portion of the output is labeled "Test of Homogeneity of Variances." Levene's statistic (discussed in Chapter 5) is nonsignificant because the *p*-value is .451 (above our α-level of .05), indicating that homogeneity of variance is present. Note that Levene's test is

Table 7-4	SPSS OUTPUT FROM A ONE-WAY ANOVA

MDVisits — Descriptives

	N	Mean	Standard Deviation	Standard Error	95% Confidence Interval for Mean Lower Bound	Upper Bound	Minimum	Maximum
1 None	30	2.57	1.455	.266	2.02	3.11	0	6
2 Private	28	4.46	2.009	.380	3.69	5.24	1	9
3 Medicare	26	4.19	1.767	.346	3.48	4.91	1	8
4 TRICARE	24	4.08	1.816	.371	3.32	4.85	1	8
Total	108	3.79	1.904	.183	3.42	4.15	0	9

Test of Homogeneity of Variances

MDVisits

Levene Statistic	df1	df2	Significance
.886	3	104	.451

(Continued)

Table 7-4	SPSS OUTPUT FROM A ONE-WAY ANOVA *(Continued)*

Analysis of Variance

MDVisits

	Sum of Squares	df	Mean Square	f	Significance
Between groups	63.899	3	21.300	6.833	.000
Within groups	324.203	104	3.117		
Total	388.102	107			

Multiple Comparisons

Dependent variable: MDvisits

Bonferroni

Multiple Comparisons

MDVisits

Bonferroni

					95% Confidence Interval	
(*I*) Insure	(*J*) Insure	Mean Difference (*I − J*)	Standard Error	Significance	Lower Bound	Upper Bound
1 None	2 Private	−1.898[a]	.464	.001	−3.15	−.65
	3 Medicare	−1.626[a]	.473	.005	−2.90	−.35
	4 TRICARE	−1.517[a]	.484	.013	−2.82	−.22
2 Private	1 None	1.898[a]	.464	.001	.65	3.15
	3 Medicare	.272	.481	1.000	−1.02	1.57
	4 TRICARE	.381	.491	1.000	−.94	1.70
3 Medicare	1 None	1.626[a]	.473	.005	.35	2.90
	2 Private	−.272	.481	1.000	−1.57	1.02
	4 TRICARE	.109	.500	1.000	−1.24	1.45
4 TRICARE	1 None	1.517[a]	.484	.013	.22	2.82
	2 Private	−.381	.491	1.000	−1.70	.94
	3 Medicare	−.109	.500	1.000	−1.45	1.24

[a]The mean difference is significant at the .05 level.

less impacted by departures from normality and therefore more precise than the test computed by hand.

The third portion of the output presents the ANOVA table. Note that SPSS shows the entire ANOVA table and that it is identical to the one computed by hand. The important thing to view is the actual *p*-value of the computed *f*-statistic. The computed *f*-statistic is 6.833 (almost identical to what was computed by hand). Because the *p*-value associated with it is .000, which is less than .05, it can be concluded that at least one of the group means is different from the others.

The fourth portion of the output presents the results of the Bonferroni *post hoc* test, which can be somewhat confusing to read. In the *post hoc* table, each row presents one group contrasted against all of the others. For example, the first row shows the comparison of the group with no insurance (none) with the other three groups. The first column shows the mean difference between each pair, the second column shows the standard error of the difference, and the third column shows the *p*-value for the post hoc test. The fourth and fifth columns show the 95% confidence interval around the mean difference scores.

From the third column, it is possible to tell which pairs of means are significantly different from each other with a *p*-value of <.05. The mean difference between those with no insurance and those with private insurance has a *p*-value of .001 and thus is statistically significant. The difference between those with no insurance and Medicare is also significant (*p* = .005) as is the difference between those with no insurance and TRICARE (*p* = .013). No other differences between means are significant.

KRUSKAL-WALLIS *H*-TEST

The Kruskal-Wallis *H*-test is a nonparametric test used to determine whether a relationship exists between two variables when one variable is nominal (or ordinal with a limited number of categories) and the other variable is ordinal, interval, or ratio (Kruskal & Wallis, 1952). In particular, the test is used to determine whether a difference exists in the distribution of values among three or more groups. The nominal variable is used to divide the sample into "*k*" groups ("*k*" being the number of possible values or categories of the nominal variable). To determine whether the distributions of these "*k*" groups are different from each other, the sums of the rankings for each of the groups are compared to see the degree to which the sums differ from what would be expected under the null hypothesis. Because the Kruskal-Wallis *H*-test is a nonparametric test, it can be used in situations in which the assumptions for the one-way ANOVA are not met (e.g., small sample sizes, nonnormally distributed data, no homogeneity of variance, or noncontinuous data).

Step-by-Step Procedure for Computing the Kruskal-Wallis *H*-Test

The study question that will be used to illustrate the computation of the Kruskal-Wallis *H*-test is "Is there a difference in how health science students in different programs evaluate a campus magazine?" This question is answered by using data from a study of 21 students who attend a local university. Seven students, each from three

Putting It All Together

After the mean number of visits to the physician for each group, the one-way ANOVA, and the *post hoc* tests have been computed, the conclusions can be stated. In this study, community health fair attendees had an average of 3.79 (standard deviation, 1.90) physician visits per year. A one-way ANOVA revealed that the type of insurance was significantly associated with the number of physician visits per year. Further analysis with a Bonferroni *post hoc* test showed that participants with no insurance made significantly fewer physician visits (2.57 a year) than did those with private insurance (4.46 visits a year), Medicare (4.19 visits a year), or TRICARE (4.08 visits a year), and no other differences were found between the groups in the number of physician visits.

Table 7-5	MAGAZINE RATINGS BY HEALTH SCIENCES STUDENTS							
Nursing			**Physical Therapy**			**Dental Hygiene**		
Person ID	Rating Score	Rank	Person ID	Rating Score	Rank	Person ID	Rating Score	Rank
11	25	16.0	21	23	14.0	30	12	2.0
12	26	17.0	22	28	19.0	31	13	3.0
13	27	18.0	23	29	20.0	32	14	4.0
14	21	12.0	24	19	9.5	33	20	11.0
15	18	8.0	25	22	13.0	34	15	5.0
16	19	9.5	26	9	1.0	35	17	7.0
17	24	15.0	27	30	21.0	36	16	6.0
Sum of ranks:	95.5	Sum of ranks	97.5	Sum of ranks	38.0			

majors (i.e., nursing, physical therapy, and dental hygiene), were randomly selected to evaluate the magazine. Each student was given a 1-year set of the magazine and asked to rate it on a scale of 1 to 30, where a higher score means higher quality. The data are shown in Table 7-5. A summary of the ranking process is shown in Table 7-6. The procedure for computing the test using SPSS is shown in Box 7-4, and the SPSS output is shown in Table 7-7.

Step 1: State the Null and Alternative Hypotheses

- H_0: There will be no difference in the rating of the magazine among students in the different majors.
- H_A: Students in at least one discipline will rate the magazine differently from students in the other majors.

Step 2: Define the Significance Level (a-Level) and Find the Critical Value for the Kruskal-Wallis H-Statistic

In this study, an α-level of .10 is used, meaning that we are willing to have a probability of .10 in making a type I error—rejecting the null hypothesis when it is actually true. When using the Kruskal-Wallis H-statistic, one of two tables is chosen to determine whether the two groups are significantly different. If each group contains at least five subjects, the chi-square table is used with a $k - 1$ degree of freedom (see Appendix G). If each group contains fewer than five subjects, the Kruskal-Wallis H-table is used to obtain an exact p-value (see Appendix G). In this case, because each group contains seven subjects, the critical value is taken from the chi-square table (Appendix G). There are $k - 1$ degrees of freedom, with k representing the number of groups. For this test, therefore, there are $3 - 1 = 2$ degrees of freedom. The critical value for the chi-square statistic at $\alpha = .10$ and 2 degrees of freedom is 4.61. Thus, the computed value of the Kruskal-Wallis H-test must exceed this value to be able to state that differences exist among the groups.

Step 3: Make Sure That the Data Meet All the Necessary Assumptions

The data appear to meet all the assumptions of the Kruskal-Wallis H-test. The data constitute an independent random sample. The level of measurement of the dependent variable,

Table 7-6	RANKING THE DATA		
Group	Actual Score	Position Number	Rank of Score
2	9	1	1
3	12	2	2
3	13	3	3
3	14	4	4
3	15	5	5
3	16	6	6
3	17	7	7
1	18	8	8
1	19	9	9.5 (9 + 10)/2
2	19	10	9.5
3	20	11	11
1	21	12	12
2	22	13	13
2	23	14	14
1	24	15	15
1	25	16	16
1	26	17	17
1	27	18	18
2	28	19	19
2	29	20	20
2	30	21	21

1.List all scores from lowest to highest. Keep track of which group each score comes from.
2.List the position numbers (from 1 to *n*; in this case, from 1 to 21). There should be as many position numbers as there are participants in the study.
3.Compute the ranks. Tied scores get the average rank of all the positions that they occupy.

"magazine rating," is ordinal, and the grouping variable, "major," has three categories.

Step 4: Compute the Median and Interquartile Range for Each Group

The actual data are shown in Table 7-5. Because three distributions are compared, the first piece of information that is necessary is a measure of central tendency and variation for each group. Since the data are not normally distributed, we will use the medians and the interquartile ranges because they are more robust measures than the mean and standard deviation. In this example, the median magazine ratings were 24 (interquartile range, 7) for the student nurses, 23 (interquartile range, 10) for the physical therapy students, and 15 (interquartile range, 4) for the dental hygiene students. Overall, the dental hygiene students seemed to rate the magazine lower than the other two groups, and so a Kruskal-Wallis *H*-statistic is computed to see whether this difference is truly statistically significant.

Step 5: Compute the Kruskal-Wallis *H*-Statistic and Perform Post Hoc Tests if Necessary

The first step in computing the Kruskal-Wallis *H*-statistic is to rank all the data points from all the groups in one table (see Table 7-6). The size of the number is used, beginning with the smallest and keeping track of which numbers are in which group. The smallest number gets a rank of 1; the second smallest, a rank of 2; and so on. Where there are two or more measures with the same value, they will be "tied for rank," in which case the average rank of all the positions with the same value is assigned to each measure. For example, if two data points are tied for fifth place, the rank of 5.5 is assigned [(5 + 6)/2]. R_i represents the sum of the ranks for the *i*th group, which are obtained by summing the ranks of the data points in each group. Table 7-5 shows the sum of the ranks. In this example, the sum of ranks is computed as follows:

For nursing students:

$$R_1 = 16 + 17 + 18 + 12 + 8 + 9.5 + 15.0 = 95.5$$

For physical therapy students:

$$R_2 = 14 + 19 + 20 + 9.5 + 13 + 1 + 21 = 97.5$$

For dental hygiene students:

$$R_3 = 2 + 3 + 4 + 11 + 5 + 7 + 6 = 38$$

BOX 7-4 **COMPUTING THE KRUSKAL-WALLIS *H*-STATISTIC USING SPSS**

Step 1: The data are entered into an SPSS data set.

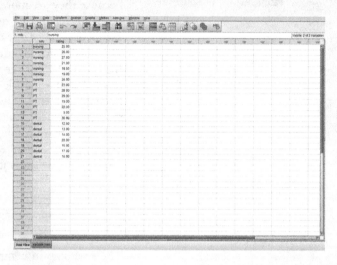

Step 2: The menu bar is used to click on "Analyze" and to select "Nonparametric Tests" and "Independent Samples."

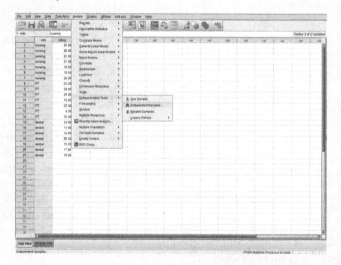

BOX 7-4 COMPUTING THE KRUSKAL-WALLIS *H*-STATISTIC USING SPSS *(Continued)*

Step 3: When the "Nonparametric tests: two of more independent samples" popup box appears, click on "Fields." Move "rating" into the "TestFields" box; the variable "edu" is then selected and moved over to the slot labeled "Groups." Note that edu must be identified as a nominal variable and rating as a scale variable in your data (in the "Data View" window, the variable edu should have "Nominal" listed and rating should have "Scale" indicated under "Measure").

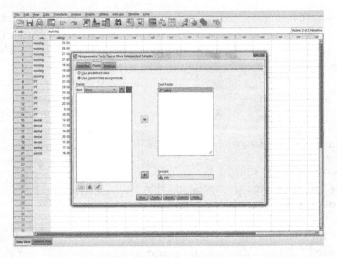

Step 4: Click on "Settings" in the popup box. Select "Customize tests," then "Kruskal-Wallis one-way ANOVA (*k* samples)." Make sure that in the box next to "Multiple comparisons," it says "All pairwise."

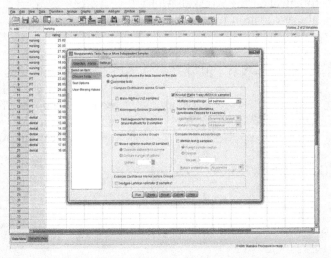

Step 5: When "Run" is clicked, the results appear in the output window (shown in Table 7-7).

Table 7-7	SPSS OUTPUT FROM THE KRUSKAL-WALLIS *H*-TEST

Hypothesis Test Summary

Null Hypothesis	Test	Significance	Decision
1 The distribution of MDVisits is the same across categories of insure.	Independent samples Kruskal-Wallis test	.014	Reject the null hypothesis.

Note. Asymptotic significances are displayed. The significant level is .05.

After the ranks have been assigned and summed for each group, the Kruskal-Wallis *H*-statistic can be computed. The basic formula for the Kruskal-Wallis *H*-statistic is

$$H = \frac{12 \sum_{i=1}^{k} R_i^2 / n_i}{n(n+1)} - 3(n+1)$$

where n is the number of participants in the study, and $\sum_{i=1}^{k} R_i^2$ is the sum of the squared sums of ranks for all groups (k represents the total number of groups). There is one complication, however. If there are any ties in ranks (i.e., if two or more ranks are identical), this statistic must be corrected for ties. Although the hand computation of this correction is beyond the scope of this book, please note that SPSS will automatically compute the correction.

In this case, to calculate the Kruskal-Wallis *H*-statistic, the above equation is used, substituting the appropriate numbers:

$$H = \left[\left(\frac{12}{N(N+1)} \right) \frac{\sum R_i^2}{n_i} \right] - 3(21+1)$$

$$H = \left[\left(\frac{12}{21(21+1)} \right) \left(\frac{95.5^2}{7} + \frac{97.5^2}{7} + \frac{38^2}{7} \right) \right]$$
$$- 3(21+1)$$

$$H = \left[\left(\frac{12}{462} \right) (1,302.89 + 1,358.04 + 206.29) \right]$$
$$- 66$$

$$H = [.02957 \times 2,867.22] - 66$$

$$H = 74.47 - 66$$

$$H = 8.473$$

Because the computed Kruskal-Wallis *H*-statistic of 8.473 is greater than the critical value of 4.605, it can be concluded that a significant difference exists at $p < .10$ between the groups in how they rate the magazine. However, as with ANOVA, a *post hoc* test is needed to determine which of the groups differ from one another.

To determine which of the groups differ from each other, *post hoc* tests need to be conducted. Glantz (1997) presents a nonparametric post hoc (the Dunn *Q*) test suitable for both equal and unequal sample sizes. The test statistic is as follows:

$$Q = \frac{\overline{R}_1 - \overline{R}_2}{\sqrt{\left(\frac{N(N+1)}{12} \right) \left(\frac{1}{n_1} + \frac{1}{n_2} \right)}}$$

where $\overline{R}_1$ is the average of the ranks in the first group being compared, $\overline{R}_2$ is the average of the ranks in the second group being compared, and n_1 and n_2 are the number in the first and second groups, respectively. The resulting statistic is compared with the critical value in the *Q*-table (see Appendix H).

The critical value for the Dunn's *Q*-test at $\alpha = .10$ and $k = 3$ is 2.394. Equation 7-12 is used to compare the ratings of the student nurses and physical therapy students by substituting the relevant numbers.

$$Q = \frac{(95.5/7) - (97.5/7)}{\sqrt{\left(\frac{21(21+1)}{12} \right) \left(\frac{1}{7} + \frac{1}{7} \right)}}$$

$$Q = \frac{-0.289}{\sqrt{38.5 \times 0.286}} = \frac{-0.289}{3.32}$$

$$Q = -0.087$$

Because –0.087 is less than 2.39, these two distributions are not significantly different from each other.

Equation 7-12 is also used to compare the ratings of the student nurses and dental hygiene students by substituting the relevant numbers.

$$Q = \frac{(95.5/7) - (38/7)}{\sqrt{\left(\frac{21(21+1)}{12}\right)\left(\frac{1}{7} + \frac{1}{7}\right)}}$$

$$Q = \frac{13.64 - 5.43}{\sqrt{38.5 \times 0.286}} = \frac{8.21}{3.32}$$

$$Q = 2.47$$

Because 2.47 is greater than 2.39, these two distributions are significantly different from each other.

Equation 7-12 is used to compare the ratings of the physical therapy and dental hygiene students by substituting the relevant numbers.

$$Q = \frac{(97.5/7) - (38/7)}{\sqrt{\left(\frac{21(21+1)}{12}\right)\left(\frac{1}{7} + \frac{1}{7}\right)}}$$

$$Q = \frac{13.92 - 5.43}{\sqrt{38.5 \times 0.286}} = \frac{8.49}{3.32}$$

$$Q = 2.56$$

Because 2.56 is greater than 2.39, these two distributions are significantly different from each other.

Step 6: Determine Statistical Significance and State a Conclusion

Significant differences were found in the distribution of ratings of the campus magazine by the three student groups as tested by the Kruskal-Wallis ANOVA at $\alpha = .10$. Further examination

with Dunn's Q *post hoc* test revealed that the dental hygiene students rated the magazine significantly worse than did the nursing or physical therapy students and that no significant difference existed in the ratings between the nursing and the physical therapy students.

Step-by-Step Procedure for Using SPSS to Compute the Kruskal-Wallis *H*-Statistic

To use SPSS to compute a Kruskal-Wallis *H*-statistic, the data must be entered into the data editor (see Box 7-4). After the data have been entered, the menu system can be used as shown to obtain the Kruskal-Wallis *H*-statistic. The SPSS output (Table 7-7) appears in the output window.

The SPSS output provides the Kruskal-Wallis *p*-value (see Table 7-7). Because the *p*-value in our example is .014 and well below the α-level of .10, it can be concluded that a significant difference exists in how the students in the three majors rated the campus magazine. SPSS will not compute the *post hoc* tests, and so, if needed, these should be done by hand.

SUMMARY

One-way ANOVA and the Kruskal-Wallis test are used to compare the distribution of two or more groups. When the overall *f* for the ANOVA test or the *H* for a Kruskal-Wallis test is significant and more than two groups are being compared, *post hoc* tests are necessary to determine which groups differ from each other. Also, with ANOVA, when directional hypotheses are appropriate, *a priori* contrasts may be specified and tested.

Putting It All Together

The conclusions are stated as follows: A significant difference exists in how the students in the three majors rated the campus magazine at $p \leq .014$ by the Kruskal-Wallis *H*-test. *Post hoc* tests indicate that dental hygiene students rated the magazine significantly lower than either nursing students or physical therapy students.

CHAPTER REVIEW

Multiple-Choice Concept Review

1. The Kruskal-Wallis test is
   a. a type of *t* test.
   b. a parametric test.
   c. a nonparametric test.
   d. a and b only.

2. The Kruskal-Wallis test is used to determine whether the distributions of which of the following are different from each other?
   a. Two independent measures
   b. Three or more independent measures
   c. Repeated measures from a case and a matched control
   d. Repeated measures from three or more groups

3. The one-way ANOVA is best used when the measurement scale of the characteristic of interest is
   a. nominal.
   b. ordinal.
   c. interval or ratio.
   d. any of the above.

4. The Kruskal-Wallis *H*-test can be used when
   a. the total sample size is unknown.
   b. the measurement scale is ordinal.
   c. the data are paired.
   d. all of the above are true.

5. The one-way ANOVA determines whether the means of the groups are different by comparing the
   a. within-group variance of the groups to each other.
   b. within-group variance to the between-group variance.
   c. ranks of the raw data.
   d. the between groups variance against the *f*-table.

6. The one-way ANOVA test tells you
   a. whether the mean of one or more groups is different from the others.
   b. which group mean is different from the others.
   c. if the groups differ in their variance.
   d. which group has the biggest variance.

7. The Kruskal-Wallis test would be better than a one-way ANOVA when
   a. the grouping variable has more than two categories.
   b. the dependent variable is not normally distributed.
   c. you want to know whether there is a difference in means between the groups.
   d. the sample size within each group is large.

8. If the ANOVA test is significant, the next step would be to
   a. conclude that the group with the biggest mean is significantly different from the other groups.
   b. conduct a *post hoc* test to determine which mean(s) are significantly different from the others.
   c. conduct a test of homogeneity of variance.
   d. conduct a nonparametric test.

9. The situation in which an independent samples *t* test would be used instead of an ANOVA is
   a. when the independent variable is normally distributed.
   b. when the groups have difference variances.
   c. when the sample size is small.
   d. when there are only two categories in the grouping variable.

10. Nonparametric tests such as the Kruskal-Wallis and the Mann-Whitney *U*-test should be used when
    a. the data do not meet the distribution requirements for a parametric test.
    b. the question is specifically about differences in the mean.
    c. there are more than three groups to compare.
    d. a *post hoc* test is required.

Choosing the Best Statistical Test

For each of the following scenarios (1 to 10), pick the most appropriate test (a to f) from the following choices:
   a. Independent *t* test
   b. Mann-Whitney *U*-test
   c. Paired *t* test
   d. Wilcoxon matched-pairs test
   e. One-way ANOVA
   f. Kruskal-Wallis *H*-test

1. Determine whether a relationship exists between race (i.e., White, Black, Asian/Pacific Islander, other) and satisfaction with the economy (on a scale of 1 to 10, where 1 = extremely unhappy and 10 = ecstatic). Satisfaction is not normally distributed, and the sample contains 47 people.

2. Determine the relationship between preschoolers' scores on a fluency assessment and having older siblings (yes/no). The sample contains 22 preschoolers, and the data (fluency) are normally distributed.

3. A weight-loss program enrolled 45 heterosexual couples. Did the husbands lose more weight than their wives? The data (weight loss) are normally distributed.

4. What is the average number of times per month people exercised before and after a 3-hour exercise orientation program? The study includes 17 participants, and the data (number of times people exercised) are not normally distributed.

5. In a study of 72 women, a researcher wants to know whether cholesterol level is related to the women's highest attained degree (no degree, high school diploma,

associate's degree, and bachelor's degree). The data (cholesterol levels) are normally distributed.

6. Do significant differences exist between husbands and wives regarding holiday depression? There is an ordinal measure of depression, which is not normally distributed. The sample contains 47 couples.

7. A group of researchers is interested in determining whether a relationship exists between geographic area (i.e., rural, suburban, and urban) and SAT math scores. The data include 2,100 scores, which are normally distributed.

8. Among entering kindergarten students, does a relationship exist between the number of letters of the alphabet recognized and the type of dwelling in which the child lived (i.e., house, apartment, and mobile home)? The sample contains 48 children, and the data (letters) are not normally distributed.

9. Do the ounces of alcohol consumed in a week by undergraduate and graduate students differ? The sample contains 130 students, and the data (ounces of alcohol) are normally distributed.

10. How much money was paid for a prescription of azithromax (Zithromax) by each type of insurance (i.e., Medicare, Medicaid, Blue Cross, and Cigna)? The sample contains 2,230 people, and the data (amount paid) are normally distributed.

Critical Thinking Concept Review

1. Develop five hypotheses that could be tested with a one-way ANOVA or Kruskal-Wallis H-test.

2. Find the critical value of the one-way ANOVA and Kruskal-Wallis H-test for each of the following α-values and degrees of freedom.

α-Value	Degrees of Freedom (Numerator)	Degrees of Freedom (Denominator)	One-Way Analysis of Variance
.01	2	30	
.05	2	30	
.01	3	25	
.05	3	25	

3. Complete the following ANOVA table.

Source of Variance	Sum of Squares (SS)	Degrees of Freedom (df)	Mean Square (MS)	f-ratio	p-Value
Between groups		2			
Within groups	12.3	62			
Total	109.7				

Computational Problems

For each of the following four exercises, state the most likely hypothesis and compute the one-way ANOVA to determine whether a statistically significant difference exists between the groups in question. Use an α-level of .05. Do a Bonferroni *post hoc* test to determine which of the means are significantly different from each other. For problems 1 to 4, perform the computations both by hand and by using SPSS. Note that exercises 1 and 2 may not meet all the assumptions to use the one-way ANOVA, but they are included to start you off with problems that are easy to compute. For problem 5, use SPSS only.

Repeat the above for problems 1 to 5 using the Kruskal-Wallis *H*-test instead. Perform the computations in problems 1 to 4 by hand and using SPSS. Use SPSS only for problem 5.

1. An elementary school teacher wants to compare the differences in the reading speed among three groups in her class. The reading speed (words per minute) of the three groups is shown in the following table.

Group I	Group II	Group III
25	17	9
16	21	11
18	13	12
10	14	8
9		

2. A city official wants to know whether any difference exists in the number of traffic accidents in three cities. The number of traffic accidents in a typical day in the three cities is shown in the following table.

City A	City B	City C
20	18	9
12	14	13
11	7	15
16	6	4
19	10	3
10	8	2
17	5	8

3. A health sciences researcher wants to study the self-esteem of domestic violence victims. She wants to know whether self-esteem is associated with education level. The education level and self-esteem scores (higher indicates higher self-esteem) of the victims are shown in the following table.

Less than High School Diploma	High School Diploma	Some College	Bachelor's Degree and Above
17	22	24	26
15	23	25	27
14	24	26	28
16	25	24	29
17	26	28	30
26	27	29	31
15	28	27	32
18	20	26	33
19	18	25	34
21	20	23	35

4. A researcher wants to compare the salaries of the assistant professors at five universities. The salaries of the assistant professors (US dollars per month) at each university are shown in the following table.

University A	University B	University C	University D	University E
1,689	5,206	2,970	3,745	6,091
1,630	4,455	2,611	3,511	5,999
1,620	4,380	2,754	3,068	5,891
1,757	4,235	2,810	3,524	6,015
2,776	5,015	2,913	3,754	5,789
1,721	5,225	2,596	3,333	5,842
1,866	4,631	2,688	3,901	5,546
1,764	4,776	2,013	3,102	5,329
1,835		2,001		
1,952				

5. A researcher wants to compare the total blood cholesterol levels in patients from four different census tracts in a major city. The cholesterol levels are shown in the following table.

Area A	Area B		Area C		Area D	
96	120	224	138	222	101	191
126	122	230	139	224	104	192
166	128	242	140	230	104	193
168	131	250	140	231	107	194
173	132	251	141	232	108	195
178	147		159	233	122	200
190	148		166	237	125	206
194	149		172	243	136	207
195	151		176	245	139	207
198	160		180	263	149	209
212	160		182	274	160	210
212	162		185	294	162	212
213	164		188	307	162	215
215	165		188	327	168	221
216	174		192		171	224
227	184		194		173	227
	185		194		174	229
	188		200		175	231
	192		202		180	239
	194		203		182	241
	197		206		182	248
	198		210		184	262
	201		215		184	317
	221		220		190	

Differences Among Group Means: N-Way ANOVA and MANOVA

OBJECTIVES

After studying this chapter, you should be able to:

1. Determine when N-way ANOVA is appropriate to use.

2. Discuss the advantages of testing for interactions.

3. Compute a two-way ANOVA using SPSS and correctly interpret the results.

4. Explain the appropriate use of multivariate analysis of variance (MANOVA).

5. Correctly interpret the SPSS output of a one-factor MANOVA with two dependent variables.

OVERVIEW OF N-WAY ANALYSIS OF VARIANCE AND MANOVA

We introduced analysis of variance (ANOVA) models in Chapter 7 with a one-way ANOVA; that is, an ANOVA model with one independent variable (referred to as a factor) and one dependent variable. This chapter discusses the use of ANOVA with more than one independent variable (N-way ANOVA). N-way ANOVA is used to test for the differences in the mean value of a dependent variable among different groups defined by two or more independent variables (factors). In the literature, this is commonly referred to as a "between-subjects factorial ANOVA." We then extend the discussion to an analysis that includes more than one dependent variable. Such an analysis, usually called multivariate analysis of variance (MANOVA), allows the researcher to look for relationships among multiple dependent and independent variables simultaneously.

There are great advantages in having more than one independent and/or more than one dependent variable in an ANOVA. One advantage is economy: Many hypotheses can be tested without an increased risk of type I errors due to multiple comparisons. The other key advantage is the ability to test for interactions, also called effect modifications. Although it is interesting and valuable to learn whether one approach works better than another, it may be even more important to find out whether the effect of one independent variable on a dependent variable is modified by the presence of other variables. In other words, is the association between the independent and dependent variable different depending on the value of some third variable, the effect modifier? Testing for an interaction allows us to determine whether the results of a treatment vary depending on the groups or conditions in which it is applied.

RESEARCH QUESTION FOR N-WAY ANOVA

Remember that all ANOVA models answer basically the same question, namely, "Is there a difference in the means of different groups?" The important thing to understand about N-way ANOVA models is that the factors are used to define the groups whose means we are comparing. We begin by discussing examples of a two-way ANOVA (two factors/one independent variable) from the literature and then expand the discussion with an example of a three-way ANOVA (three factors/one independent variable). Note that N-way ANOVA, just like one-way ANOVA, can only tell us whether differences between the means exist. *Post hoc* tests (covered in Chapter 7) are necessary to determine which means differ from one another.

In general, two-way ANOVAs help us to address these questions:

1. Does the mean of the dependent variable differ for the different levels (or categories) of Factor A (in other words, is there a main effect from Factor A)?

2. Does the mean of the dependent variable differ for the different levels (or categories) of Factor B (in other words, is there a main effect from Factor B)?

3. Is there an interaction effect from the intersection of Factors A and B on the mean of the dependent variable? In other words, does the difference in the mean of the dependent variable across levels of Factor A vary depending on the level of Factor B (or does the difference in the mean across levels of Factor B differ depending on the level of Factor A)?

Obviously, these questions can be extended to three or more factors.

Does Heavy Alcohol Consumption Increase the Risk of Heart Disease for People with Diabetes than for Those Without Diabetes? An Example of a Two-Way ANOVA

This study examines the risk factors for heart disease in people with diabetes and those without diabetes (Sakuta, Suzuki, Katayama, Yasuda & Ito 2005); in particular, it asks whether heavy alcohol consumption would have a different effect on the cardiac health of people with diabetes compared with those without diabetes. It employs a marker for heart disease called "plasma total homocysteine" (abbreviated tHcy); higher levels of tHcy indicate greater risk. In this study, the two independent factors are diabetic status (Type 2 diabetic or not) and alcohol consumption (high vs. low) and the dependent variable is tHcy level, which is assumed to be continuous and normally distributed. In essence, this study asks three questions:

1. Do people with Type 2 diabetes have different mean tHcy levels than people without diabetes?

2. Does mean tHcy level differ by level of alcohol consumption (high vs. low)?

Table 8-1	**GROUPS DEFINED BY TWO INDEPENDENT FACTORS**			
	Factor 2: Drinking Status			
Factor 1: Diabetes Status	Abstainer	Moderate Drinker	Heavy Drinker	Row Total
Diabetes status				
Does not have diabetes	112	302	398	*812*
Has Type 2 diabetes	28	41	71	*140*
Column total	*140*	*343*	*469*	*TOTAL N = 952*

Note: The numbers are the number of people in each group. There are a total of 952 participants in this study. Note that each study participant is in one and only one group. *Source*: Data from Sakuta H, Suzuki T, Katayama Y, Yasuda H, Ito T. (2005). Heavy Alcohol Intake, Homocysteine and Type 2 Diabetes. Diabetic Medicine. 22:1359–1363.

3. Is there an interaction effect of diabetes and alcohol consumption on tHcy levels? In other words, does the difference in mean tHcy level between those with high versus low alcohol consumption vary depending on Type 2 diabetes status?

Table 8-1 shows how the two factors define different groups that we want to compare.

This is an example of a 2 × 3 design, often called a 2 × 3 factorial design. The first factor is diabetes status and it has two levels (Type 2 diabetic patient vs. not Type 2 diabetic patient). The second factor is drinking status, with three levels (an abstainer group, a moderate drinker group, and a heavy drinker group). The intersection of the two factors defines six groups (2 levels × 3 levels) and each subject can be in one and only one of these groups.

If the study authors analyzed each independent variable separately, they would not derive the information that is provided by studying the interaction effect in the two-way ANOVA.

In fact, these authors found that there was no significant difference in mean tHcy levels for diabetic patients ($p = .929$, so no main effect for diabetes status), but there was a main effect of heavy drinking on mean tHcy levels ($p = .010$). More importantly, however, they found that there was a significant interaction effect ($p = .009$). Those who were both diabetic and heavy drinkers had a significantly higher mean level of tHcy than the heavy drinkers who were not diabetic.

Is Drivers' Reaction Time for Braking Affected by Cell Phone Usage, Time of Day, and Distance Between Cars? An Example of a Three-Way ANOVA

Al-Darrab, Khan & Ishrat (2009) examine how cell phone use and other driving conditions might affect a driver's reaction time. The study has three factors (independent variables). Factor A is the distance between cars and it has three levels (10, 15, and 20 m). Factor B is the cell-phone call duration and has three levels (30, 60, and 90 seconds). Factor C is time of day while driving and has two levels (day and night). This study asks the following set of questions:

1. Does the distance between cars affect the mean reaction time for braking (e.g., is there a main effect of Factor A)?
2. Does cell-phone call duration affect the mean reaction time for braking (e.g., is there a main effect of Factor B)?
3. Does time of day affect the mean reaction time for braking (e.g., is there a main effect of Factor C)?
4. Is there an interaction effect of distance between cars and cell-phone call duration on the mean braking time (e.g., is there an interaction effect of Factors A and B)?
5. Is there an interaction effect of distance between cars and time of day on the mean reaction time for braking (e.g., is

there an interaction effect of Factors A and C)?

6. Is there an interaction effect of cell-phone call duration and time of day on the mean reaction time for braking (e.g., is there an interaction effect of Factors B and C)?

7. Is there an interaction effect of distance between cars, cell-phone call duration, and time of day on the mean reaction time for braking (e.g., is there a three-way interaction between Factors A, B, and C)?

The results of this study are presented in Table 8-2. This is an ANOVA table similar to the ones presented in Chapter 7. However, instead of a single factor, the sums of squares from all three factors and the interaction terms are shown. Note that there is no effect of Factor A (distance to the next car) but that there is a significant effect of cell-phone call duration and time of day on the mean reaction to braking time. In addition, all interaction effects are significant. Overall, this study found that mean reaction time is significantly slower with longer cell-phone calls, that it is significantly slower at night, and that all three factors interact to affect reaction time as well.

TYPE OF DATA REQUIRED

N-way ANOVA is simply an extension of the one-way ANOVA. The independent variables are nominal (categorical), and the dependent variable is of ordinal or ratio measurement scale.

ASSUMPTIONS

The assumptions for an N-way ANOVA are similar to those for the one-way ANOVA. The independent variables must be made up of mutually exclusive groups. The dependent variable must be normally distributed and must demonstrate homogeneity of variance across the groups defined by the levels of each factor and by the interaction of the factors. However, ANOVA has been shown to be fairly robust. This means that even if the variables do not rigidly adhere to the assumptions required for the test, the results may still be close to the truth. The risk of error is lower if the sample size is

Table 8-2	RESULTS OF THREE-WAY ANOVA					
Source	Sum of Squares	df	Mean Square	F Value	p-Value	
Model	1.802	17	.106	22.12	<.0001	Significant
A	.018	2	.009	1.92	.1612	
B	.640	2	.320	66.73	<.0001	
C	.394	1	.394	82.12	<.0001	
A × B	.137	4	.034	7.12	.0002	
A × C	.063	2	.031	6.52	.0038	
B × C	.380	2	.190	39.59	<.0001	
A × B × C	.172	4	.043	8.98	<.0001	
Pure Error	.173	36	.005			
Cor Total	1.975	53				

Source: Reproduced with permission from Al-Darrab, I. A., Khan, Z. A., & Ishrat, S. I. (2009). An experimental study on the effect of mobile phone conversation on drivers' reaction time in braking response. *Journal of Safety Research, 40* (3), 185–189.

large, the design is balanced (i.e., the groups are of roughly the same size), and the data are not badly skewed.

COMPUTING THE N-WAY ANOVA

The ANOVA Table

The results of the calculations for the N-way ANOVA test are best summarized in a table format. This presentation of the results is similar to that for one-way ANOVA; the format for a two-way ANOVA is displayed in Table 8-3. This can simply be expanded for three-way and higher order ANOVAs.

This table displays all the elements necessary to compute the f-ratio between the within-group variance and the between-group variance for each of the factors and for the interaction term. The sums of squares for Factor A, Factor B, and the interaction (AB) are all computed. The sums of squares treatment (SSTr) are simply the sums of squares of Factor A, Factor B, and the interaction (AB) combined. This can be regarded as a measure of all the variance in

the data due to the two factors. The remaining variance, sums of squares error, is the residual and can be obtained from SST–SSTr. Once the sums of squares are obtained and the degrees of freedom determined, the mean square and the f-ratios for each factor and the interaction can be computed. SPSS determines the exact p-values for each of these tests from the computed f-ratios. The obtained p-values are then compared to the investigator-defined α-level to determine the statistical significance.

Step-by-Step Procedure for Computing the N-Way ANOVA with SPSS

We build upon the example that we used in Chapter 7, in which we asked the research question "Does type of health insurance have a significant effect on the number of physician visits?" We add a variable, "gender," to the analysis and then ask the following questions:

1. Does the mean number of physician visits differ for the different levels of type of insurance?

Table 8-3	TWO-WAY ANOVA TABLE				
Source of Variation	Sum of Squares (SS)	Degrees of freedom (df$_x$)	Mean Square (MS)	f (Variance Ratio)	p-Value
Factor A	SSA	df$_a$ = a – 1	SSA/df$_a$	MSA/MSE	p-value
Factor B	SSB	df$_b$ = b – 1	SB/df$_b$	MSB/MSE	p-value
Interaction (AB)	SSAB	df$_{ab}$ = (a – 1) (b – 1)	SSAB/df$_{ab}$	MSAB/MSE	p-value
Treatments	SSTr	df$_{tr}$ = ab – 1	(this is just the total effect of the factors)		
Residual (error)	SSE	df$_e$ = ab(n – 1)	SSE/df$_e$	(this is the total variation from all nonmeasured sources)	
TOTAL	SST	df$_t$ = abn – 1	(this is the total variation)		

2. Does the mean number of physician visits differ for the different levels of gender?
3. Is there an interaction effect from the intersection of type of insurance and gender on the mean of the dependent variable? In other words, does the difference in mean number of physician visits by type of insurance vary depending on the person's gender?

The factors that are of interest in this analysis are "type of insurance," with four categories (no insurance, Medicare, TRICARE, and private insurance), and gender, with two categories (male or female). The dependent variable, "number of physician visits in the past year," is of ratio measurement scale.

The data are shown in Table 8-4, and a summary of the computational process is shown in Box 8-1. The text follows along with these tables.

Step 1: State the Hypotheses

- H_0: Mean number of physician visits does not differ by type of insurance.

Table 8-4	GENDER, HEALTH INSURANCE, SATISFACTION WITH PROVIDER, AND NUMBER OF ANNUAL VISTS							
Gender	Insurance	#MD Visits	Satcare	Gender	Insurance	#MD Visits	Sat
Data for those with no Insurance				Data for those with Medicare			
0	1	0	87	0	3	1	91
0	1	0	92	0	3	2	70
0	1	1	83	0	3	2	82
0	1	1	84	1	3	2	86
0	1	1	93	0	3	2	91
0	1	1	94	0	3	3	82
0	1	1	94	0	3	3	83
0	1	2	78	0	3	3	87
1	1	2	82	0	3	3	89
1	1	2	84	1	3	4	74
0	1	2	85	0	3	4	74
0	1	2	85	1	3	4	76
0	1	2	85	1	3	4	79
0	1	2	86	1	3	4	81
0	1	2	91	0	3	4	81
1	1	3	77	0	3	4	85
0	1	3	77	1	3	5	68
0	1	3	78	1	3	5	69
1	1	3	80	1	3	5	75
1	1	3	82	1	3	5	77
1	1	3	86	0	3	5	81

(Continued)

Table 8-4	GENDER, HEALTH INSURANCE, SATISFACTION WITH PROVIDER, AND NUMBER OF ANNUAL VISTS *(Continued)*						
Gender	Insurance	#MD Visits	Satcare	Gender	Insurance	#MD Visits	Sat
Data for those with no Insurance				Data for those with Medicare			
1	1	3	87	1	3	6	80
1	1	3	89	1	3	6	72
1	1	4	76	1	3	6	82
1	1	4	77	1	3	7	62
1	1	4	78	0	3	7	63
1	1	4	79	1	3	8	87
1	1	5	84				
1	1	6	79				
Data for Those with Private Insurance				Data for Those with TriCare			
0	2	1	88	0	4	1	87
0	2	1	90	0	4	1	90
0	2	2	83	0	4	1	1
0	2	2	86	0	4	2	75
1	2	2	87	0	4	2	85
0	2	3	81	0	4	3	80
1	2	3	81	1	4	3	83
0	2	3	82	0	4	3	84
0	2	3	90	0	4	3	85
0	2	4	72	0	4	4	72
0	2	4	78	0	4	4	76
0	2	4	80	1	4	4	78
0	2	4	81	0	4	4	82
0	2	4	90	1	4	4	89
1	2	5	67	0	4	5	62
1	2	5	68	1	4	5	64
1	2	5	70	1	4	5	66
1	2	5	71	1	4	5	75
0	2	5	73	1	4	5	79
1	2	5	75	1	4	6	69
0	2	6	90	0	4	6	78
1	2	6	65	1	4	6	81
1	2	6	73	1	4	7	75

(Continued)

Table 8-4	GENDER, HEALTH INSURANCE, SATISFACTION WITH PROVIDER, AND NUMBER OF ANNUAL VISTS *(Continued)*						
Gender	Insurance	#MD Visits	Satcare	Gender	Insurance	#MD Visits	Sat
Data for those with no Insurance				Data for those with Medicare			
1	2	6	75	1	4	8	94
1	2	7	95				
1	2	7	65				
1	2	8	92				
1	2	9	95				

- H_a: At least one of the four insurance groups has a different mean number of physician visits than the other groups.
- H_0: Mean number of physician visits does not differ by gender.
- H_b: The mean number of physician visits is different for males and females.
- H_0: There is no interaction effect of gender and insurance type on the mean number of physician visits.
- H_c: There is an interaction effect of gender and insurance type on physician visits. In other words, the difference in the mean number of physician visits by insurance category is different depending on gender.

Step 2: Define the Significance Level (α-Level)

To be able to say that a statistically significant difference between the means exists, the *p*-value of the computed *f*-statistic (obtained from SPSS) must be less than the α-level that is chosen. Note that each factor (and the interaction) is tested separately.

In this example, an α-level of .05 is used.

Note: For Steps 3 to 5, You Will Need to Obtain and Use the Output From SPSS

It is fairly easy to compute a two-way ANOVA using SPSS. Box 8-1 illustrates the process with images from the SPSS program. After the data have been entered, the menu system is used to obtain the two-way ANOVA by clicking on "Analyze" and then selecting "General Linear Models." Choose "Univariate," and follow the instructions given in Box 8-1 to obtain the output.

Step 3: Make Sure That the Data Meet All the Necessary Assumptions

The data, as shown in Table 8-4, meet all the necessary assumptions. The people in this study constitute an independent random sample because they were randomly selected from among those attending the community health fair. The total sample size is fairly large ($N = 108$) so that any minor deviations from normality and homogeneity should not substantively affect the results. As discussed in Chapter 7, the dependent variable is approximately normally distributed (see the stem-and-leaf plots in Table 7-3) and is of a ratio measurement scale.

To test for homogeneity of variance between the groups, the Levene's test is used. This appears in the SPSS output (Table 8-5) and is labeled "Levene's Test of Equality of Variances." As the Levene's test is nonsignificant ($p = .735$), we conclude that there is homogeneity of variance (i.e., we fail to reject

(Text continues on page 195)

BOX 8-1   **OBTAINING A TWO-WAY ANOVA USING SPSS**

Step 1: The data are entered into an SPSS data set, and the menu bar is used to click on "Analyze" and then to select "General Linear Models" and "Univariate."

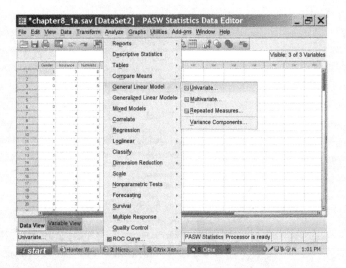

Step 2: When the "Univariate" popup box appears, "mdvisits" is moved to the "Dependent List" and "insure" and "gender' are moved to the "Fixed Factor" box.

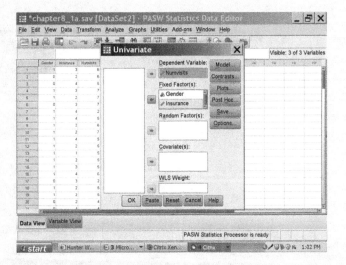

(Continued)

BOX 8-1 OBTAINING A TWO-WAY ANOVA USING SPSS *(Continued)*

Step 3: Click on "Options." In the "Display" section, select "Descriptive Statistics" and Homogeneity tests. Click "Continue."

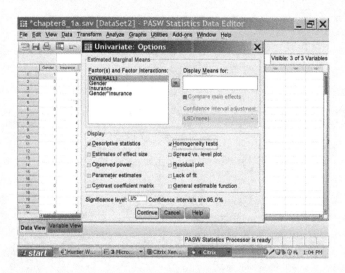

Step 4: Click on "*Post hoc.*" Move both "insure" into the "*Post hoc* Tests For" window and select the *post hoc* test "Bonferroni." Note that "Gender" does not need a *post hoc* test as it has only two categories. Now click the "Continue" button.

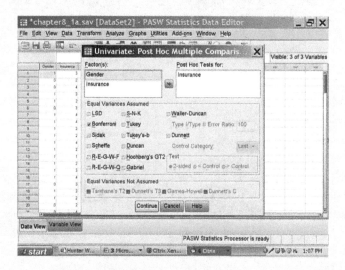

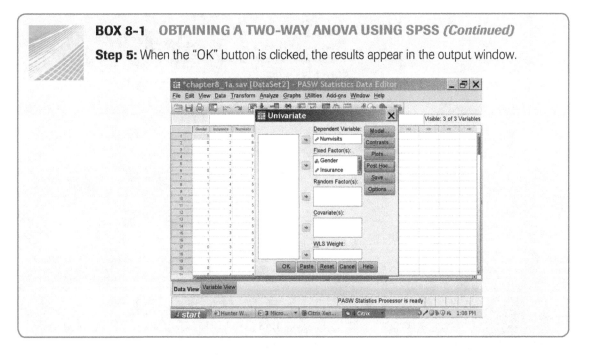

BOX 8-1 OBTAINING A TWO-WAY ANOVA USING SPSS (Continued)

Step 5: When the "OK" button is clicked, the results appear in the output window.

the null hypothesis that there is no difference in variance by group).

Step 4: Obtain the Mean and Standard Deviation for Each Group

The first portion of the SPSS output is labeled "Descriptive Statistics." This is where the mean and standard deviation of each group and subgroup can be found. These should be put into a table for the convenience of your reader (see Table 8-5).

As shown, people with private insurance made the most visits to their physicians in the previous year (mean, 4.46; standard deviation, 2.01), followed by those with Medicare (mean, 4.19; standard deviation, 1.77) and TRICARE (mean, 4.08; standard deviation, 1.82), with the least number of visits being made by those with no insurance (mean, 2.57; standard deviation, 1.46). Regarding gender, men made an average of 2.78

visits (standard deviation, 1.54), and women made an average of 4.80 visits (standard deviation, 1.70). Although it appears that the "no insurance" group is different from the others and that women made more visits than men, the two-way ANOVA must be performed, followed by *post hoc* tests, to confirm these impressions.

Step 5: Complete the Two-Way ANOVA Table

The two-way ANOVA table labeled "Tests of Between-Subjects Effects" can be found in the printout.

Step 6: Determine Statistical Significance and State a Conclusion

Remember, our α-level is .05. Since both gender and insurance type have p-values of much less than this ($p < .001$ for each), it is clear that they both have a significant effect on the number of

(*Text continues on page 198*)

Table 8-5	OUTPUT FROM SPSS UNIVARIATE PROCEDURE (TWO-WAY ANOVA)

Between-Subjects Factors

		N
Gender	0	54
	1	54
Insurance	1	30
	2	28
	3	26
	4	24

Univariate Analysis of Variance
Descriptive Statistics
Dependent Variable: Numvisits

Gender	Insurance	Mean	Standard Deviation	N
0	1	1.53	.915	15
	2	3.29	1.437	14
	3	3.31	1.548	13
	4	3.17	1.528	12
	Total	2.78	1.538	54
1	1	3.60	1.121	15
	2	5.64	1.823	14
	3	5.08	1.553	13
	4	5.00	1.651	12
	Total	4.80	1.698	54
Total	1	2.57	1.455	30
	2	4.46	2.009	28
	3	4.19	1.767	26
	4	4.08	1.816	24
	Total	3.79	1.904	108

Levene's Test of Equality of Error Variances[a]
Dependent Variable: Numvisits

F	df1	df2	Sig.
.624	7	100	.735

Tests the null hypothesis that the error variance of the dependent variable is equal across groups.
[a] Design: Intercept + Gender + Insurance + Gender × Insurance.

(Continued)

| Table 8-5 | **OUTPUT FROM SPSS UNIVARIATE PROCEDURE (2-WAY ANOVA)** *(Continued)* |

Tests of Between-Subjects Effects
Dependent Variable: Numvisits

Source	Type III Sum of Squares	df	Mean Square	F	Significance
Corrected Model	175.338[a]	7	25.048	11.773	.000
Intercept	1,570.575	1	1,570.575	738.178	.000
Gender	107.964	1	107.964	50.744	.000
Insurance	63.899	3	21.300	10.011	.000
Gender × Insurance	1.430	3	.477	.224	.880
Error	212.764	100	2.128		
Total	1,937.000	108			
Corrected Total	388.102	107			

[a]$R^2 = .452$ (adjusted $R^2 = .413$).

Post Hoc Tests Insurance
Multiple Comparisons
Numvisits
Bonferroni

(I) Insurance	(J) Insurance	Mean Difference (I − J)	Standard Error	Significance	95% Confidence Interval	
					Lower Bound	Upper Bound
1	2	−1.90[a]	.383	.000	−2.93	−.87
	3	−1.63[a]	.391	.000	−2.68	−.57
	4	−1.52[a]	.399	.002	−2.59	−.44
2	1	1.90[a]	.383	.000	.87	2.93
	3	.27	.397	1.000	−.80	1.34
	4	.38	.406	1.000	−.71	1.47
3	1	1.63[a]	.391	.000	.57	2.68
	2	−.27	.397	1.000	−1.34	.80
	4	.11	.413	1.000	−1.00	1.22
4	1	1.52[a]	.399	.002	.44	2.59
	2	−.38	.406	1.000	−1.47	.71
	3	−.11	.413	1.000	−1.22	1.00

Note. Based on observed means.
The error term is Mean Square (Error) = 2.128.
[a]The mean difference is significant at the .05 level.

Putting It All Together

In this study, community health fair attendees had an average of 3.79 (standard deviation, 1.90) physician visits per year. An N-way ANOVA revealed that type of insurance and gender were both significantly associated with the number of physician visits per year. Further analysis with a Bonferroni *post hoc* test showed that participants with no insurance made significantly fewer physician visits (mean, 2.57 a year) than did those with other types of insurance and that women made more visits than men (mean, 4.80 compared with 2.78). No significant interaction between insurance type and gender was found.

physician visits. It is also clear that there is no interaction effect ($p = .880$). An examination of the *post hoc* tests (look under multiple comparisons) shows us that it is the uninsured group that is significantly different from the other three groups. Because gender has only two categories, we do not need *post hoc* tests for it.

MULTIVARIATE ANALYSIS OF VARIANCE

A multivariate analysis of variance (MANOVA) allows the researcher to look for relationships among multiple dependent and independent variables simultaneously. It is used when there are at least two dependent variables that are of interval/ratio measurement scale and one or more factors (independent variables). It is an extension of ANOVA and tests whether the mean difference among groups with a combination of the dependent variables is statistically significant. Technically, this combination of the dependent variables is referred to as the "joint distribution." Figure 8-1 provides a visual representation of what the joint distribution of two variables looks like.

RESEARCH QUESTIONS

The research question that MANOVA asks is "Is the joint distribution of two or more dependent variables significantly related to one or more factors?" In general, MANOVA is used for one of three reasons: to avoid the problem of multiple comparisons, to answer

intrinsically multivariate questions, or (less commonly) as an alternative to repeated-measures ANOVA (covered in Chapter 9). The first reason, which is to avoid the problem of multiple comparisons, is the most common. For example, if we have several related dependent variables, such as resting heart rate, blood pressure, and respiration rate, we could analyze the effects of our independent variable on them using a series of ANOVAs. However, we would increase the chance of falsely rejecting the null hypothesis (type I error) because of the many tests that we would be performing. By performing a single MANOVA instead, this problem is minimized.

A second reason to use MANOVA is to address questions that are intrinsically multivariate. For example, we may want to know

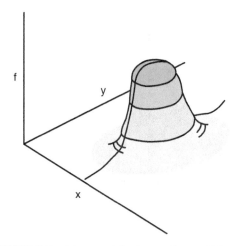

FIGURE 8-1 Joint normal distribution of two variables.

how our study participants differ on several measures as a whole. One example is the testing of multiple measures of responses that should be consistent. A third reason to use MANOVA is as an alternative to repeated-measures ANOVA (O'Brien & Kaiser, 1985), although this is not commonly done.

In general, MANOVA is more powerful than separate ANOVAs, and the interpretation of the results may be improved by considering the outcome measures simultaneously. If the outcome measures are not correlated, however, there is no advantage to conducting a MANOVA.

The following studies provide examples of how MANOVA is used in practice. The first study sought to explore the factors associated with job satisfaction and intention to leave among hospice nurses. The second study examined the effect of coconut fragrance on cardiovascular responses to stress and used MANOVA in lieu of repeated-measures ANOVA.

What Factors Are Associated with Job Satisfaction and Intention to Leave Among Hospice Nurses?

This is a question that researchers addressed in a study of 777 hospice nurses working for a for-profit corporation (Miller, 2008). The two dependent variables of interest were "job satisfaction," as measured by the Minnesota Satisfaction Questionnaire, and "intention to leave," as measured by the Anticipated Turnover Scale. The independent variables were hospice nurse age, level of education, ethnicity, tenure in nursing, and tenure in current job; note that these were all categorical variables (e.g., age was coded to lower than 30, 30 to 39, 40 to 49, 50 to 59, 60). Using MANOVA, the authors concluded that none of the hospice nurse characteristics were significantly related to job satisfaction or intention to leave.

Does Coconut Fragrance Alter the Cardiac Response to Stress?

This question was examined in a study comparing the cardiac responses while under stress of 17 subjects who had inhaled coconut fragrance as compared with those of 15 subjects who had inhaled air (Mezzacappa et al., 2010). A "stress" condition was created by having the subjects conduct mental arithmetic. One dependent variable of interest was heart rate. The heart rate was measured at baseline, during the task, and after the task was over. The independent factor was air (coconut scent vs. regular air). MANOVA was used to see whether there was a significant difference in heart rate at baseline, during the task, and after the task was over between the two groups. The results indicated that the heart-rate response was significantly greater in subjects breathing nonfragrant air as compared with those breathing coconut-scented air.

TYPE OF DATA REQUIRED

In order to conduct a MANOVA, we need at least two dependent variables that are moderately correlated (an r of at least .30) and at least one independent factor. The dependent variables should be of interval/ratio measurement scale. The independent variables should be of nominal measurement scale.

ASSUMPTIONS

For ANOVA, the assumptions include random sample, normal distribution, and equal variances across the groups on the dependent variable. MANOVA also requires that these assumptions, as well as some additional assumptions, be met. Some of these additional assumptions are as follows:

- **No outliers:** MANOVA is sensitive to outliers.
- **Linearity of dependent variable:** Moderately correlated dependent variables are preferred; if the dependent

variables are independent of each other, then we have to sacrifice the degrees of freedom, and it will decrease the power of the analysis.

- **Multivariate normality:** The dependent variables should have a multivariate normal distribution with the same variance covariance matrix in each group (SPSS, 1999a). This is tested using Box's M test.
- **Homogeneity of the variance–covariance matrix:** This is tested using the Box's M test. As this test is very sensitive to deviations from Normality, the significance for this test is typically defined as $\alpha <$ .001. Box's M tests with p-values that are greater than .001 are considered nonsignificant (in other words, the data meet this assumption if the Box's M test is nonsignificant) (Winer, 1971).
- **Homogeneity of variance among the independent groups for each dependent variable:** This is tested with the Levene's test.

COMPUTING A MANOVA

To demonstrate a MANOVA analysis, we will use all the data given in Table 8-4. Earlier in this chapter, we demonstrated how to compute an N-way ANOVA with the number of physician visits as the dependent variable. Now we are going to provide an example of a MANOVA by adding satisfaction with medical care as a second independent variable. The variable "Sat" is "satisfaction with the health care provider" and is measured by a scale that ranges from 0 to 100. "0" indicates no satisfaction with the health care provider at all, and "100" indicates perfect satisfaction. As shown in Table 8-6, these two dependent variables are significantly and moderately correlated at Pearson $r = -.375$ ($p \leq .000$). The three research questions that this analysis will address are as follows:

Table 8-6	**SPSS PRINTOUT: CORRELATION OF NUMBER OF VISITS TO PHYSICIAN WITH SATISFACTION WITH HEALTH CARE**	

Correlations

		Numvisits	Satcare
Numvisits	Pearson correlation	1	-.375[a]
	Sig. (two-tailed)		.000
	N	108	108
Satcare	Pearson correlation	-.375[a]	1
	Sig. (two-tailed)	.000	
	N	108	108

[a]Correlation is significant at the .01 level (two-tailed).

1. Do men and women differ significantly from each other in their satisfaction with their health care provider and the number of visits they made to a doctor in the past year?
2. Do the four insurance groups differ significantly from each other in their satisfaction with their health care provider and the number of visits they made to a doctor in the past year?
3. Is there an interaction between gender and insurance status in relation to satisfaction with their health care provider and the number of visits they made to a doctor in the past year?

Box 8-2 contains the step-by-step directions for obtaining a MANOVA by using SPSS.

Table 8-7 contains the output (to save space, we have eliminated some of the tables that we will not use, in the printout). Comments have been added to increase clarity. In the next section, we will take you through the six-step process to test a set of hypotheses with MANOVA, referring to Box 8-2 and Table 8-7 as we do so.

(*Text continues on page 205*)

BOX 8-2   OBTAINING A MANOVA USING SPSS

Step 1: The data are entered into an SPSS data set, and the menu bar is used to click on "Analyze" and then to select "General Linear Models" and "Multivariate."

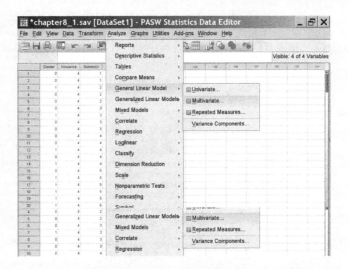

Step 2: When the "Multivariate" popup box appears, "Numvisits and "Satcare" are moved to the "Dependent List" and "Gender" and "Insurance" are moved to the "Fixed Factor" box.

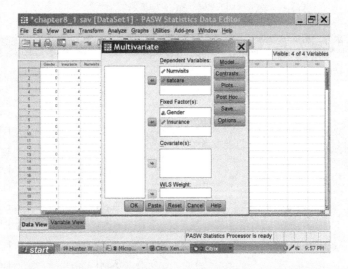

(Continued)

BOX 8-2 **OBTAINING A MANOVA USING SPSS** *(Continued)*

Step 4: Click on "Options." In the "Display" section, select "Descriptive Statistics" and Homogeneity tests. Click "Continue."

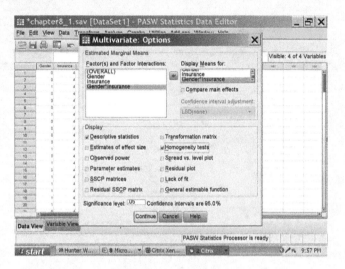

Step 5: Click Continue.
Step 6: When the "OK" button is clicked, the results appear in the output window.

Table 8-7	SPSS MANOVA OUTPUT

Descriptive Statistics

	Gender	Insurance	Mean	Standard Deviation	N
Numvisits	0	1	1.53	.915	15
		2	3.29	1.437	14
		3	3.31	1.548	13
		4	3.17	1.528	12
		Total	2.78	1.538	54
	1	1	3.60	1.121	15
		2	5.64	1.823	14
		3	5.08	1.553	13
		4	5.00	1.651	12
		Total	4.80	1.698	54

Author's Note: This section (Descriptive Statistics) is where we obtain the means of the different groups that we are comparing.

(Continued)

Table 8-7	**SPSS MANOVA OUTPUT** *(Continued)*

Descriptive Statistics

	Gender	Insurance	Mean	Standard Deviation	N
	Total	1	2.57	1.455	30
		2	4.46	2.009	28
		3	4.19	1.767	26
		4	4.08	1.816	24
		Total	3.79	1.904	108
Satcare	0	1	86.13	5.755	15
		2	83.14	6.163	14
		3	81.46	8.232	13
		4	79.67	7.691	12
		Total	82.80	7.178	54
	1	1	80.53	5.249	15
		2	77.07	10.979	14
		3	76.92	6.849	13
		4	76.33	9.736	12
		Total	77.83	8.371	54
	Total	1	83.33	6.116	30
		2	80.11	9.267	28
		3	79.19	7.772	26
		4	78.00	8.748	24
		Total	80.31	8.151	108

Author's Note: **Box's M test is used to test** *the equality of covariance between the groups. The null hypothesis is that observed covariance matrices of the dependent variable are equal across groups. The α-level used is typically $\alpha < .001$. Because the reported p-value here is .003 (which is larger than .001), we conclude that the covariance matrices are not significantly different from one another.*

Box's Test of Equality of Covariance Matrices[a]

Box's M	45.877
F	2.040
df1	21
df2	3,3264.264
Sig.	.003

[a]*Author's Note: This section (Multivariate Tests) is where we assess the statistical significance of the factors and the interaction term. The α-level we have chosen is $\alpha \leq .05$. The multivariate tests are presented first. Remember that rather than one statistic (F in ANOVA), we get four multivariate tests. Although they are all similar, it is best to report Pillai's trace, as this is the most robust and conservative measure of the four. The results show that gender and insurance type are both related to the joint distribution of the dependent variables but that there is no interaction effect.*

(Continued)

Multivariate Tests[a]

Effect		Value	F	Hypothesis df	Error df	Sig.
Intercept	Pillai's Trace	.993	6,816.432[b]	2.000	99.000	.000
	Wilks' Lambda	.007	6,816.432[b]	2.000	99.000	.000
	Hotelling's Trace	137.706	6,816.432[b]	2.000	99.000	.000
	Roy's Largest Root	137.706	6,816.432[b]	2.000	99.000	.000
Gender	Pillai's Trace	.354	27.129[b]	2.000	99.000	.000
	Wilks' Lambda	.646	27.129[b]	2.000	99.000	.000
	Hotelling's Trace	.548	27.129[b]	2.000	99.000	.000
	Roy's Largest Root	.548	27.129[b]	2.000	99.000	.000
Insurance	Pillai's Trace	.261	4.998	6.000	200.000	.000
	Wilks' Lambda	.744	5.266[b]	6.000	198.000	.000
	Hotelling's Trace	.339	5.529	6.000	196.000	.000
	Roy's Largest Root	.319	10.649[c]	3.000	100.000	.000
Gender × Insurance	Pillai's Trace	.010	.168	6.000	200.000	.985
	Wilks' Lambda	.990	.167[b]	6.000	198.000	.985
	Hotelling's Trace	.010	.166	6.000	196.000	.986
	Roy's Largest Root	.009	.301[c]	3.000	100.000	.825

[a]Design: Intercept + Gender + Insurance + Gender × Insurance.
[b]Exact statistic.
[c]The statistic is an upper bound on F that yields a lower bound on the significance level.
Author's Note: This section (Levene's Test) tests the assumption of homogeneity of variance for each of the independent groups separately for each dependent variable. The nonsignificant values of the Levene's test show equal variance between groups and give us confidence in the individual ANOVA models.

Levene's Test of Equality of Error Variances[a]

	F	df1	df2	Sig.
Numvisits	.624	7	100	.735
Satcare	2.117	7	100	.048

Note. Tests the null hypothesis that the error variance of the dependent variable is equal across groups.
[a] Design: Intercept + Gender + Insurance + Gender × Insurance.
Author's Note: Since the multivariate results are significant, we now examine the relevant univariate results. The univariate results tell us whether the significant multivariate results apply to one or both dependent variables. In this case, we would examine the univariate results for the two factors: gender and type of insurance. We do not pay attention to the printout for the univariate effects for the interaction, because the multivariate results were not significant. These results tell us that gender has an effect on both the number of MD visits and satisfaction with health care while insurance type has an effect only on the number of visits (the p-value for satisfaction with health care is .07 and is not statistically significant).

(Continued)

Tests of Between-Subjects Effects *(Continued)*

Source	Dependent Variable	Type III Sum of Squares	df	Mean Square	F	Sig.
Corrected Model	Numvisits	175.338[a]	7	25.048	11.773	.000
	Satcare	1,129.700[b]	7	161.386	2.699	.013
Intercept	Numvisits	1,570.575	1	1,570.575	738.178	.000
	Satcare	68,9155.784	1	68,9155.784	11,525.121	.000
Gender	Numvisits	107.964	1	107.964	50.744	.000
	Satcare	640.080	1	640.080	10.704	.001
Insurance	Numvisits	63.899	3	21.300	10.011	.000
	Satcare	435.913	3	145.304	2.430	.070
Gender × Insurance	Numvisits	1.430	3	.477	.224	.880
	Satcare	28.750	3	9.583	.160	.923
Error	Numvisits	212.764	100	2.128		
	Satcare	5,979.597	100	59.796		
Total	Numvisits	1,937.000	108			
	Satcare	703,760.000	108			
Corrected Total	Numvisits	388.102	107			
	Satcare	7,109.296	107			

[a]$R^2 = .452$ (adjusted $R^2 = .413$).
[b]$R^2 = .159$ (adjusted $R^2 = .100$).

Step 1: State the Null and Alternative Hypotheses

- H_0: There is no association between gender and number of visits to a physician or gender and satisfaction with health care provider.
- H_A: Gender is associated with the number of visits to a physician and/or satisfaction with the health care provider.
- H_0: There is no association between insurance type and the number of visits to a physician or between gender and satisfaction with the health care provider.
- H_A: Insurance group is associated with the number of visits to a physician and/

or gender and satisfaction with the health care provider.

- H_0: There is no interaction between gender and insurance type in predicting the number of visits to a physician and/or satisfaction with the health care provider.
- H_A: There is interaction between gender and insurance type in predicting the number of visits to a physician and/or satisfaction with the health care provider.

Step 2: Define the Significance Level (α-Level)

In this example, an α-level of .05 is used.

Step 3: Make Sure That the Data Meet All the Necessary Assumptions

The data, as we discussed earlier, meet all the necessary assumptions for N-way ANOVA (if you run a histogram on the variable "Sat," you will see that it is roughly normally distributed). To test the assumptions related to MANOVA, we need to look at the printout in Tables 8-6 and 8-7. Table 8-6 shows that our dependent variables are moderately correlated with one another (Pearson $r = -.375$). Table 8-7 is where the MANOVA results can be found. Examine the Box's M test and the Levene's test. The Box's M test ($p = .003$) is not significant at $\alpha < .001$ (note that it is common to use $\alpha = .001$ instead of $\alpha = .05$ for this test), and so we note that the assumption of the equality of the covariance matrices has been met. Although the Levene's test is significant for one of the dependent variables (SATCARE), it is close to .05 (.048), and so we will run the MANOVA anyway.

Step 4: Compute the Mean, Standard Deviation, and Variance for Each Group

The means and standard deviations of the dependent variables for each of the subgroups and overall can be found at the start of the printout, in the box labeled "Descriptive Statistics." Look at these numbers, and see whether you can spot any patterns. It appears that people with no insurance have fewer doctor visits than do others and that women have more visits than men. It also appears that those with Medicare or TriCare are less satisfied with their care and that women are less satisfied than men with their care. However, until we examine the MANOVA results, we will not know whether any of these relationships are statistically significant.

Step 5: Examine the Printout to Assess the Significance of the MANOVA

The section labeled "Multivariate Tests" is where we start to assess the statistical significance of the factors and the interaction term. Remember, the α-level we have chosen is $\alpha = .05$. The multivariate tests are presented first. Note that rather than getting one statistic (F in ANOVA), we get four multivariate tests: Pillai's trace, Wilks' lambda, Hotelling's trace, and Roy's largest root.

1. Wilks' lambda represents the product of the unexplained variances—that is, the error variance. Thus, a small value indicates significance.
2. Pillai's trace (or Pillai-Bartlett trace) is the sum of the explained variances; therefore, a large value indicates significance.
3. Roy's greatest characteristic root is based on the first discriminant variate.
4. Hotelling-Lawley trace is the sum of the ratio of the between and within sums of squares for each of the discriminant variates.

Any of these statistics can be used to test the overall multivariate hypothesis. Although they are all similar, it is best to report Pillai's trace, as this is the most robust and conservative measure of the four. However, Wilks' lambda is historically the most widely used.

If the overall MANOVA is significant, we will want to determine where the differences lie: Do the groups differ on all the dependent variables or only one? Generally, the investigator will conduct univariate analyses after a multivariate significant result; that is, he or she will conduct an ANOVA for each dependent variable. The danger of type I error is "protected" by the overall significant MANOVA.

The univariate results are labeled "Between-Subjects Effects." There are two dependent variables: "Numvisits" and "Satcare." The univariate results tell us that gender is significantly associated with both the number of visits and satisfaction with care ($p = .000$ and $p = .001$, respectively) and that insurance status is only significantly associated with the number of visits ($p = .000$). There are no interaction effects ($p = .880$ for number of physician visits, and $p = .923$ for satisfaction with care). Note that we can also request *post hoc* tests on the individual univariate tests.

Step 6: State a Conclusion

It can be concluded that gender is significantly associated with both the number of physician visits and satisfaction with care and that insurance status is only significantly associated with the number of physician visits. There are no interaction effects.

SUMMARY

ANOVA is a powerful, robust test that allows us to test for relationships between categorical independent variables and a continuous (measured at the interval or ratio level) dependent variable. Testing for interactions between the independent variables is particularly useful when we want to determine whether the effects of some intervention will be the same for all types of people or conditions. ANOVA may be extended to the use of more than one dependent variable in a given analysis. This analysis, usually called MANOVA, allows the researcher to look for relationships among dependent and many independent variables.

CHAPTER REVIEW

Multiple-Choice Concept Review

1. All ANOVA models determine whether there is a difference in the _____ of different groups.
   a. medians
   b. means
   c. ranges
   d. interquartile ranges

2. N-way ANOVA models require that independent variables generally are
   a. ordinal.
   b. ratio.
   c. interval.
   d. nominal.

3. The main difference between N-way ANOVA and MANOVA is
   a. that ANOVA models have only one independent variable.
   b. that ANOVA models have only one dependent variable.
   c. that MANOVA models can have more than one independent variable.
   d. b and c.

4. All of the following are outcome measures for MANOVA *except*
   a. Wilks' lambda,
   b. F,
   c. Roy's greatest characteristic root,
   d. Pillai-Bartlett trace,

5. Conducting a MANOVA is advantageous to an ANOVA if the outcome measures are
   a. correlated.
   b. not correlated.
   c. categorical.
   d. normally distributed.

6. All the following are assumptions for the N-way ANOVA *except*
   a. homogeneity of variance.
   b. heterogeneity of variance.
   c. Independent variables must be made up of mutually exclusive groups.
   d. Dependent variable must be normally distributed.

7. Statistical significance of an ANOVA test is obtained by comparing
   a. the p-value to the α-level.
   b. the p-value to the f-ratio.
   c. the f-ratio to the α-level.
   d. the p-value to the degrees of freedom

8. All the following are elements needed to compute the f-ratio for each of the factors and for the interaction term in an N-way ANOVA *except*
   a. sums of squares for each factor.
   b. sums of squares error.
   c. p-value.
   d. degrees of freedom.

9. Consider a two-way ANOVA. Factor A has three categories and Factor B has four categories. How many groups are defined by these two factors?
   a. 2
   b. 4
   c. 7
   d. 12

10. Consider a three-way ANOVA. Factor A has three categories, Factor B has four categories, and Factor C has two categories. How many interaction effects are there in all?
    a. 4
    b. 9
    c. 14
    d. 24

Choosing the Best Statistical Test

For each of the following scenarios (1 to 10), choose the most appropriate test (a to h).

a. Independent t test
b. Mann-Whitney U test
c. Paired t test
d. Wilcoxon matched-pairs test

e. One-way ANOVA

f. Kruskal-Wallis *H*-test

g. N-way ANOVA

h. MANOVA

1. A smoking cessation program enrolled 48 father–son pairs. Did the fathers smoke fewer cigarettes than their sons in the month after the program (number of cigarettes smoked is normally distributed)?

2. Among 15 attendees of a 2-hour weight-loss program, were the number of calories consumed the day before and the day after the program different (calories are not normally distributed)?

3. How are alcohol consumption (heavy, moderate, and none) and gender (male and female) related to body mass index (BMI) ($n = 420$, BMI is normally distributed)?

4. A researcher wants to compare two groups of people receiving federal assistance (Medicare vs. Medicaid) on number of physician visits (normally distributed, $n = 215$).

5. Do the number of hours spent online in a week by undergraduate, graduate, and postdoctoral students differ? The sample contains 170 students, and the data (number of hours spent online) are not normally distributed.

6. A group of researchers is interested in determining whether a relationship exists between the nine US census regions (e.g., Northeast and Midwest), type of school graduated from (public vs. private college) and MCAT scores ($n = 4,012$ scores, which are normally distributed).

7. Does a relationship exist between race (White, Black, Asian/Pacific Islander, other) and satisfaction with the health care system (on a scale of 1 to 10, where 1 = very unhappy and 10 = ecstatic)? Satisfaction is not normally distributed ($n = 44$).

8. What is the relationship between preschoolers' scores on an IQ assessment and their having been breast-fed (yes/no)? The sample contains 24 preschoolers, and the data (IQ) are not normally distributed.

9. How are residence (urban, suburban, or rural) and gender (male and female) related to the number of physician visits in a year ($n = 90$, number of visits is normally distributed)?

10. Are depression and anxiety levels (both measured on normally distributed ordinal scales) related to urban residence (urban vs. other), education level (less than high school, high school only, and college graduate), and gender ($n = 750$)?

Critical Thinking Concept Review

1. Develop three hypotheses that could be tested with an N-way ANOVA.

2. Develop three hypotheses that could be tested with a MANOVA.

3. Complete the following N-way ANOVA table, and interpret the table. The dependent variable is "worry about the future" and is normally distributed. Factor A is smoking history (never smoked, quit smoking, or still smokes), and Factor B is "experiences depressive symptoms" (never vs. ever). The Levene's test is not significant.

Two-Way Analysis of Variance Table

Source of Variation	Sum of Squares (SS)	Degrees of Freedom (df$_x$)	Mean Square (MS)	F (Variance Ratio)	Significant at $\alpha = .05$ (compare F to the Tcrit)?
Factor A	11.6	2			
Factor B	98.9	1			
Interaction (AB)					
Treatments					
Residual (error)	1,746.8	688			
TOTAL	1,948.7				

Computational Problems

Computational Problems for Chapter 8: Use SPSS to answer the following questions:

1. Low birth weight is a significant public health problem in the United States. Research shows that there are many maternal demographic factors that are associated with low birth weight in their infants. Data are presented below on the demographic characteristics at 60 months of age and the weight of the infant at birth. Specifically, we have data on race/ethnicity, which has three categories (1 = Black/African-American, 2 = White/Caucasian, and 3 = Hispanic); maternal age, which has three categories (1 = less than 18, 2 = 18 to 34, and 3 = greater than 34 years); and maternal smoking status, which has two categories (1 = ever smoked vs. 0 = never smoked). Use the appropriate ANOVA techniques to answer the following questions:
a. Is maternal race/ethnicity associated with low birth weight in their infants?
b. Is maternal age (categorized) associated with low birth weight in their infants?
c. Is maternal smoking status associated with low birth weight in their infants?
d. Do any of these variables interact with respect to the outcome?

ID	Race/Ethnicity	Maternal Age	Smoking	Birth Weight in grams
1	1	1	0	1,646
2	1	1	1	1,986
3	1	1	1	1,986
4	1	1	0	2,838
5	1	1	0	2,979

ID	Race/Ethnicity	Maternal Age	Smoking	Birth Weight in grams
6	1	1	0	1,873
7	1	1	0	2,951
8	1	1	1	2,440
9	2	1	0	2,412
10	2	1	0	3,405
11	2	1	0	3,008
12	2	1	0	3,320
13	2	1	1	3,433
14	2	1	0	3,490
15	2	1	0	4,739
16	3	1	1	3,519
17	3	1	0	3,575
18	3	1	1	3,462
19	3	1	1	3,519
20	1	2	1	1,078
21	1	2	1	1,334
22	1	2	1	1,759
23	1	2	0	2,071
24	1	2	0	2,440
25	1	2	0	2,951
26	1	2	0	3,065
27	1	2	0	4,058
28	2	2	0	4,341
29	2	2	1	3,263
30	2	2	1	2,752
31	2	2	1	3,320
32	2	2	1	4,483
33	2	2	1	2,951
34	3	2	0	2,979
35	3	2	0	3,547
36	3	2	0	4,256
37	3	2	0	3,433
38	3	2	0	3,235
39	3	2	0	3,746
40	3	2	0	3,831

(Continued)

ID	Race/Ethnicity	Maternal Age	Smoking	Birth Weight in grams
41	1	3	1	2,497
42	1	3	0	2,923
43	1	3	1	3,433
44	1	3	0	2,497
45	2	3	1	3,916
46	2	3	0	2,525
47	2	3	0	2,611
48	2	3	1	3,774
49	2	3	0	4,341
50	2	3	1	4,200
51	2	3	0	3,433
52	3	3	0	2,355
53	3	3	1	2,838
54	3	3	1	2,838
55	3	3	0	3,235
56	3	3	1	3,320
57	3	3	0	3,405
58	3	3	1	3,490
59	3	3	0	3,433
60	3	3	1	3,973

2. A researcher is interested in the impact of a dietary intervention and/or exercise intervention on weight loss and cholesterol level. Study participants are randomly assigned to receive the dietary intervention and/or the exercise intervention. The data are given in the following table. Use MANOVA to evaluate the impact of the two interventions on the two outcomes, and determine whether there is an interaction effect.

ID	Diet	Exercise	Pounds Lost	Cholesterol
1	0	0	1	96
2	0	0	4	126
3	0	0	1	166
4	0	0	2	168
5	0	0	4	173
6	0	0	3	178
7	0	0	6	190
8	0	0	4	194

ID	Diet	Exercise	Pounds Lost	Cholesterol
9	0	0	2	195
10	0	0	4	198
11	0	0	4	212
12	0	0	5	212
13	0	0	2	213
14	0	0	5	215
15	0	0	6	216
16	1	0	6	227
17	1	0	9	120
18	1	0	8	122
19	1	0	6	128
20	1	0	5	131
21	1	0	11	132
22	1	0	5	147
23	1	0	7	148
24	1	0	6	149
25	1	0	7	151
26	1	0	8	160
27	1	0	6	160
28	1	0	9	162
29	1	0	12	164
30	1	0	6	165
31	0	1	7	174
32	0	1	8	184
33	0	1	7	185
34	0	1	8	188
35	0	1	6	192
36	0	1	5	194
37	0	1	8	197
38	0	1	10	198
39	0	1	7	201
40	0	1	3	221
41	0	1	6	224
42	0	1	8	230
43	0	1	9	242
44	0	1	5	250

(Continued)

ID	Diet	Exercise	Pounds Lost	Cholesterol
45	0	1	6	251
46	1	1	5	138
47	1	1	7	139
48	1	1	5	140
49	1	1	4	140
50	1	1	5	141
51	1	1	6	159
52	1	1	7	166
53	1	1	4	172
54	1	1	5	176
55	1	1	6	180
56	1	1	7	182
57	1	1	8	185
58	1	1	3	188
59	1	1	5	188
60	1	1	6	192

Comparing the Means of Three or More Related Groups: Repeated-Measures ANOVA and Friedman's ANOVA by Rank

OBJECTIVES

After studying this chapter, you should be able to:

1. Describe the purpose of repeated-measures analysis of variance (ANOVA) and Friedman's ANOVA by rank.

2. Choose between the repeated-measures ANOVA statistic and the Friedman's ANOVA by rank statistic.

3. Compute the repeated-measures ANOVA statistic and the Friedman's ANOVA by rank statistic and determine whether group means and medians are significantly different from each other.

4. Understand and interpret *post hoc* tests with repeated-measures ANOVA or Friedman's ANOVA by rank.

5. Use SPSS to compute the repeated-measures ANOVA and the Friedman's two-way ANOVA by rank and correctly interpret the output.

6. Write up the results of the repeated-measures ANOVA and the Friedman's ANOVA by rank.

OVERVIEW OF THE REPEATED-MEASURES ANOVA AND THE FRIEDMAN'S ANOVA BY RANK

The repeated-measures analysis of variance (ANOVA) statistic is a parametric test that allows researchers to determine whether the means of three or more measures from the same person or matched controls are similar or different. The computation of a repeated-measures ANOVA is similar to that of a one-way ANOVA, and many of the assumptions are shared. The difference between a one-way ANOVA and a repeated-measures ANOVA is that the repeated-measures ANOVA also controls for the between-subjects variance by removing it from the error term and measuring it separately. In this chapter, a single-factor repeated-measures ANOVA, the most basic of the repeated-measures models, is presented. More complicated models that incorporate aspects of both the one-way ANOVA and the repeated-measures ANOVA can be used as well. The more complex models are typically used in analyses that seek to control for both repeated measures over time and fixed factors that do not change over time (e.g., gender).

The Friedman's ANOVA by rank is a non-parametric test that is analogous to single-factor repeated-measures ANOVA. It ascertains whether the medians of the measures being compared are different by examining the distributions of the rankings of the repeated measures (similar to the Kruskal-Wallis *H* test). It has fewer assumptions and can be used with a variety of data. It is, however, a less sensitive test and is less likely to find significant differences.

Related Measures

There are three main types of repeated-measures designs (also called within-subjects designs). One type involves taking repeated measures of the same variable(s) over time on a group or groups of subjects. For example, if we were studying hypertension, we would probably want more than one blood pressure reading on our subjects. The second type involves exposing the same subjects to all levels of the treatment. This is often called using subjects as their own controls. Finally, the same measures may be taken from a "case" and two or more matched controls, although this design is more often used in randomized, controlled studies involving animals than in those involving humans.

Advantages of Repeated-Measures Designs

Suppose we wanted to test medications to reduce nausea during chemotherapy. We could randomly assign patients to one of the following three conditions: medication 1, medication 2, or control. However, if our subjects varied widely in the amount of nausea they experienced, the within-subject variability would be large. Because the *f*-statistic is based on the ratio of between-group variance to within-group variance, there would have to be a very large between-group difference to attain a significant result. That is, the large variability among the subjects could obscure any real differences between the groups. This would be particularly true if the groups were small.

One way to remove these individual differences would be to assign each subject to all treatments. Each subject would be exposed to medication 1, medication 2, and the control condition in random order. Each subject would serve as his or her own control, and the within or error variance would be decreased. This would result in a more powerful test and would decrease the number of subjects needed for the study. Because repeated measures generally reduce the error term, they enhance the power of the analysis, resulting in the need for fewer subjects. Both repeated-measures ANOVA and Friedman's ANOVA by rank can be used to analyze the data from within-subjects designs.

Problems with the Use of Repeated Measures

Carryover effects occur when some or all of the effects of a treatment given at one time are still evident at the time of the second treatment. In drug trials, for example, time is allowed for one drug to "wash out" before a second drug is tested. Adequate time should be allowed to prevent carryover effects. When subjects are exposed to more than one treatment, we need to consider that previous treatments may still be having an effect.

Position effects occur when the order in which the treatments are given affects the outcome. For example, participants may be excited to be in the study at the start (e.g., for the first experimental treatment) but may become bored and less attentive by the third or fourth treatment. Repeated exposure to measures may result in an increase in the outcome measure that is related to the subject learning about the measure, rather than a real change. Because subjects are measured repeatedly, such things as sensitization to the instruments may cause difficulties. Scores on an anxiety scale may vary because of repeated exposure to the scale rather than to real changes in anxiety. Even physiologic measures may reflect this. For example, vital signs may increase with a new situation, then decrease with repeated measures. Practice with previous tests may increase scores on later tests. Subjects may become bored by repeated measures and be careless with later tests. Investigators often randomize the order in which the subjects are exposed to the treatments to eliminate effects due to the order of treatment.

RESEARCH QUESTION

The research question that repeated-measures ANOVA asks is "Are the means of the three or more related groups significantly different from one another?" In particular, we are testing the null hypothesis that the means of the three or more groups are equivalent. The Friedman's ANOVA by rank test is a nonparametric test that is similar to repeated-measures ANOVA and can be used when the data do not meet the assumptions. It asks the following question: "Are the distributions of three or more dependent groups significantly different from one another?" In this case, we are testing the null hypothesis that the distribution of the three or more groups is equivalent. Typically, we report the median when using the Friedman's ANOVA by rank, rather than reporting the mean.

The following studies provide examples of how these two methods are used in practice. The first study uses repeated-measures ANOVA to examine different sources of stress in emergency department (ED) staff. The second

study uses the Friedman's ANOVA by rank to examine taste preferences for medicine, and the third uses repeated-measures ANOVA to examine the effect of immersing in water after exercising on calorie intake.

Which Factors Cause the Most Work-Related Stress for Emergency Department Staff?

Laposa, Alden & Fullerton (2003) examined this question in a study of work-related stress among 51 ED personnel. This was an observational, cross-sectional study conducted in a large urban ED. The self-administered survey included items related to work history and sociodemographic characteristics; the dependent variable was a measure of work stress, the Health Professionals Stress Inventory (HPSI). The HPSI measures three different sources of work stress: organizational characteristics, patient care, and interpersonal conflict. Each person had a score for each of the three measures. The three stress scores were compared using repeated-measures ANOVA to see which source of stress contributed the most to work stress. In this case, three different but related variables (organizational characteristics, patient care, and interpersonal conflict) were measured in the same study participant at one point in time. Overall, the study reported that all three workplace factors cause similar amounts of stress.

Are There Significant Differences in the Taste of Commonly Used Liquid Steroid Preparations Given to Children?

Mitchell & Counselman (2003) explored this question in a double-blind study. The researchers employed 86 medical students and residents as taste testers of three commonly used liquid steroids: prednisone, prednisolone, and dexamethasone. Each volunteer was asked to drink 5 ml of each steroid (labeled A, B, and C) and to rate it on four aspects: taste, texture, smell, and aftertaste. A saltine cracker and water were given between the different steroids. In this study, different items were rated by the same person (e.g., the rating of taste of the three different medicines). The ratings of these three steroid preparations were compared. A Friedman's ANOVA by rank was used because the data were ordinal and not normally distributed. The investigators concluded that dexamethasone was the most palatable and that prednisolone was more palatable than prednisone.

Does Postexercise Immersion in Cold Water Affect Postexercise Calorie Consumption?

Halse, Wallman & Guelfi (2011) addressed this question in a study of 10 physically active men. In this study, each man participated in three randomized, counterbalanced trials consisting of 40 minutes of treadmill running, followed by 20 minutes of either cold-water immersion, neutral-water immersion, or a resting control time with no water immersion. Afterward, the participants were given access to a buffet-type breakfast and allowed to eat as much as they wanted to. This study used repeated-measures ANOVA to compare the calorie consumption of the men under these three conditions and concluded that the men consumed significantly more energy after both the cold-water immersion and the neutral-water immersion (as compared with the control state with no water immersion).

TYPE OF DATA REQUIRED

To use either a repeated-measures ANOVA or a Friedman's ANOVA by rank, it is necessary to make sure that there are at least three related measures of the characteristic of interest. These measures can be either of the same variable at multiple points in time or of three related variables. To decide on which test to use, it is necessary to know the measurement scale of the variable measuring the characteristic of interest

and whether it is normally distributed. It is also necessary to know whether there is correlated symmetry, which is a combination of homogeneity of variance between each set of measures and similar correlations across all of the measures of the dependent variable. Finally, it is necessary to know the total sample size.

Dependent and Independent Variables in Repeated-Measures Designs

In this design, the dependent variable is explicitly measured. However, the independent variable is implicit (e.g., not actually measured as a number that is used in computation) and is defined by one of four general situations. The simplest situation is when the same measurement is taken on the same subject at different points in time. In this case, the independent variable is time, and each time at which data are collected is another level. The second situation is when the same measurement is taken under different experimental conditions, such as comparing the taste of three different medicines or examining the effects of different dosages of a drug. In the case of comparing the taste of three different medicines, the independent variable is "type of medicine" and has three levels, one for each type of medicine. The third situation is when similar, but not identical, constructs are measured on the same scale at the same time, as was done in the study comparing the intensity of different types of work stress. The independent variable is "type of work stress" and has three levels: organizational characteristics, patient care, and interpersonal conflict. The fourth situation is when a study has a case and multiple matched control groups in which each group is a level of the independent variable.

Choosing between the Two Tests

If the repeated-measures ANOVA is used when one or more of its assumptions are not met, there is a threat to internal validity (i.e., to the statistical conclusions that are drawn) because the computed p-value may not be accurate. However, similar to the one-way ANOVA, the repeated-measures ANOVA is robust to violations of normality. This means that it can be used even when one or more of the variables are nonnormally distributed to obtain essentially the correct p-value. There is a lower risk of error when doing so if there is a large sample size. However, the repeated-measures ANOVA is very sensitive to violations of the assumption of correlated symmetry. In this case, the Friedman's ANOVA by rank or an adjustment to the repeated-measures ANOVA with the Greenhouse–Geisser procedure should be used.

REPEATED-MEASURES ANOVA

The repeated-measures ANOVA table is similar to that of a one-way ANOVA, with the addition of an extra row (labeled "Blocks") to show the variation in the dependent variable that can be attributed to each individual in the study (Table 9-1). The single-factor repeated-measures ANOVA table has six columns and four rows. The first column lists the sources of variance, as described by the three rows (i.e., treatments, blocks, and error) with a summary row, "Total," which displays the total variation.

The next three columns contain the numbers that are needed to compute the f-ratio. These are the sums of squares, the degrees of freedom, and the mean square for each source of variation. The fifth column contains the actual value of the f-ratio, and the sixth column lists whether it is a statistically significant value. This table displays all the computational elements necessary to compute the f-ratio between the within-groups variance and the between-groups variance. Just as with a one-way ANOVA, the computed value of the ANOVA is compared with the critical value (obtained from the f-tables in Appendix F) to see whether the different means are significantly different from each other.

Post Hoc Tests Used with Repeated-Measures ANOVA

After a significant f test has been obtained for repeated-measures ANOVA, the null hypothesis is rejected, and it can be said that at least one of the group means is different from the others. However, similar to a one-way ANOVA, it is necessary to perform post hoc tests to determine which of the means are different. Post hoc tests are performed only when there is a significant overall f test for the repeated-measures ANOVA. Several post hoc tests that are appropriate for the repeated-measures ANOVA are available

Table 9-1	REPEATED-MEASURES ANOVA TABLE				
Source of Variation	**Sum of Squares**	**Degrees of Freedom**	**Mean Square**	**Variance Ratio (f Test)**	**p-Value**
Treatments	SS_{tr}	$(k - 1)$	$SS_{tr}/(k - 1)$	MS_{tr}/MS_e	
Blocks	SS_{bl}	$(n - 1)$	$SS_{bl}/(n - 1)$		
Error	SS_e	$(k - 1)(n - 1)$	$SS_e/(k - 1)(n - 1)$		
Total	SS_t	$(k \times n) - 1$			

Note. Treatments refer to the variation caused by the different experimental conditions (i.e., the different levels of the independent variable). *Blocks* refer to the variation that results from the variation between subjects. *Error* is the variation due to random error, and *Total* is the total variation.
k, number of treatments; MS_e, mean square error; MS_{tr}, mean square treatment; n, number of people in the study; SS_{bl}, block sum of squares; SS_e, error sum of squares; SS_t, total sum of squares; SS_{tr}, treatment sum of squares.

to researchers. Tests that are commonly used include the least significant difference (LSD) test, modified Bonferroni *t* test, and Sidak test. The LSD test does not adjust for multiple comparisons and carries a high risk of making a type I error (i.e., saying a finding is significant when it really is not). The modified Bonferroni test is much more conservative; with smaller numbers of comparisons (e.g., three-way), this is not an issue, but with larger numbers of groups to compare, the risk of a type II error (i.e., saying a finding is not significant when it really is) increases greatly. The Sidak test is somewhat less conservative and is a better choice when comparing larger numbers of groups (Clark, 2003). The modified Bonferroni *t* test is presented here.

Step-by-Step Procedure for Computing Repeated-Measures ANOVA

We illustrate computing a single-factor repeated-measures ANOVA by addressing the following question: Do different laboratory instruments return the same laboratory values for hemoglobin A_{1c} (HbA$_{1c}$)? The values of HbA$_{1c}$ are used to monitor glycemic control in diabetic patients. According to clinical guidelines from the American Diabetes Association, a value of 7 or less is desirable (American Diabetes Association, 2007). The question of the reliability of laboratory instruments is a critical one for individuals with diabetes, who need to have their HbA$_{1c}$ values monitored regularly to control their blood glucose levels. If different laboratory instruments do not return a consistent HbA$_{1c}$ value, the information given to people with diabetes may be inconsistent over time if a hospital changes instruments or uses different instruments in the same lab.

To answer this question, we have taken and tested blood samples from 30 patients with diabetes with three instruments commonly used to test for HbA$_{1c}$ values (coded as A, B, and C). The dependent variable is "HbA$_{1c}$ level." The independent variable is "type of instrument" and

has three levels: instrument A, instrument B, and instrument C. The data are shown in Table 9-2, the hand-computation is shown in Box 9-1, and the SPSS analysis is shown in Box 9-2.

Step 1: State the Null and Alternative Hypotheses

The first step is to state a hypothesis about the expected findings (see Box 9-1).

- H_0: There will be no difference in the mean value of HbA$_{1c}$ between the instruments.
- H_A: The mean value of HbA$_{1c}$ will be significantly different with at least one of the instruments.

Step 2: Define the Significance Level (α-Level) and Obtain the Critical Value for the f Test

In this example, an α-level of $p < .05$ is used. We obtain the critical value from the *f*-table (Appendix F). We will need the degrees of freedom for the treatment variance (df$_{tr}$) and for the error (df$_e$). The degrees of freedom for the treatment variance are the number of levels of the independent variable minus 1, and the degrees of freedom for the error are $(n - 1) \times (k - 1)$. The df$_{tr}$ = 2 and the df$_e$ = 58. The critical value of the *f*-statistic is found in the *f*-table at α = .05. In the *f*-table, the df$_e$ is the denominator. The critical value for $f_{2,58}$ at .05 is approximately 3.15. The computed *f*-statistic must exceed this value to reject the null hypothesis and to be able to say that the means are significantly different from each other.

Step 3: Make Sure That the Data Meet All the Necessary Assumptions

We can tell that the data, as shown in Tables 9-2 and 9-3, meet most of the assumptions for the repeated-measures ANOVA. The people in this study constitute an independent random sample because they were randomly selected

(*Text continues on page 229*)

BOX 9-1   HAND COMPUTING THE REPEATED-MEASURES ANOVA

Step 1: State the null and alternative hypotheses:

- H0: There will be no difference in the mean value of HbA_{1c} between the three instruments.
- HA: The mean value of HbA_{1c} will be significantly different in at least one of the three instruments.

Step 2: Determine the significance level (α-level) and obtain the critical value for the f test.

- The α-level $= .05$.
- The degrees of freedom treatments (df_{tr}) = the number of levels of the treatment variable minus 1 ($3 - 1 = 2$).
- The degrees of freedom for error (df_e) $= (n - 1)(k - 1) = (29) \times (2) = 58$.
- The critical value from the f-table for $f_{2,58}$ at α-level $= .05$ is 3.15. (Use the value at $f_{2,60}$, which is as close as you can get in the f-table.)

Step 3: Make sure that the data meet the necessary assumptions.

- The measures constitute an independent random sample.
- There are at least three measures of the dependent variable.
- The dependent variable is somewhat normally distributed.
- The dependent variable is of an interval or a ratio measurement scale.
- There is no potential for a position or carryover effect.
- There is no compound symmetry (see the SPSS printout), which means that it is necessary to proceed with caution and to use the Greenhouse–Geisser procedure in SPSS.

Step 4: Present the mean and standard deviation for each group.

Measure	Instrument A	Instrument B	Instrument C
Mean HbA_{1c}	7.17	7.07	8.33
Standard deviation	2.71	2.25	1.95

Computations for the means and standard deviations:

Means Standard Deviation

$$\bar{x} = \frac{\sum x}{N} \qquad s = \sqrt{\frac{\sum x^2 - \frac{\left(\sum x\right)^2}{N}}{N - 1}}$$

Instrument A: $\bar{x} = \dfrac{215.2}{30} = 7.17 \qquad s = \sqrt{\dfrac{1756.14 - \dfrac{(215.2)^2}{30}}{29}} = 2.71$

(Continued)

BOX 9-1   HAND COMPUTING THE REPEATED-MEASURES ANOVA
(Continued)

Instrument B:
$$\bar{X} = \frac{212.2}{30} = 7.07 \qquad s = \sqrt{\frac{1647.64 - \frac{(212.2)^2}{30}}{29}} = 2.25$$

Instrument C:
$$\bar{X} = \frac{250.0}{30} = 8.33 \qquad s = \sqrt{\frac{2193.00 - \frac{(250.0)^2}{30}}{29}} = 1.95$$

Step 5: Perform the computations to complete the repeated-measures ANOVA table and *post hoc* tests.

Calculate the sum of squares:

Correction factor (C)

$$C = \frac{\left(\sum\sum X_{ij}\right)^2}{k \times N}$$

$$C = \frac{(215.2 + 212.2 + 250.0)^2}{3 \times 30}$$

$$C = \frac{(677.4)^2}{90}$$

$$C = 5098.564$$

Total sum of squares (SS_t):

$$SS_t = \sum\sum X_{ij}^2 - C$$

$$SS_t = (1757.14 + 1647.64 + 2193.0) - 5098.564$$

$$SS_t = 499.216.$$

Treatment sum of squares (SS_{tr}):

$$SS_{tr} = \frac{\sum T_j^2}{N} - C$$

BOX 9-1 HAND COMPUTING THE REPEATED-MEASURES ANOVA
(Continued)

$$SS_{tr} = \frac{215.2^2 + 212.2^2 + 250.0^2}{30} - 5098.564$$

$$SS_{tr} = \frac{153839.88}{30} - 5098.564$$

$$SS_{tr} = 29.432$$

Block sum of squares (SS_bl):

$$SS_{bl} = \frac{\sum T_j^2}{k} - C$$

$$SS_{bl} = (44.1^2 + 24^2 + 24.5^2 + 18.5^2 + 18.8^2 + 21.4^2 + 23.6^2 + 29.0^2 + 21.9^2 + 19.6^2$$
$$+ 25.2^2 + 17.3^2 + 17.1^2 + 24.2^2 + 27.9^2 + 24.3^2 + 15.6^2 + 35.2^2 + 14.8^2 + 16.4^2 +$$
$$23.1^2 + 24.6^2 + 17.5^2 + 19.2^2 + 28.7^2 + 26.0^2 + 16.4^2 + 20.4^2 + 19.7^2 + 18.4^2)/3$$
$$- 5098.564$$

$$SS_{bl} = \frac{6413.24}{3} - 5098.564$$

$$SS_{bl} = 372.516.$$

Error sum of squares (SS_e):

$$SS_e = SS_t - SS_{tr} - SS_{bl}$$
$$SS_e = 499.216 - 372.516 - 29.432$$
$$SS_e = 97.268$$

Calculate the mean squares:

Mean square treatment (MS_tr):

$$MS_{tr} = \frac{SS_{tr}}{df_{tr}}$$

$$MS_{tr} = \frac{29.43}{2}$$

$$MS_{tr} = 14.716$$

Mean square blocks (MS_bl):

$$MS_{bl} = \frac{SS_{bl}}{df_{bl}}$$

$$MS_{bl} = \frac{372.53}{29}$$

$$MS_{bl} = 12.845$$

(Continued)

BOX 9-1 HAND COMPUTING THE REPEATED-MEASURES ANOVA
(Continued)

Mean square error (MS$_e$):

$$MS_e = \frac{SS_e}{df_e}$$

$$MS_e = \frac{97.27}{58}$$

$$MS_e = 1.677$$

Compute the f-statistic (f_{ratio}):

$$f_{ratio} = \frac{MS_{tr}}{MS_e}$$

$$f_{ratio} = \frac{14.716}{1.677}$$

$$f_{ratio} = 8.775$$

Create the repeated-measures ANOVA table:

Repeated-Measures ANOVA Table

Source of Variation	Sum of Squares	Degrees of Freedom	Mean Square	Variance Ratio (*f* Test)	*p*-Value
Treatments	29.432	2	14.716	8.775	≤.05
Blocks	372.516	29	12.845		
Error	97.268	58	1.677		
Total	499.216				

Assess the statistical significance of the findings:
The critical value is 3.15. Because 8.775 is greater than 3.15, at least some of the means are significantly different from some of the other means.

Compute the *post hoc* tests (modified Bonferroni *t* test) to determine which means are significantly different from each other.

$$\text{Modified Bonferroni } t \text{ test} = \frac{\bar{X}_1 - \bar{X}_2}{\sqrt{\dfrac{2 \times MS_e}{n}}}$$

The critical value for the Bonferroni *t* test is in the two-tailed *t* test chart at: $t_{/k}$ and df_e

$$\frac{\alpha}{k} = \frac{.05}{3} = .016$$

$$df_e = 58$$

BOX 9-1 HAND COMPUTING THE REPEATED-MEASURES ANOVA
(Continued)

The critical value for t at .016, df $= 58$ is approximately 2.66.
(Use the value in the chart at $\alpha = .01$ and df $= 60$.)

Bonferroni t test: A versus B:

$$\text{Bonferroni } t \text{ test} = \frac{7.173 - 7.073}{\sqrt{\dfrac{2 \times 1.677}{30}}}$$

$$\text{Bonferroni } t \text{ test} = \frac{0.10}{\sqrt{\dfrac{3.354}{30}}}$$

Bonferroni t test: A versus B $= 0.2991$. The two means are not significantly different because .2291 $<$ 2.66.

Bonferroni t test: A versus C:

$$\text{Bonferroni } t \text{ test} = \frac{8.333 - 7.173}{\sqrt{\dfrac{2 \times 1.677}{30}}}$$

$$\text{Bonferroni } t \text{ test} = \frac{8.333 - 7.173}{0.3343}$$

Bonferroni t test: A versus C $= 3.47$. The two means are significantly different because 3.47 $<$ 2.66.

Bonferroni t test: B versus C:

$$\text{Bonferroni } t \text{ test} = \frac{8.333 - 7.073}{\sqrt{(2 \times 1.677)/30}}$$

$$\text{Bonferroni } t \text{ test} = \frac{1.26}{.3343}$$

Bonferroni t test: B versus C $= 3.77$. The two means are significantly different because 3.77 is greater than 2.66.

Step 6: Determine the statistical significance and state a conclusion.

At least some of the measures of HbA_{1c} obtained with the different instruments differ significantly from each other. In particular, *post hoc* tests reveal that the scores obtained with instrument C differ significantly from those obtained with the other two instruments. However, the scores obtained with instrument A and instrument B do not differ significantly from each other.

BOX 9-2 COMPUTING THE REPEATED-MEASURES ANOVA USING SPSS

Step1: The data are entered into an SPSS data set, and the menu bar is used to click on "Analyze" and then to select "General Linear Model" and then "Repeated Measures."

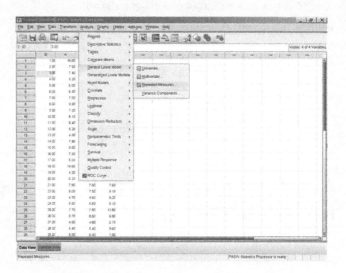

Step 2: In the "Repeated Measures Define Factor(s)" popup box, "hba1c" is typed over the word "factor1" in the "Within-Subject Factor Name" slot, a "3" is put in "Number of Levels," slot, and the "Add" button is clicked.

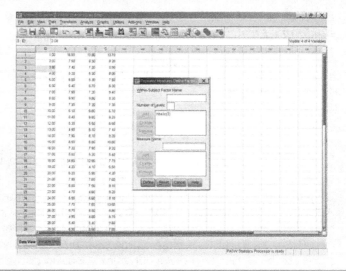

BOX 9-2   COMPUTING THE REPEATED-MEASURES ANOVA USING SPSS
(Continued)

Step 3: The "Define" button is clicked. The variables "A," "B," and "C" are moved into the slots labeled "__?__ (1)," "__?__ (2)," and "__?__ (3)." The "Between-Subjects Factors" and "Covariates" boxes are left empty. The "Options" button is then clicked.

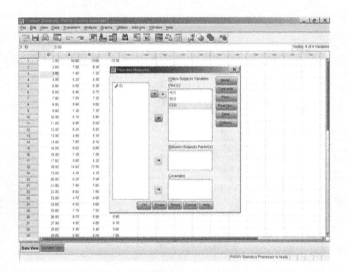

Step 4: In the "Options" popup box, the "Descriptive Statistics" box is selected and "hba1c" is moved over to the "Display Means for" box. The "Compare main effects" box is clicked, and "Bonferroni" is selected from the dropdown menu. Then the "Continue" button is clicked. After the "OK" button is clicked, the output appears in the output window.

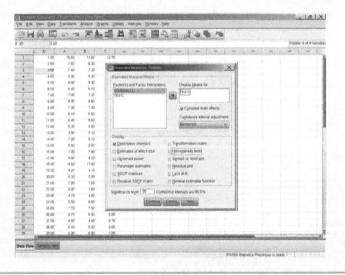

Table 9-2	HbA$_{1c}$ LEVELS AS MEASURED BY THREE INSTRUMENTS				
Person ID	Instrument A	Instrument B	Instrument C	Block (Row) Total (T_j)	Block (Row) Total Squared
1	16.6	13.8	13.7	44.1	653.69
2	7.5	8.3	8.2	24	192.38
3	7.4	7.2	9.9	24.5	204.61
4	5.2	5.3	8	18.5	119.13
5	6	5.3	7.5	18.8	120.34
6	6.4	6.7	8.3	21.4	154.74
7	7	7.2	9.4	23.6	189.2
8	9.9	9.8	9.3	29	280.54
9	7.3	7.3	7.3	21.9	159.87
10	6.1	6.8	6.7	19.6	128.34
11	8.4	8.6	8.2	25.2	211.76
12	5.2	5.5	6.6	17.3	100.85
13	4.9	5.1	7.1	17.1	100.43
14	7.9	8.1	8.2	24.2	195.26
15	8.5	8.8	10.6	27.9	262.05
16	7.2	7.9	9.2	24.3	198.89
17	5	5.2	5.4	15.6	81.2
18	14.6	12.9	7.7	35.2	438.86
19	4.2	4.1	6.5	14.8	76.7
20	6.2	5.9	4.3	16.4	91.74
21	7.9	7.6	7.6	23.1	177.93
22	8	7.5	9.1	24.6	203.06
23	4.7	4.6	8.2	17.5	110.49
24	5.5	5.6	8.1	19.2	127.22
25	7.7	7.5	13.5	28.7	297.79
26	8.7	8.5	8.8	26	225.38
27	4.9	4.8	6.7	16.4	91.94
28	5.4	5.4	9.6	20.4	150.48
29	5.9	6	7.8	19.7	131.65
30	5	4.9	8.5	18.4	121.26
Column Total (T_j)	215.2	212.2	250	677.4	5597.78

Note. The numbers listed in plain type are the data, and the numbers in italics are computed values from the data used to obtain the repeated-measures ANOVA.

from among a large group of patients with diabetes and were not related to one another. There are three measures of the dependent variable. The dependent variable is not grossly skewed. There is a good range of values, and the dependent variable is of a ratio measurement scale. We can only gauge compound symmetry from the SPSS output (Table 9-4). There is no compound symmetry, but SPSS can adjust for this, and we can still use repeated-measures ANOVA. There is no potential for either a position effect or a carryover effect because all the blood samples were taken at one time.

Table 9-3	STEM AND LEAF PLOTS OF HbA$_{1c}$ AS MEASURED BY EACH INSTRUMENT
	Each Leaf: 1 Case
	Instrument A Stem-and-Leaf Plot
Frequency	Stem-and-Leaf Plot
4.00	4.2799
7.00	5.0022459
4.00	6.0124
8.00	7.02345799
4.00	8.0457
1.00	9.9
2.00 Extremes	(≥14.6)
	Instrument B Stem-and-Leaf Plot
4.00	4.1689
8.00	5.12334569
3.00	6.078
7.00	7.2235569
5.00	8.13568
1.00	9.8
2.00 Extremes	(≥12.9)
	Instrument C Stem-and-Leaf Plot
1.00 Extremes	(≤4.3)
1.00	5.4
4.00	6.5677
6.00	7.135678
9.00	8.012222358
6.00	9.123469
1.00	10.6
2.00 Extremes	(≥13.5)

Step 4: Compute the Means and Standard Deviations for Each Group

The means and standard deviations are computed using the totals shown in Table 9-2. Note that instrument C gives a higher mean value of HbA$_{1c}$ (8.33; standard deviation, 1.95) than does instrument A (7.17; standard deviation, 2.71) or instrument B (7.07; standard deviation, 2.25). However, we need to run a repeated-measures ANOVA with a *post hoc* test to confirm the initial impression that instrument C returns a significantly different value compared to the other two instruments.

Step 5: Perform the Computations Necessary to Complete the ANOVA Table and Perform Post Hoc Tests to Determine Which Group Means are Significantly Different

The next step is to complete the ANOVA table, as shown in Table 9-1. First, the four sums of squares must be computed: the total sum of squares (df_t), treatment sum of squares (df_{tr}), block sum of squares (df_{bl}), and error sum of squares (df_e). The totals are put into the appropriate place in the ANOVA table. To compute the sums of squares, "C," a correction factor, must be computed first. The necessary formulas and computations are shown in Box 9-1.

In this case, the overall *f*-statistic is significant, which means that at least one of the means is significantly different from the others. We need to conduct *post hoc* tests to find out which of the means are really different. We will use a modified Bonferroni *t* test (Glantz, 1997).

Table 9-4	SPSS OUTPUT FROM REPEATED-MEASURES ANOVA ANALYSIS OF VARIANCE

General Linear Model

Descriptive Statistics

	Mean	Standard Deviation	N
A	7.1733	2.71292	30
B	7.0733	2.24897	30
C	8.3333	1.94464	30

Note. This part of the printout is where we find the mean HbA_{1c} and its standard deviation as measured by each of the three different machines.

Mauchly's Test of Sphericity[a]

Measure: MEASURE_1

Within-Subjects Effect	Mauchly's W	Approx. X^2	df	Significance	Epsilon[b] Greenhouse–Geisser	Huynh–Feldt	Lower-bound
hba1c	.212	43.420	2	.000	.559	.566	.500

Tests the null hypothesis that the error covariance matrix of the orthonormalized transformed dependent variables is proportional to an identity matrix.

Note. This part of the output provides "Mauchly's test of sphericity." This is the test that determines whether there is compound symmetry. If the p-value of this test is significant (look at the "Significance" column), then there is no compound symmetry and it is necessary to look at the areas of the printout where the Greenhouse–Geisser adjusted procedure is presented to obtain accurate information. In this case, there is no compound symmetry because the p-value for the Mauchly's test of sphericity is well under .05.

[a]Design: Intercept Within-Subjects Design: hba1c.

[b]May be used to adjust the degrees of freedom for the averaged tests of significance. Corrected tests are displayed in the Tests of Within-Subjects Effects table.

Tests of Within-Subjects Effects

Measure: MEASURE_1

Source		Type III Sum of Squares	df	Mean Square	f	Significance
hba1c	Sphericity Assumed	29.432	2	14.716	8.775	.000
	Greenhouse–Geisser	29.432	1.119	26.311	8.775	.004
	Huynh–Feldt	29.432	1.132	26.002	8.775	.004
	Lower-bound	29.432	1.000	29.432	8.775	.006
Error (hba1c)	Sphericity Assumed	97.268	58	1.677		
	Greenhouse–Geisser	97.268	32.440	2.998		
	Huynh–Feldt	97.268	32.825	2.963		
	Lower-bound	97.268	29.000	3.354		

Note. This part of the printout is labeled "Tests of Within-Subjects Effects." The treatment sum of squares (SS_{tr}) can be found in the first column. If there was compound symmetry, the values in the first row, labeled "Sphericity Assumed," would be used. Note that these values correspond exactly to the values in the ANOVA table computed earlier (see Box 9-1, Step 5). Because there is no compound symmetry, the values in the second row, labeled "Greenhouse–Geisser," are used to put together the ANOVA table. The sum of squares error (SS_e) is also found in this portion. The two most important pieces of information in this part of the output are the value of the computed f test (8.775) and its p-value (.004). Note that the p-value is obtained from the row labeled "Greenhouse–Geisser," which says that significant differences exist in the means of the three groups that were compared.

Table 9-4	**SPSS OUTPUT FROM REPEATED-MEASURES ANOVA ANALYSIS OF VARIANCE** *(Continued)*

Tests of Between-Subjects Effects

Measure: MEASURE_1

Transformed Variable: Average

Source	Type III Sum of Squares	df	Mean Square	f	Significance
Intercept	5098.564	1	5098.564	396.918	.000
Error	372.516	29	12.845		

Note. This portion of the output contains two useful pieces of information. The first, labeled "Intercept," provides the value of the correction factor that was hand computed. The second, labeled "Error," provides the value of the sum of square blocks (SS_{bl}).

Pairwise Comparisons

Measure: MEASURE_1

(I) hba1c	(J) hba1c	Mean Difference (I − J)	Standard Error	Significance[a]	95% Confidence Interval for Difference[a]	
					Lower Bound	Upper Bound
1	2	.100	.125	1.000	−.218	.418
	3	−1.160[b]	.426	.032	−2.242	−.078
2	1	−.100	.125	1.000	−.418	.218
	3	−1.260[b]	.372	.006	−2.206	−.314
3	1	−1.160[b]	.426	.032	.078	2.242
	2	1.260[b]	.372	.006	.314	2.206

Note. This portion of the output contains the post hoc tests. Under the heading "Estimated Marginal Means," there is a box labeled "Pairwise Comparisons." This box shows the results of the Bonferroni comparisons. From this, it can be seen that the third mean (machine "C") is significantly different from the other two means (machine "A" and machine "B").

Based on estimated marginal means.

[a]Adjustment for multiple comparisons: Bonferroni.

[b]The mean difference is significant at the .05 level.

Two things are needed to compute the modified Bonferroni *t* test: the formula and the correct critical value of the *t* test. The formula is the same *t* test formula discussed earlier in Chapter 5. The difference is that the error variance (SS_e) from the ANOVA table is used as the denominator for the *t* test. The formula and computations are shown in Box 9-1.

The correct critical value of the *t* test is a little tricky to compute. To keep the total probability of making a type I error below .05, the computed *t*-statistic must exceed the value required for α/k (Glantz, 1997). In this example, three measures are compared ($k = 3$) so that the α-level for the

critical value for the *post hoc* Bonferroni *t* test will be .05/3, which equals .016.

Step 6: Determine Statistical Significance and State a Conclusion

Overall, we find that at least some of the measures of HbA$_{1c}$ differ significantly from each other as tested with the repeated-measures ANOVA at $p \leq .05$. On further examination with the modified Bonferroni *post hoc* test, it is clear that instrument C returns significantly higher scores than either of the other instruments and that the other two instruments do not differ from each other.

Step-by-Step Procedure for Using SPSS to Compute the Repeated-Measures ANOVA

It is somewhat complicated to compute a repeated-measures ANOVA using SPSS, because SPSS uses that particular function to compute several different types of ANOVA models. Thus, the directions must be followed exactly as shown to be sure that the correct information is obtained from the printout. It is critical to read the printout carefully. Box 9-2 illustrates the process with screen shots from the SPSS program, and Table 9-4 contains an annotated printout to show where all of the necessary information can be found.

Using SPSS to Conduct the Analysis

First, data need to be entered into the data editor. The four variables are the person ID and the three different machines "A," "B," and "C." After the data have been entered, the menu system is used to obtain the repeated-measures ANOVA. First, click on "Analyze" and then select "General Linear Model" and "Repeated Measures." When the "Repeated Measures Define Factor(s)" popup box appears, the name "hba1c" is typed in the "Within-Subject Factor Name" slot. A "3" is put in the "Number of Levels" slot because there are three levels of

the independent variable (i.e., A, B, C), and then the "Add" button is clicked. In general, a descriptive name should be used for the "Within-Subject Factor Name" (but not a variable name already used in the SPSS data set). The number of levels is the number of measures of the dependent variable that are compared. Then the "Define" button is clicked. When the "Repeated Measures" popup box appears, the variables "A," "B," and "C" are moved into the three spots in the "Within-Subjects Variables" box. Then, the "Options" button is clicked. In the "Options" popup box, the "Descriptive Statistics" box is selected. The variable "hba1c" is moved to the "Display Means for" box. Then, the "Compare main effects" box is clicked and "Bonferroni" is selected from the dropdown menu. The "Continue" button is clicked, followed by the "OK" button. The output appears in the output window.

Interpreting the Output

The SPSS output is shown in Table 9-4. Some parts of this printout are not relevant to repeated-measures ANOVA, and in this table, we show only the relevant sections. The table is annotated so that you can find the relevant information and construct the repeated-measures ANOVA table.

Putting It All Together

This study found that there were significant differences in the mean values of HbA$_{1c}$ as measured by the three different instruments, according to the repeated-measures ANOVA, using the Greenhouse–Geisser procedure (Greenhouse & Geisser, 1959). Modified Bonferroni *post hoc* tests (Glantz, 1997) revealed that the "C" instrument differed from both the "A" and the "B," but that the "A" and the "B" were not significantly different from each other.

FRIEDMAN'S ANOVA BY RANK

Friedman's ANOVA by rank is a nonparametric test that is similar to the repeated-measures ANOVA (Friedman, 1937, 1939). It is used to test the differences in the median value of an ordinal, interval, or ratio variable with repeated measures of the dependent variable. It is useful in cases in which a repeated-measures ANOVA cannot be used because one or more of the assumptions are violated. It is often used to examine differences in ratings or preferences for similar items (e.g., different flavors of medicine).

In this approach, the independent variable is used to divide the sample into the "k" groups (k being the number of possible values or levels of the nominal variable). To determine whether the medians of the "k" groups are different from each other, the sums of the rankings for each of the groups are compared to see the degree to which the sums differ from what would be expected under the null hypothesis.

Table 9-5	SATISFACTION OF PATIENTS WITH DIFFERENT TYPES OF HEALTH CARE PROVIDERS					
	Satisfaction			Rank		
Patient ID	NP	MD	PA	NP	MD	PA
1	9	7	6	3	2	1
2	9.5	6.5	8	3	1	2
3	5	7	4	2	3	1
4	8.5	8.5	6	2.5	2.5	1
5	9.5	5	7	3	1	2
6	7.5	8	6	2	3	1
7	8	6.5	6.5	3	1.5	1.5
8	7	6.5	4	3	2	1
9	8.5	7	6.5	3	2	1
10	6	7	3	2	3	1
	Rank Totals			26.5	21	12.5

MD, medical doctor; NP, nurse practitioner; PA, physician's assistant.

Step-by-Step Procedure for Computing the Friedman's ANOVA by Rank

The computation of the Friedman's ANOVA is illustrated by answering the following question: Is the type of health care provider related to the patient's satisfaction with care? Data are from a study of 10 patients seen for health care at an Health Maintenance Organization (HMO). The data are shown in Table 9-5. Each patient had three different urgent care visits. On one visit, the patient was seen by a physician (MD); at another visit, by a nurse practitioner (NP); and at the third visit, by a physician's assistant (PA). After each visit, the patient completed a patient satisfaction survey. Satisfaction was measured by a 10-item scale, which returns scores from 0 to 10, with 0 indicating the least satisfied and 10 indicating the most satisfied. The data and the ranking are shown in Table 9-5. The procedure for computing the test by hand is shown in Box 9-3 and by using SPSS in Box 9-4. The SPSS output is shown in Table 9-6.

Step 1: State the Null and Alternative Hypotheses

- H_0: There will be no significant differences in the satisfaction of patients seeing an MD, NP, or PA.
- H_A: There will be significant differences in the satisfaction of patients seeing an MD, NP, or PA.

Step 2: Define the Significance Level (α-Level) and Obtain the Critical Value for the f Test

In this study, an α-level of less than or equal to .05 is used. To be able to say that the two groups are significantly different from each other when using the Friedman's ANOVA by rank statistic, it is necessary to choose from one of two tables (SPSS does this automatically). When the group sizes are small, the Friedman's ANOVA by rank

BOX 9-3   COMPUTING FRIEDMAN'S ANALYSIS OF VARIANCE BY HAND

Step 1: State the null and alternative hypotheses.

- **H_0:** There will be no significant differences in the satisfaction of patients seeing an MD, NP, or PA.
- **H_A:** There will be significant differences in the satisfaction of patients seeing an MD, NP, or PA.

Step 2: Define the significance level (α-level) and obtain the critical value for the f test.

- The α-level $= .05$.
- There are 2 degrees of freedom ($k - 1 = 3 - 1 = 2$).
- There are three groups and 10 subjects; the critical value is obtained from the chi-square table (see Appendix L).
- The critical value for the chi-square statistic at $p \le .05$ and 2 degrees of freedom is 5.991.

Step 3: Make sure that the data meet all the necessary assumptions.

- The measurement scale is ordinal.
- There are three measures of the dependent variable for each participant.
- There are no expected participant–treatment interactions.
- The study participants are independent of each other.
- The data appear to meet all the assumptions.

Step 4: Compute the median and the interquartile range.
The median satisfaction rating and interquartile ranges are as follows:

- The MDs received a median satisfaction rating of 7.00 (interquartile range, 6.5 to 7.25)
- The NPs received a median satisfaction rating of 8.25 (interquartile range, 6.75 to 9.125)
- The PAs received a median satisfaction rating of 6.00 (interquartile range, 4.0 to 6.625)

Step 5: Compute Friedman's ANOVA by rank statistic.

$$\chi_f^2 = \frac{12}{nk(k+1)} \times \sum (R_j)^2 - 3n(k+1)$$

$$\chi_f^2 = \frac{12}{10 \times 3 \times (3+1)} \times \sum (26.5^2 + 21^2 + 12.5^2) - 3 \times 10 \times (3+1)$$

$$\chi_f^2 = 129.95 - 120.00 = 9.95$$

Because 9.95 is greater than 5.991, the computed value exceeds the critical value, and so the Friedman's ANOVA by rank is statistically significant.

Compute the *post hoc* tests:
NP with MD ($p = 2$; this is comparing two adjoining rank sums):

$$q = \frac{26.5 - 21}{\sqrt{[2 \times 10 \times (2+1)]/12}}$$

$$q = \frac{5.5}{\sqrt{60/12}}$$

$$q = \frac{5.5}{2.236} = 2.46$$

BOX 9-3   COMPUTING FRIEDMAN'S ANALYSIS OF VARIANCE BY HAND
(Continued)

Because the critical value is 2.772 (from the SNK q-table), it can be concluded that this difference is not statistically significant.

NP with PA ($p = 3$; this is spanning 3 rank sums):

$$q = \frac{26.5 - 12.5}{\sqrt{[3 \times 10 \times (3+1)]/12}}$$

$$q = \frac{14}{\sqrt{120/12}}$$

$$q = \frac{14}{3.16} = 4.43$$

Because the critical value is 3.314 (from the SNK q-table), this difference is statistically significant.

MD with PA ($p = 2$; this is comparing two adjoining rank sums):

$$q = \frac{21.0 - 12.5}{\sqrt{[2 \times 10 \times (2+1)]/12}}$$

$$q = \frac{8.5}{\sqrt{120/12}}$$

$$q = \frac{8.5}{2.23} = 3.801$$

Because the critical value is 2.772 (from the SNK q-table), this difference is statistically significant.

---

has an exact distribution (Appendix G). However, when the group sizes are large, that distribution becomes very similar to the chi-square distribution. Therefore, for analyses with three groups of nine or fewer participants and four groups of four or fewer participants, the Friedman's ANOVA by rank should be used (see Appendix G). For all other situations (five or more groups or more

than nine participants), the chi-square table (see Appendix L) is used with $k - 1$ degrees of freedom to obtain the critical value.

Because this study uses three groups and 10 subjects, the critical value is obtained from the chi-square table (see Appendix L). Note that there are 2 degrees of freedom ($k - 1 = 3 - 1 = 2$). The critical value for the chi-square statistic at

Table 9-6	SPSS OUTPUT FROM FRIEDMAN'S ANOVA BY RANK			
		Hypothesis Test Summary		
	Null Hypothesis	**Test**	**Significance**	**Decision**
1	The distributions of NP, MD, and PA are the same.	Related-samples Friedman's two-way analysis of variance by Ranks	.005	Reject the null hypothesis.

Asymptotic significances are displayed. The significant level is .05.

BOX 9-4 COMPUTING FRIEDMAN'S ANOVA WITH SPSS

Step 1: The data are entered into an SPSS data set, and the menu bar is used to click on "Analyze" and then to select "Nonparametric tests" and "*K*-Related Samples."

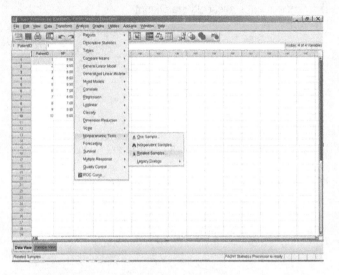

Step 2: Click on the "Objective" table, and select "Customize Analysis."

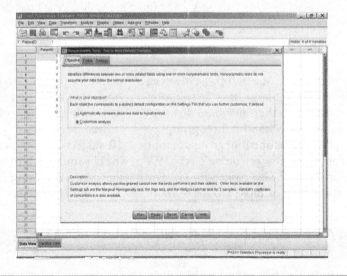

BOX 9-4　COMPUTING FRIEDMAN'S ANOVA WITH SPSS *(Continued)*

Step 3: Click on the "Fields" Tab; then select the variables NP, MD, and PA and move them over to the slot labeled "Test Variables."

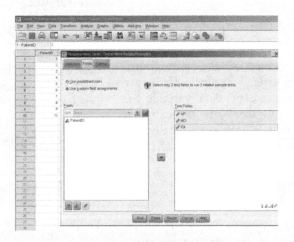

Step 4: Click on the "Settings" Tab. Select the "Customize Tests" box in the upper left-hand corner. Then select "Friedman's ANOVA By Rank" and select "all pairwise" comparisons. Click on "Run," and the output will appear in the output window **(Table 9-6).**

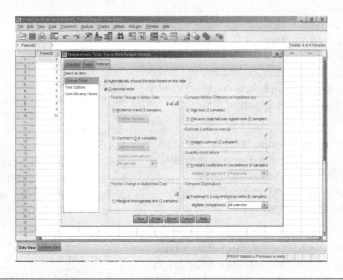

$p \leq .05$ and 2 degrees of freedom is 5.991. Thus, the computed value of the Friedman's ANOVA by rank must exceed this value to be able to say that differences exist between the groups.

Step 3: Make Sure That the Data Meet All the Necessary Assumptions

The data appear to meet all the assumptions. The measurement scale is ordinal. There are three measures of the dependent variable for each participant, and there are no expected participant–treatment interactions. Finally, the study participants are independent of each other.

Step 4: Compute the Medians and Interquartile Ranges

The actual data are shown in Table 9-5. The median satisfaction rating and interquartile ranges are as follows: the MDs received a median satisfaction rating of 7.00 (interquartile range, 6.5 to 7.25), the NPs received a median satisfaction rating of 8.25 (interquartile range, 6.75 to 9.125), and the PAs received a median satisfaction rating of 6.00 (interquartile range, 4.0 to 6.625) (see Table 8-7). Although it appears that NPs received the highest satisfaction ratings and PAs received the lowest ratings, the Friedman's ANOVA by rank is needed to test this apparent finding.

Step 5: Perform the Computations Necessary to Compute Friedman's ANOVA by Rank and Perform Post Hoc Tests to Determine Which Group Medians are Significantly Different

To compute a Friedman's ANOVA by rank statistic, it is necessary to compute the sum of ranks (rank sums) for each of the measures of the dependent variable. The first step is to rank the data in the same way that we did for the Wilcoxon matched-pairs test. The data are ranked across each participant (e.g., rank across the rows). For example, the values for the first participant are 9, 7, and 6. The ranks are 3, 2, and 1. See Table 9-6 for the rankings for each of the 10 study participants. The second step is to compute the sum of the ranks for each measure of the dependent variable (e.g., sum the columns). When the respondents have already ranked the data, this part can be skipped and just the ranks summed. This is shown in Box 9-3. After the $\sum (R_i)$ has been computed, Friedman's ANOVA by rank statistic can be computed. The basic formula for the Friedman's ANOVA by rank statistic is

$$x_r^2 = \frac{12}{nk(k+1)} \sum (R_i)^2 - 3n(k+1)$$

where n is the number of study participants (subjects), k is the number of levels of the independent variable (e.g., the number of measures of the dependent variable), and $\sum (R_i)^2$ is the sum of the squared ranks. When values are tied for rank, a correction for ties is performed. The hand computation for this goes beyond the scope of this book. However, SPSS does correct for ties, and so hand-computed answers will not exactly match the SPSS printout in cases with ties. For this particular study, the statistic is computed using the basic formula as shown in Box 9-3.

Because there is a significant overall Friedman statistic, at least one of the medians is significantly different from the others. *Post hoc* tests must be conducted to find out which medians are truly different. An adaptation of the Student-Newman-Keuls (SNK) test can be used for multiple comparisons following Friedman's ANOVA by rank (Glantz, 1997). The first step is to put the rank sums in order from smallest to largest. In this case, it would be 12.5 (PA), 21.0 (MD), and 26.5 (NP). The next step is to compute the SNK statistic for each pair of ranks to determine which are statistically significantly different from each other.

The SNK test statistic is computed as follows per Glantz (1997):

$$q = \frac{R_a - R_b}{\sqrt{[pn\,(p+1)]/12}}$$

where R_a and R_b are the rank sums for the two groups being compared, p is the number of groups spanned by the comparison, and n is the number of participants in the study. The resulting value of q is compared with the critical value of q for p comparisons with an infinite number of degrees of freedom (see Appendix I). In this example, it is necessary to make three comparisons: NP with MD, NP with PA, and MD with PA. The three values of q should be computed as shown in Box 9-3.

Step 6: Determine Statistical Significance and State a Conclusion

The final step is to state the results and to draw conclusions. Overall, this study found that significant differences existed in the satisfaction of patients with NPs, MDs, and PAs, as tested by Friedman's ANOVA by rank. Further examination with modified SNK tests (Glantz, 1997) indicated that patients are significantly less satisfied with PAs than with MDs or NPs. No other differences were found.

Step-by-Step Procedure for Using SPSS to Compute Friedman's ANOVA by Rank

Box 9-4 shows the process for obtaining a Friedman's ANOVA by rank with SPSS. The four variables are the person ID, patient satisfaction with NPs (NP), patient satisfaction with MDs (MD), and patient satisfaction with PAs (PA). After the data have been entered, the menu system can be used to obtain Friedman's statistic as shown. When the "OK" button is clicked, the SPSS output appears in the output window (see Table 9-6).

The SPSS output (see Table 9-6) provides the computed Friedman statistic (called the chi-square here) and the p-value associated with that statistic.

CHAPTER REVIEW

Multiple-Choice Concept Review

1. The Friedman's ANOVA by rank is
   a. a type of t test.
   b. a parametric test.
   c. a nonparametric test.
   d. a and b only.

2. The means of which of the following are determined to be different by the repeated-measures ANOVA test?
   a. Two independent measures
   b. Three or more independent measures
   c. Two repeated measures from a case and a matched control
   d. Three or more repeated measures

3. The repeated-measures ANOVA is best used when the measurement scale of the characteristic of interest is
   a. nominal.
   b. ordinal.
   c. interval or ratio.
   d. any of the above.

4. The carryover effect best describes the situation in which
   a. the total sample size numbers less than 30.
   b. the experiences of an earlier trial affect the results of a later trial.
   c. the test subjects remember experiences from earlier in their life.
   d. the order used to test the interventions affects the outcome.

5. The repeated-measures ANOVA is
   a. a parametric test.
   b. a nonparametric test.
   c. a type of descriptive statistic.
   d. a way to deal with data that is not normally distributed.

6. Friedman's ANOVA by rank has which of the following characteristics?
   a. It is very useful for comparing ranked data.
   b. It is appropriate in situations in which the data are not suitable to repeated-measures ANOVA.
   c. It is analogous to a paired *t* test.
   d. Both a and b are true.

7. The position effect occurs under which of the following circumstances?
   a. The total sample size is less than 30.
   b. The experiences in an earlier trial affect the results of a later trial.
   c. The subjects remember experiences from earlier in their life.
   d. The order used to test the interventions affects the outcome.

8. A study is conducted to examine the effect of three different anxiety-reduction techniques for dental patients. Each patient experiences a different technique in three different preventive (e.g., tooth cleaning) visits, which are spaced 6 months apart. These data include
   a. three independent measures of the same variable.
   b. three related measures taken at the same time.
   c. three repeated measures over time from the same participant.
   d. a and c only.

9. A study is conducted to see whether physicians' attitudes toward child abuse victims, adult victims of sexual assault, and adult victims of domestic violence are related to each other. Data are collected by a single survey conducted during a medical conference. These data include
   a. three independent measures of the same variable.
   b. three related measures taken at the same time.
   c. three repeated measures over time from the same participant.
   d. three repeated measures taken from matched patients.

10. A study is conducted to see whether back pain is best treated by chiropractic interventions, medication, surgery, or no intervention. The chiropractic intervention group has 24 people, the medication group has 17 people, the surgery group has 14 people, and the no intervention group has 18 people. These data include
    a. four independent measures of the same variable.
    b. four related measures taken at the same time.
    c. four repeated measures over time from the same participant.
    d. four repeated measures taken from matched patients.

Choosing the Best Statistical Test

For each of the following scenarios (1 to 10), pick the most appropriate test (a to h) from the following choices:

a. Independent *t* test
b. Mann-Whitney *U* test
c. Paired *t* test
d. Wilcoxon matched-pairs test
e. One-way ANOVA
f. Kruskal-Wallis *H* test
g. Repeated-measures ANOVA
h. Friedman ANOVA by rank

1. What are the preferences for contraceptive methods among college freshmen (i.e., no contraception, condoms, injected medoxyprogesterone (Depo-Provera), or birth control pills)? Each student ranks the methods from 1 to 5, with 5 being the most desirable. The sample contains 22 students.

2. What is the relationship between the number of years a person is married and whether he or she dies by suicide or homicide? The data are from a study of premature mortality. The sample contains 121 people, and the data (marital duration) are not normally distributed.

3. Is there a difference in length of stay between two types of surgery to repair hernias in young children? The sample contains 25 children, and the data (length of stay) are normally distributed.

4. Does marijuana smoking increase the appetite of cancer patients? Compare three smoking groups (i.e., never, less than once a week, weekly or more) on the number of calories consumed in a week. Each group contains 14 people, and the data (calorie consumption) are normally distributed.

5. How do people rate their mood (1 to 10, with 1 = very unhappy to 10 = ecstatic) while sitting in five differently colored rooms (i.e., blue, orange, green, purple, and red)? Each person sits in each room and then rates his or her mood. The sample contains 16 people, and the data (mood rating) are not normally distributed.

6. Does type of news media affect the level of stress a story causes? These data on the level of stress are rated 1 to 5, with 5 being the highest reported by people who see a war-related story on television or read about it in the newspaper. The television group contains 21 people, the newspaper group contains 15 people, and the data (stress rating) are not normally distributed.

7. Do workplace wellness programs increase exercise rate? A workplace wellness program enrolls 452 participants. The number of minutes a week that the participants exercise is measured weekly for the 6-week program. The data (minutes of exercise) are normally distributed.

8. Do sixth-graders differ in their knowledge of healthy eating before and after an intervention to teach good nutrition? Knowledge is measured by a 20-item quiz. The sample contains 102 students, and the data (knowledge of healthy eating) are not normally distributed.

9. Does test anxiety change during the first year of college? The sample contains 15 people, and anxiety is measured at four points in time: entry, end of first semester, end of second semester, and end of summer semester. The data (anxiety level) are normally distributed.

10. Do women diagnosed with gestational diabetes consume fewer grams of carbohydrates each day than do other pregnant women? A study was conducted with 130 women with gestational diabetes and 130 nondiabetic pregnant women. The women were matched on age, ethnicity, and number of prior pregnancies. Data on grams of carbohydrate consumed in the week before the 7-month prenatal visit were obtained from both groups. The data (grams of carbohydrate consumed) are roughly normally distributed.

Critical Thinking Concept Review

1. Develop five hypotheses that could be tested with a repeated-measures ANOVA or a Friedman's ANOVA by rank.

2. Give an example of each of the following types of studies:
   a. A study that provides repeated measures on the same person taken over time
   b. A study that provides related measures on the same person taken at one time
   c. A study that provides related measures taken from a case and at least two matched controls

3. Complete the following ANOVA table and write up the results.

Source of Variation	Sum of Squares	Degrees of Freedom	Mean Square	Variance Ratio (f Test)	p-Value
Treatments		2			
Blocks	163.42	11			
Error	16.83	22			
Total	204.75				

Computational Problems

For each of the following four problems, state the most likely hypothesis and compute a repeated-measures ANOVA to determine whether a statistically significant difference exists between the groups in question. Use an α-level of .05. Do a *post hoc* test to determine which of the means are significantly different from each other. For problems 1 to 4, perform the computations both by hand and by using SPSS. Problems 1 and 2 may not meet all the assumptions for the repeated-measures ANOVA. They are included to start you off with problems that are easy to compute. For problem 5, use SPSS only. Repeat the above for problems 1 to 5 but compute Friedman's ANOVA by rank instead. Perform the computations both by hand and by using SPSS for problems 1 to 4 and use SPSS only for problem 5.

1. A pilot study is conducted to measure the effectiveness of four different techniques for reducing test anxiety in students. Each student tries a different technique before taking an examination (spaced 3 weeks apart), and the order that the techniques were used is randomly assigned to each student. Anxiety is measured by a scale that generates sum scores ranging from 0 to 20, with 0 indicating the least anxiety and 20 indicating the most anxiety. Which technique appears to work the best?

Subject	Trial 1	Trial 2	Trial 3	Trial 4
1	18	14	12	6
2	19	12	8	4
3	14	10	6	2
4	16	12	10	4
5	12	8	6	2
6	18	10	5	1
7	16	10	8	4
8	18	8	4	1
9	16	12	6	2
10	19	16	10	8
11	16	14	10	9
12	16	12	8	8

2. A physical therapist wants to know which of three exercise machines increases heart rate the most. She recruits a group of cardiac rehabilitation patients into her study. The participants' heart rates are recorded after they use three types of exercise equipment for 10 minutes. Each piece of equipment is tried on a different visit, and the order of use is randomized for each person. Is there a difference between the three pieces of exercise equipment in terms of the effect on heart rate?

Person	Machine 1	Machine 2	Machine 3
1	111	165	214
2	110	165	224
3	88	131	188
4	94	133	185
5	65	108	149
6	68	118	176
7	124	176	240
8	84	116	185
9	96	136	184

(Continued)

Person	Machine 1	Machine 2	Machine 3
10	92	150	216
11	76	121	177
12	77	118	172
13	80	133	204
14	87	132	179
15	87	156	223
16	57	98	130
17	84	131	185
18	77	109	163

3. An instructor wants to know whether taking the statistics series improved students' inherent math abilities as measured by a 100-point assessment. Students complete the assessment before they take the first statistics course, after they take the basic course, and again after they take the advanced math course. The scores are shown in the following table. What should the instructor conclude?

Subject	Baseline	Basic Course	Advanced Course
1	75	77	80
2	76	78	81
3	83	85	87
4	89	91	93
5	60	62	64
6	63	65	67
7	89	91	94
8	79	81	83
9	91	93	93
10	87	89	91
11	71	75	75
12	72	76	76
13	75	79	79
14	82	86	86
15	82	86	86
16	52	66	64
17	79	83	83
18	72	76	76
19	66	70	71
20	90	91	95
21	80	81	85
22	92	93	92

Subject	Baseline	Basic Course	Advanced Course
23	88	89	93
24	72	73	77
25	73	74	78
26	76	79	81
27	63	66	68
28	59	62	64
29	55	58	60
30	80	83	85

4. The laboratory at a local hospital purchased new coolers for transporting the clinical test samples. It is important to keep the cooler at a constant temperature. The laboratory technicians decide to test the coolers' ability to keep a constant temperature using a standardized sample. A sample of 20 coolers is used. A test sample is put in each cooler, and the inside temperature is measured at baseline (when the sample is put in) and 1, 2, 3, and 4 hours afterward. The temperatures at different points in time are shown below. Can the coolers keep a constant temperature? Temperature is measured in Fahrenheit (Celsius).

Cooler Number	Baseline	Hour 1	Hour 2	Hour 3	Hour 4
1	32.00 (0)	31.90 (–0.05)	31.90 (–0.05)	32.40 (0.22)	34.00 (1.11)
2	30.00 (–1.11)	30.00 (–1.11)	30.10 (–1.05)	30.50 (–0.83)	33.50 (0.83)
3	23.60 (–4.67)	23.70 (–4.61)	23.70 (–4.61)	24.00 (–4.44)	28.10 (–2.17)
4	27.30 (–2.61)	27.30 (–2.61)	27.40 (–2.56)	28.00 (–2.22)	32.30 (0.16)
5	25.50 (–3.61)	25.50 (–3.61)	25.40 (–3.66)	28.20 (–2.11)	30.20 (–1.00)
6	36.00 (2.22)	36.10 (2.28)	36.20 (2.33)	36.50 (2.50)	39.40 (4.11)
7	32.00 (0)	32.10 (0.06)	32.10 (0.06)	32.30 (0.16)	36.40 (2.44)
8	39.10 (3.94)	38.90 (3.83)	38.90 (3.83)	39.90 (4.39)	43.80 (6.56)
9	40.90 (4.94)	41.00 (5.00)	41.10 (5.05)	41.20 (5.11)	47.90 (8.83)
10	34.50 (1.39)	34.50 (1.39)	34.60 (1.44)	34.80 (1.56)	40.60 (4.78)
11	20.90 (–6.16)	20.90 (–6.16)	21.00 (–6.11)	21.40 (–5.89)	25.00 (–3.89)
12	30.00 (–1.1)	29.90 (–1.17)	29.80 (–1.22)	30.50 (–0.83)	35.40 (1.89)
13	27.80 (–2.33)	27.80 (–2.33)	27.90 (–2.28)	28.30 (–2.05)	32.90 (0.50)
14	31.80 (–0.11)	31.90 (–0.05)	31.90 (–0.05)	32.30 (0.17)	37.50 (3.06)
15	31.80 (–0.11)	31.80 (–0.11)	31.90 (–0.05)	32.00 (0)	37.50 (3.06)
16	30.90 (–0.61)	31.00 (–0.56)	31.00 (–0.56)	31.20 (–0.44)	36.40 (2.44)
17	29.10 (–1.61)	29.00 (–1.67)	29.20 (–1.56)	29.50 (–1.39)	34.30 (1.28)
18	25.50 (–3.61)	25.50 (–3.61)	25.60 (–3.56)	25.90 (–3.39)	30.20 (–1.00)
19	27.30 (–2.61)	27.40 (–2.56)	27.40 (–2.56)	27.90 (–2.78)	32.30 (0.17)
20	29.10 (–1.61)	29.10 (–1.61)	29.00 (–1.67)	29.50 (–1.39)	34.30 (1.28)

5. The pulse rates of 30 patients are monitored during an operation. The data below show the pulses (6 seconds) taken every 5 minutes. Are the pulse rates significantly different during the course of the operation?

Subject	Minute 0	Minute 5	Minute 10	Minute 15	Minute 20	Minute 25	Minute 30	Minute 35
1	7.3	8	7.1	7.7	7.2	7.2	7	7.6
2	7.8	8.7	7.2	8.4	7.5	8.1	7.3	7.1
3	7.2	7.4	7.1	7.5	7.2	7.1	7	7
4	7.3	8.4	7.2	7.9	7.5	8.5	7.3	7.1
5	7.7	7.8	7.2	8.4	7.6	7.4	7.1	7.1
6	7.3	7.6	7.2	8.1	7.3	7.2	7	7
7	8.3	8.3	7.7	8.5	7.8	7.8	7.2	7.8
8	9.6	9.8	9.3	9.8	8.8	9.9	9.4	10
9	9.1	8.8	8.6	9.1	7.8	9.3	8.5	8.5
10	9.5	9.7	9	9.6	8.9	9.8	9.2	10
11	7.8	8.5	8.3	9.1	8	9.5	7.6	7.9
12	8.6	8.9	7.8	9	8	8.7	7.8	7.8
13	8.5	9.1	8.1	9.3	8	8.3	7.8	8.5
14	9.2	9.1	8	9.4	8.5	9.6	8.6	8.9
15	8.2	9.2	7.9	9.1	7.8	8.3	7.5	8.2
16	7	7.5	7.1	7.4	7.1	7.1	7	7.7
17	9.7	9.9	9.1	9.7	9	10	9.6	9.9
18	9.8	9.9	9.5	9.8	9	10	9.7	9.9
19	8.6	9.4	8.2	9.5	8.7	9.8	8.3	9.5
20	8.8	9	7.9	8.5	8.1	9.3	8	9.8
21	9.3	9.8	9.3	9.8	8.7	10	9.3	9.3
22	7.5	7.9	7.2	8.1	7.3	7.7	7.1	7.2
23	9	9.3	7.8	9.1	8.2	9.4	8.1	8.5
24	8.9	9.7	8.9	9.5	8.6	9.7	9.4	9.2
25	9.9	10	9.7	9.9	9.4	10	9.9	9.9
26	7.2	7.2	7	7.9	7.1	7.1	7	7.3
27	7	7.1	7	7.2	7	7	7	7
28	7.3	7.5	7.1	7.6	7.3	7.9	7.1	7.6
29	9	9	8.1	9.1	7.8	9.3	7.7	7.1
30	7.5	8.5	7.2	8.5	8	8.9	7.2	7.6

Comparing Means and Controlling for Covariates: ANCOVA

OBJECTIVES

After studying this chapter, you should be able to:

1. Determine when analysis of covariance (ANCOVA) is appropriate to use.

2. Discuss the assumptions, interpretations, and limitations of analysis of covariance.

3. Conduct an ANCOVA using SPSS and interpret the results.

OVERVIEW OF ANCOVA

In the preceding chapters, the statistical methods of analysis of variance (ANOVA)—one-way, N-way, and multivariate analysis of variance (MANOVA)—are described as techniques used to investigate differences among group means. These tests are used when we are interested in the effects of categorical (independent) variables on the means of continuous (e.g., dependent) measures.

This chapter presents another ANOVA technique: the analysis of covariance (ANCOVA). This technique combines ANOVA with linear regression (Chapter 14) to measure the differences among group means when we also want to control for one or more continuous variables that might affect the outcome.

These other continuous variables of interest are referred to as the "covariates" and are considered to be neither a dependent variable nor an independent variable. When we are controlling for the variance in the dependent variable that comes from this covariate, what we are doing is removing that variance from the error term. The effect is the reduction of error variance and therefore an increase in the power of the analysis. Power is the likelihood of correctly rejecting the null hypothesis. With ANCOVA, the control of the extraneous variation also provides a more accurate estimate of the real difference among groups.

For example, if we were going to compare two different programs to help patients with diabetes adhere to a diet, we would want to be able to control for the length of time since diagnosis of the patients in each group. Because we know that the length of time since diagnosis has an effect on adherence to treatment regimen, the effect of time on adherence could be measured and the variation in the outcome due to time since diagnosis could then be accounted for before the two programs were compared.

RESEARCH QUESTIONS

In general, ANCOVA answers the same research question as ANOVA: Do the groups differ in terms of the outcome to a greater degree than we would expect by chance alone? However, with ANOVA, two sets of variables are involved in the analysis: the independent variables and the dependent variable. With ANCOVA, a third type of variable is included: the covariate. The covariate may be entered because it is known to have an effect on the dependent variable, and the removal of its effect decreases the error term. It may also be used in study designs with control groups to account for preexisting conditions that may differ between the intervention and control groups. When subjects are not randomly assigned to groups, it is very important to ensure that the groups are equal on factors that may affect the value of the dependent variable. Even with random assignment, one cannot necessarily assume group equality, particularly when the groups are small. ANCOVA has been used when random assignment has not been sufficient to measure and control for initial differences.

The following studies provide examples of how ANCOVA is used in practice. The first study uses ANCOVA to "equate" two test groups that were not randomly assigned in a study of the effect of an educational intervention on knowledge about breast self-examinations (BSEs). The second study looks at the effect of three interventions (Tai Chi, resistance exercise, and a no-exercise control group) on bone mineral density (BMD) in the elderly. In this study, the study participants were randomly assigned to groups. ANCOVA is used here to both control for the effect of age and to adjust for some pretest differences in the groups.

Note that although ANCOVA has been widely used for such statistical equalization of groups, it is not a cure-all and should be used with caution. Some authors condemn its use for anything but the intent to remove another source of variation from the dependent variable; they do not believe that it should be used to equate groups. To use ANCOVA with dissimilar groups, they claim one would have to be able to assert that the groups were essentially equivalent except for differences in the prevalence of the variable(s) being included as covariate(s). This is virtually impossible to know for certain. For more information, see the article by Owen & Froman (1998).

What Is the Effect of an Educational Intervention on Breast Self-Examination?

Wood, Duffy, Morris, & Carnes (2002) tested an educational intervention to promote BSE in older women. In their quasi-experimental design, subjects were not randomly assigned to groups, and it was found that prior to the intervention, the control group differed significantly from the experimental group with respect to knowledge and skill related to BSE. Therefore, those variables were entered into the analyses as covariates so as to statistically control for this difference and isolate the effect of the intervention on the outcome. If the investigators had not done that, they could not have determined whether the significant differences between the two groups after the intervention were due to the intervention or due to the initial differences between the groups in terms of knowledge and skill.

Do Tai Chi Exercises Increase Bone Mineral Density in Women More than Resistance-Band Exercises or No Exercise?

Woo, Hong Lau, & Lynn (2007) examined the effect of different types of exercise on, among other things, bone mineral density (BMD) in a group of community-dwelling elderly women. In this study, the women were assigned to one of three conditions: no exercise, Tai Chi classes three times per week, or resistance-band exercises three times per week. At baseline, there were differences in quadriceps strength and spine BMD (but not hip BMD) in the three groups. At 12 months, the mean change in BMD at the hip was examined for the three groups. Using ANCOVA to control for age, pretest quadriceps strength, and pretest spine BMD, the researchers found a modest positive effect in the exercise groups as compared with the control group.

TYPE OF DATA REQUIRED

As with ANOVA, one or more categorical variables are independent variables, and the dependent variable is continuous and meets the requirements of normal distribution and equality of variance across groups. In addition, the covariate should be a continuous variable. This is discussed in further detail in the following section.

ASSUMPTIONS

To ensure a valid interpretation of ANCOVA results, several assumptions should be met. These assumptions are based on requirements necessary for the validity of the regression and the ANOVA components of the test. The first three assumptions are those associated with ANOVA:

1. The groups should be mutually exclusive.
2. The variances of the groups should be equivalent (homogeneity of variance).
3. The dependent variable should be normally distributed.

There are three additional assumptions for ANCOVA:

1. The covariate should be a continuous variable.

If a variable is at the nominal level, it cannot be used as a covariate. (However, a nominal variable may be included as an additional independent variable in ANOVA, rather than as a covariate.)

2. The covariate and the dependent variable must show a linear relationship.

When this assumption is violated, the analysis will have little benefit, because there will be little reduction in error variance. The test is most effective when that relationship lies above Pearson $r = 0.30$. The stronger the linear correlation, the more effective the ANCOVA analysis will be. That is, the more the two variables are related in a linear way, the greater is the reduction in error variance by controlling for the covariate. If the relationship between the covariate and the dependent variable is not linear, one appropriate test would be N-way ANOVA; the covariate would have to be transformed into a categorical variable and then simply included as another independent variable.

3. The direction and strength of the relationship between the covariate and the dependent variable must be similar in each group.

We call this requirement *homogeneity of regression across groups*. When there is homogeneity of regression, the regression lines will be parallel. When this assumption is violated, the chance of a type I error is increased. This assumption can be expressed in another way: The independent variable should not have an effect on the relationship between the covariate and the dependent variable (i.e., no interaction effect between the covariate and the independent variable on the dependent variable). Another way to say this is that the covariate should have the same effect on the dependent variable in all the groups.

STEP-BY-STEP PROCEDURE FOR COMPUTING ANCOVA USING SPSS

Low BMD is a clinical and public health concern because it is a risk factor for medical conditions such as osteopenia and osteoporosis. Previous research has shown that both exercise and increased daily fruit and vegetable servings can be beneficial in combating low BMD. We also know that exercise habits and diet are often associated with each other such that those who exercise tend to also eat more fruit and vegetables.

The research question that will be used to illustrate the use of ANCOVA is "Is the level of exercise related to BMD in a group of healthy community-dwelling women once fruit and vegetable intake is controlled for?" We will use the data in Table 10-1 to answer this question. "ID" is the participant ID (we have data from 100 women), "BMD" is bone mineral density (measured as the amount of matter per square centimeter of bones), "Produce" is the number of servings of produce (fruits and vegetables) consumed daily, and "Exercise" is whether the woman exercises at least three times a week. The data are shown in Table 10-1, the tests of the assumptions are shown in Table 10-2, and the results are shown in Table 10-3.

Table 10-1	DATA ABOUT EXERCISE, NUTRITION, AND BMD						
ID	Exercise	Produce	BMD	ID	Exercise	Produce	BMD
1	0	6.00	1.00	51	0	7.00	1.08
2	1	3.00	.87	52	1	7.00	1.04
3	0	3.00	.51	53	0	3.00	.66
4	1	7.00	.95	54	1	3.00	.39
5	0	3.00	1.03	55	0	3.00	.41
6	1	7.00	1.04	56	1	5.00	.49
7	0	5.00	.40	57	1	10.00	1.05
8	0	9.00	.90	58	1	5.00	.61
9	1	5.00	.61	59	1	17.00	.81
10	1	8.00	1.34	60	1	1.00	.40
11	0	5.00	.62	61	0	3.00	.36
12	0	12.00	1.23	62	0	6.00	.52
13	1	5.00	.75	63	0	7.00	1.18
14	1	9.00	1.34	64	1	4.00	1.14
15	1	1.00	.60	65	0	7.00	.85
16	1	6.00	.62	66	0	7.00	.54
17	1	12.00	1.35	67	1	3.00	.96
18	1	5.00	.97	68	1	4.00	.90

Table 10-1	DATA ABOUT EXERCISE, NUTRITION, AND BMD *(Continued)*						
ID	Exercise	Produce	BMD	ID	Exercise	Produce	BMD
19	0	3.00	.82	69	0	4.00	.42
20	1	2.00	.47	70	0	2.00	.60
21	1	5.00	1.31	71	1	9.00	.97
22	1	6.00	1.18	72	0	6.00	.98
23	1	11.00	1.49	73	1	8.00	.94
24	1	8.00	1.29	74	1	6.00	.57
25	0	2.00	.51	75	0	9.00	.99
26	0	2.00	.34	76	1	8.00	1.27
27	0	8.00	1.14	77	0	3.00	.49
28	0	8.00	.61	78	1	14.00	.82
29	0	10.00	.69	79	1	4.00	.88
30	0	.0	.34	80	1	6.00	.94
31	0	12.00	.81	81	0	2.00	.40
32	1	7.00	1.17	82	1	9.00	1.24
33	1	9.00	.88	83	0	1.00	.34
34	0	12.00	.79	84	1	8.00	1.21
35	1	7.00	.68	85	0	7.00	.88
36	0	4.00	.79	86	0	7.00	.52
37	0	3.00	.79	87	0	6.00	.75
38	0	4.00	.90	88	1	4.00	.86
39	0	4.00	.74	89	0	10.00	.59
40	1	10.00	1.30	90	1	10.00	1.33
41	0	7.00	1.39	91	0	2.00	.38
42	1	5.00	.52	92	1	10.00	.80
43	0	11.00	1.22	93	1	8.00	1.34
44	1	5.00	.61	94	1	7.00	.56
45	0	1.00	.38	95	1	3.00	.60
46	0	6.00	1.08	96	0	4.00	.91
47	0	1.00	.35	97	1	5.00	.58
48	1	8.00	1.06	98	0	11.00	1.14
49	0	4.00	.97	99	1	8.00	.94
50	0	2.00	.44	100	0	4.00	.90

Step 1: State the Null and Alternative Hypotheses

- H_0: The two exercise groups do not differ on mean BMD.
- H_A: Once produce consumption is controlled for, there will be a significant difference in the BMD of the two exercise groups.

Step 2: Define the Significance Level (α-Level)

To be able to say that a statistically significant difference between the means exists, the p-value of the computed f-statistic must exceed the critical value for the α-level that is chosen. In this example, an α-level of .05 is used. We will

BOX 10-1 OBTAINING AN ANCOVA USING SPSS

Step 1: The data are entered into an SPSS data set.

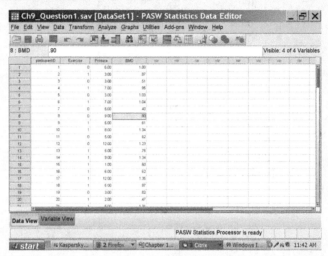

Step 2: The correlation between the covariate and the dependent variable is obtained. Click on "Analyze," and then select "Correlate" and "Bivariate."

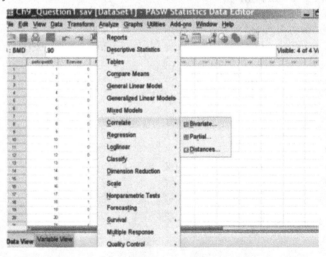

BOX 10-1 OBTAINING AN ANCOVA USING SPSS *(Continued)*

Move over Produce and BMD to the Variable Box and click "OK." The correlation will appear in the output window (Table 10-2).

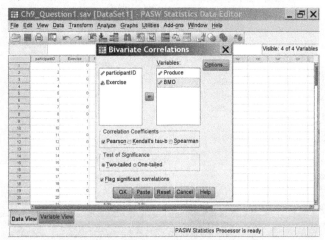

Step 3: The assumption of homogeneity of regression is tested by obtaining an analysis of covariance (ANCOVA) with an interaction term between the covariate and the factor (independent variable).

First, select "Analyze menu," then "General Linear Model," and then "Univariate."

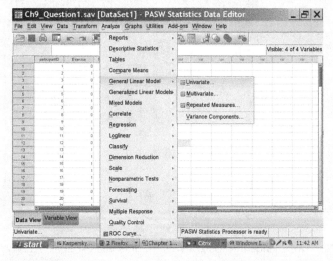

BOX 10-1   OBTAINING AN ANCOVA USING SPSS *(Continued)*

Next, move over "BMD" to the dependent varible slot, "Exercise" to the "Fixed Factors" slot and "Produce" to the "Covariate" slot.

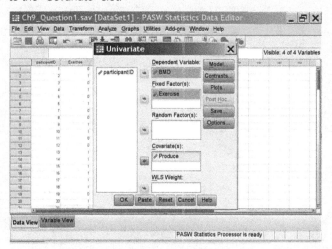

Now, select "Model" and, within this menu, select "Custom." Under "Build Terms," we select "Main Effects." We click on "Exercise" and "Produce" and move them to the space for the model on the right side.

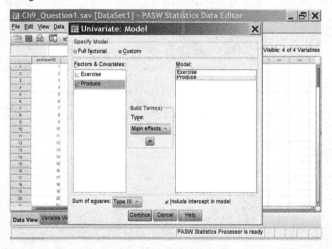

Next, we change the "Build Terms" to "Interaction," again highlight "Exercise" and "Produce," and move them over together as an interaction term.

We then click "Continue" and then click "OK." Table 10-2 contains the results of this analysis as well. Of interest is the interaction between the main effect, "BMD," and the covariate, "Produce." The *F* associated with the interaction is .148 (*p* = .701). Because the *p*-value is

BOX 10-1   OBTAINING AN ANCOVA USING SPSS *(Continued)*

greater than .05, there is no significant interaction between the independent variable and the covariate. Thus, the assumption is met, and it is appropriate to conduct the ANCOVA.

Step 4: The ANCOVA is obtained.

First, select the "Analyze menu," then "General Linear Model," and then "Univariate." Click on "Model" (as in the previous step), and make sure it is set on "Full Factorial" and not on "Custom."

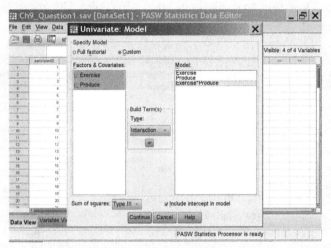

Next, choose "Options." In the Options Box, select "Display Means" for "Exercise" and click on the boxes for "Descriptive Statistics" and "Homogeneity tests." Click on "Continue." Click on "OK." The output will appear in the output window (Table 10-3).

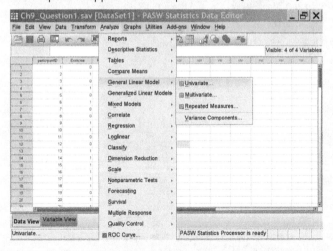

obtain the exact p-value of the ANCOVA from the SPSS printout.

Step 3: Make Sure That the Data Meet All the Necessary Assumptions

In order to complete steps 3 to 6, the ANCOVA analysis must be run. Box 10-1 explains how to do this in SPSS. Once this analysis is run, the output (Table 10-3) is examined to complete steps 3 to 6.

As shown in the printout, the data meet the necessary assumptions. The people in this study constitute an independent random sample as the data are drawn from a large national study. The groups are mutually exclusive because participants are in only one of the two exercise groups. The total sample size is fairly large

Table 10-2	TESTING SOME ASSUMPTIONS OF ANCOVA: SPSS PRINTOUT FROM TWO PROCEDURES

Correlations

		BMD	Produce
BMD	Pearson correlation	1	.576[a]
	Significant (two-tailed)		.000
	N	100	100
Produce	Pearson correlation	.576[a]	1
	Significant (two-tailed)	.000	
	N	100	100

[a]Correlation is significant at the .01 level (two-tailed).
Author's note: Examine the correlation between the covariate (Produce) and the dependent variable (BMD). Note, from the Correlation Table that follows, that they are significantly ($p = .000$) and strongly ($r = .576$) correlated with each other.

Tests of Between-Subjects Effects

Dependent Variable: BMD

Source	Type III Sum of Squares	df	Mean Square	F	Significance
Corrected model	3.424[a]	3	1.141	18.583	.000
Intercept	5.777	1	5.777	94.070	.000
Exercise	.124	1	.124	2.017	.159
Produce	2.534	1	2.534	41.264	.000
Exercise × Produce	.009	1	.009	.148	.701
Error	5.896	96	.061		
Total	77.766	100			
Corrected total	9.320	99			

[a]$R^2 = .367$ (Adjusted $R^2 = .348$).
Author's note: Examine the ANCOVA with the interaction term included. See whether there is an interaction effect between exercise and servings of fruits/vegetables on BMD. Note from the Tests of Between-Subjects Effects table below that there is not. The p-value of the interaction (Exercise × Produce) equals .701 and is not significant.

(N = 100) so that any minor deviations from normality and homogeneity should not substantively affect the results. The dependent variable, BMD, is of ratio measurement scale. It is not quite normally distributed, but we will proceed as ANOVA models are robust to violations of normality. There is homogeneity of variance, as shown by the nonsignificant Levene's test. The covariate, "Produce," is continuous, and it is moderately correlated with the dependent variable ($r = .576$, $p \leq .000$). As shown, there is no interaction effect of Exercise and Produce on BMD. The data meet all the assumptions, and so an ANCOVA will be used.

Step 4: Compute the Mean and Adjusted Means for Each Group

The actual means are the means that we can compute straight from the data. The mean BMD in the no exercise group is .7341 (standard deviation, .288) and the mean BMD in the exercise group is .9206 (standard deviation, .299). However, these means do not take into account the differences in the BMD of the groups that may be due to produce consumption. The adjusted means tell us what the difference in the two groups would be if the produce

consumption was equal. The adjusted mean BMD is .769 in the no-exercise group and .886 in the exercise group. The difference between the two of .117 (e.g., .886 – .769) is what we report. We can see from the difference in these two sets of means that some of the difference we are observing in BMD is likely due to produce consumption and not to exercise (Table 10-3).

Step 5: Examine the ANCOVA Table

The ANCOVA table (Table 10-3) shows the significance of the covariate (Produce) and the factor (Exercise). The covariate, as we expect, is significant. The factor, exercise, has a p-value of .023.

Step 6: Determine Statistical Significance and State a Conclusion

As the p-value of .023 is less than our α-level of .05, we determine that exercise is significantly associated with BMD. We can conclude that after controlling for produce consumption, women who exercise regularly have a significantly higher BMD when compared with women who do not exercise regularly. In particular, the difference in BMD between the two groups, once produce consumption is controlled for, is .117.

Table 10-3	ANCOVA PRINTOUT		
Levene's Test of Equality of Error Variances[a]			
Dependent Variable: BMD			
F	df1	df2	Significance
.783	1	98	.378

Tests the null hypothesis that the error variance of the dependent variable is equal across groups.

[a]Design: Intercept + Produce + Exercise.
Author's note: In the ANCOVA printout, check to make sure that there is homogeneity of variance. As shown in the following table, the Levene's test is not significant (p = .378), and so the assumption of homogeneity of variance is met and ANCOVA can be used.

(Continued)

Table 10-3	ANCOVA PRINTOUT *(Continued)*

Univariate Analysis of Variance

Descriptive Statistics

Dependent Variable: BMD

Exercise		Mean	Standard Deviation	*N*
dimension	0	.7341	.28848	50
	1	.9206	.29870	50
	Total	.8273	.30682	100

Author's note: Check the significance of the ANCOVA. Ignore the descriptive statistics here; we will report the adjusted means in the following table. Note that exercise has a significant effect on BMD.

Tests of Between-Subjects Effects

Dependent Variable: BMD

Source	Type III Sum of Squares	df	Mean Square	F	Significance
Corrected model	3.415[a]	2	1.707	28.047	.000
Intercept	5.811	1	5.811	95.458	.000
Produce	2.545	1	2.545	41.803	.000
Exercise	.325	1	.325	5.343	.023
Error	5.905	97	.061		
Total	77.766	100			
Corrected total	9.320	99			

[a]$R^2 = .366$ (Adjusted $R^2 = .353$).

Author's note: Compare the adjusted means and state a conclusion. The mean BMD among those who exercise (mean = .89) is significantly higher than that of people who do not exercise (mean = .77), after adjusting for servings of fruits/vegetables ($p = .000$).

Estimated Marginal Means

Meets Exercise Guidelines

Dependent Variable: BMD

Meets Exercise Guidelines		Mean	Standard Error	95% Confidence Interval	
				Lower Bound	Upper Bound
dimensionl	0	.769[a]	.035	.699	.839
	1	.886[a]	.035	.816	.956

[a]Covariates appearing in the model are evaluated at the following values: Produce = 6.0500.

CONCEPTUAL UNDERSTANDING OF ANOVA AND REGRESSION TO ANCOVA

To understand the rationale behind the mathematical operations involved in ANCOVA, it is necessary to understand the concept of the residual. In the chapter on correlation (Chapter 11), we explain that squaring the Pearson correlation coefficient results in a quantity, r^2, known as a *coefficient of determination*. This coefficient is often used as a measure of the meaningfulness of r because it is a measure of the variance shared by the two variables. To calculate the proportion of variance that is not shared by the two variables, we would subtract r^2 from 1. For example, if the correlation between two variables is 0.50, then r^2 is 0.25, and 1 minus r^2 is 0.75. We could then state that 25% of the variance was shared by the two variables and 75% was not shared. This 75% is called the *variance of the residual*. Regression analysis is concerned with the regression sum of squares and the residual sum of squares. With ANOVA, the within sum of squares, or the error term, is analogous to the residual sum of squares in regression. Thus, the residual variance is the variation in the outcome not explained by the variables (independent and covariates) in the study. With ANCOVA, we use the residuals to determine whether groups differ *after* the effect of some other variable has been removed.

SUMMARY

ANCOVA is an extension of ANOVA that allows us to remove additional sources of variation, from a continuous variable and from the error term, thus enhancing the power of our analysis. This technique is not a cure-all for difficulties with unequal groups and should be used only after careful consideration has been given to meeting the underlying assumptions. It is particularly important to check for homogeneity of regression (i.e., lack of interaction), because if that assumption is violated, ANCOVA can lead to improper interpretation of results.

CHAPTER REVIEW

Multiple-Choice Concept Review

1. Which type of variable is included in ANCOVA but not in ANOVA?
   a. independent variable
   b. dependent variable
   c. covariate
   d. categorical

2. Power is the likelihood of
   a. correctly accepting the alternate hypothesis.
   b. correctly accepting the null hypothesis.
   c. correctly rejecting the alternate hypothesis.
   d. correctly rejecting the null hypothesis.

3. Which of the following is *not* an assumption of ANCOVA?
   a. The covariate should be a nominal variable.
   b. The covariate and the dependent variable must show a linear relationship.
   c. The covariate should be a continuous variable.
   d. The direction and strength between the covariate and dependent variable must be similar in each group.

4. If an interaction between the covariate and the independent variable exists, then
   a. it can be controlled for by using the common regression coefficient (b).
   b. the p-value will be significant.
   c. the correlation coefficient will equal 1.
   d. ANCOVA should not be used.

5. ANCOVA uses residuals to determine
   a. whether groups differ after the variance of some variable has been removed.
   b. whether groups differ after the effect of some variable has been removed.
   c. the power of the analysis.
   d. the significance of the analysis.

6. With ANCOVA, the effect of the covariate is
   a. subtracted from 1 and then included in the comparison of means.
   b. squared and then included in the comparison of means.
   c. factored into the comparison of means.
   d. removed before the means are compared.

7. Statistical significance of an ANCOVA test is obtained by comparing
   a. the p-value to the α-level.
   b. the p-value to the f-ratio.
   c. the f-ratio to the α-level.
   d. the p-value to the degrees of freedom.

8. If the correlation between two variables is 0.40, what is its r^2 (coefficient of determination)?
   a. 0.16
   b. 0.25
   c. 0.40
   d. 1.00

9. If the correlation between two variables is 0.30, what is its $1 - r^2$?
   a. 0.09
   b. 0.30
   c. 0.70
   d. 0.91

10. If the correlation between two variables is 0.60, the variance of the residual is
    a. 36%.
    b. 40%.
    c. 60%.
    d. 64%.

Choosing the Best Statistical Test

For each of the following scenarios (1 to 10), choose the most appropriate test (a to i).
   a. Independent t test
   b. Mann-Whitney U test
   c. Paired t test
   d. Wilcoxon matched-pairs test

    e. One-way ANOVA
    f. Kruskal-Wallis H test
    g. N-way ANOVA
    h. MANOVA
    i. ANCOVA

1. Are happiness and quality of life (both measured on normally distributed ordinal scales) related to coastal residence (west coast vs. east coast), education level (less than high school, high school only, college graduate), and gender ($n = 750$)?

2. How are self-reported stress levels (high, low, or none) and gender (male or female) related to resting heart rate ($n = 560$, heart rate is normally distributed)?

3. What is the average number of cigarettes smoked the day before as compared with the day after a meeting among 18 members of a smoking cessation program (number of cigarettes smoked is not normally distributed)?

4. Do the number of hours spent in a week by an undergraduate and graduate watching television differ? The sample contains 510 students, and the data (number of hours of television watched) are not normally distributed.

5. A researcher wants to compare two groups of asthmatic children, those who received the flu vaccine versus those who did not, on number of emergency department visits in the past year (not normally distributed, $n = 345$).

6. A group of researchers is interested in determining whether a relationship exists between the nine US census regions (i.e., Northeast or Midwest), breast-feeding status (yes/no), and IQ scores ($n = 6,500$ scores, which are normally distributed).

7. What is the relationship between a toddler's scores on an IQ assessment and being an only child (yes/no)? The sample contains 90 toddlers, and the data (IQ scores) are normally distributed.

8. Does a relationship exist between race (White, Black, Asian/Pacific Islander, other) and satisfaction with the primary care provider (on a scale of 1 to 10, where 1 = completely unsatisfied and 10 = extremely satisfied)? ($n = 52$, satisfaction is not normally distributed).

9. A researcher is interested in examining the efficacy of an intervention to teach people preventive measures to reduce the risk of contracting influenza. After controlling for years of education, do four groups of people (defined by neighborhood of residence and treatment) differ in their knowledge of preventive measures? (It is assumed that years of education is related to knowledge of these measures; years of education is measured from 0 to 20 years and is normally distributed, $n = 400$.)

10. How are race (White, Black, Asian/Pacific Islander, other) and type of occupation (blue collar vs. white collar) related to the number of annual mental health services received ($n = 90$, number of visits is normally distributed)?

Critical Thinking Concept Review

1. Write three hypotheses that could be tested with ANCOVA.

2. Locate an article in your area of interest that uses ANCOVA. Write a brief review of the purpose of the article, the methods, and the findings. Can you identify the dependent variable? The covariate(s)? The independent variable(s)? Why were the covariates chosen? How were they measured?

3. Define the concept of "covariates." Identify how the ANCOVA accounts for covariates, as well as *how* and *why* we adjust for covariates in research.

Computational Problems

1. Research suggests that both maternal smoking history and maternal BMI are associated with the delivery of a low-birth-weight infant. In the data set provided, smoking status is coded as 1 = never smoked, 2 = past smoker, and 3= current smoker. BMI and birth weight are continuous variables. Use the data to
   a. determine whether infant birth weight and maternal BMI are correlated with each other.
   b. determine whether the assumption of homogeneity of regression (i.e., no interaction between birth weight and maternal BMI) is met such that ANCOVA can be used.
   c. conduct an ANCOVA to assess whether the mean birth weight differs by maternal smoking status after taking maternal BMI into account.

2. HITS, a domestic-violence screening tool, has been used in clinical settings to identify women who are currently experiencing intimate partner violence (IPV). HITS consists of four questions, each with an answer ranging from 1 to 5, for a total potential point value of 20. Research has shown that a history of experiencing IPV is associated with experiencing violence in a current relationship. In addition, drug use and age have been found to be associated with experiencing IPV. Using ANCOVA, determine whether these factors (history of IPV and substance abuse) are associated with a score on the HITS scale after taking age into account. Be sure to check that the assumptions necessary for ANCOVA are met.

Correlation Coefficients: Measuring the Association of Two Variables

OBJECTIVES

After studying this chapter, you should be able to:

1. Explain when to use correlational techniques to answer research questions or test hypotheses.

2. Choose between the Pearson and the Spearman correlation coefficients.

3. Hand compute the Pearson and the Spearman correlation coefficients and determine whether they are statistically significant.

4. Use SPSS to compute the Pearson and the Spearman correlation coefficients and correctly interpret the output.

5. Report a correlation coefficient in terms of the direction and strength of association and its statistical significance.

6. Be able to identify and know when it is appropriate to use multiple correlation, partial correlation, and semipartial correlation.

OVERVIEW OF CORRELATION COEFFICIENTS

The term correlation is used in everyday language to indicate association. In this chapter, it concerns a specific type of relation that is measured mathematically; we can calculate a number representing the strength of the relationship. However, a correlation that shows that two variables are related does not necessarily mean that one variable caused the other. It is a mistake to infer causation from correlation alone. For example, there is a relation between the number of alarms in a fire and the extent of the damage. However, the fire alarms themselves did not cause the damage, rather the fire did. Therefore, although a relationship may exist, other factors also may affect the variables under study.

In mathematical terms, a correlation coefficient provides a measure of the strength and direction of the relationship between two variables. This is displayed in graphic terms using a *scatter plot*. A scatter plot shows the relationship between two variables by plotting the data points on a two-dimensional grid. The independent variable is put on the x-axis, and the dependent variable is put on the y-axis. Figure 11-1 displays several scatter plots (graphs A to D). Graph A shows a *positive correlation*, which means that as the first variable (x) increases, the second variable (y) also increases. Graph B shows a *negative correlation* (sometimes called an *inverse correlation*), which means that as x increases, y decreases. Graph C shows two variables that are not correlated with each other in any way. Graph D shows a *nonlinear (curvilinear) relationship*. It is clear from the scatter plots that x and y are related to each other, but it is not a linear relationship. Note that the Pearson correlation coefficient only measures linear (i.e., straight-line)

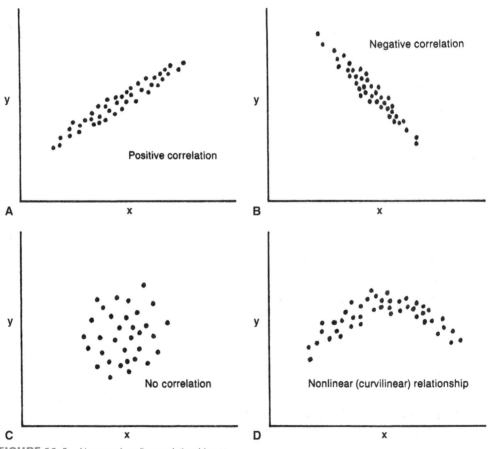

FIGURE 11-1   Linear and nonlinear relationships.

relationships, while the Spearman correlation coefficient measures monotonic relationships, or relationships that are always in the same direction (positive for all values of x and y or negative for all values) but do not have to be precisely linear.

Difference between the Pearson and Spearman Correlation Coefficients

The Pearson correlation coefficient is a parametric test that allows researchers to determine whether an association exists between two variables of interval or ratio measurement scale. The Spearman correlation coefficient is the nonparametric alternative that can be used with ordinal-level data, as well as interval- and ratio-level variables. Sometimes, the Pearson correlation coefficient is estimated for ordinal-level data as well, but in these cases, the Spearman correlation coefficient would be the more appropriate option and the Pearson correlation might lead to incorrect conclusions because the variables do not fulfill the distribution requirements of the test. The main difference between the two tests is that whereas the Pearson correlation coefficient is a parametric test that requires both variables to be normally distributed, the Spearman correlation coefficient does not.

Assessing the Strength and Direction of Relationships with Correlation Coefficients

The Pearson and Spearman correlation coefficients, which are denoted by r, provide a number that indicates both the *strength* and the *direction* of the relationship between the two values. Correlation coefficients can range from –1 to +1. When r equals –1, it indicates a perfect *negative* or *inverse relationship*; when r equals 0, it indicates *no relationship*; and when r equals +1, it indicates a perfect *positive relationship*. The closer a correlation coefficient

is to 0, the weaker the relationship is between the two variables. The amount of variance in the dependent variable that is explained by the independent variable is assessed with a statistic called the *coefficient of determination*. The coefficient of determination is obtained by squaring the Pearson r value, which is simply represented by r^2.

The r^2 ranges between 0 and 1, with a higher value meaning that more of the variance is shared. A visual depiction of shared variance is shown in Figure 11-2. If the first circle in the figure represents all of the variance in x and the second circle represents all of the variance in y, then the extent to which the two circles overlap is the shared variance (r^2). Another way to view this is to say that r^2 represents the amount of variance in the dependent variable y as explained by the independent variable x.

There is some debate about the way the relative value of r should be interpreted in terms of the strength of the association. In part, the interpretation of r should depend on whether researchers are studying the relationship of two different variables to each other (e.g., hours studied and test score) or two measures of the same variable across time or individuals (e.g., an assessment of test–retest reliability). When examining the relationship of two different variables, several authors have suggested the following: if the absolute value of r is around ±.10, it should be regarded as *weak to nonexistent*, meaning that $.10^2$, or about 1%, of the variance is shared; if the absolute value of r is around .30, it should be regarded as *moderate or typical*, meaning that $.3^2$, or about 9%,

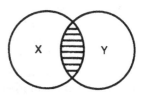

FIGURE 11-2 Shared Variance of X and Y.

of the variance is shared; and if the absolute value of r is ±.50, it should be regarded as *substantial*, meaning that $.5^2$, or 25%, or more of the variance is shared (Cohen, 1988; Gliner, Morgan, & Harmon, 2002; Kraemer et al., 2003). When examining the relationship of two variables that are essentially measuring the same thing, a much higher correlation would be expected, and the interpretation would be adjusted accordingly.

RESEARCH QUESTION

Correlational techniques are used to study the relationship of two different variables, or the same variable can be measured at two different points in time. In exploratory studies, one intent is to determine whether relationships exist; in hypothesis-testing studies, they are used to test a hypothesis about a particular relationship. They may also be used to answer the questions about the reliability and validity of variables.

The studies presented here illustrate different uses of the Pearson and the Spearman correlation coefficients. In the first two studies, the extent to which one variable is associated with another is determined using correlation coefficients. In the third study, the correlation coefficient is used to assess the test–retest reliability of a scale. In the fourth study, the concurrent validity of a measurement scale is assessed. The questions asked in all of these studies can be answered using either the Pearson or the Spearman correlation coefficient.

Is Maternal Competence Associated with Social Support?

This question was addressed by Tarkka (2003) in her study of the predictors of maternal competence in first-time mothers of 8-month-old infants. The study used data from the third wave of a longitudinal observational study conducted with 248 first-time mothers who had given birth in a large urban hospital. Maternal competence was measured with a 10-item scale (an ordinal measure), and social support was measured with an 18-item social support scale (an ordinal measure). Using the Spearman correlation coefficient, the researchers found that functional social support had a strong positive correlation with self-perceived maternal competence ($r = .45, p < .0001$).

Is Weight Loss in Patients with Alzheimer's Disease Associated with Behavioral Problems?

White, McConnel, Bales, and Kuchibhatla (2004) considered this question in a study of 32 patients with Alzheimer's disease residing in the skilled nursing or assisted-living facilities in two retirement communities. This longitudinal, observational study assessed the association between body mass index (BMI; a ratio measure) and behavioral symptoms as measured with the Neuropsychiatric Inventory: Nursing Home Version (an ordinal measure), at baseline, at 12 weeks, and again at 24 weeks. Using the Spearman correlation coefficient, the researchers found that baseline BMI had a strong negative relationship to higher levels of behavioral symptoms ($r = -.52, p < .01$). In other words, the more behavioral symptoms a patient had, the less he or she was likely to weigh at baseline. The study also found that change in weight loss over 24 weeks was moderately negatively correlated with change in the behavioral symptoms of agitation and aggression ($r = -.37, p < .05$) and more strongly negatively correlated with change in the behavioral symptoms of disinhibition ($r = -.45, p < .05$).

Is a Patient Satisfaction Score Stable Over Time?

A study by Miles, Penny, Power, and Mercey (2003) compared patient satisfaction with nurse-led and physician-led care. To ensure that the patient satisfaction scale used had test–retest reliability, the researchers administered the test to a group of patients and then readministered it approximately 2 weeks later. The Pearson correlation coefficient showed that there was a high correlation between the two scores ($r = .95$, $p < .001$), indicating that the scale had good test–retest reliability.

Does the Groningen Orthopedic Social Support Scale Have Good Concurrent Validity?

The concurrent validity of the Groningen Orthopedic Social Support Scale was examined in this cross-sectional study of 199 arthroplasty patients recruited from one hospital in the Netherlands (van der Akker-Scheek, Stevens, Spriensma, & van Horn, 2004). Concurrent validity is the extent to which the scale being tested correlates with other accepted measures of the same or closely related constructs. This study used a general social support scale, the Social Support List 12, as the closely related construct for comparison. Using a Pearson correlation coefficient, the study found that the Groningen Scale had good concurrent validity, with a correlation of $r = .72$ ($p < .001$).

TYPES OF DATA REQUIRED

The two tests of correlation (Pearson and Spearman) have slightly different requirements in terms of the variable types and distributions, as well as their relationships.

Pearson Correlation

For the Pearson test of correlation to be valid, the following conditions must apply:

- The two variables are on either the interval measurement scale or the ratio measurement scale.

- The two variables are normally distributed.
- The two variables are related to each other in a linear fashion (straight line).
- There are no outliers (variables that fall outside of the pattern of the rest of the data).

The Spearman test of correlation is valid under all the conditions in which the Pearson test of correlation is valid. In addition, the Spearman test of correlation is valid when

- One or both of the variables are on the ordinal measurement scale.
- One or both of the intervals are not normally distributed.
- The two variables are related to each other in a monotonic way (e.g., the direction of the relationship does not change) even if not linear.
- The Spearman test of correlation is less influenced by outliers.

ASSUMPTONS

The relationship between x and y must be linear for the Pearson correlation to be valid; that is, when the two scores for each individual are graphed, they should tend to form a straight line. In practice, the points will not all fall on this line, but they should be scattered closely around it. For the Spearman correlation, the relationship between x and y need not be linear, but it must be monotonic. This means that the direction of correlation between x and y must always be in the same direction, either positive or negative, and cannot be positive in one range of values and then negative in another range of values (e.g., the graph of the two variables cannot be shaped as a parabola). The technique for graphing the relationship between two variables is demonstrated in the next section of this chapter. Other assumptions for the Pearson and Spearman correlation coefficients are shown in Box 11-1.

BOX 11-1   CHOOSING BETWEEN THE PEARSON AND THE SPEARMAN CORRELATION COEFFICIENTS

The Pearson correlation coefficient can be used when the following assumptions are met:

- The study participants constitute an independent random sample.
- There are two variables to be compared.
- The two measures are normally distributed.
- The two measures are of interval or ratio measurement scale. (There are some cases in which the Pearson correlation coefficient may be computed with ordinal data.)
- The two variables have a linear relationship.
- There are not influential outliers.
- For each value of one variable, the distribution of the other variable is normal.
- For every value of the first measure (x), the distribution of the second measure (y) must have equal variance, and for every value of y, the distribution of x must have equal variance. This is called the assumption of homoscedasticity.

The Spearman correlation coefficient can be used when the following assumptions are met:

- The study participants constitute an independent random sample.
- There are two variables to be compared.
- The two measures are of ordinal, interval, or ratio measurement scale.
- The two variables have a monotonic relationship.
- Outliers are less likely to have a major impact on the test.

COMPUTING THE PEARSON CORRELATION COEFFICIENT

The Pearson correlation coefficient is a parametric test used to determine whether a linear association exists between two normally distributed measures of an interval or ratio measurement scale. These measures can be two independent variables, the same variable measured at two different points in time, or two variables that are expected to be closely related (e.g., two different versions of a depression scale).

Step-by-Step Procedure for Computing the Pearson Correlation Coefficient

To illustrate how to compute the Pearson correlation coefficient, we consider the following question: Can a screening test predict success in a statistics class? This question was answered by examining data from 10 graduate students. Each student took the screening test before starting the statistics class. They each completed the class; their final grades are shown in Table 11-1. The details for how to compute the Pearson correlation coefficient are shown in Box 11-2.

Step 1: State the Null and Alternative Hypotheses

First, the null and alternative hypotheses are stated.

- **H$_0$:** The test scores of the screening test taken before the statistics class will not be associated with the final grades.

Table 11-1	SCREENING TEST SCORES AND FINAL GRADES				
Student ID	Pretest Score (*x*)	Final Course Grade (*y*)	x^2	y^2	*xy*
1	39	84	1,521	7,056	3,276
2	22	84	484	7,056	1,848
3	49	92	2,401	8,464	4,508
4	45	82	2,025	6,724	3,690
5	33	78	1,089	6,084	2,574
6	20	77	400	5,929	1,540
7	14	74	196	5,476	1,036
8	31	87	961	7,569	2,697
9	35	88	1,225	7,744	3,080
10	51	83	2,601	6,889	4,233
Total	339	829	12,903	68,991	28,482

Note. The numbers listed in roman (plain) type are the data; the numbers in italics are computed values from the data used to obtain the Pearson correlation coefficient.

BOX 11-2   STEP-BY-STEP COMPUTING OF THE PEARSON CORRELATION COEFFICIENT

Step 1: State the null and alternative hypotheses.

- **H₀:** There is no association between the screening test and the final grades in statistics.
- **Hₐ:** There is an association between the screening test and the final grades in statistics.

Step 2: Define the significance level (α-level), and obtain the critical value for *r*.

- The α-level = .05. The degrees of freedom equal 10 − 2 = 8.
- The critical value from the Pearson *r* table at 8 degrees of freedom and α = .05 (two-tailed) is .632.

Step 3: Make sure that the data meet all of the necessary assumptions.

- The measures constitute an independent random sample.
- There are at least two measures to compare.
- The measures are both normally distributed.
- The measures are both of interval or ratio measurement scale.
- A linear relationship appears to exist between the two variables.

Step 4: Present a scatter plot.

- See Figure 11-3.

Step 5: Perform the computations necessary to obtain a Pearson correlation coefficient.

- Pearson correlation coefficient:

(Continued)

BOX 11-2   STEP-BY-STEP COMPUTING OF THE PEARSON CORRELATION COEFFICIENT *(Continued)*

$$r = \frac{\sum xy - \frac{\sum x \sum y}{N}}{\sqrt{\left(\sum x^2 - \frac{(\sum x)^2}{N}\right) \times \left(\sum y^2 - \frac{(\sum y)^2}{N}\right)}}$$

- The numbers from Table 11-1 are then plugged into the above equation:

$$r = \frac{28,482 - \frac{339 \times 829}{10}}{\sqrt{\left(12,903 - \frac{339^2}{10}\right)\left(68,991 - \frac{829^2}{10}\right)}}$$

$$r = \frac{28,482 - 28,103}{\sqrt{(1,411) \times (267)}}$$

$$r = \frac{379}{614}$$

$$r = .617$$
$$r^2 = .381$$

- The critical value is .632.
- The computed r of .617 is less than .632, so no significant association exists between the two variables.

Step 6: Determine the statistical significance and state a conclusion.

- The screening score is not a significant predictor of the final grade in the statistics class at $\alpha = .05$ (two-tailed).

- H_A: The test scores of the screening test taken before the statistics class will be associated with the final grades.

Step 2: Define the Significance Level (α-Level) and Find the Critical Value

To be able to say that a statistically significant association between the two variables

exists, the computed value of the correlation coefficient (r) must exceed the critical value for the α-level that is chosen. The computed value is the r that is computed by hand or using SPSS, and the critical value is the value of r that is obtained from the table of critical values for the Pearson correlation coefficient (Appendix J). The critical value is that value at which the probability of obtaining that value or one more extreme is at or below the predetermined α.

In this example, we choose an α-level of .05. The degrees of freedom for r are computed as the number of participants minus 2 ($n - 2$). In this case, there are 10 graduate students, so the degrees of freedom equal 8. Because this test is using a nondirectional hypothesis, a two-tailed test is used to illustrate how this procedure is done. (The default in SPSS is a two-tailed test.) The critical value for r with 8 degrees of freedom for a two-tailed test is .632 (see Appendix J). Thus, any correlation coefficient with an absolute value greater than .632 will be considered statistically significant.

Step 3: Make Sure That the Data Meet All of the Necessary Assumptions

The data, as shown in Table 11-1, meet all the assumptions necessary to compute the Pearson correlation coefficient. The people in this study constitute an independent random sample: they are part of the larger group of students taking statistics, selected randomly, and they are not related to each other. There are two variables to compare, and both are normally distributed, as shown in the stem-and-leaf plots (Table 11-2). Both measures are of a ratio measurement scale, and a linear relationship appears to exist between them (see the scatter plot in Figure 11-3). It is assumed that they have a joint normal distribution and that the assumption concerning the distributions and the variance of the subpopulations hold. Because all of the necessary assumptions appear to be met, computation of a Pearson correlation coefficient can proceed.

Step 4: Present a Scatter Plot

The scatter plot is obtained by plotting each point on a graph. The plot is shown in Figure 11-3.

Table 11-2	STEM-AND-LEAF PLOTS FOR THE SCREENING TEST AND FINAL GRADES

Screening Test Stem-and-Leaf Plot

Frequency	Stem-and-Leaf Plot
1.00	1.4
2.00	2.02
4.00	3.1359
2.00	4.59
1.00	5.1

Stem width: 10;

Each leaf: 1 case(s)

Final Grade Stem-and-Leaf Plot

Frequency	Stem-and-Leaf Plot
1.00	7.4
2.00	7.78
4.00	8.2344
2.00	8.78
1.00	9.2

Stem width: 10;

Each leaf: 1 case(s)

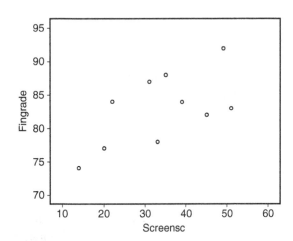

FIGURE 11-3 Scatter plot.

Step 5: Perform the Computations Necessary to Compute the Pearson Correlation Coefficient (r) and the r² and Obtain the Associated p-Value

The equation used to compute the Pearson correlation coefficient (r) is

$$r = \frac{\sum xy - \dfrac{\sum x \sum y}{N}}{\sqrt{\left(\sum x^2 - \dfrac{(\sum x)^2}{N}\right) \times \left(\sum y^2 - \dfrac{(\sum y)^2}{N}\right)}}$$

The Σxy is the cross-product of x and y. To obtain this value, the value of x is multiplied by its corresponding value of y for each data point and then the individual cross-products are summed (see Table 11-1 for computations). The other quantities shown should be familiar by now. Their computations are also shown in Table 11-1. After all of these values have been plugged into the equation as shown in Box 11-2, the resulting r-value of .617 does *not* exceed the critical value of .632. It can be concluded that the correlation is not significant at $\alpha = .05$ (two-tailed).

Step 6: State a Conclusion

The final step is to state a conclusion. Overall, this study found that the correlation (r) between the screening score and the final grade is not significant.

Step-by-Step Procedure for Using SPSS to Compute the Pearson Correlation Coefficient

It is fairly straightforward to compute a Pearson correlation coefficient using SPSS. Box 11-3 illustrates the process with screen shots from the SPSS program. First, the data are entered into the data editor (Step 1). After the data have been entered, the menu system is used to obtain a scatter plot and the Pearson correlation coefficient. To obtain a scatterplot, click on "Graphs" and then "Legacy Dialogs" and select "Scatter/Dot" and follow the steps in Box 11-3. After the scatter plot has been obtained, click on "Analyze" and then follow the steps in Box 11-3 to obtain the Pearson correlation coefficients. Once you have done this, the SPSS output should appear in the output window.

The SPSS output (see Table 11-3) provides the mean and standard deviation of each group as well as all the information needed to obtain r and r^2 and to determine whether they are statistically significant. The first part of the output is labeled "Graph" and contains the scatter plot. The second part of the output is labeled "Correlations." In the "Descriptive Statistics" section, the means and standard deviations are listed for each variable. The mean screening score is 33.9 (standard deviation, 12.5), and the mean final grade is 82.9 (standard deviation, 5.45).

Table 11-3	**SPSS OUTPUT FROM A PEARSON CORRELATION COEFFICIENT**

Descriptive Statistics

	Mean	Standard Deviation	N
Screensc	33.90	12.521	10
Fingrade	82.90	5.446	10

Correlations

		Screensc	Fingrade
Screensc	Pearson correlation	1	.617
	Significance (two-tailed)		.057
	N	10	10
Fingrade	Pearson correlation	.617	1
	Significance (two-tailed)	.057	
	N	10	10

BOX 11-3   OBTAINING A PEARSON CORRELATION COEFFICIENT USING SPSS

Step 1: The data are entered into the SPSS data window.

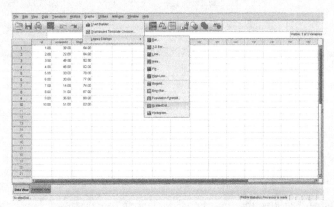

Step 2: The menu system is used to click on "Graphs" and then to select "Scatter."

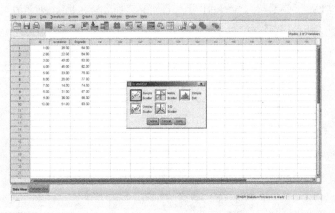

Step 3: When the "Scatterplot" popup box appears, "Simple" and then "Define" are selected.

(Continued)

Step 4: When the "Simple Scatterplot" popup box appears, "fingrade" is moved to the "Y Axis" variable slot and "screensc" is moved to the "X Axis" variable slot. When "OK" is clicked, the scatter plot appears in the output window.

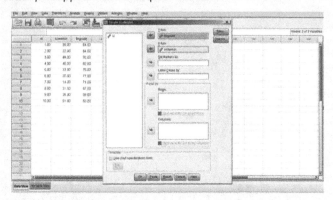

Step 5: The menu system is used to click on "Analyze" and then to select "Correlate" and "Bivariate."

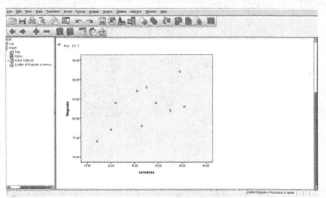

Step 6: When the "Bivariate Correlations" popup box appears, the variables "screensc" and "fingrade" are moved to the "Variables" slot. Then the boxes labeled "Pearson" and "Two-tailed" are checked. The "Options" button is then clicked.

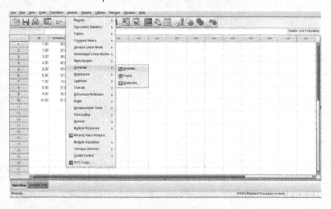

BOX 11-3   OBTAINING A PEARSON CORRELATION COEFFICIENT USING SPSS *(Continued)*

Step 7: When the "Bivariate Correlations: Options" popup box appears, the box "Means and standard deviations" is checked, and then the "Continue" button is clicked. When the "Bivariate Correlations" popup box reappears, the "OK" button is clicked, and the output appears in the output window.

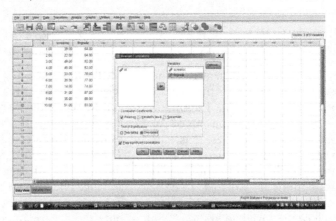

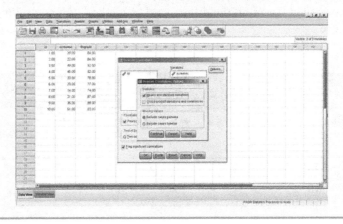

In the box labeled "Correlations," the *r*-value and the associated *p*-value (one-tailed) can be found. The correlation coefficient (*r*) must be squared by hand because it is not provided in the output.

The output is a *symmetrical correlation matrix*. You only have to look at the top half of the matrix. The correlation of "screensc" (screening score) and "fingrade" (final grade) is found in the box where the two intersect. (There are two places where the variables intersect and the correlations are equal.) The *r* value is .617 with an associated *p*-value of .057. Because the actual *p*-value (.057) is greater than the previously set α-level (.05), it is concluded that the two variables do not have a statistically significant linear association.

Putting It All Together

The final step is to state the results and state a conclusion. Overall, this study found that the screening score was strongly positively associated with final grade ($r = .617$), with the screening score explaining 38.1% of the variance in the final statistics grade. However, this association is not statistically significant because $p = .057$, which is greater than .05.

THE SPEARMAN CORRELATION COEFFICIENT

The Spearman correlation coefficient is a nonparametric test that is similar to the Pearson correlation coefficient (Spearman, 1904). It is used to test the monotonic relationship of two ordinal, interval, or ratio variables. It is especially useful in cases in which a Pearson correlation coefficient cannot be used because one or more of the assumptions are violated. To determine if these two variables are correlated, the rankings for each of the variables are used, and a statistic is computed based on the differences in the rank scores.

Step-by-Step Procedure for Computing the Spearman Correlation Coefficient

To illustrate how to compute the Spearman correlation coefficient, the following question is considered: Is the fat content of a cake related to its calorie content? This question is answered by using data from 10 different prepackaged cakes. There is the "calorie content for each cake" and the "percent of calories from fat" in a single serving. The data for this example are shown in Table 11-4, as are the numbers needed to compute the Spearman correlation coefficient. The method for computing the Spearman correlation coefficient using SPSS is found in Box 11-4.

Table 11-4	FAT CONTENT AND CALORIES IN A SINGLE SERVING OF DIFFERENT CAKE BRANDS						
Cake No.	Fat (%) (x)	Calories (y)	Ranking of x	Ranking of y	Rank Differences (d_i)	Squared Rank Differences (d_i^2)
1	20	290	7	8	−1	1
2	10	270	2	7	−5	25
3	11	190	3	5	−2	4
4	12	160	4	1	3	9
5	25	180	9	3	6	36
6	8	175	1	2	−1	1
7	13	185	5	4	1	1
8	22	310	8	10	2	4
9	30	295	10	9	1	1
10	14	210	6	6	0	0
Sums	165	2,275	—	—	—	82

$\sum x_i$

BOX 11-4 COMPUTING THE SPEARMAN RANK CORRELATION COEFFICIENT USING SPSS

Step 1: The data are entered into the SPSS data window. The menu system is used to click on "Analyze" and then to select "Correlate" and "Bivariate."

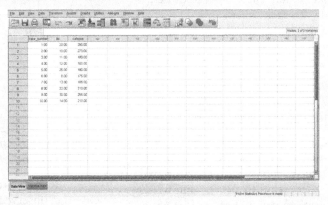

Step 2: In the "Bivariate Correlations" pop-up box, the variables "fat" and "calories" are moved to the "Variables" slot. The box labeled "Spearman" in the "Correlation Coefficients" section is checked. The box labeled "Two-tailed" in the "Test of Significance" section is also checked. When the "OK" button is clicked, the output appears in the output window.

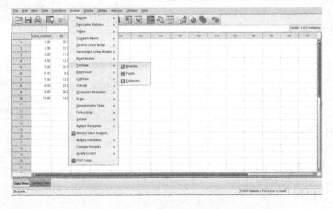

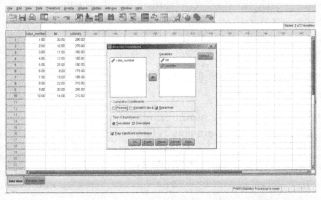

Step 1: State the Null and Alternative Hypotheses

- H_0: Fat content and calories will not be associated with each other.
- H_A: There will be an association of fat content with calories.

Step 2: Determine Statistical Significance (α-Level) and Find the Critical Value for the Spearman Correlation Coefficient (r_s)

In this study, an α-level of .05 and a two-tailed test is used. To be able to say that the two groups are correlated, the computed Spearman rank correlation coefficient needs to exceed the critical value. The critical value is found in one of two tables. When n is between 4 and 30, the critical value is found in the table of critical values of the Spearman test statistic (Appendix K) for the critical values of r_s. When n is greater than 30, a z-score is computed using the formula below, and the actual p-value is obtained by looking up the computed z-score in the z-table (Daniel, 2005) (see Appendix B).

$$z = r_s \times \sqrt{x - n}$$

In this example, because n equals 10, the critical value is obtained from the Spearman rank table (Appendix K). The critical value for the Spearman rank correlation coefficient at α = .05 (two-tailed) and n = 10 is .6364. Thus, if the computed Spearman rank correlation coefficient is either greater than .6364 or less than −.6364, it is statistically significant.

Step 3: Make Sure That the Data Meet All of the Necessary Assumptions

The data appear to meet all of the assumptions of the Spearman correlation coefficient. The measurement scale for both variables is "ratio." There are two variables, and the relationship of these two variables is of interest. Finally, the study participants are independent of each other.

Step 4: Present a Scatter Plot

The scatter plot is shown in Table 11-5 (SPSS output). The relationship appears to be weak and not really linear, but it is monotonic.

Step 5: Perform the Computations Necessary to Compute the Spearman Rank Correlation Coefficient

To compute a Spearman rank correlation coefficient, the observed values for each variable must be ranked separately and then a difference of the ranks for each subject is computed (all computations are shown in Table 11-4). The first step is to rank the fat content from smallest to largest. The smallest number gets a rank of "1," the second smallest a rank of "2," and so

Table 11-5	SPSS SCATTER PLOT EXAMINING FAT CONTENT AND CALORIES IN PACKAGED CAKES

SPSS Output From a Spearman Correlation Coefficient

Correlations

			Fat	Calories
Spearman rho (γ)	Fat	Correlation Coefficient	1.000	.503
		Significance (two-tailed)		.138
		N	10	10
	Calories	Correlation Coefficient	.503	1.000
		Significance (two-tailed)	.138	
		N	10	10

on. When there are two or more measures with the same value, they are "tied for rank." In that case, the ranks of all the positions that have identical measures are averaged. For example, if two data points are tied for fifth place, the rank 5.5 should be assigned to both:

$$5.5 = \frac{5+6}{2}$$

The second step is to rank the calories per slice from smallest to largest in the same way. The third step is to compute the rank difference score for each pair of rankings by subtracting the rank of the second variable from the rank of the first variable for each cake. The set of difference scores is referred to as the $d_i's$. The fourth step is to square each difference score. The last step is to sum the squared differences. In this case, the sum of the squared difference score is

$$\sum d_i^2 = 1 + 25 + 4 + 9 + 36 + 1 + 1 + 4 + 1 + 0$$

$$\sum d_i^2 = 82$$

After the Σd_i^2 has been computed, the Spearman rank correlation coefficient is computed. The basic formula for the Spearman rank correlation coefficient is

$$r_s = 1 - \frac{6\sum d_i^2}{n(n^2 - 1)}$$

where n is the number of study participants (types of cake in this example) and Σd_i^2 is the sum of the squared differences in rank scores between the two variables (x and y).

When there are values that are tied for rank, a correction for ties is performed. The hand computation of a correction for ties goes beyond the scope of this book, but SPSS does it automatically. Interested readers can learn more in the

text by Daniel (2005). The correction for ties does not greatly change the computed value of the computed correlation coefficient unless the number of ties is very large. In this example, the Spearman rank correlation coefficient is computed as follows:

$$r_s = 1 - \frac{6\sum d_i^2}{n(n^2 - 1)}$$

$$r_s = 1 - \frac{6 \times 82}{10(10^2 - 1)}$$

$$r_s = 1 - \frac{492}{990}$$

$$r_s = 1 - .497$$

$$r_s = .503$$

Because the computed value does not exceed the critical value, r is not statistically significant (.503 is less than .6364).

Step 6: State a Conclusion

The final step is to state the results and to draw a conclusion. No significant correlation exists between fat content and calories in a serving of commercially available cakes.

Step-by-Step Procedure for Using SPSS to Compute the Spearman Correlation Coefficient

To use SPSS to compute a Spearman rank correlation coefficient, the data need to be entered into the data editor (see Box 11-4). Then, the scatter plot that shows the relationship between the two variables must be obtained. The same method used earlier in the chapter to obtain a scatter plot of the screening score (screensc) with the final grade (fingrade) is used to obtain a scatter plot. After the scatter plot has been obtained, the menu system is used to obtain the Spearman correlation coefficient. Click on "Analyze" and then follow the directions in

Putting It All Together

Overall, this study found no significant correlation between the percentage of fat in a serving of cake and the calories in that serving (at $\alpha = .05$ level).

Box 11-4. When the "OK" button is clicked, the output appears in the output window (see Table 11-5).

The SPSS output (see Table 11-5) provides the Spearman correlation coefficient and its significance level (p-value). The computed Spearman correlation coefficient is .503, with a p-value of .138. Because .138 is larger than the established α-level of .05, it is concluded that the correlation coefficient is not statistically significant.

OTHER TYPES OF CORRELATION

There are measures other than the Pearson and Spearman r for measuring relationships. An overview is given here, but computational formulas are not presented.

Phi

When both variables being correlated are dichotomous (i.e., each has only two values), a shortcut version of r can be used. Examples of dichotomous variables include gender (male and female), questions that elicit a yes or no response choice, and pass or fail. When using SPSS to analyze your data, you can get Phi by clicking on "Analyze," "Descriptive Statistics," "Crosstabs," "Statistics," and clicking the box next to "Phi and Cramer's V."

Kendall's Tau

This is a nonparametric measure and was developed as an alternative procedure for the Spearman correlation. It is sometimes used when measuring the relationship between two ranked (ordinal) variables. Kendall's Tau might be an alternative if your data seriously violated the assumptions underlying r. It can be calculated in SPSS by checking the "Kendall's Tau-b" box instead of "Pearson" or "Spearman" when running a bivariate correlation test.

Contingency Coefficient

This is a nonparametric technique that can be used to measure the relationship between two nominal-level variables. The variables need not be dichotomous but may have two or more categories. For example, this technique could be used to determine the relationship between ethnicity and political affiliation. To calculate this coefficient in SPSS, you select "Analyze," Descriptive Statistics," "Cross-tabs," "Statistics," and then "Contingency Coefficient."

"Universal" Measure

We have been discussing the monotonic relationship between two variables. Although the relationship may be positive or negative, it is the same across all the observed values. An example of a nonlinear relationship is seen in Figure 11-1D. In this case, low scores on the x variable are related to low scores on the y variable, but high scores on x also are related to low scores on y. Such a relationship is called curvilinear. An example might be the possible relationship between anxiety and test scores. In this graph, those with moderate anxiety could perform the best on tests; those with very low or very high anxiety perform poorly. There is a real advantage to having data plotted to determine whether a nonmonotonic relationship exists, because Pearson and Spearman r cannot be used to test such a relationship.

Eta, sometimes called the correlation ratio, is used to measure a nonlinear relationship. The range of values for Eta is 0 to +1. It can be used with all variables, whether nominal or continuous. Eta is closely related to r and has been called a "universal" relationship because it can be used regardless of the form of the relationship (Nunnally & Bernstein, 1994). When it is used with two continuous variables that have a linear relationship, it reduces to r.

Partial Correlation

When discussing research design, we confront the notion of control. How do we control variance that will distract or mislead us? There are several ways. If we are concerned about the impact of a variable, such as age, we might use random assignment of subjects to groups as a method of control, we might select only one age group, or we might match subjects by age before assigning them to groups. There also are statistical measures of control: We can record the age of the subjects and controls and adjust for that as a variable in the analysis.

One method of statistical control is partial correlation. This technique also allows us to describe the relationship between two variables (or more, if you go to multiple partial correlation) after statistically controlling for the influence of some third variable. When studying research design, you learned that the relationship between two variables may be unclear because of the confounding influence of another variable. For example, if you calculate the correlation between mental age and height in children 1 to 10 years of age, you will find a high correlation. Does that mean that height causes intelligence? The key factor is age, not height. Once you control for age, the relationship between height and mental age becomes trivial.

Semipartial Correlation

This is the correlation of two variables with the effect of a third variable removed from only one of the variables being correlated. It is closely tied to multiple correlation, as is discussed in the next section. Semipartial correlation may be written as $r1(2.3)$ or $ry(1.2)$. The first way indicates the correlation between variables 1 and 2 with the effect of variable 3 removed from 2 alone; the second way indicates the correlation between the dependent variable, y, and an independent variable, 1, with the effect of variable 2 removed from 1 alone.

Multiple Correlation

We have been discussing correlation as measuring the relationship between two variables. This concept can be extended to one in which the relationship is measured between one variable and a combination of other variables. When discussing r, we were talking about one independent variable (x) and one dependent variable (y). In multiple correlation (r), we are talking about more than one independent variable (x_1, x_2, x_3, and so on) and one dependent variable (y). It is also possible to have more than one dependent variable (y_1, y_2, y_3, and so on); this is called canonical correlation.

The multiple correlation, r, can range from 0 to 1. There are no negative r's because the method of least squares is used to calculate r, and squaring numbers eliminates negatives. r^2 is the amount of variance accounted for in the dependent variable by the combination of independent variables. When reporting multiple correlations, r^2 rather than r is often presented.

As we demonstrated in the discussion of semipartial correlation, the calculation of the squared multiple correlation, r^2, may require more than simply adding the squared correlation of each independent variable with the dependent variable because of the confounding effect of one independent variable on the relationship between the dependent variables and another independent variable.

SUMMARY

Correlation is a procedure for quantifying the relationship between two or more variables. It measures the strength and indicates the direction of the relationship. There are a number of different measures of correlation. Which measure you use depends on the number of variables, their characteristics, and their relationship with each other. Multiple correlation measures the relationship between one variable and a weighted composite of the other variables. Partial correlation is a statistical method for describing the relationship between two variables, with the effect of another confounding variable removed. In semipartial correlation, the influence of a third variable is removed from only one of the variables being correlated.

CHAPTER REVIEW

Multiple-Choice Concept Review

1. The Pearson correlation test is best described as
   a. a type of ANOVA.
   b. a parametric test.
   c. a nonparametric test.
   d. none of the above.

2. The Pearson correlation coefficient is best used to determine the association of
   a. two ratio variables to each other.
   b. three or more ratio variables to each other.
   c. two nominal variables to each other.
   d. three or more ordinal variables to each other.

3. The Pearson correlation coefficient is most appropriate to use when
   a. neither of the variables is normally distributed.
   b. one of the variables is normally distributed.
   c. both of the variables are normally distributed.
   d. none of the above.

4. The Pearson correlation coefficient provides a measure of
   a. U-shaped relationships.
   b. the strength of curvilinear relationships.
   c. the strength of linear relationships.
   d. all of the above.

5. Correlation coefficients measure
   a. positive relationships.
   b. inverse relationships.
   c. curvilinear relationships.
   d. a and b only.

6. The Spearman correlation coefficient is best used to examine the relationship of
   a. three or more ratio variables to each other.
   b. two nonnormally distributed ordinal or interval or ratio variables to each other.
   c. two nominal variables to each other.
   d. a nominal variable to a ratio variable.

7. The Spearman correlation coefficient should be used instead of the Pearson correlation coefficient when
   a. neither of the variables is normally distributed.
   b. one of the variables is normally distributed.
   c. both of the variables are normally distributed.
   d. both a and b.

8. A perfect inverse relationship would have an *r* of
   a. −1.
   b. 0.
   c. +1.
   d. 100.

9. The r^2 measures
   a. the variance not shared by the two variables.
   b. strength of the positive relationship of the two variables.
   c. the variance shared by the two variables.
   d. none of the above.

10. The Pearson and Spearman correlation coefficients can be used to measure
    a. the relationship of two independent variables to each other.
    b. the relationship of two related variables to each other.
    c. test–retest reliability.
    d. all of the above.

Choosing the Best Statistical Test

For each of the following scenarios (1 to 10), pick the most appropriate test (a to h) from the following choices:
   a. Independent *t* test
   b. Mann-Whitney *U*-test
   c. Paired *t* test
   d. Wilcoxon matched-pairs test
   e. One-way ANOVA
   f. Kruskal-Wallis H-test
   g. Repeated-measures ANOVA
   h. Friedman ANOVA by rank
   i. Pearson correlation coefficient
   j. Spearman correlation coefficient
   k. Chi-square statistic

1. Is there a difference in the average number of hours per week of homework reported by 60 nursing graduate students taking a required class, with one section taught by an associate professor and the other section taught by an adjunct professor? There are 30 students in each section, and number of hours is not normally distributed.

2. Do students who take *Ginkgo biloba* (for memory enhancement) for the 12 months leading up to the doctoral candidacy examination perform better than students who only take *Ginkgo biloba* for 6 months leading up to the examination? Eighty-eight students participate in the study, and grades are normally distributed.

3. The body mass indexes (BMIs) of 32 same-sex identical twins are assessed at the National Twins Conference. BMI is normally distributed. Is there a difference in BMI of the twins?

4. Sixty-two Alzheimer's patients are studied regarding their cigarette smoking history. Smoking history is coded as never smoked, smoked for 10 years or less, or smoked for 10 or more years. Is there a difference in the mean reaction time the participants have when catching a yardstick dropped vertically between the thumb and index finger of the dominant hand? Reaction time is normally distributed.

5. Dr Sneezie, an allergist, decides to do an in-office test of whether average hours of exercise per week are related to the number of times a patient uses an inhaler in a week. Neither variable is normally distributed in his patient population.

6. Does job satisfaction differ between salaried workers and hourly employees who are ineligible for overtime? Job satisfaction is measured on a five-point Likert scale ($n = 75$).

7. Are adolescent girls who receive the human papillomavirus vaccination at age 12 years more likely to engage in sexual behaviors at a younger age than adolescent girls who receive the vaccine at age 14 or 16 years? The three groups ($n = 150$ each) are questioned 1 year after vaccination regarding how many times in the past month they engaged in sexual activity. Sexual activity is not normally distributed.

8. Is civic engagement related to age in years? Civic engagement is measured on a seven-point Likert scale from minimal involvement to high involvement. Civic engagement and age are both normally distributed ($n = 7{,}567$).

Critical Thinking Concept Review

1. Develop five hypotheses that could be tested with the Pearson or Spearman correlation coefficient.

2. Find the critical value of the Pearson correlation coefficients for each of the following p-values and sample sizes. In each case, assume that a two-tailed test is conducted.
   a. $\alpha = .05$; sample size = 18
   b. $\alpha = .01$; sample size = 45
   c. $\alpha = .10$; sample size = 102
   d. $\alpha = .05$; sample size = 29
   e. $\alpha = .10$; sample size = 8

Computational Problems

For problems 1 to 4, state the most likely hypothesis and compute both a Pearson correlation coefficient and a Spearman correlation coefficient. For problems 1 and 2, perform the computations for all problems both by hand and using SPSS. For problems 3 and 4, use SPSS only. In each case, consider which test, Pearson or Spearman, is the more appropriate choice.

1. An HMO administrator wants to examine the relationship of self-rated health to the number of physician visits made in 1 year. The self-rated health is rated on a scale of 1 to 5, where 1 = poor health and 5 = excellent health; the number of physician visits made in the past year is shown in the table below:

Patient ID	Self-Rated Health	No. of Physician Visits in the Past Year
1	5	2
2	4	1
3	4	2
4	5	3
5	4	3
6	3	4
7	3	4
8	4	4
9	2	5
10	2	5
11	3	5
12	1	4

2. A nurse manager wants to examine the relationship between age in years and the number of poor mental health days that cancer patients report experiencing in the past month. Age is in years, and the number of poor mental health days in the past month is self-rated by the patient.

Patient ID	Age (Years)	No. of Poor Mental Health Days
1	21	30
2	47	30
3	52	30
4	48	20
5	43	14
6	32	7
7	72	6
8	23	5
9	39	5
10	41	5
11	22	3
12	34	3
13	37	3
14	39	3
15	68	3
16	19	2
17	22	2
18	42	2
19	41	1
20	48	1
21	19	0

3. A researcher wants to see if a relationship exists between satisfaction with health care and the number of physician visits made in a year among women. Data from 31 women interviewed by telephone are shown in the table below.

Patient ID	No. of Physician Visits	Satisfaction with Physician
1	1	1
2	1	1
3	1	3
4	1	1
5	1	2

Patient ID	No. of Physician Visits	Satisfaction with Physician
6	2	1
7	2	1
8	2	3
9	2	3
10	2	4
11	3	1
12	3	3
13	3	1
14	3	2
15	3	2
16	4	3
17	4	1
18	4	4
19	4	1
20	4	1
21	4	2
22	4	2
23	4	2
24	5	1
25	5	2
26	6	3
27	7	2
28	10	1
29	10	3
30	11	1
31	12	1

4. A study seeks to examine the relationship between physician–patient communication and patient satisfaction with the physician. Physician–patient communication is measured on a scale from 1 to 16 (higher scores mean better communication). Patient satisfaction is measured on a scale from 1 to 5 (higher scores mean greater satisfaction). Data from 36 patients interviewed after their primary care visits are shown in the table below.

Patient ID	Physician Communication	Satisfaction with Physician
1	11	5
2	12	5

(Continued)

Patient ID	Physician Communication	Satisfaction with Physician
3	12	5
4	12	5
5	13	5
6	16	5
7	10	4
8	10	4
9	10	4
10	10	4
11	11	4
12	11	4
13	13	4
14	13	4
15	4	3
16	6	3
17	6	3
18	8	3
19	9	3
20	9	3
21	9	3
22	10	3
23	12	3
24	14	3
25	4	2
26	5	2
27	5	2
28	6	2
29	8	2
30	9	2
31	13	2
32	4	1
33	4	1
34	4	1
35	5	1
36	9	1

Examining Cross-Tabulations: The Chi-Square and Associated Statistics

OBJECTIVES

After studying this chapter, you should be able to:

1. Compute and interpret odds ratios from a cross-tabulation table.

2. Describe the statistics available to assess the statistical significance of a cross-tabulation table (e.g., chi-square test, Yates' continuity correction, Fisher's exact test, McNemar test) and choose the correct one to use.

3. Hand compute a chi-square statistic from a 2 × 2 cross-tabulation table and interpret the results.

4. Use SPSS to obtain a cross-tabulation table, compute the associated statistics (e.g., chi-square statistic, Fisher's exact test), and interpret the results.

5. Use SPSS to obtain a McNemar test and interpret the results.

6. Write up the results of a cross-tabulation analysis for presentation and publication.

OVERVIEW OF THE CROSS-TABULATION TABLES AND RELATED STATISTICS

Cross-tabulation tables provide a graphical display of the relationship of two categorical variables to each other. These tables show the joint probability distribution of the two variables and are used when both variables are nominal (or ordinal, with a very limited set of categories). As we discussed in Chapter 3, marginal, joint, and conditional probabilities and unadjusted odds ratios can be obtained from a cross-tabulation table. These numbers provide different measures of how an independent variable (e.g., "obesity") affects the chance of having a condition (e.g., "postsurgical mortality").

The statistical significance of a contingency table can be assessed using the chi-square statistic, a similar statistic called the Fisher's exact test, or the McNemar test. The choice between these tests depends on several factors, including the relationship of the two variables to each other (Box 12-1). When the two variables are independent of each other, one of three statistics is most commonly used: a chi-square statistic, a chi-square statistic with a Yates' correction, or a Fisher's exact test. When the two variables are not independent of each other (e.g., two measures on the same person or on paired subjects), then the McNemar test is used.

The chi-square statistic is the most commonly reported nonparametric statistic and is used when the two variables are independent of one another. It compares the actual number (or frequency) in each group with the expected number if the two variables were completely independent of one another. The expected number in each group is computed from the data. The question is whether the expected number in each group under the conditions of independence differs significantly from the actual number in each group.

Sometimes, the data do not meet the assumptions for a chi-square test. In this case, there are two options, the chi-square test with the Yates' correction or the Fisher's exact test. Both of these are discussed in more detail below.

When the cross-tabulation table is composed of paired, or nonindependent, observations, such as before and after measurements on the same individuals or observations of individuals who are in some way related (e.g., twins), the

---

BOX 12-1   CHOOSING BETWEEN THE CHI-SQUARE TEST AND THE McNEMAR TEST

A chi-square test or related test can be used when the following assumptions are met:

- The study participants constitute an independent random sample.
- There are two variables to be compared, and the variables are independent of each other.
- The two measures are nominal or ordinal (with a limited number of categories).
- In 2 × 2 tables, each cell has at least 10 expected frequencies in each cell.
- If there are five to nine expected cases in each cell, the Yates' continuity correction of the chi-square is used.
- If there are fewer than five expected cases in any cell, a Fisher's exact test is used.
- In large 2 × 2 tables, no more than 20% of the cells should have expected frequencies of less than 5. If they do, a Fisher's exact test should be used.
- There are no cells with an expected frequency of 0.

A McNemar test can be used when the following assumptions are met:

- The study participants constitute a paired or matched sample.
- There are two variables to be compared.
- The variables represent paired or matched data.
- There are sufficient cell sizes.

McNemar test is used instead of the chi-square. This test takes the lack of independence in the observations into account when estimating the probability of the observed data (p-value).

RESEARCH QUESTIONS

As discussed in Chapter 3, a cross-tabulation table allows a comparison of the proportion of subjects in different groups who experience an outcome. The research question that we can ask with the associated statistics when we have data on the number of total cases of condition C is "Does the proportion of people in group 'A' who **have** condition 'C' differ significantly from the proportion of people in group 'B' who **have** condition 'C.'" In addition, it is possible to calculate the odds ratio, which compares the odds of having or getting condition "C" in those in group "A" to that of those in group "B."

The statistic that is chosen to test the statistical significance of the relationships depicted in the cross-tabulation table depends on the type of comparison that is being made and the number of participants in the study. For example, in the first two studies below, the researchers compare unrelated groups of people and use tests for independent subjects. In the first study, a group of smokers who received an intervention is compared with an unmatched group that did not receive the intervention; the numbers are fairly large, and a chi-square test can be used. In the second study, the researchers compare patients with non-Hodgkin's lymphoma (NHL) with patients who do not have NHL; because the numbers in some cells are small, the researchers use the Fisher's exact test (similar to the chi-square test). In the third study, the researchers compare two measurements taken on the same woman under different conditions. Because these are repeated measures on the same individuals, the researchers chose the McNemar test, which is appropriate to use when comparing proportions that are paired.

Does Telephone Counseling Increase Smoking Cessation Rates Among Young Adult Smokers?

As part of a study on smoking cessation, the American Cancer Society addressed the following question: Does telephone counseling increase smoking cessation rates among young adult smokers (Rabius, McAlister, Geiger, & Huang, 2004)? In this study, 420 young adult smokers (ages 18 to 25 years) called the American Cancer Society hotline seeking assistance with quitting smoking. All study participants received three booklets on smoking cessation; additionally, half were offered up to five telephone counseling sessions. The independent variable was "receipt of telephone counseling (yes/no)," and the dependent variable was "abstinent from smoking (yes/no)." The study found that those who were offered the telephone counseling were significantly more likely to be abstinent from smoking 3 months later than those who were not offered the telephone counseling (19.6% vs. 9% $p < .005$) as tested by the chi-square test.

Is Autoimmune Disease a Risk Factor for the Development of Non-Hodgkin's Lymphoma?

A case-control study of 278 patients with NHL and a control group of 317 patients with other hematologic disorders considered the following question: Is autoimmune disease a risk factor for NHL (Cuttner, Spiera, Troy, & Wallenstein, 2005)? The independent variable was autoimmune disease (yes/no), and the dependent variable was NHL (yes/no). Overall, 13% of the NHL patients had a prior autoimmune disease compared with 5% of the controls. This was a statistically significant difference as tested by the Fisher's exact test ($p = .001$). The Fisher's exact test was used instead of the chi-square test because of the small cell sizes in the cross-tabulation table.

Does a Woman's Position During Labor Have an Effect on Her Perception of Labor Pain Intensity?

A study of 58 women in Japan who chose natural childbirth was conducted in an obstetrics clinic to answer this question (Adachi, Shimada, & Usui, 2003). The study had women alternately assume the sitting and supine (lying down) positions for 15 minutes during cervical dilatation from 6 to 8 cm and then compared the self-reported labor pain of the women when in each position. Pain was measured by a visual analogue scale that asked women to rate the pain on a scale from 0 to 100. Pain ratings of 30 or greater were classified as "moderate/high." The independent variable was position (sitting vs. supine) and the dependent variable was pain (low vs. moderate/high). Overall, women were significantly more likely to report continuous moderate or higher lumbar pain while in the supine position (34.5%) than while in a sitting position (10.3%). This difference was statistically significant as tested by the McNemar test ($p = .001$). The McNemar test was used because the variable was a repeated measure on the same participants.

TYPE OF DATA REQUIRED

Cross-tabulations are used when both of the variables are nominal (categorical). The type of data required is the same for the chi-square test, the Fisher's exact test, and the McNemar test. Although the most common cross-tabulation

presents data on two dichotomous variables (two variables each of which has two categories), in some cases, one or both variables have more than two categories. The conventions for presenting a 2 × 2 (2 categories by 2 categories) cross-tabulation table are presented in Table 12-1. The details of constructing cross-tabulation tables are explained in detail in Chapter 3. We present a brief review here using the same data that we will use to illustrate computing a chi-square statistic.

Constructing a 2 × 2 Cross-Tabulation Table from Data

We will use data adapted from a study on the exercise habits of graduate students to illustrate how to create a cross-tabulation table. The study asked the following question: "Are male graduate students more likely to exercise frequently (three times a week or more) than female graduate students?" The two variables are students' gender and exercise frequency. The variable "gender" defines the two groups (male and female), and the variable "exercise frequency" defines the two possible outcomes (exercises three or more times a week vs. exercises less than three times a week). The data to help answer this question are shown in Table 12-2. The cross-tabulation table that was constructed from these data is presented in Table 12-3.

The cross-tabulation of these two variables defines four categories; each study participant fits into one and only one category. There are

Table 12-1	CONVENTIONS FOR PRESENTING A 2 × 2 CROSS-TABULATION TABLE		
	Has Condition (+)	Does Not Have Condition (−)	Total
Group 1 (+)	Cell A	Cell B	A + B
Group 2 (−)	Cell C	Cell D	C + D
Total	A + C	B + D	A + B + C + D

Table 12-2	GENDER AND EXERCISE FREQUENCY: RAW DATA				
ID	Gender	Exercise Three Times a Week or More	ID	Gender	Exercise at Least Three Times a Week
101	Female	Yes	201	Male	Yes
102	Female	Yes	202	Male	Yes
103	Female	Yes	203	Male	Yes
104	Female	Yes	204	Male	Yes
105	Female	Yes	205	Male	Yes
106	Female	Yes	206	Male	Yes
107	Female	Yes	207	Male	Yes
108	Female	Yes	208	Male	Yes
109	Female	Yes	209	Male	Yes
110	Female	Yes	210	Male	Yes
111	Female	Yes	211	Male	Yes
112	Female	Yes	212	Male	Yes
113	Female	No	213	Male	Yes
114	Female	No	214	Male	Yes
115	Female	No	215	Male	Yes
116	Female	No	216	Male	Yes
117	Female	No	217	Male	Yes
118	Female	No	218	Male	Yes
119	Female	No	219	Male	Yes
120	Female	No	220	Male	No
121	Female	No	221	Male	No
122	Female	No	222	Male	No
123	Female	No	223	Male	No
124	Female	No	224	Male	No
125	Female	No	225	Male	No
126	Female	No	226	Male	No
127	Female	No	227	Male	No
128	Female	No	228	Male	No
129	Female	No	229	Male	No
130	Female	No	230	Male	No
131	Female	No	231	Male	No
132	Female	No	232	Male	No
133	Female	No			
134	Female	No			
135	Female	No			
136	Female	No			

Table 12-3	GENDER AND EXERCISE FREQUENCY CROSS-TABULATION		
	Exercise Three Times a Week or More	Exercise Less Than Three Times a Week	Total
Women	(A) 12	(B) 24	A + B = 36
Men	(C) 19	(D) 13	C + D = 32
Total	A + C = 31	B + D = 37	A + B + C + D = 68

68 participants in this study: 12 are women who exercise three times a week or more (Cell A), 24 are women who exercise less than three times a week (Cell B), 19 are men who exercise three times a week or more (Cell C), and 13 are men who exercise less than three times a week (Cell D).

Obtaining Marginal Probabilities

The first set of numbers that can be obtained from Table 12-3 is the marginal probabilities. The group membership (row) marginal probabilities are computed below.

The probability of being a woman is computed as follows:

$$\frac{A + B}{A + B + C + D} = \frac{36}{68} = .529$$

The probability of being a man is computed as follows:

$$\frac{C + D}{A + B + C + D} = \frac{32}{68} = .471$$

The outcome (column) marginal probabilities are computed below.

The probability of exercising three times a week or more is computed as follows:

$$\frac{A + C}{A + B + C + D} = \frac{31}{68} = .456$$

The probability of exercising less than three times a week is computed as follows:

$$\frac{B + D}{A + B + C + D} = \frac{37}{68} = .544$$

Obtaining Conditional Probabilities and the Unadjusted Odds Ratio

The probability of exercising three times or more a week *given* membership in each group is computed below.

The probability of exercising three or more times a week in the group of women is computed as follows:

$$\frac{A}{A + B} = \frac{12}{36} = .333$$

The probability of exercising three or more times a week in the group of men is computed as follows:

$$\frac{C}{C + D} = \frac{19}{32} = .594$$

The unadjusted odds ratio gives the odds of women exercising relative to men and is computed as follows:

$$\frac{A \times D}{B \times C} = \frac{12 \times 13}{24 \times 19} = \frac{156}{456} = .342$$

To find the odds of men exercising relative to women, the inverse of the odds ratio is taken:

$$\left(\frac{1}{0.342} = 2.92 \right)$$

In this case, the odds of men exercising are 2.92 times greater than those of women exercising. The above probabilities and odds ratios describe the difference between male and female students in terms of their exercising three or more times a week. However, we do not yet know if these differences are greater than what we would expect to find due to chance. For that, we need to conduct a test of statistical significance, such as the chi-square test.

ASSUMPTIONS UNDERLYING THE CHI-SQUARE TEST

There are three assumptions underlying the chi-square test:

1. The data are frequency data.
2. There is an adequate sample size.
3. The measures are independent of each other.

The *first assumption* is that the data are frequency data, that is, a count of the number of subjects in each condition under analysis. The chi-square test cannot be used to analyze the difference between scores or their means. If the variables are not categorical, they must be categorized before being used in a chi-square test. Whether to categorize depends on the data and the question to be answered.

If the data are not normally distributed and violate the assumptions underlying the appropriate parametric technique, for continuous variables, then categorization might be appropriate. The categories developed must adequately represent the data and must be based on sound rationale. If you had the ages of subjects, you could categorize them as 20 to 29, 30 to 39, and 40 to 49. However, through categorization, you are treating all people within one of your three categories as being equal in age. Does a 29-year-old belong in the same group as a 20-year-old, or is he or she more like a 30-year-old? Specificity and variability are decreased through this categorization, and as a result, the analysis will be less powerful.

The question addressed affects the categorization of subjects. Suppose the researcher was interested in whether being in school affects some categorical outcome measure. Then grouping children as preschool age versus elementary school age would make sense, rather than using

their actual ages. When categories have clinical relevance, statistical analyses that preserve these categories are more likely to provide useful interpretations. They are less likely to provide "differences that do not make a difference."

The *second assumption* is that the sample size is adequate. In cross-tabulation procedures, cells are formed by the combination of measures. None of the cells should be empty. Expected frequencies of less than five in any cells of the 2 × 2 table present problems. In larger tables (more than two categories for one or both variables), many researchers use the rule of thumb that not more than 20% of the cells should have frequencies of less than five (SPSS, 1999a, p. 67). If the cells do not contain adequate numbers, then the variables should be restructured to have fewer categories. It is very important to look at the frequencies of variables before running analyses to ascertain whether adequate numbers of subjects exist. Even with that, however, low numbers in particular cells may not be obvious until the cross-tabulation is run. Most statistical programs print a warning when cell sizes are inadequate. If the cell sizes are problematic, then the researcher should consider restructuring the variable to have fewer categories.

The *third assumption* is that the measures are independent of each other. This means that the categories created are mutually exclusive; that is, no subject can be in more than one cell in the design, and no subject can be used more than once. It also means that the response of one subject cannot influence the response of another. This seems relatively straightforward, but difficulties arise in clinical research situations when data are collected for a period of time. If you are testing subjects in a hospital or clinic, you must be sure that a person who is readmitted is not enrolled in the study for a second time. You also must be sure that subjects in one condition are not communicating with subjects in their own or different conditions in such a way that responses are contaminated.

COMPUTING A CHI-SQUARE STATISTIC

The logic behind the chi-square test is that it compares the "expected frequencies" with the observed frequencies in each cell. By "expected frequencies," we mean the number of observations in each cell of the 2 × 2 table that you would expect to see if the two variables are not associated with each other (are independent). Expected frequencies are computed from the data based on the null hypothesis of no differences between the two groups. The chi-square statistic is then computed using both the observed and the expected frequencies to determine the extent to which they differ. The size of the chi-square statistic depends on the magnitude of these differences. If the differences are large enough to generate a chi-square value that exceeds the critical value, the null hypothesis is rejected, and it can be stated that the relationship between the two variables is statistically significant.

Step-by-Step Procedure for Computing the Chi-Square Statistic for a 2 × 2 Table by Hand

The chi-square statistic is computed with the following formula:

$$X^2 = \sum_{i=1}^{n} \frac{(f_o - f_e)^2}{f_e}$$

where f_o is the observed frequency in the cell and f_e is the expected frequency in each cell. For each of the n cells (four cells for a 2 × 2 table), the following computation should be done:

$$\frac{(f_o - f_e)^2}{f_e}$$

The chi-square statistic is computed by adding together the results of these computations for each cell. The observed frequencies are the actual frequencies (number of observations) in each cell. For a 2 × 2 table, the expected frequencies are computed as follows:

Expected frequencies for cell A are computed as follows:

$$f_{eA} = (A + B)\frac{A + C}{A + B + C + D}$$

Expected frequencies for cell B are computed as follows:

$$f_{eB} = (A + B)\frac{B + D}{A + B + C + D}$$

Expected frequencies for cell C are computed as follows:

$$f_{eC} = (C + D)\frac{A + C}{A + B + C + D}$$

Expected frequencies for cell D are computed as follows:

$$f_{eD} = (C + D)\frac{B + D}{A + B + C + D}$$

The computed chi-square statistic is then compared with the critical value to ascertain statistical significance. The critical value is obtained from the chi-square table (see Appendix L). The critical value is the number that is at the intersection of the α-level that is being used and the degrees of freedom. The degrees of freedom for the chi-square statistic are computed as (# rows − 1) × (# columns − 1); this equals 1 for a 2 × 2 table. Thus, from Appendix L, the critical value for the chi-square statistic for a 2 × 2 table and $\alpha = .05$ is 3.841.

To illustrate how to compute the chi-square statistic, the cross-tabulation table constructed in the previous section is used (Table 12-3). This study considers the following question: Is there a difference in the exercise habits of male and female graduate students? Details of each step and the accompanying computations can be found in Box 12-2.

BOX 12-2   STEP-BY-STEP COMPUTING: A CHI-SQUARE STATISTIC

Step 1: State the null and alternative hypotheses.

• H_0: Gender will not be significantly related to exercise frequency.

• H_A: Gender will be significantly related to exercise frequency.

Step 2: Define the significance level (α-level), determine the degrees of freedom, and obtain the critical value for the chi-square statistic.

The α-level is .05, and the degrees of freedom are $(2 - 1) \times (2 - 1) = 1$. The critical value from the chi-square table at degrees of freedom equal to 1 and an $\alpha = .05$ is 3.841.

Step 3: Make sure that the data meet all of the necessary assumptions.

• The measures constitute an independent random sample.
• There are at least two measures to compare.
• The two measures are independent of each other.
• The measures are both nominal.
• The expected cell sizes are sufficient.

Step 4: Create a cross-tabulation table, obtain the relevant probabilities, and obtain the unadjusted odds ratio

• The cross-tabulation table is shown in Table 12-4. The associated probabilities are shown below:

Group	Proportion Who Exercise Three or More Times Per Week
Women	$\dfrac{A}{A+B} = \dfrac{12}{36} = .333$
Men	$\dfrac{C}{C+D} = \dfrac{19}{32} = .594$
Odds ratio of women exercising relative to men:	$\dfrac{A \times D}{B \times C} = \dfrac{12 \times 13}{19 \times 24} = \dfrac{156}{456} = 0.342$
Odds ration of men exercising relative to women:	$\dfrac{456}{156} = 2.92$

Step 5: Perform the computations necessary to obtain the chi-square statistic.

Step 5A. The expected frequencies for each cell are computed as follows:

Cell A (female exercisers) $f_{eA} = (A+B)\dfrac{A+C}{A+B+C+D}$ $f_{eA} = 36 \times (31/68)$
$f_{eA} = 16.41$

Cell B (female nonexercisers) $f_{eB} = (A+B)\dfrac{B+D}{A+B+C+D}$ $f_{eB} = 36 \times (37/68)$
$f_{eB} = 19.59$

(Continued)

BOX 12-2   STEP-BY-STEP COMPUTING: A CHI-SQUARE STATISTIC
(Continued)

Cell C (male exercisers) $f_{eC} = (C+D)\dfrac{A+C}{A+B+C+D}$ $f_{OC} = 32 \times (31/68)$
$f_{OC} = 14.59$

Cell D (male nonexercisers) $f_{eD} = (C+D)\dfrac{B+D}{A+B+C+D}$ $f_{OD} = 32 \times (37/68)$
$f_{OD} = 17.41$

Step 5B. The proportion of deviation from the expected frequency for each cell is computed using the following formula: $\dfrac{(f_o - f_e)^2}{f}$

Cell A $\dfrac{(f_{oA} - f_{eA})^2}{f_{eA}}$ $= \dfrac{(12 - 16.41)^2}{16.41}$
$= 1.185$

Cell B $\dfrac{(f_{oB} - f_{eB})^2}{f_{eB}}$ $= \dfrac{(24 - 19.59)^2}{19.59}$
$= 0.993$

Cell C $\dfrac{(f_{eC} - f_{eC})^2}{f_{eC}}$ $= \dfrac{(19 - 14.59)^2}{14.59}$
$= 1.33$

Cell D $\dfrac{(f_{oD} - f_{eD})^2}{f_{eD}}$ $= \dfrac{(13 - 17.41)^2}{17.41}$
$= 1.117$

Step 5C. The chi-square statistic is computed as follows:

$$X^2 = \sum \frac{(f_o - f_e)^2}{f_e} = 1.185 + .993 + 1.33 + 1.117 = 4.628$$

Step 6: Determine the statistical significance and state a conclusion.
The relationship between the two variables is statistically significant. The critical value is 3.84, and the computed value is 4.628. Because the computed value of the chi-square statistic is greater than the critical value (4.628 > 2.841), it can be concluded that gender is significantly associated with exercise frequency.

Step 1: State the Null and Alternative Hypothesis

- H_0: There will be no difference in the proportion of male and female graduate students who exercise three or more times a week.
- H_A: There will be a difference in the proportion of male and female graduate students who exercise three or more times a week.

Step 2: Define the Significance Level (α-Level) and Find the Critical Value for the Chi-Square Statistic

To say that a statistically significant difference exists in the groups, the computed value of the chi-square statistic must exceed the critical value for the α-level that is chosen. The computed value of the chi-square statistic is computed by hand or using SPSS, and the critical value is obtained from the chi-square table (see Appendix L). The critical value is that value at which the probability of obtaining that value or higher is below the predetermined α-level.

In this example, an α-level of .05 is used. The degrees of freedom are $(2 - 1) \times (2 - 1) = 1$. The critical value of 3.841 is obtained from the chi-square table (see Appendix L). Thus, computed chi-square values of greater than 3.841 or above will be considered statistically significant. When using SPSS, you will be given the p-value itself to compare to your alpha level and you will not need to compare the chi-square statistic to the critical value.

Step 3: Make Sure That the Data Meet All of the Necessary Assumptions

The data, as shown in Table 12-2, meet all of the necessary assumptions. The participants are from an independent random sample, the measures are independent of each other, and both measures are nominal. As shown in Step 5, the expected size of each cell is greater than 10, so the chi-square test can be used.

Step 4: Create a Cross-Tabulation Table, Obtain the Relevant Probabilities, and Obtain the Unadjusted Odds Ratio

The cross-tabulation table is shown in Table 12-3. Overall, as shown by the conditional probabilities, 33.3% of female and 59.4% of male graduate students report exercising three or more times per week. The odds ratio indicates that the odds of exercising three or more times a week among female students are 0.342 times lower than those of male students.

Alternately, the odds of exercising three or more times a week among male students are $(1/0.342 = 2.92)$ 2.92 times greater than those of female students.

Step 5: Perform the Computations Necessary to Compute the Chi-Square Statistic

The expected frequencies for each cell are computed in Step 5A of Box 12-2. After these are known, the proportion of deviation from the expected frequency for each cell can be computed as in Step 5B of Box 12-2. Finally, the chi-square formula, which is used to sum these together, can be computed as in Step 5C of Box 12-2 to obtain the chi-square value of 4.628.

Step 6: Determine the Statistical Significance and State a Conclusion

The final step is to state the results and draw a conclusion. Because the computed value of the chi-square statistic (4.628) is larger than the critical value (3.841), it can be concluded that gender is significantly related to exercise frequency and specifically that male students are more likely to exercise three times a week or more than female students.

Step-by-Step Procedure for Using SPSS to Create a Cross-Tabulation Table and Compute the Associated Statistics

It is fairly straightforward to compute a chi-square statistic using SPSS. Box 12-3 illustrates the process. First, the data are entered into the data window (Step 1). The three variables are the student ID ("ID"), gender ("Gender"), and exercise ("Exercise"). After the data have been entered, the menu system can be used to obtain the cross-tabulation table and associated statistics by clicking on "Analyze" and then selecting "Descriptive Statistics" and "Cross-tabs" and following the directions in Box 12-3. In particular, when the "Cross-tabs: Cell Display" pop-up box appears, be sure to check the "Observed" button and all of the boxes under "Percentages" (i.e., "Row," "Column," and "Total"). You can also check the "Expected" box to get expected cell counts in case you want to calculate the chi-square statistic yourself.

The SPSS output provides the cross-tabulation table and all the information necessary to assess the statistical significance of the findings (Table 12-4). The first part of the output is labeled "Case Processing Summary," which shows whether any of the data are missing (none are in this case). The second part of the output contains the cross-tabulation table. In this table, the cell, marginal totals, and all the associated probabilities can be found. For example, in the row labeled "Female" with the column labeled "Yes" (Cell A), there are four numbers in the first cell. The first number is the observed number in that cell ($n = 12$). The second number is the conditional probability of having the outcome (exercising three or more times a week) given that the participant is a woman. A total of 33.3% of the women do exercise three or more times a week. The third number is the conditional probability of being a woman among those (given that) who exercise three or more times a week. About 38.7% of the people who exercise three or more times a week are women.

BOX 12-3 OBTAINING A CROSS-TABULATION TABLE AND ASSOCIATED CHI-SQUARE STATISTIC USING SPSS

Step 1: The data are entered into an SPSS data set.

BOX 12-3   OBTAINING A CROSS-TABULATION TABLE AND ASSOCIATED CHI-SQUARE STATISTIC USING SPSS *(Continued)*

Step 2: A cross-tabulation table is obtained by first clicking on "Analyze" and then selecting "Descriptive Statistics" and "Cross-tabs."

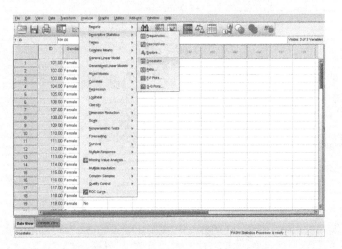

Step 3: When the "Cross-tabs" pop-up box appears, the variable "Gender" is moved to the "Row" slot, and the variable "Exercises 3×/week or more" is moved to the "Column" slot. The "Cells" button is then clicked.

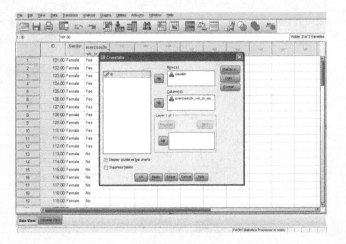

(Continued)

BOX 12-3 OBTAINING A CROSS-TABULATION TABLE AND ASSOCIATED CHI-SQUARE STATISTIC USING SPSS *(Continued)*

Step 4: In the "Cross-tabs: Cell Display" pop-up box, the "Observed" box is checked, and then all the boxes under "Percentages" are checked ("Row," "Column," and "Total"). The "Continue" button is then clicked.

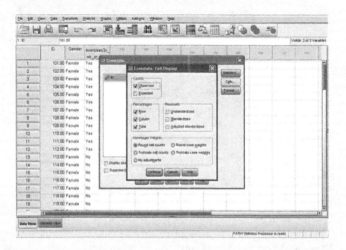

Step 5: In the "Cross-tabs" pop-up box, the "Statistics" button is clicked. In the "Cross-tabs: Statistics" pop-up box, the boxes labeled "Chi-square," "Phi and Cramer's V," and "Risk" are checked, and then the "Continue" button is clicked. When the "Cross-tabs" pop-up box appears, the "OK" button is clicked, and the output appears in the output window.

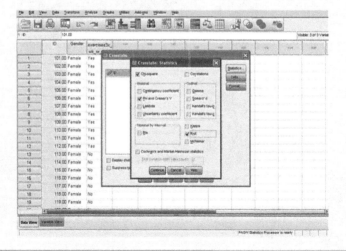

Table 12-4	**SPSS OUTPUT FROM A CROSS-TABULATION TABLE**

Case Processing Summary

	Cases					
	Valid		Missing		Total	
	N	Percent	N	Percent	N	Percent
Gender* exercises3x_wk_or_more	68	100.0	0	.0	68	100.0

Gender* exercises3x_wk_or_more Cross-Tabulation

			exercises3x_wk_or_more		
			No	Yes	Total
Gender	Female	Count	24	12	36
		% within gender	66.7	33.3	100.0
		% within exercises3x_wk_or_more (%)	64.9	38.7	52.9
		% of total	35.3	17.6	52.9
	Male	Count	13	19	32
		% within gender	40.6	59.4	100.0
		% within exercises3x_wk_or_more	35.1%	61.3%	47.1%
		% of total	19.1	27.9	47.1
Total		Count	37	31	68
		% within gender	54.4	45.6	100.0
		% within exercises3x_wk_or_more	100.0	100.0	100.0
		% of total	54.4	45.6	100.0

Chi-Square Tests

	Value	df	Asymptotic Significance (Two-Sided)	Exact Significance (Two-Sided)	Exact Significance (One-Sided)
Pearson chi-square	4.632[a]	1	.031		
Continuity correction[b]	3.641	1	.056		
Likelihood ratio	4.679	1	.031		
Fisher's exact test				.050	.028
Number of valid cases	68				

[a]Zero cells (.0%) have expected count less than 5. The minimum expected count is 14.59.
[b]Computed only for a 2 × 2 table.

(Continued)

| Table 12-4 | SPSS OUTPUT FROM A CROSS-TABULATION TABLE *(Continued)* |

Risk Estimate

		95% Confidence Interval	
	Value	Lower	Upper
Odds ratio for gender (female/male)	2.923	1.087	7.858
For cohort exercises3x_wk_or_more = No	1.641	1.017	2.648
For cohort exercises3x_wk_or_more = Yes	.561	.326	.967
Number of valid cases	68		

Finally, the fourth row provides the joint probability of being both a woman and exercising three or more times a week (17.6% of the total group are women who exercise three or more times a week).

The third part of the printout provides different measures of statistical significance. As shown in the footnote, the box that provides the p-values of the computed statistics, the minimum expected count is 14.59. Because this is above 10, the Pearson chi-square value can be used. The computed chi-square value is 4.632 with an associated p-value of .031. If the minimum expected count was between 5 and 9, the continuity correction chi-square (Yates' continuity correction) would be used instead. If the minimum count was below 5, the two-tailed Fisher's exact test would be used, which SPSS automatically generates for all 2 × 2 tables. You can buy an optional module that will allow you to compute a Fisher's exact test for larger tables.

The fourth and fifth parts of the printout provide information about the strength of the relationship between the two variables. The fourth part, "Symmetric Measures," provides Phi (for 2 × 2 tables) and Cramer's V (for large tables), which are rough measures of the strength of the association between the two variables. Note that these measures are not commonly used anymore, although you may see them in older articles. The fifth part of the printout, "Risk Estimate," provides the odds ratio and the 95% confidence interval around the odds ratio. In this case, Phi is −261, indicating a moderate inverse relationship. The unadjusted odds ratio is .342 with a 95% confidence interval of (.127, .920).

ALTERNATIVE TESTS TO THE CHI-SQUARE TEST

When the data do not quite meet the assumptions of the chi-square statistic, we can use either the Fisher's exact test or the continuity correction.

Putting It All Together

A total of 68 graduate students participated in the study; 52.9% were women and 47.1% were men. Overall, 33.3% of the women and 59.4% of the men exercised three times or more each week. The odds of exercising three or more times a week among women were 0.342 times lower than those of men; alternatively, it could be said that men had an odds of exercising three or more times a week that were 2.92 times higher than those of women. This gender difference in the probability of exercising three or more times a week was statistically significant at $\alpha = .05$ based on the chi-square test.

SPSS provides both of these automatically. The *continuity correction* (also called the Yates' correction) is sometimes used because when the expected frequency in any of the cells in a 2×2 table is less than 10 but greater than 5, the sampling distribution of chi-square for that analysis may depart substantially from normal (Hinkle, Wiersma, & Jurs, 1998). In those cases, the continuity correction can be used to adjust for this departure. The correction consists of subtracting .5 from the difference between each pair of observed and expected frequencies.

The *Fisher's exact test* is an alternative to the Pearson chi-square for the 2×2 table that should be used when any expected cell counts are <5. The Fisher's exact test is considered a more precise method of estimating the *p*-value for contingency tables than the continuity correction and is valid even when expected cell counts are extremely small (<5). The Fisher's exact test assumes that the marginal counts remain fixed at the observed values and calculates exact probabilities of obtaining the observed results if the two variables are independent (SPSS, 1999a). The basic SPSS modules will compute the Fisher's exact test for a 2×2 table, but you will need to purchase specialized modules to compute the Fisher's exact test for larger tables.

THE McNEMAR TEST

The McNemar test is a variation on the chi-square statistic that tests the statistical significance of changes of two paired or otherwise nonindependent measures of dichotomous variables (e.g., variables that can only take on two values). The observations can be paired either because they are multiple measures over time on the same person (e.g., pretest–posttest) or because they are measures taken on a case and a matched control (e.g., twin studies) (McNemar, 1969). Also, some authors recommend using the McNemar test to measure the statistical significance of interrater agreement (Ludbrook, 2004).

Step-by-Step Procedure for Using SPSS to Compute the McNemar Test

To illustrate the use of SPSS to compute a McNemar test, a subset of data adapted from a study of 35 female clients from a battered women's shelter was used (Table 12-5). Among other outcomes, this study assessed whether there were changes in screening positive for depression from shelter entry to shelter exit. The Center for Epidemiologic Studies Depression Scale (CES-D) (Radloff, 1977) was used as the screening tool; as recommended to maximize sensitivity and specificity, a cutoff score of 27 was used (Schulberg, Saul, Ganguli, Christy, & Frank, 1985). Those with scores above 27 were coded as screened positive for depression (further clinical work would be necessary to make a definitive diagnosis). Those with scores of 27 and below were coded as screened negative for depression. The CES-D was administered twice: once upon entry into the shelter and again at discharge from the shelter.

To use SPSS, the data are entered into the SPSS data window (Box 12-4, Step 1). The three variables are the participant ID ("ID"), the dichotomous pretest depression measure ("CESD27P0": 1 = screened positive for depression, 0 = did not screen positive), and the dichotomous posttest depression measure ("CESD27P1": 1 = screened positive for depression, 0 = did not screen positive). In this analysis, the dichotomous pretest depression measure (CESD27P0) is compared with the dichotomous posttest depression measure (CESD27P1). Then, a cross-tabulation table is obtained by using the menu system to click on "Analyze" and then to select "Descriptive Statistics" and "Crosstabs." When the "Cross-tabs" pop-up box appears, the variable "CESD27P0" is moved to the "Row" slot, and "CESD27P1" is moved to the "Column" slot. Then, the "Cells" button is clicked. When the "Cross-tabs: Cell Display" pop-up box appears, "Observed" is checked, as

Table 12-5	PRESHELTER AND POSTSHELTER DEPRESSION LEVELS IN BATTERED WOMEN				
ID	Preshelter Depression (1 = Yes)	Postshelter Depression (1 = Yes)	ID	Preshelter Depression (1 = Yes)	Postshelter Depression (1 = Yes)
101	0	0	119	1	0
102	0	0	120	1	0
103	0	0	121	1	0
104	0	0	122	1	0
105	0	0	123	1	0
106	0	0	124	1	0
107	0	0	125	1	0
108	0	0	126	1	0
109	0	0	127	1	0
110	0	0	128	1	0
111	0	0	129	1	0
112	0	0	130	1	0
113	0	0	131	1	1
114	0	1	132	1	1
115	1	0	133	1	1
116	1	0	134	1	1
117	1	0	135	1	1
118	1	0			

are all of the boxes under "Percentages." The "Continue" button is then clicked. To obtain the statistics of interest in the "Cross-tabs" pop-up box, the "Statistics" button is clicked. In the "Cross-tabs: Statistics" pop-up box, the box labeled "McNemar" is checked, and then the "Continue" button is clicked. Finally, in the "Cross-tabs" pop-up box, when "OK" is clicked, the cross-tabulation table appears in the output window.

The SPSS output (Table 12-6) provides the cross-tabulation table and the p-value of the McNemar test. The first part of the output is labeled "Case Processing Summary," which shows if any of the data are missing (none

are in this case). The second part of the output contains the cross-tabulation table. In this table, the cell, marginal totals, and all the associated probabilities (percents) can be found. The ones of interest in this case are primarily the marginal probabilities. As shown in the table, at entry into the shelter, 60% (21 of 35) of the women screened positive for depression. However, at shelter exit, only 17.1% (6 of 35) screened positive for depression. The p-value of the McNemar test is listed as being .000, so it can be concluded that there is a statistically significant decrease in the proportion of shelter women screening positive for depression between entering and leaving the shelter.

BOX 12-4 **OBTAINING A CROSS-TABULATION TABLE AND ASSOCIATED McNEMAR STATISTIC USING SPSS**

Step 1: The data are entered into an SPSS data set.

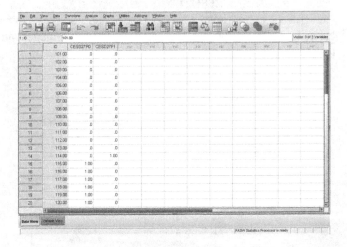

Step 2: A cross-tabulation table can be obtained by clicking on "Analyze" and then selecting "Descriptive Statistics" and "Cross-tabs."

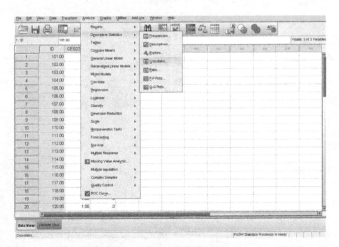

(Continued)

BOX 12-4 OBTAINING A CROSS-TABULATION TABLE AND ASSOCIATED McNEMAR STATISTIC USING SPSS *(Continued)*

Step 3: In the "Cross-tabs" pop-up box, the variable "CESD27P0" is moved to the "Row" slot, and the variable "CESD27P1" is moved to the "Column" slot. The "Cells'" button is then clicked. In the "Cross-tabs: Cell Display" pop-up box, "Observed" is clicked, and all the boxes ("Row," "Column," and "Total") under "Percentages" are checked. The "Continue" button is then clicked.

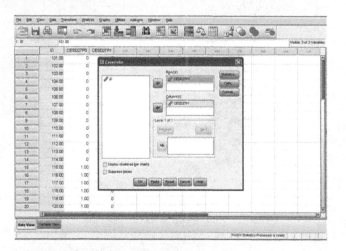

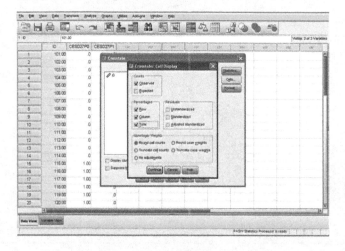

BOX 12-4   OBTAINING A CROSS-TABULATION TABLE AND ASSOCIATED McNEMAR STATISTIC USING SPSS *(Continued)*

Step 4: In the "Cross-tabs" box, the "Statistics" button is clicked. In the "Cross-tabs: Statistics" pop-up window, the box labeled "McNemar" is checked. The "Continue" button is then clicked. In the "Cross-tabs" pop-up box, when the "OK" button is clicked, the output appears in the output window.

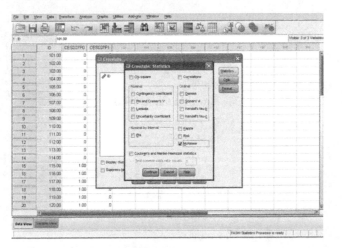

Putting It All Together

A total of 35 women who sought refuge at a battered women's shelter participated in this study. At entry into the shelter, the majority (60%) screened positive for depression using the CES-D. At exit from the shelter, only 17.1% screened positive for depression. This decrease was statistically significant based on the McNemar test with a $p = .000$ (or $p < .001$).

Table 12-6	SPSS OUTPUT FROM A McNEMAR TEST

Case Processing Summary

	Cases					
	Valid		Missing		Total	
	N	Percent	N	Percent	N	Percent
CESD27P0 * CESD27P1	35	100.0	0	.0	35	100.0

CESD27P0 * CESD27P1 Cross-Tabulation

			CESD27P1		
			.00	1.00	Total
CESD27P0	.00	Count	13	1	14
		% within CESD27P0	92.9	7.1	100.0
		% within CESD27P1	44.8	16.7	40.0
		% of total	37.1	2.9	40.0
	1.00	Count	16	5	21
		% within CESD27P0	76.2	23.8	100.0
		% within CESD27P1	55.2	83.3	60.0
		% of total	45.7	14.3	60.0
Total		Count	29	6	35
		% within CESD27P0	82.9	17.1	100.0
		% within CESD27P1	100.0	100.0	100.0
		% of total	82.9	17.1	100.0

Chi-Square Tests

	Value	Exact Significance (two-sided)
McNemar test Number of valid cases 35		.000[a]

[a]Binomial distribution used.

CHAPTER REVIEW

Multiple-Choice Concept Review

1. The chi-square test is best described as
   a. a type of correlation.
   b. a parametric test.
   c. a nonparametric test.
   d. none of the above.

2. The chi-square test is used to determine if the proportions are different among
   a. two groups only defined by one variable.
   b. three groups only defined by one variable.
   c. four groups only defined by one variable.
   d. four or more groups defined by two variables.

3. The McNemar test is used to determine if the proportions are different among
   a. a pretest measure and a posttest measure.
   b. a measure on a case group and a matched control group.
   c. two distinct groups.
   d. a and b only.

4. The Fisher's exact test is used when
   a. the observed frequency in a cell is less than five.
   b. the expected frequency in a cell is less than five.
   c. more precision in the computation is warranted.
   d. none of the above is true.

5. The Yates' continuity correction is used when
   a. the total sample size is at least 30.
   b. the grouping variable is dichotomous.
   c. the expected frequency in at least one cell is less than 10.
   d. all of the above are true.

6. A cross-tabulation is an appropriate way to display data that are
   a. ratio.
   b. interval.
   c. ordinal (with many values).
   d. nominal.

7. In a cross-tabulation table, what does "A + B + C + D" represent?
   a. The number of people with the condition
   b. The number of people without the condition
   c. The total sample
   d. None of the above

8. The McNemar test is used to
   a. compare pretest–posttest proportions on the same person.
   b. compare proportions on a case and matched control.
   c. assess interrater agreement.
   d. do all of the above.

9. Which of the following tests should be used to answer the question: Are men or women more likely to use seatbelts?
   a. Chi-square test
   b. McNemar test
   c. *t* test
   d. a and b only

10. Which of the following tests should be used to answer the question: Are teenagers more likely to use a seat belt after viewing a graphic highway safety video?
    a. Chi-square test
    b. McNemar test
    c. *t* test
    d. a and b only

Choosing the Best Statistical Test

For each of the following scenarios (1 to 10), choose the most appropriate test (a to l).
   a. Independent *t* test
   b. Mann-Whitney *U*-test
   c. Paired *t* test
   d. Wilcoxon matched-pairs test
   e. One-way analysis of variance (ANOVA)
   f. Kruskal-Wallis *H*-test
   g. Repeated-measures ANOVA
   h. Friedman ANOVA by rank
   i. Pearson correlation coefficient
   j. Spearman correlation coefficient
   k. Chi-square test
   l. McNemar test

1. Determine if a relationship exists between ethnic identity (African American, Asian American, White, Hispanic, or Latino) and type of health insurance such as private insurance, Medicaid, or no insurance ($n = 47$).

2. Determine the relationship between BMI, which is normally distributed, and minutes of exercise a week, which is not ($n = 12$).

3. A weight-loss program enrolled 45 pairs of twins. One twin in each pair walked for 15 minutes a day. Did the walking twin lose more weight than the other twin? Weight loss is normally distributed.

4. Determine whether mothers of young children engage in lead poisoning prevention behaviors (yes/no) before and after a nursing education intervention ($n = 126$).

5. In a study of 84 elderly men, a researcher wants to know if systolic blood pressure, which is normally distributed, is related to men's marital status, which is single, married, divorced, or widowed.

6. A study of mentally disabled adults seeks to find out if having a visit from a therapy pet (yes/no) significantly reduces feelings of social isolation. Social isolation is measured on an investigator-developed scale and is not normally distributed ($n = 35$).

7. Determine the relationship between current smoking (yes/no) and excessive snoring as rated by the wives (yes/no) in a group of 122 men.

8. Determine the relationship between the average number of days in a month that people wore a seatbelt, which is not normally distributed, before and after viewing a graphic highway safety DVD ($n = 17$).

9. Determine the relationship between the year in school (freshman, sophomore, junior, and senior) and having a car on campus ($n = 1,058$ students).

10. Determine whether two raters agree on the diagnosis of psoriasis (present or absent) using newly developed criteria ($n =$ ratings of 32 cases by the two raters).

Critical Thinking Concept Review

1. Find the critical value for the chi-square test for all of the following situations:

Situation	Critical Value
2×2 table; $\alpha = .10$	
2×2 table; $\alpha = .05$	
2×2 table; $\alpha = .01$	
2×3 table; $\alpha = .05$	
3×3 table; $\alpha = .01$	

2. Write three hypotheses that could be tested with the chi-square test.

3. Write three hypotheses that could be tested with the McNemar test.

4. Locate an article in your area of interest that uses the chi-square test. Write a brief review of the purpose of the article, the methods, and the findings. Try to reproduce the cross-tabulation table if it is not given.

5. Locate an article in your area of interest that uses the McNemar test. Write a brief review of the purpose of the article, the methods, and the findings. Try to reproduce the cross-tabulation table if it is not given.

Computational Problems

Hand Computation Only

For problems 1 to 5, state the most likely hypothesis, complete the cross-tabulation table, compute the appropriate probabilities (i.e., marginal and conditional), and calculate the chi-square statistic by hand.

1. A new type of steroid cream for the prevention of psoriasis flare-ups is being tested. The cross-tabulation table presents the relationship between the occurrence of flare-ups and use of the steroid cream. What is the relationship between the usage of the cream and the occurrence of flare-ups?

	Flare-Ups		
Uses Steroid Cream	Yes	No	Total
Yes		2	14
No		10	18
Total			

2. A new drug for preventing nasal cancer is tested among experimental rabbits. The data are shown in the table below. Is occurrence of nasal cancer different between the oral and injection groups?

	Nasal Cancer		
Drug Delivery	Yes	No	Total
Oral	52	19	
Injection		5	
Total	91		

3. A study is conducted to examine the relationship between type of health insurance and having or not having an annual physical examination among senior citizens attending a health fair. The data are shown in the table below.

	Annual Physical Examination		
Type of Health Insurance	Yes	No	Total
Traditional Medicare	133		352
Medicare HMO	201	247	
Total			

4. A study is conducted to examine whether education level is related to having regular exercise (30 minutes three times a week) among adults.

	Regular Exercise		
Education Level	Yes	No	Total
Less than high school degree		92	144
High school degree only	44		131
College degree (2 or 4 years)		100	
Total	152		

5. A study is conducted to determine if age is related to happiness over the winter holidays. Happiness is measured by a question asking if the respondent is generally happy during the holidays. The responses include always happy, sometimes happy, and unhappy.

	Happy During the Winter Holidays			
Age (Years)	Always	Sometimes	Rarely	Total
21–30	28	22		81
31–40	17		25	62
41–50		16		
Total	64			213

Using SPSS Only

6. For this problem, please state the most likely hypothesis and then use SPSS to create a cross-tabulation table, obtain the appropriate probabilities, and calculate the appropriate statistic. Sample data from 30 women adapted from a national survey of women's health are presented in the table below. Enter the data for these 30 women, obtain a cross-tabulation table with statistics, and use the SPSS printout to answer the following questions:

    a. Is living at or below 200% of the poverty level associated with not having a medical home (whether or not the person has a usual place to get medical care)?

    b. Is living at or below 200% of the poverty level associated with having an unmet need for medical care?

ID	At 200% of the Poverty Level (1 = At or Below; 0 = Above 200% of Poverty)	Medical Home (1 = Has Regular Source of Care; 0 = Does Not Have Care)	Unmet Need for Care (1 = Hadunmet Need in Past Year; 0 = Does Not Have Unmet Need)
101	0	1.00	.00
102	0	.00	.00
103	0	.00	.00
104	0	1.00	.00
105	0	1.00	1.0
106	0	1.00	.00
107	0	1.00	1.0
108	0	1.00	.00
109	0	1.00	1.0
110	0	1.00	.00
111	0	1.00	1.0
112	0	.00	.00
113	0	.00	.00
114	0	.00	.00
115	0	1.00	.00
116	0	1.00	.00
117	0	1.00	.00
118	1	.00	1.0
119	1	1.00	1.0
120	1	1.00	1.0
121	1	.00	1.0
122	1	1.00	1.0
123	1	1.00	.00

ID	At 200% of the Poverty Level (1 = At or Below; 0 = Above 200% of Poverty)	Medical Home (1 = Has Regular Source of Care; 0 = Does Not Have Care)	Unmet Need for Care (1 = Had unmet Need in Past Year; 0 = Does Not Have Unmet Need)
124	1	1.00	1.0
125	1	.00	.00
126	1	1.00	.00
127	1	1.00	1.0
128	1	1.00	1.0
129	1	.00	.00
130	1	.00	.00

7. A pilot study is conducted to examine the extent to which the self-ratings of nursing students agree with the ratings given to them by standardized patients (trained actors posing as patients). Presented in the table below are data from 17 nursing student–standardized patient pairs. The nursing students performed a physical examination on the standardized patient. The standardized patient and the nursing student both rated whether they believed the examination was complete. Are the two in agreement?

ID	Student Nurse Rating (1 = Complete; 0 = Incomplete)	Standardized Patient Rating (1 = Complete; 0 = Incomplete)
11	0	0
12	1	0
13	1	0
14	1	1
15	1	1
16	1	1
17	0	0
18	1	1
19	1	1
20	1	0
21	0	0
22	0	1
23	1	0
24	1	0
25	1	1
26	1	1
27	0	0

Model Building and Presentation

Statistical Model Building and Logistic Regression

OBJECTIVES

After studying this chapter, you should be able to:

1. Describe the use of models in health research.
2. Explain the advantages of examining several independent variables in the same model.
3. Determine when it is appropriate to use logistic regression.
4. Interpret a computer printout of a logistic regression analysis.
5. Evaluate research reports using this technique.

INTRODUCTION TO MODEL BUILDING

A model is a representation of reality, usually greatly simplified. Models can be physical (e.g., model cars and models of buildings) or conceptual (e.g., organizational charts, blueprints, and mathematical equations). In either case, a good model contains the most essential elements of the phenomena that are represented and allows visualization of the way that the different parts of the model are related. In health sciences research, we build and test conceptual models of biological, health, and social systems to gain an understanding of how these systems function and to make predictions about future activity.

The conceptual models used in health sciences research are typically built around a specific outcome (i.e., the dependent variable) and involve an exploration of how other factors (i.e., the independent variables) are related to the outcome. Model building in health sciences research relies heavily on multivariate statistical techniques. These techniques include several

319

we have already covered, such as *n*-way analysis of variance (ANOVA) and *n*-way analysis of covariance (ANCOVA), as well as multiple linear regression, multiple logistic regression, nonlinear regression models, survival analysis, path analysis, structural equation modeling, and factor analysis. Many of these techniques are complicated to use and interpret. A basic overview of one of the most commonly used techniques, multiple logistic regression, is provided in this chapter.

Regression models are used extensively by researchers. They allow us to determine the strength and direction of an association between two variables after adjusting for the influence of other variables, and they also allow us to identify the best fitting and most parsimonious model to describe the relationship between the dependent variable and a set of independent or predictor variables. There are various types of regression that can be used, including logistic regression, linear regression, polytomous regression, and Poisson regression. The appropriate form of regression to use is determined by the distribution of the outcome, or dependent variable, being modeled.

UTILITY OF MULTIVARIATE REGRESSION MODELS

By multivariate we mean that the model includes more than one predictor variable. Although it is possible, and common, to conduct simple regression in which the association between one dependent and one independent variable is assessed, it is usual to then add additional independent variables to the model, which is referred to as multivariate regression. Multivariate regression models allow researchers to consider the effects of several independent variables on one dependent variable of interest simultaneously. This is important for several reasons:

1. Almost any health outcome (e.g., health status and use of health services) is affected by more than one variable.

2. Many independent variables may be related to each other as well as to the outcome of interest (i.e., have shared variance or are collinear), and multivariate regression models can help researchers to determine which factors are the most important. For example, education level and employment are often linked because people with more education are also more likely to be employed. With multivariate regression, we can determine which variable is more strongly associated with the outcome.

3. Sometimes simple (bivariate) statistics can lead to spurious results. For example, an analysis of food consumption and drowning patterns may indicate that ice cream consumption is significantly associated with drowning, but it is really the season (summer) that is associated with both events. This situation is referred to as confounding, and unless the model controlled for the season, false results would be reported.

4. It is also possible for one variable to mask the relationship of two other variables to each other, which is another type of confounding. In a bivariate analysis, an independent variable may not appear to be significantly associated with a dependent variable and the true relationship may only emerge in a multivariate analysis that takes into account the effect of other independent variables.

STEPS IN CONDUCTING A MULTIVARIATE REGRESSION ANALYSIS

Building a multivariate model is a complex process that requires careful planning. The model is only as good as the thinking processes and the data that are put into it. Although the details differ from technique to technique, the general procedure outlined in Box 13-1 for performing a regression analysis works well for almost any multivariate analysis. This process is a standard one, and variants are found in numerous statistics textbooks that discuss multivariate analysis (Daniel, 2005; Tabachnick & Fidel, 2006). The most important part of conducting a multivariate analysis is planning the whole study; these steps are written with the understanding that they are part of a larger study plan (as discussed in Chapter 1).

The first step is to state the hypothesis being tested. A multivariate hypothesis is more complex than the types of hypotheses discussed in other chapters. Specifically, a multivariate hypothesis states which of the independent variables are expected to remain statistically significant when considered together; it also specifies what the strongest predictors of the dependent variable are expected to be. The second and third steps involve preparing the data for the multivariate analysis. It is critical that the data are clean and free from errors and that the bivariate relationships among the variables in the model are well understood. These steps are necessary to engage in the fourth and fifth steps, that is, the actual building and refining of the model. In general, the building of a multivariate model is an iterative process. It may take a number of different formulations of the model until the correct or best-fitting model is established.

CONCEPTUAL UNDERSTANDING OF LOGISTIC REGRESSION: ODDS RATIOS, ADJUSTED ODDS RATIOS, RISK RATIOS, AND RELATIVE RISKS

Before applying logistic regression, we need to explain, in detail, some of the terms used with this analysis. An *odds* is defined as the probability of occurrence (or presence) over the probability of nonoccurrence (or absence). An odds can be an incidence odds, meaning the odds of getting the outcome, if the data come from a longitudinal study in which a group at risk for the outcome is followed to identify new cases. Alternately, an odds can be a prevalence odds, if both old and new cases are included, as would be the case in a cross-sectional study. An incidence odds would be interpreted as the odds of *getting* the outcome, while a prevalence odds would be interpreted as the odds of *having* the outcome. The *odds ratio* is the odds of the outcome in one group (e.g., those exposed to some hypothesized cause) divided by the odds in another group (those not exposed).

We can illustrate the relationship between relative risk and odds ratios with data from a study on the abuse of pregnant women (Hawkins et al., 1996). Data were collected from 3,055 pregnant women. Of those, 220 had a baby that weighed less than 2,500 g (low birth weight [LBW]), and 2,835 did not. Seven hundred and forty-six of the women reported smoking during their pregnancy, and 2,309 did not. Because the participants in this study were recruited while pregnant and therefore exposure was determined before the outcome occurred, this study can estimate the incidence odds.

Computing an Odds Ratio

Table 13-1 contains probabilities based on the data in Table 13-2. The probability of having a normal weight infant when the mother does not smoke during pregnancy is calculated as the number of normal weight infants in the group with nonsmoking mothers over the total number who did not smoke during pregnancy (2,165/2,309). The resulting probability is .94. In the same way, the probability of an LBW baby with a nonsmoking mother is the number of LBW babies (144) over the total number of nonsmoking mothers (2,309). Therefore, for nonsmoking women, the probability of having a normal weight baby is 2,165/2,309 = .94 and that of having an LBW infant is 144/2,309 = .06. For the smoking mothers, the probabilities are 670/746 = .90 for normal weight and 76/746 = .10 for LBW.

BOX 13-1   **STEPS IN CONDUCTING A MULTIVARIATE ANALYSIS**

Step 1: Define the specific hypothesis that is being tested.

- Specify the dependent variable and the independent variables.
- State the expected bivariate relationships between each independent variable and the dependent variable.
- State the expected relationships among the independent variables.
- State the multivariate hypothesis.
- Choose an α-level.

Step 2: Run univariate frequencies and obtain the appropriate descriptive statistics.

- Ensure that the data are clean: check for out-of-range codes and outliers and correct as necessary.
- Ascertain that sufficient variation is present among the independent variables.
- Describe the distribution of the dependent and independent variable in the sample.
- Make sure that the dependent variable is of the correct form for the model (i.e., nominal with two categories for logistic regression models).
- Recode the variables as needed.

Step 3: Run the bivariate analyses.

- Test the bivariate relationships between each independent variable and the dependent variable as stated in Step 1, noting those that are significant and those that are not.
- Examine the relationships between the independent variables, noting those that are highly intercorrelated ($r^2 \geq .85$) or that seem to be almost identical in cross-tabulation.

Step 4: Choose the initial variables for the multivariate analysis.

- This is the step in which the hypothesis is operationalized.
- Choose the dependent variable in a form that is appropriate to the model.
- Choose the independent variables based on the theory and on the bivariate results. Note that the independent variables identified in Step 3, which are highly intercorrelated or that are almost identical, cannot be in the same model because they are essentially measuring the same thing. By including highly correlated variables in the model, you will find the association of each with the outcome after adjusting for the other, which may leave very little association left over. In general, choose one of the two variables for inclusion, perhaps the one most strongly related to the dependent variable in the simple model.
- Almost always plan to include some sociodemographic measures in the model as these are often important confounding variables.

Step 5: Run the full model.

- You may want to enter independent variables in blocks in order to compare models.
- Ensure that the data meet the assumptions of the model.
- Assess the statistical significance of the overall model and of the individual predictors.
- Conduct diagnostics to check the extent to which the model meets the assumptions.

BOX 13-1   STEPS IN CONDUCTING A MULTIVARIATE ANALYSIS
(Continued)

Step 6: Rerun the model, or compare blocks to obtain the best possible model.

- Strive for model parsimony.
- Compare different models.
- Discuss the practical significance of the results.

The odds of an event are the probability of occurrence over the probability of nonoccurrence. The odds of these events are presented in Table 13-3. The odds of having an LBW infant for smoking mothers are .1/.9 = .11 and for nonsmoking mothers are .06/.94 = .06. The odds ratio is calculated as .11/.06 = 1.83 in Table 13-4. We can say that the odds of having an LBW infant are almost two times greater (1.83 times) in a smoker than in a nonsmoker.

Risk Ratios and Relative Risk

Odds ratios are often used to approximate what epidemiologists call the *risk ratio* or the *relative risk*. A risk is the number of occurrences out of the total. In our example, the risk of LBW among smokers is 76/746 = .1 and the risk of LBW among nonsmokers is 144/2,309 = .06. The risk ratio is the risk of getting the outcome given one condition divided by the risk given another condition. Thus, the risk of LBW is .1/.06 =1.67 times higher for women who smoke compared to those who do not smoke.

The odds ratio is at least equal to relative risk but often overestimates it, especially if the occurrence of the event is not rare. Here the odds ratio was 1.85, and the risk ratio was 1.67, so the odds ratio only slightly overestimates the risk ratio because LBW is not a common occurrence (it is rare). Table 13-5 contains the calculation of the risks of LBW with and without smoking. Table 13-6 contains a calculation of the risk ratio. It is important to note

Table 13-1	PROBABILITIES

Probability of Normal Birth Weight with No Smoking

Normal weight $\dfrac{2165}{2309} = 0.94$
No smoking

Probability of Low Birth Weight (LBW) with No Smoking

LBW $\dfrac{144}{2309} = 0.06$
No smoking

Probability of Normal Birth Weight with Smoking

Normal weight $\dfrac{670}{746} = 0.90$
Smoking

Probability of LBW with Smoking

LBW $\dfrac{76}{746} = 0.10$
Smoking

Table 13-2	THE RELATIONSHIP BETWEEN SMOKING DURING PREGNANCY AND LOW BIRTH WEIGHT		
	Low Birth Weight		
Smoking	No	Yes	Total
No	2,165	144	2,309
Yes	670	76	746
Total	2,835	220	3,055

Source: Data from Hawkins, J. W., Pearce, C. W., Kearney, M. H., Munro, B. H., Haggerty, L. A., Dwyer, J., et al. (1996). *Abuse, women's self-care, and pregnancy outcomes.* Funded by the National Institute for Nursing Research, National Institutes of Health AREA grant 1 R15 NRO4246-01.

Table 13-3	**ODDS**

Odds of low birth weight (LBW) infant, when no smoking:

$$\frac{\text{Probability of occurrence}}{\text{Probability of nonoccurrence}} = \frac{.06}{.94} = .06$$

Odds of LBW infant, with smoking:

$$\frac{\text{Probability of occurrence}}{\text{Probability of nonoccurrence}} = \frac{.10}{.90} = .11$$

Table 13-4	**ODDS RATIO**

Ratio of one probability to the other:

$$\frac{.11}{.06} = 1.85$$

that the incidence odds ratio approximates the risk ratio. If this study design had been cross-sectional in nature and included both old and new cases of the outcome, the odds ratio would be a prevalence odds ratio and would not be a good estimation of the risk ratio.

Odds Ratios Versus Risk Ratios

So the question is: why would we calculate an odds ratio and use this parameter to estimate the risk ratio when we could just calculate a risk ratio? The answer is essentially that we have a statistical technique, logistic regression, that allows us to calculate an odds ratio while simultaneously adjusting for other factors. Because odds ratios are generated by the logistic regression procedure, it is important to understand what they are and not confuse them with actual measures of risk. Also note that the odds ratio from a simple logistic regression model is the crude, or unadjusted, odds ratio. The odds ratio from a multivariate logistic regression model is the odds ratio adjusted for, or removing the confounding due to all the other independent variables in the model.

Understanding Adjusted and Unadjusted Odds Ratios

An example of the difference between unadjusted and adjusted odds ratios can be found in a study of preeclampsia and stroke in young women by Brown, Dueker, and Jamieson (2006). In this study, the researchers asked the following question: Does having preeclampsia during pregnancy increase the odds of having a stroke after the postpartum period has ended? They also asked the following question: Does the increase in odds from preeclampsia remain after adjusting for other factors related to stroke, such as age, race, smoking, body mass index (BMI), diabetes, high cholesterol, and prepregnancy high blood pressure? To answer these two questions, researchers used data from the Stroke Prevention in Young Women Case Control Study. This particular analysis included 261 women who had had a stroke along with 421 neighborhood controls of a similar age who had not had a stroke. The researchers then determined if the women in each group had a history of preeclampsia.

The results of this study are shown in Table 13-7. First, the cross-tabulation table

Table 13-5	**RISKS OF LOW BIRTH WEIGHT**

Without smoking:

$$\frac{144}{2309} = .06$$

With smoking:

$$\frac{76}{746} = .10$$

Table 13-6	**RELATIVE RISK**

$$\frac{.10}{.06} = 1.67$$

examines the relationship between preeclampsia and stroke. The unadjusted odds ratio for stroke is 1.59, which is statistically significant (as tested by the chi-square). This means that women who had preeclampsia had an odds ratio of stroke that was 1.59 times higher (e.g., 59% higher) than that of women without preeclampsia. From the unadjusted odds only, it appears that a significant ($p < .05$) relationship exists between the two variables. However, many other factors related to both stroke and preeclampsia might also explain the relationship between the two variables. This study built three different logistic regression models to account for the effect of some of these variables.

In two of the three models, preeclampsia was a significant predictor of stroke. In the first model (Model A), researchers controlled for age, race, education, and the number of pregnancies. In this model, the adjusted odds of stroke caused by preeclampsia are statistically significant and are also slightly higher than are the unadjusted odds. In other words, when controlling for the effect of age, race, education, and the number of pregnancies, it appears that those with preeclampsia are 1.63 (or 63%) more likely to have a stroke.

In the second model (Model B), researchers controlled for all of the variables in Model A; additionally, they controlled for smoking, BMI, diabetes, elevated cholesterol, and angina or myocardial infarction. After these variables are added to the model, the adjusted odds of having

Table 13-7	**ADJUSTED AND UNADJUSTED ODDS RATIO OF PREECLAMPSIA AS A RISK FACTOR FOR ISCHEMIC STROKE AMONG YOUNG WOMEN**			
Cross-Tabulation Table				
	Stroke		No Stroke	Total
Preeclampsia	40		43	83
No preeclampsia	221		378	599
Total	261		421	682
Odds Ratio Model				
			Value	Significance
Crude odds ratio				
Crude odds ratio computation	$\dfrac{A \times D}{B \times C} = \dfrac{40 \times 378}{221 \times 43}$		1.59	$p < .05$
Adjusted odds ratios				
Model A	Controls for age, race, education, and number of pregnancies		1.63	$p < .05$
Model B	Controls for age, race, education, number of pregnancies, smoking, BMI, diabetes, elevated cholesterol level, and angina or MI		1.58	$p \geq .05$ (not significant)
Model C	Controls for age, race, education, number of pregnancies, smoking, BMI, diabetes, elevated cholesterol level, angina or MI, and prepregnancy hypertension		1.38	$p \geq .05$ (not significant)

BMI, body mass index; CI, confidence interval; MI, myocardial infarction; ns, not significant.
Source: Adapted with permission from Brown D. W., Dueker, N., & Jamieson, D. J., et al. (2006). Preeclampsia and the risk of ischemic stroke among young women. *Stroke, 37,* 1–5. (http://www.strokeaha.org).

a stroke because of preeclampsia are not significant. A similar effect is seen in Model C, which controlled for everything in Model B as well as preexisting hypertension. This study clearly indicates the importance of using adjusted odds ratios. Although it initially appeared that preeclampsia was a risk factor for future stroke, further exploration with logistic regression models indicated that other factors are likely to be responsible for what caused the apparent increase in odds of stroke caused by preeclampsia.

OVERVIEW OF LOGISTIC REGRESSION

Logistic regression models are used when the dependent variable is dichotomous (two categories), but the independent variable can be of any measurement scale. They are fairly straightforward to understand and so we will start the application of multivariate model building with this technique. Studies that lend themselves to logistic regression are those that address the occurrence or nonoccurrence of a disease, mortality (dead or alive), and so forth. It is a good practice to code a dichotomous outcome variable as 1, indicating the presence of the outcome, or 0, indicating the absence of the outcome, and run a logistic regression model. For dependent variables with more than two distinct outcome categories (i.e., polytomous outcomes), logistic regression cannot be used; instead, a different form of regression, called polytomous or multinomial regression, is used.

RESEARCH QUESTION FOR LOGISTIC REGRESSION

Logistic regression models ask the following question: "What is the increase or decrease in odds of getting an outcome, controlling for a number of variables simultaneously, given someone has a risk or protective factor for that outcome?" This question is answered with the adjusted odds ratios that are the central part of the logistic regression results. An odds ratio measures how much more likely (or less likely) an outcome is to be present given certain conditions or exposures. The odds ratio is the ratio of the odds of the outcome among those with a certain characteristic or exposure over (i.e., divided by) the odds of the outcome among those without that characteristic or exposure. Statistical significance of the odds ratio can be determined by the p-value or by looking to see if the value for the odds ratio under the null hypothesis (which would be 1, because if the odds in those exposed equaled the odds in those unexposed, then the odds ratio equals 1) is not included within the 95% confidence interval.

We can use the risk of lung cancer in cannabis smokers and nonsmokers as an illustrative example of odds ratios (Berthiller et al., 2008). When looking at the probability of getting lung cancer in cannabis smokers and nonsmokers, this study found that the odds ratio for lung cancer was 2.4 for ever smoking cannabis. This means that cannabis smokers had odds of getting lung cancer that were over twice that of nonsmokers. In other words, cannabis smokers have approximately (since odds and risk are not exactly the same) 2.5 times the risk of getting lung cancer compared to the nonsmokers. The odds ratio approximates another indicator called the risk ratio (or relative risk), which is the ratio of the probability of getting an outcome (i.e., the proportion that gets the outcome) in those exposed to that of those not exposed. We discussed unadjusted odds ratios in some detail in Chapter 12.

The advantage of multiple logistic regression models (two or more independent variables) is that they allow us to compute adjusted odds ratios, that is, odds ratios that are adjusted to account for the effect of other variables on both the risk factor and the outcome. In the example above, the researchers found that the increased odds of lung cancer remained for cannabis smokers even after adjusting for country of origin, age, tobacco smoking, and occupational exposure. The following two studies both illustrate the utility of these models in obtaining these adjusted odds ratios.

What are the Predictors of Taking Action to Lose Weight among Obese Adolescents?

Using data from the 2002 Youth Risk Behavioral Survey, Bittner Fagan et al. (2008) examined predictors of taking action to lose weight among obese adolescents in Delaware. "Taking action" was defined as the participants modifying their diet and/or increasing the amount of exercise in the past 30 days. The researchers used multivariate logistic regression to look at the association of the following independent variables—age, gender, reported intention to lose weight, and having an accurate perception of their weight (i.e., accurately reporting that they are overweight)—with taking action. They found that the adjusted odds ratio for intending to lose weight was 11.6 (with a p-value $\leq .05$)—this means that the odds of having taken action to lose weight in the past 30 days was 11.6 times higher among those who reported having an intention to lose weight compared to those who did not and that this was statistically significant. None of the other variables examined were significantly associated with taking action to lose weight.

What are the Predictors of Seroconversion After Hepatitis B Vaccination among HIV-Infected Patients?

A study by Pettit et al. (2010) looked at predictors of seroconversion after vaccination against hepatitis B among human immunodeficiency virus (HIV) infected individuals. HIV infection is known to impact response to vaccination. The researchers used multivariate logistic regression and found that a higher CD4 count was associated with higher odds of seroconversion (odds ratio = 1.13, $p = .02$). Because CD4 count was not categorized, the results suggest that for each additional unit of CD4 count, the odds of seroconversion are 1.13 times higher (or is 13% higher), and this association is statistically significant at the $\alpha = .05$ level.

TYPE OF DATA REQUIRED

In logistic regression, the independent variables may be at any level of measurement from nominal to ratio. Nominal-level variables that have two categories must be coded before entry (i.e., assign numeric codes to represent the categories instead of entering the text), and nominal-level variables with more than two categories must be recoded into dummy variables (see section below on creating dummy variables). The dependent variable is categorical and must have only two categories. There should be at least a 95% to 5% split in the data distribution between the two categories of the dependent variable; at least 5%—but no more than 95%—of the participants should have the outcome. Additionally, for all nominal and ordinal independent variables, there needs to be at least some cases in all combinations of the dependent and independent variables (e.g., in the bivariate cross-tabulations, there should be no empty cells). Finally, although a discussion of power analysis for logistic regression is beyond this text, it is recommended that there be at least 10 cases per independent variable (Garson, 2006).

Dummy Variables

If an independent variable is categorical but has more than two categories, it is necessary to create dummy variables. Using dummy variables is a way to express a nominal variable with multiple categories by a series of dichotomous variables that compare one category to a different category that serves as the reference. For example, if you were looking at a variable for race/ethnicity, you might have four categories with the following numeric labels: non-Hispanic White (1), non-Hispanic Black (2), non-Hispanic Asian (3), and Hispanic (4). The reason why we need dummy variables is that numerical values assigned to represent the categories need to make sense. In this example, the numeric difference of two points between non-Hispanic White (code = 1) and non-Hispanic Asian (code = 3) has no valid interpretation. However, if dummy variables are created, statements about the differences in the outcome for each ethnic group relative to one of the groups (which we set as the "reference category") can be made.

Creating Dummy Variables

The first step in creating dummy variables is to determine the number of variables that are needed. This will be one less than the number of categories of the variable. Because the race/ethnicity variable in our example has four levels, three dummy variables are needed to represent these four categories. The second step is to determine which of the categories will serve as the "reference" category. The choice of reference category is up to the researcher. In this case, non-Hispanic White is used as the reference category. Therefore, three dummy variables are created to represent the comparison of each race/ethnicity (non-Hispanic Black, non-Hispanic Asian, and Hispanic) to that reference category (non-Hispanic White):

- Black (1 = person is non-Hispanic Black; 0 = person is any other race/ethnicity.)
- Asian (1 = person is non-Hispanic Asian; 0 = person is any other race/ethnicity.)
- Hispanic (1 = person is Hispanic; 0 = person is any other race/ethnicity.)

The final step is to include the dummy variables as independent variables in the regression model **instead of** the original four-category race/ethnicity variable and to then run the regression model.

HOW DOES LOGISTIC REGRESSION WORK?

Logistic fits a shape (referred to as a line) to the data using a method called "maximum likelihood estimation" (Kleinbaum & Klein, 2002). In logistic regression, the dependent variable is dichotomous (only has two values), and the independent variables may be of any measurement scale (note that the independent variables are easiest to interpret if they are also dichotomous). The dependent variable is transformed using a logit transformation (SPSS does this calculation), and the probability that the dependent variable will equal 1 is modeled. The coefficients (the betas) of a multivariate logistic regression represent the log of the adjusted odds ratios for each of the dependent variables. To obtain the adjusted odds ratios and obtain the confidence interval around the odds ratios, the each beta coefficient is exponentiated (the antilog is taken) (Ostir & Uchida, 2000). Most statistics packages, including SPSS, provide both the adjusted odds ratios and the confidence intervals around those ratios when requested.

INFORMATION OBTAINED FROM LOGISTIC REGRESSION MODELS

Several important pieces of information can be obtained from the multivariate logistic regression model, including (1) the statistical significance of the overall model, (2) the overall fit of the model to the data, (3) a rough estimate of the overall amount of variation in the dependent variable explained by all of the independent variables, (4) the adjusted odds ratios (e.g., the increase or decrease in odds that the dependent variable will occur given the value of the independent variable), (5) the confidence intervals around the adjusted odds ratios, and (6) the statistical significance of each of the adjusted odds ratios.

As shown in the example below, the SPSS printout provides information about all of these items. The statistical significance of the overall model is assessed with the model chi-square. The overall fit of the model to the data is measured by the Hosmer-Lemeshow goodness-of-fit test. Whereas a nonsignificant result indicates that the model is a good fit, a significant result indicates that the logistic regression model does not fit well. Note that a poorly fitted model can still have significant predictors in it. A rough estimate of the overall amount of variation in the dependent variable explained by the model is estimated by two methods: the Cox and Snell R^2 and the Nagelkerke R^2. There is still some debate in the literature about the extent to which the amount of variance explained by a logistic regression can be measured and assigned meaning to the R^2. The best practice is to report both values and to be cautious in their interpretation. The last three items, the adjusted odds ratios, the confidence intervals around the adjusted odds ratios, and the statistical significance of the adjusted odds ratios, can be found in the last part of the printout.

Computer Analysis Example

The data in this example come from the 2004 New York City Health and Nutrition Examination Survey (NYCHANES), which was a cross-sectional survey of 1,999 New York City residents. In this example, we are using data on a random subset of 489 study participants to look at the association of eating out in restaurants often (five times per week on average) with trying to lose weight. The thinking is that those trying to lose weight will have reduced their frequency of eating out. In addition, we include gender in the model since both the outcome (eating out) and the exposure (trying to lose weight) likely vary by participant gender. The outcome variable is dichotomous with two groups: those who eat out five times per week on average (coded as 1) and those who eat out less than 5 times per week on average (coded as 0). The predictor or independent variables are as follows:

1. Loseweight—a dichotomous variable where those who have not tried to lose weight in the past year = 0 and those who have tried to lose weight in the past year = 1.
2. Gender—male = 0, female = 1.

Coding

Categorical independent variables that have more than two categories need to be recoded into dummy variables, as described above. The computer program will produce the dummy variables for you. You tell it which variable needs recoding and tell it what type of coding you want. Interaction terms also may be entered into the equation. For example, you could include an interaction term to assess whether the association between eating out in restaurants and trying to lose weight differs depending on participant gender. You would do this by adding an interaction term, lose-weight × gender, as an independent variable to the model.

Interpreting a Logistic Regression Conducted in SPSS

Box 13-2 shows the steps in SPSS needed to obtain this model, and Figure 13-1 contains the output from the model. The dependent variable, restaurant_dicho, was entered as 0 = no (do not eat out ≥5 times per week) and 1 = yes (eat out ≥5 times per week). This is appropriate coding for the logistic regression procedure. If the data had been entered as no = 1 and yes = 2, for example, the variable would have to be recoded before analysis for ease of interpretation.

The Statistical Significance of the Overall Model: The Model Chi-Square

The model chi-square is what we use to determine the statistical significance of the overall model. It is estimated from –2 × the log likelihood (–2LL). To estimate –2LL, the log likelihood of the alternate model (with all the independent variables you included) is compared to the log likelihood of the null model (with no variables included). Because the addition of variables will explain either the same or more variation compared to the null model,

BOX 13-2 USING SPSS TO OBTAIN A MULTIPLE LOGISTIC REGRESSION MODEL

Step 1: The data are opened in SPSS (File, Open, Data).

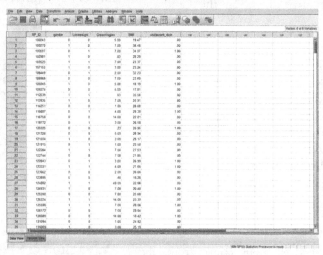

Step 2: The menu system is used to obtain the regression model by first clicking on "Analyze" and then selecting "Regression" and "Binary Logistic."

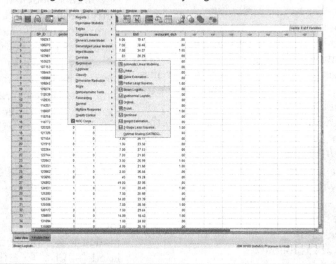

BOX 13-2   USING SPSS TO OBTAIN A MULTIPLE LOGISTIC REGRESSION MODEL *(Continued)*

Step 3: In the "Logistic Regression" pop-up box, the dependent variable "Restaurant_Dicho" is moved into the "Dependent" variable slot, and the independent variables are moved into the "Covariates" box. The method is selected (e.g., we use "Enter") in the "Method" box, and then the "Options" button is clicked.

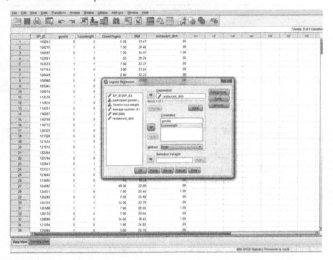

Step 4: In the "Logistic Regression: Options" pop-up box, under "Statistics and Plots," the box for "Hosmer-Lemeshow goodness-of-fit" is checked. The box for "CI for exp(B)" is checked, and the confidence interval is entered, which, in this case, is a 95% confidence interval. The box next to "Iteration History" is checked. The "Continue" button is clicked. When the "Logistic Regression" pop-up box reappears and "OK" is clicked, the output appears in the output window.

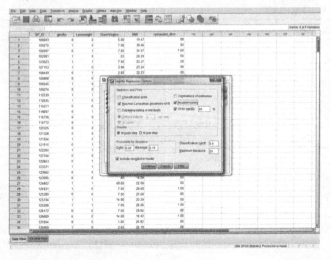

Logistic Regression

DEPENDENT VARIABLE ENCODING

ORIGINAL VALUE	INTERNAL VALUE
Eat out <5 times per week	0
Eat out at least 5 times per week	1

ITERATION HISTORY [a,b,c]

Iteration		−2 Log Likelihood	Coefficients Constant
Step 0	1	518.490	−1.101
	2	516.861	−1.233
	3	516.860	−1.238
	4	516.860	−1.238

[a]Constant is included in the model.
[b]Initial −2 Log Likelihood: 516.860.
[c]Estimation terminated at iteration number 4 because parameter estimates changed by less than .001.

OMNIBUS TESTS OF MODEL COEFFICIENTS

		Chi-Square	df	Significance
Step 1	Step	25.524	2	.000
	Block	25.524	2	.000
	Model	25.524	2	.000

MODEL SUMMARY

Step	−2 Log Likelihood	Cox & Snell R^2	Nagelkerke R^2
1	491.336[a]	.051	.078

[a]Estimation terminated at iteration number 4 because parameter estimates changed by less than .001.

HOSMER AND LEMESHOW TEST

Step	Chi-Square	df	Significance
1	.358	2	.836

FIGURE 13-1 Full logistic regression model.

VARIABLES IN THE EQUATION

		B	SE	Wald	df	Significance	Exp(*B*)	95% CI for Exp(*B*) Lower	Upper
Step 1[a]	Loseweight	−.030	.229	.017	1	.896	.970	.620	1.519
	Gender	−1.111	.228	23.675	1	.000	.329	.210	.515
	Constant	−.644	.172	13.995	1	.000	.525		

[a]Variable(s) entered on step 1: loseweight, gender.

FIGURE 13-1   (*Continued*) Full logistic regression model.

when you subtract the log likelihood of the alternate model from that of the null model, you will get either zero (if the additional variables add nothing to the model) or a negative number (if the additional variables create a better model than the null). By multiplying this by −2, the −2LL becomes positive. In our example, the −2LL for the null model is 516.86 (stated in the iteration history table) and for the full model (with both lose weight and gender) compared to the null model is 491.34. The difference between the two is the model chi-square.

The model chi-square is found in the part of the printout labeled "omnibus tests of model coefficients." The omnibus tests of model coefficients table gives the chi-square statistic and its *p*-value for the comparison of the −2LL for the various models you defined. As you can see in the table (Fig. 13-1), there are three chi-squares, one for step, one for block, and one for model. In this analysis, the variables were entered all together, not in blocks, so the values for step, block, and model are the same throughout. If we had entered the variables in a stepwise fashion within each block, these values would vary.

The Overall Fit of the Model to the Data

This is determined by the Hosmer-Lemeshow goodness-of-fit statistic. This statistic compares the observed probabilities to those predicted by the model. In other words, it examines the residuals. When the significance is large for the test of −2 LL or the goodness-of-fit statistic, you do not reject the null hypothesis that the model fits. In other words, a nonsignificant result indicates that the model fits; a significant result indicates that it does not fit. We see in Figure 13-1 that the chi-square is .358 with 2 df, and the *p*-value is .836. This indicates that the model does fit the data.

Estimate the Overall Amount of Variation in the Dependent Variable Explained by All of the Independent Variables

In the model summary table (Fig. 13-1), there are values for Cox & Snell and Nagelkerke R^2. The variance explained thus far is 5.1% to 7.8%.

Obtain the Adjusted Odds with Confidence Intervals and Statistical Significance

The part of the printout labeled "variables in the equation" shows the regression coefficients (*B* or beta), statistical significance, and confidence intervals. The *regression coefficient (or beta)* associated with each independent variable and the constant term is given in the first column, which is labeled "*B*." The *beta* in multiple regression can be used to create a prediction equation; that is, knowing a person's code on each variable, we can use the regression coefficients and the constant term to predict the individual's outcome. We explain more about this in Chapter 14. In logistic regression, these betas are used to determine the odds ratios.

The next column contains the standard errors for the predictors and the constant. In general, a statistic is divided by its standard error to give the value that is tested for significance. The column after this is the Wald statistic, which essentially gives the same information, albeit in a different form, as does the statistical significance.

The column labeled Exp(B) is a critical column, as it provides us with the adjusted odds ratios. Mathematically, this is e (the base of the natural logarithm, 2.718) raised to the power of *beta*. In this example, 2.718 raised to the power of −.03 (*beta* for loseweight) is .97. Remember that the odds ratio is the ratio of one probability to the other. In this example, it is the odds of eating out often among those who have tried to lose weight in the past year over the odds of eating out often among those who have not tried to lose weight in the past year.

The confidence intervals around the odds ratios were requested and are .62 to 1.52. We can see that the odds ratio under the null hypothesis (H_0: the odds of eating out often among those who have tried to lose weight is the same as that among those who have not tried to lose weight; in other words, the odds ratio = 1) falls between the lower and upper confidence interval. Therefore, the difference in the odds of eating out for those who have tried to lose weight compared to those who have not is not statistically significant. In addition, we can see that the *p*-value is .896, which is greater than .05 and therefore the odds ratio is not significant.

On the other hand, we can see from the regression results that the odds ratio for gender is .33 and the *p*-value is .000. This means that the odds of eating out among women is .33 times lower than that of men, adjusting for trying to lose weight in the past year. Furthermore, because the *p*-value is .000, this difference in the odds of eating out often by gender is statistically significant at the $\alpha = .05$ level.

SUMMARY

Logistic regression is commonly reported when the outcome measure is dichotomous. As with all methods of regression, it is of utmost importance to select variables for inclusion in the model based on a clear scientific rationale. After we assess the fit of the model, we need to verify the importance of each variable to the model. Variables that do not contribute to the model should be eliminated and a new model fit. The new model should be compared with the old model through the likelihood ratio test. Once you have obtained a model that you believe contains the essential variables, you should consider whether to add interaction terms.

CHAPTER REVIEW

Multiple-Choice Concept Review

1. Multivariate logistic regression models are useful because
   a. they allow one to simultaneously consider the effects of several independent variables on the dependent variable of interest.
   b. they minimize the risk of obtaining spurious results.
   c. most health outcomes have multiple causes.
   d. all of the above are true.

2. Multivariate logistic regression models are best used with
   a. a dichotomous dependent variable.
   b. any ratio-level variable.
   c. a normally distributed ratio-level variable.
   d. all of the above.

3. The odds ratio predicted by the null hypothesis
   a. is greater than 1.
   b. is less than 1.
   c. is equal to 1.
   d. cannot be answered without more information.

4. An odds ratio of 0.7 is interpreted as
   a. the odds of the outcome among those with the exposure (independent variable) are 0.7 times *greater* than that of those without the exposure.
   b. the odds of the outcome among those with the exposure (independent variable) are 0.7 times *smaller* than that of those without the exposure.
   c. the association between the outcome and the independent variable is statistically significant at the $\alpha = .05$ level.
   d. the null hypothesis is true.

5. A logistic regression model was run looking at the association between gender (male = 0, female = 1) and diabetes (yes = 1, no = 0). The odds ratio was 3.4, and the 95% confidence interval around the odds ratio was 2.9 to 4.6. This means that
   a. the association between gender and diabetes is statistically significant at the $\alpha = .05$ level.
   b. the association between gender and diabetes is not statistically significant at the $\alpha = .05$ level.
   c. women have a lower odds of diabetes but we cannot tell if that difference is statistically significant.
   d. the *p*-value is greater than .05.

6. Which of the following is/are true about the Hosmer-Lemeshow test?
   a. The null hypothesis is that the data do not fit the model.
   b. If the *p*-value for this test is less than .05, we conclude that the model does not fit the data.
   c. This test tells us that all of the independent variables in the model are significantly associated with the outcome.
   d. Both a and b.

7. The relationship between an odds ratio and a risk ratio is
   a. that the odds ratio usually underestimates the risk ratio.
   b. that the risk ratio is a good estimation of the odds ratio when the outcome is common.
   c. that the odds ratio is approximately the same as the risk ratio when the outcome is rare.
   d. all of the above.

8. The antilog of the regression coefficient (βs) in a multiple logistic regression model gives information about
   a. the strongest predictor of the dependent variable.
   b. the change in the dependent variable per unit increase in the independent variable.
   c. the difference (ratio) in the odds of having the condition represented by the dependent variable among those with an exposure compared to those without that exposure.
   d. a and b only.

9. Dummy variables are used to
   a. recode the dependent variable.
   b. represent ratio variables in regression models.
   c. represent dichotomous (two categories) nominal variables in regression models.
   d. represent polytomous (more than two categories) nominal variables in regression models.

10. An odds ratio of 1 means that the
   a. event is more likely to happen than the reference event.
   b. event is just as likely to happen in someone exposed as in someone not exposed.
   c. event is less likely to happen than the reference event.
   d. model is invalid.

Choosing the Best Statistical Test

For each of the following scenarios (1 to 10), choose the most appropriate test (a to l).
   a. Independent t test
   b. Mann-Whitney U-test
   c. Paired t test
   d. Wilcoxon matched-pairs test
   e. Logistic regression
   f. McNemar test
   g. One-way ANOVA
   h. Repeated-measures ANOVA
   i. Friedman's ANOVA by rank
   j. Kruskal-Wallis ANOVA
   k. Pearson correlation coefficient
   l. Spearman correlation coefficient

1. A total of 75 nursing students take a professional board preparation course, and another 73 nursing students study on their own. Which group had the higher board scores, which are normally distributed?

2. What is the relationship between the number of minutes of exercise a week and resting heart rate? There are 55 people in the study, and neither variable is normally distributed.

3. What is the relationship between having an older sibling (yes/no) and being developmentally delayed (yes/no) among preschoolers? There are 226 children in the study.

4. A weight-loss program enrolled 48 heterosexual couples. Did the husbands lose more weight than the wives? Weight loss is normally distributed.

5. In a study of 72 men, the researcher wants to know if cholesterol level, which is normally distributed, is related to the men's ethnicity (i.e., African American, White, Hispanic, and other).

6. What is the relationship between a college student's residence (lives on-campus vs. off-campus) and current smoking behavior (smokes or does not) adjusting for age? There are 114 college students in the study.

7. Patients in a critical care unit receive either experimental respiratory therapy or control respiratory therapy. Does treatment (experimental vs. control) have any effect on whether they get pneumonia after adjusting for age, gender, and race/ethnicity? There are 326 patients in the study.

8. What is the relationship between the ratio of registered nurses to certified nursing assistants in each intensive care unit (ICU) and the number of patient complications in that unit? The variables are not normally distributed, and 84 ICUs participated in the study.

9. What is the average number of minutes of television fourth graders were allowed to watch each week before and after their primary caretakers took a 3-hour parenting class? The variables are not normally distributed, and there were 37 fourth graders in the study.

10. Twenty-eight participants ranked preferences for three different types of yogurt: fat-free, low-fat, and full-fat yogurt. Is there a difference by yogurt type?

Critical Thinking Concept Review

1. Write three multivariate hypotheses that could be tested using multivariate logistic regression.

2. Locate an article of interest that uses multivariate logistic regression. Write a brief review of the purpose of the article, the methods, and the findings. Obtain all of the information that you would expect to get from a multivariate logistic regression model (adjusted odds ratios, 95% confidence intervals, and *p*-value). Write a brief conclusion.

Computational Problems

1. The 2 × 2 table below shows smoking status and participation in a sports team for 1,250 men. Calculate the odds, odds ratio, risks, and risk ratio of smoking when not on a sports team (exposed) compared to when on a sports team (unexposed).

On a Sports Team	Smokes	
	Yes	No
No	270	500
Yes	50	430

Use the SPSS data set called Chapter13 Data to answer the following questions:

2. Run a logistic regression model looking at the association of having tried to lose weight in the past year (loseweight) with gender (gender) and BMI, which is a continuous variable.
   a. Interpret the odds ratio and p-value for the association between gender and trying to lose weight after adjusting for BMI.
   b. Interpret the odds ratio and p-value for the association between BMI and trying to lose weight after adjusting for gender.
   c. Is the model a good fit to the data?

CHAPTER 14

Linear Regression

OBJECTIVES

After studying this chapter, you should be able to:

1. Know when it is appropriate to use linear regression.

2. Understand the statistics generated by the linear regression procedure.

3. Set up and solve a prediction equation.

4. Explain the difference between testing the significance of R^2 and the significance of a *regression coefficient (beta)*.

5. Discuss methods for selecting variables for entry into a linear regression model.

6. Describe testing regression assumptions.

HISTORICAL NOTE

Karl Pearson described the origin of the discovery of the regression slope in his biography of Francis Galton, *The Life, Letters and Labours of Francis Galton* (Pearson, 1930; Stanton, 2001). Galton was greatly interested in issues of heredity. In 1875, he distributed packets of sweet pea seeds (so-called mother seeds) to seven friends. Each of the friends received seeds of the same weight with significant variation across different packets. The friends planted the mother seeds and returned the daughter seeds (derived from the mother seed plants) to Galton. After plotting the weights of the daughter seeds against the weights of the mother seeds, Galton found that the median weights of daughter seeds from a particular size of mother seed roughly depicted a straight line with a positive slope less than 1.0: "Thus he naturally reached a straight regression line and the constant variability for all arrays of one character for a given character of a second. It was, perhaps, best for the progress of correlational calculus that this simple special case should be promulgated first; it is so easily grasped by the beginner." (Pearson, 1930).

OVERVIEW OF REGRESSION

We are constantly interested in predicting one thing based on another. We want to predict the weather to plan our weekend. We want to predict how well a student will do in nursing practice. We want to predict how long a patient may remain ill. Countless predictions are necessary for us to move through life. A brilliant statistical invention is regression, which permits us to make predictions from some known evidence about some unknown future events. Only about a century old, regression is the basis of many statistical methods.

Regression makes use of the correlation between variables and the notion of a straight line to develop a prediction equation. Once a relationship has been established between two variables, you can develop an equation that will allow you to predict the score of one of the variables given the scores of the others. Regression is a useful technique that allows us to predict outcomes and explain the interrelationships among variables. Linear regression models describe the linear relationship between a dependent variable and one or more independent variables by calculating a best shape to fit the data. The shape is often referred to as a regression line, but it is only truly a line when the model has two variables (one dependent and one independent variable). If the study includes three variables, the shape defined by the model is a two-dimensional plane, and if the study includes four or more variables, it is a hyperplane (which is very difficult to visualize and impossible to graph).

We can use simple linear regression to look at the association between one independent variable and one dependent variable. However, it is more common to include multiple independent variables in a multivariate linear regression model. The main advantage of a multivariate linear regression model is that it allows researchers to simultaneously examine the unique effects of several independent variables on the dependent variable. From a linear regression equation, the overall variance explained by the model as well as the unique contribution (strength and direction) of each independent variable can be obtained. In effect, linear regression models are an extension of Pearson correlation coefficients. The computations for a linear regression model are somewhat tedious and can be found in Daniel (2008).

RESEARCH QUESTIONS

How Does Socioeconomic Status Affect Age at Menarche?

James-Todd, Tahranifar, Rich-Edwards, Titievsky, and Terry (2010) analyzed data from a cohort study in which 2,138 children were followed from birth to age 7 and then contacted the participants again in adulthood and asked about their age at menarche. Data collected at birth and then again at age 7 were used to create an index (score range of 0 to 100) for childhood socioeconomic status (SES) that combined information on family income, father's education, and occupation. Multivariate linear regression was used to look at the association between change in SES between birth and age 7 and age at menarche after adjusting for a number of related factors including race/ethnicity, child's body mass index (BMI) at age 7, mother's age at menarche, mother's place of birth (United States or outside the United States), and whether the father was living with the family when the child was born. The study found that after adjusting for all these factors, a 20-point decrease in the family's SES score was associated with about a 4-month decrease in age at menarche (β = .018, 95% CI = .005, .030).

Is Maternal Depression Associated with Reduced Height in Young Children?

A study by Ertel, Koenen, Rich-Edwards, and Gillman (2010) among 872 mother–child pairs looked at the association of maternal depression midpregnancy and 6-month postpartum with child height for age and leg length at age 3. The study used multivariate linear regression to adjust for a number of potential confounders and, surprisingly, found that postpartum depression was associated with greater height for age (β = .37, 95% CI = .16, .58) and longer leg length (β = .88, 95% CI = .35, 1.41), while antenatal depression was not significantly associated with child height outcomes.

THE LINEAR REGRESSION MODEL

Types of Data Required

The primary data requirement for linear regression is that the dependent variable be of ratio scale and normally distributed. However, if the dependent variable is not normally distributed, it may be possible to do some mathematical transformations to make it more normal. One common transformation is to take the natural log (base e) of the dependent variable. The independent variables can be of any scale. Nominal independent variables that have more than two categories have to be put in the model as dummy variables, similar to what we do for multiple logistic regression models.

Assumptions

Linear regression is a parametric test, and to use it, some assumptions must be met in order for this analytic method to be valid. In addition,

certain additional assumptions must be made if we are to generalize beyond the sample statistic, that is, if we are to make inferences about the population itself. These assumptions include the following:

1. The sample must be representative of the population to which the inference will be made.
2. The dependent variable is roughly normally distributed overall and that it is normally distributed for each value of the independent variables.
3. For every value of X, the distribution of Y scores must have approximately equal variability. This is called the assumption of homoscedasticity.
4. The relationship between X and Y must be linear; that is, when the two scores for each individual are graphed, they should tend to form a straight line. The points will not all fall on this line, but they should be scattered closely around it.
5. The fifth assumption (for multiple linear regression) is that there is no multicollinearity; that is, the independent variables are not so strongly intercorrelated that they are indistinguishable from each other.

Some of these assumptions (e.g., normal distribution of the dependent variable) can be tested before the analysis begins, and some of the assumptions are assessed at the end of the analysis by a special set of statistics known as regression diagnostics. Although regression diagnostics are beyond the scope of this text, we present a brief discussion of some techniques at the end of this chapter. A more extended discussion of regression diagnostics can be found in the texts by Tabachnick and Fidel (2006) and Chatterjee and Yilmaz (1992).

SIMPLE LINEAR REGRESSION

We begin by explaining simple regression. In this method, a correlation between two variables is used to develop a prediction equation, with these predictions being based on a linear relationship between variables. If the relationship is curvilinear, other techniques, such as trend analysis, must be used.

If the correlation between two variables was perfect (+1 or −1), we could make a perfect prediction about the score on one variable, given the score on the other variable. Of course, we never get perfect correlations, so we are never able to make perfect predictions. The greater the correlation, the more accurate the prediction. If there were no correlation between two variables, knowing the score of one would be absolutely no help in estimating the score of the other. When you have no information to aid you in predicting a score, your best guess for any subject would be the mean (which is also the median for a normally distributed variable), because that is the center of the data.

To be able to make predictions, the relationship between two variables, the independent (X) and the dependent (Y), must be measured. If there is a correlation, a regression equation can be developed that will allow prediction of Y given X. For example, in the study previously mentioned, James-Todd et al. (2010) regressed age at menarche on six variables: change in SES between birth and age 7, race/ethnicity, child's BMI at age 7, mother's age at menarche, mother's place of birth (United States or outside the United States), and whether the father was living with the family when the child was born.

Regression Equation

The simple (one independent variable) regression equation is the equation for a straight line and is written as follows:

$$Y' = a + bX$$

where Y' is the *predicted score*.

Given data on X and Y from a sample of subjects, a and b can be calculated. With these two measures, Y can be predicted, given X. The letter a in the model is called the *intercept constant* and is the value of Y when $X = 0$. It is the point at which the regression line intercepts the Y axis. The letter b represents the *regression coefficient*, also referred to as *beta*, and is the rate of change in Y with a unit change in X. It is a measure of the slope of the regression line.

An example is given in Figure 14-1. The intercept constant, a, is equal to 3; you can see that it is the value of Y when $X = 0$. It is the point at which the regression line connects with the Y axis. The regression coefficient, b, is .5. This means that the value of Y goes up .5 units for every 1-unit change in X. When $X = 0$, $Y = 3$, and when X goes up to 1, Y goes up to 3.5. The regression line is the "line of best fit" and is formed by a technique called the *method of least squares*. The concept of least squares was presented in Chapter 7 with a discussion of analysis of variance (ANOVA). Because the mean is (in one sense) the center of the data, the sum of the deviations of the scores around the mean, $\sum(X - \overline{X})$, is 0. Also, if you square these deviations and add them, that number will be smaller than the sum of the squared deviations around any other measure of central tendency. In the same way, the regression line passes through the exact center of the data in the scatter diagram. Therefore, it is the "line of best fit." There are deviations around the regression line, just as there are deviations around the mean. The regression line represents the predicted scores (Y values), but because a prediction is not perfect, the actual scores (Y values) would deviate somewhat from the predicted scores. Because the regression line passes through the center of the pairs of scores, if you add the deviations from the regression line $\sum(Y - Y')$, they will equal 0. Also, if you square those deviations and add them, the sum of the squared deviations around the regression line is smaller than the sum of the

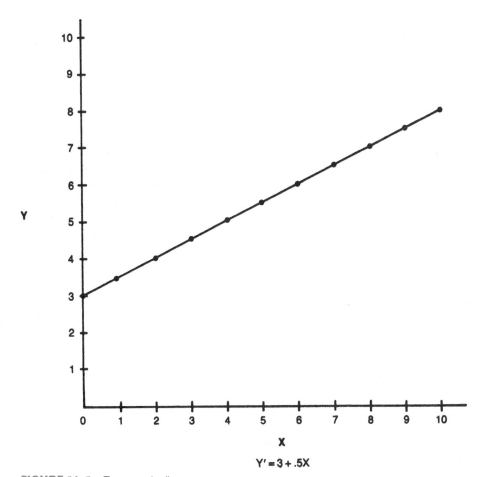

FIGURE 14-1   The regression line.

squared deviations around any other line drawn through the scatter diagram.

If James-Todd et al. (2010) had applied their prediction equation to the girl in their sample, they would find that the girl's actual age at menarche (Y) would vary from their predicted age at menarche (Y'). Because the correlations between the predictors and the outcome measure were not perfect, there is an error in the prediction. Even using the sample on which the prediction equation was calculated, there will be differences between Y and Y'. $Y - Y'$ equals the deviations from the predicted scores, just as $\overline{X} - X$ equals the deviations around the mean. The regression equation minimizes the squared differences of the predicted score from the actual score.

Given a regression equation of $Y' = 4 + 0.2X$ and three individuals with scores on X of 5, 10, and 20, respectively, the predicted scores for the three would be calculated as follows:

$a + bX = Y'$

1. $4 + (0.2)(5) = 5$
2. $4 + (0.2)(10) = 6$
3. $4 + (0.2)(20) = 8$

MULTIPLE REGRESSION

Multivariate regression looks at the association between a group of predictor variables and one dependent variable. The prediction equation is as follows:

$$Y' = a + b_1X_1 + b_2X_2 + b_3X_3 + \ldots b_kX_k$$

There is still one intercept constant, a, but each independent variable (e.g., X_1, X_2, X_3) has a separate regression coefficient. Given a prediction equation of

$$Y' = 2 + 0.5X_1 + 0.2X_2 + 0.4X_3$$

and three individuals with the following scores:

	X_1	X_2	X_3
1.	8	4	7
2.	12	3	5
3.	10	6	9

their predicted scores would be calculated as:

1. $2 + (0.5)(8) + (0.2)(4) + (0.4)(7) = 9.6$
2. $2 + (0.5)(12) + (0.2)(3) + (0.4)(5) = 10.6$
3. $2 + (0.5)(10) + (0.2)(6) + (0.4)(9) = 11.8$

If adding extra variables increases the amount of variance accounted for in the dependent variable, it will increase the accuracy of our prediction.

INFORMATION OBTAINED FROM LINEAR REGRESSION MODELS

There are two questions that we want to answer with a linear regression model. First, we want to know if the independent variables in the model, taken together, do a good job at predicting the dependent variable. We can assess this by looking at the R^2, called the *coefficient of determination*, which measures the percentage of variance explained by the model. For example, an adjusted coefficient of determination (R^2) indicates that the amount of variance in the dependent

variable explained by the model is 75.7%. It is important to use the adjusted coefficient rather than the unadjusted coefficient because the unadjusted coefficient has been shown to be positively biased (too high) when small sample sizes are used. As the sample size increases, the unadjusted and adjusted coefficients become increasingly more similar. The F-distribution with k and $(n - k - 1)$ degrees of freedom is used for testing the significance of R^2. k stands for the number of independent variables in the model, and n stands for the number of subjects (see Appendix F for the F-distribution). When using computer programs, the F-statistic and associated p-value are included in the output.

With multivariate linear regression, we are interested not only in the significance of the overall R and the amount of variance accounted for (R^2) but also in the significance of each of the independent variables. Just because R^2 is significant does not mean that all the independent variables are contributing significantly to the explained variance. In multivariate linear regression, the multiple correlation is tested for significance (R and R^2), and in addition, each of the *regression coefficients* is tested for significance. Testing the *regression coefficients* tells us whether the independent variable associated with it is contributing significantly to the variance accounted for in the dependent variable. Either the F, with 1 and $(n - k - 1)$ degrees of freedom, or t, with $(n - 2)$ degrees of freedom, distribution is used to test the significance of the *correlation coefficient*, and both are included, along with the p-value, in the output.

Step-by-Step Procedure for Explaining a Linear Regression Model

We use a study by Anderson, Isset, and McDaniel (2003) to illustrate the procedure for computing a multiple linear regression model. This study examined the following question with data obtained from the directors of nursing (DONs) in 152 nursing homes as well as from secondary data sets: Do nursing home management practices affect how nursing home residents are treated?

Note that the unit of analysis is the nursing home. One of the outcomes examined in this study was the percentage of residents who had some type of restraint (i.e., chair, vest belt, and wrist mitten) used on them in the past 4 weeks. The researchers were trying to determine if a set of eight independent variables for ownership characteristics, director characteristics, and management practices could predict the use of restraints. The multiple linear regression results from this study are shown in Table 14-1.

Step 1: State the Null and Alternative Hypotheses

- H_0: Ownership characteristics, director characteristics, and management practices are not associated with the use of restraints.

- H_A: Ownership characteristics, director characteristics, and management practices are associated with the use of restraints.

Step 2: Determine Statistical Significance Level (α-Level)

In this study, an α-level of .05 is used. The critical value for the R^2 F_{crit} with $k = 8$ and $(n - k - 1) = (152 - 8 - 1) = 143$ degrees of freedom, which we can round down to 8 and 125, is 2.01, and the F_{crit} for the regression coefficients with 1 and 143 (rounded down to 125) degrees of freedom is 3.92.

Step 3: Make Sure That the Data Meet All of the Necessary Assumptions

All of the assumptions that can be checked beforehand are met.

Table 14-1	A MULTIPLE LINEAR REGRESSION MODEL OF THE PERCENTAGE OF RESIDENTS WITH RESTRAINTS IN NURSING HOMES			
Independent Variable	B (Unadjusted)	β (SE)	β (Adjusted)	Significance of β (t Test)
Number of beds (log)	−2.102	.608	−.287	<.001
Ownership type	1.285	.715	.135	NS
DON tenure in current position	−0.411	.180	−.189	<.05
Years experience as DON	−0.481	.219	−.184	<.05
Communication openness	−1.585	.607	−.226	<.05
RN participation in decision making	−0.061	.244	−020	NS
Relationship-oriented leadership	−0.315	.525	−.049	NS
Formalization	0.212	.621	.029	NS
f-test for the whole model	4.704			
Significance level (overall)	$p < .000$			
R^2	207			
Adjusted R^2	.163			

Note. $n = 152$ nursing homes.

DON, director of nursing; NS, not significant; RN, registered nurse; SE, standard error.

Source: Adapted with permission from Anderson, R. A., Isset, L. M., & McDaniel, R. R. (2003). Nursing homes as complex adaptive systems. *Nursing Research, 52*(1), 12–21.

Step 4: Examine the Statistical Significance of the Overall Model

The first item to examine when looking at a multiple linear regression model is the significance of the overall model; this model is statistically significant with a computed *f*-value of 4.704, which is greater than our F_{crit} ($p < .000$).

Step 5: Determine the Overall Variation in the Dependent Variable Explained by the Independent Variables

The second item to examine is the overall variation in the dependent variable explained by the model (all the independent variables together) as measured by the adjusted coefficient of determination (adjusted R^2); in this model, 16.3% of the variance in restraint use is explained by the independent variables.

Step 6: Obtain the Regression Equation

The overall model equation is as follows:

Predicted % retrained = a − 2.102 (# beds) + 1.285 (ownership) − 0.411 (DON tenure)

  − 0.481 (years DON experience) − 1.585 (communication openness)

  − 0.061 (RN participation in decision making)

  − 0.315 (relationship-oriented leadership) + 0.212 (formalization).

Because the article does not provide the value of the intercept, it is left as "a." Each of these other βs (betas) tells us how we would predict the outcome to change in relation to changes in each independent variable, all other factors being held constant. So, if the number of beds increase by 1 (1 unit), and all the other variables stayed exactly the same, we would expect the % restrained to decrease by 2.102. The negative beta indicates that as the independent variable increases, the dependent variable decreases.

A positive beta would indicate a positive relationship, as the independent variable increases, so does the dependent variable.

Step 7: Determine the Relationship Between Each Independent Variable and the Dependent Variable

The independent variables that are significant predictors of the dependent variable at $\alpha = .05$ are number of beds, the tenure in the current position of the DON, the years of experience of the DON, and the level of communication openness in the facility. As described above, the unstandardized regression coefficient for each independent variable tells us how many units increase or decrease we can expect in the outcome for each unit increase in the exposure, with all other conditions held constant.

Step 8: Determine the Relative Strength of the Association of Each Independent Variable on the Dependent Variable

The relative strength of each of these predictors is ascertained by examining the adjusted regression coefficients. We use the adjusted betas in order to be able to compare the strength of the association of each independent variable with the outcome in similar units. For example, if we had age included in a model in years and income in thousands of dollars, the units are not necessarily comparable. The standardized regression coefficients are in units of standard variation and thus more comparable. The larger the absolute value of the adjusted beta, the stronger the predictor. In this model, the strongest predictor of restraint use is the number of beds, with an adjusted beta of −.287. The fact that the adjusted beta is negative indicates that as the number of beds increases, the use of restraints decreases. The second strongest predictor of restraint use is communication openness, with an adjusted beta of −.226. As communication openness increases, the use of restraints decreases. The other two predictors of restraint use, DON tenure in the current position and years of experience as a DON, each have a unique (and almost identical) effect on restraint use. Restraint use decreases both with overall DON experience and DON tenure in the current position.

Step 9: Predict the Value of the Dependent Variable

This step is not done here because the investigators were not interested in predicting the value of individual data points. However, had the investigator wanted to, the value of the dependent variable could be predicted under specified conditions for each independent variable by plugging the specified values for each independent variable into the regression equation.

Step 10: Provide a Succinct Summary of the Findings

The linear regression model predicts 16.3% of the variance in percent restrained in the past 4 weeks, and this is statistically significant using the *f*-test. The independent variables that are significant predictors of the dependent variable at $\alpha = .05$ are number of beds, the tenure in the current position of the DON, the years of experience of the DON, and the level of communication openness in the facility.

Notes on the Error Term and Regression Toward the Mean

It is useful to note that the overall regression equation can be used to predict the outcome given specific values for the independent variables. The predicted outcome will not, however, be identical to the actual outcome in the participants with those values for the independent variables. *Regression* literally means a falling back toward the mean. With perfect correlations, there is no falling back; the predicted score is

the same as the predictor. With less-than-perfect correlations, there is some error in the measurement, and we would expect that in the case of a person who received an extremely high score on the outcome, chance may have been working in his or her favor; therefore, on a second measure, his or her score would be somewhat less—it would have fallen back toward the mean. In the same way, a person with an extremely low score perhaps had all the fates against him or her and on a second measure would do better, thus moving his or her score closer to the mean.

Each prediction regresses toward the mean, depending on the strength of the correlation. If there is no correlation ($r = 0$), Y' = the mean of Y for every value of X. As the correlation rises toward 1, Y' moves proportionately outward from the mean, toward the position of the X predictor. The correlation coefficient tells us exactly what percentage of this distance Y' moves. Figure 14-2 shows predictions based on an r of .50. Note on the figure that all the predicted scores (Y' values) are halfway between the mean and the X score. This is because the correlation is .5. If the correlation had been .7, the Y' scores would have moved .7 times the distance between the mean and X. If the X score is above the mean, the predicted score will be lower than the X score and closer to the mean. With an r of .5 and an X score of +2, $Y' = (.5)(2) = 1$. With a correlation of .5, a person who was 2 standard deviations above the mean would be predicted to be 1 standard deviation above the mean on Y.

If the X score is below the mean, the predicted score is higher and closer to the mean. An X score of −3 would result in a predicted score of $(.5)(-3) = -1.5$. Remember that these are predictions based on a correlation of .5, so you would not be able to predict perfectly an individual's score. The person's actual score will differ from the predicted score. This discrepancy between predicted and actual scores reflects the error in the prediction. Because most variables will not be z-scores, we now present the more general regression equation using SPSS.

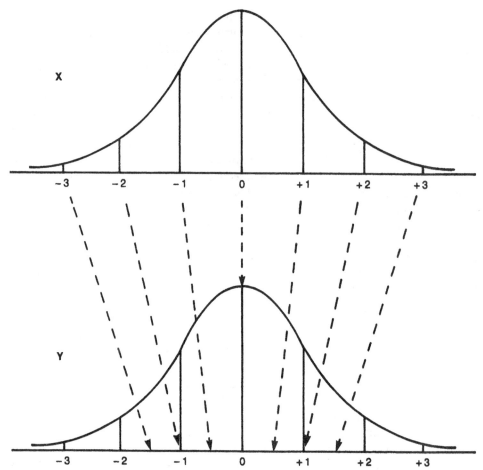

FIGURE 14-2 Predicting from X to Y with $r = .50$.

USING SPSS TO OBTAIN A MULTIPLE LINEAR REGRESSION MODEL

It is fairly straightforward to use SPSS to obtain a linear regression model. The variables need to be in the correct form for the analysis to be useful. In particular, the dependent variable needs to be of ratio measurement scale and normally distributed. The independent variables can be of any measurement scale, but special adjustments (dummy variables) need to be made for nominal variables with more than two categories.

The use of SPSS to obtain a multiple linear regression model is illustrated using data from a subset of 489 participants in the 2004 New York City Health and Nutrition Examination Survey. The question considered is "What predicts total cholesterol (mg/dl)?" This analysis provides for a discussion of several issues that may arise when conducting a multiple linear regression analysis, including the use of linear transformations and the creation of dummy variables. Box 14-1 illustrates the use of SPSS in creating a multiple linear regression model, and Table 14-2 presents the SPSS output.

BOX 14-1   USING SPSS TO OBTAIN A MULTIPLE LINEAR REGRESSION MODEL

I. Transforming the outcome

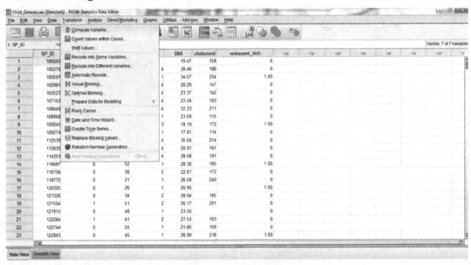

Step 1: Go to "Transform" and select "Compute Variable."

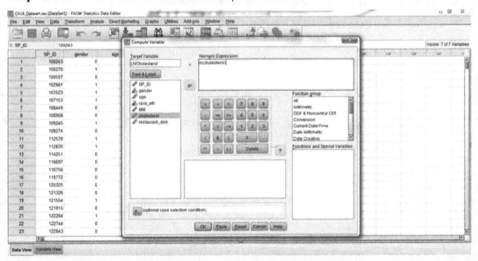

Step 2: Type the name of the new variable into the "Target Variable" box—perhaps give the variable the name "LNCholesterol."

(Continued)

BOX 14-1   USING SPSS TO OBTAIN A MULTIPLE LINEAR REGRESSION MODEL *(Continued)*

Step 3: In the "Numeric Expression" box, type "ln" and then put parentheses and move the variable "Cholesterol" over and close the parentheses, so that it reads "ln(Cholesterol)" and click on "OK."

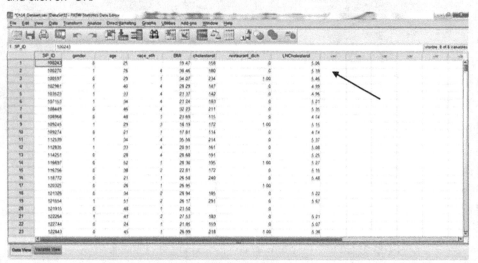

If you look in the Data View, you will see a new variable named LCholesterol added to the end of the spreadsheet.

II. Creating dummy variable

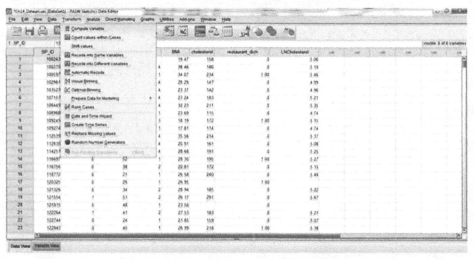

BOX 14-1   USING SPSS TO OBTAIN A MULTIPLE LINEAR REGRESSION MODEL *(Continued)*

Step 1: Select "Transform," then "Compute Variable."

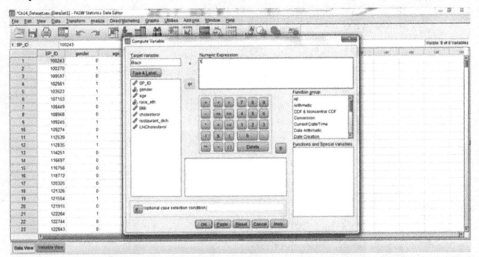

Step 2: In the "Target Variable" box, put the name of the first dummy variable "Black." In the "Numeric Expression" box put "1."

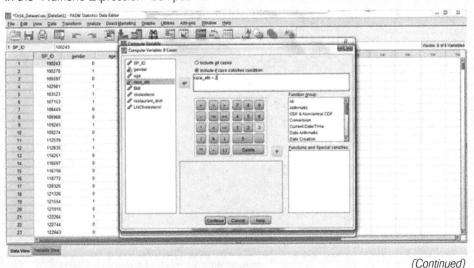

(Continued)

BOX 14-1 **USING SPSS TO OBTAIN A MULTIPLE LINEAR REGRESSION MODEL** *(Continued)*

Step 3: Click on the "If" button, click on the "If Case Satisfied Condition" button, and then move the variable "Race_Eth" into the box, after which type "=2" so that the text in the box reads "Race_eth=2." Click on Continue then "OK."

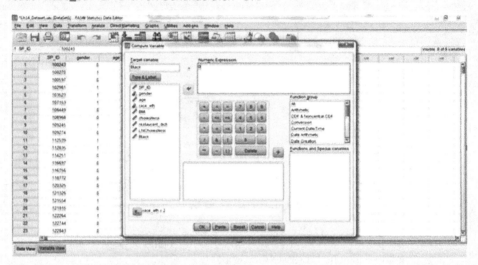

Step 4: Go back to Transform, Compute Variable, and this time set the new variable "Black" equal to 0 in the "Numeric Expression" box.

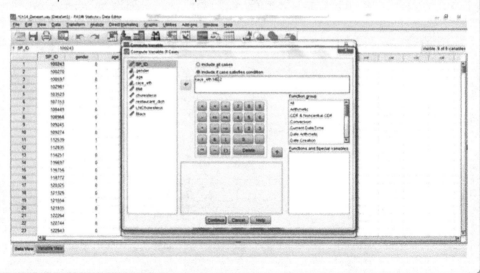

BOX 14-1 **USING SPSS TO OBTAIN A MULTIPLE LINEAR REGRESSION MODEL** *(Continued)*

Click on the "If" button and type "Race_Eth NE 2." NE stands for not equal.

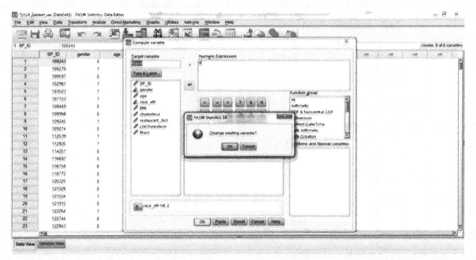

Step 5: When you get a pop-up asking if you want to change the variable, select "Yes."
Step 6: Repeat this procedure to create a dummy variable for Asian and for Hispanic.

III. Running multivariate linear regression

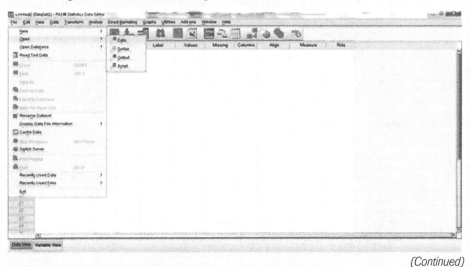

(Continued)

BOX 14-1 USING SPSS TO OBTAIN A MULTIPLE LINEAR REGRESSION MODEL *(Continued)*

Step 1: The data are opened in SPSS by clicking on "File" then "Open" and "Data." Navigate to the location of the data set in the "Look in" window, and click on the file and then click on "Open."

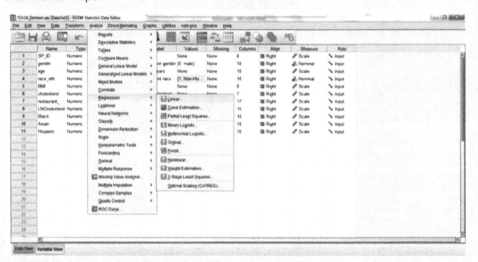

Step 2: The linear regression model is obtained by first clicking on "Analyze" and then selecting "Regression" and "Linear."

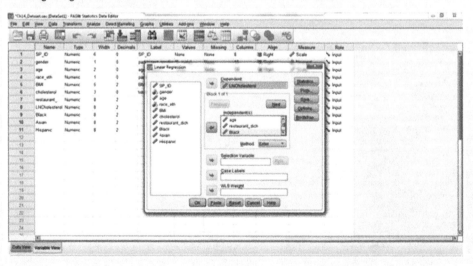

BOX 14-1 **USING SPSS TO OBTAIN A MULTIPLE LINEAR REGRESSION MODEL** *(Continued)*

Step 3: In the "Linear Regression" pop-up box, the dependent variable "lncholesterol" is moved to the "Dependent" slot, and the independent variables ("gender," "age," "restaurant_dicho," "Black," "Asian," and "Hispanic") to the "Independent" slot.

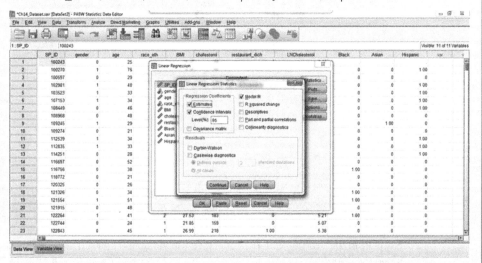

Step 4: Click on "Statistics" and check "Estimates," "Confidence Intervals," and "Model fit."

Step 5: When "OK" is clicked, the results appear in the output window.

IV. Creating an interaction term

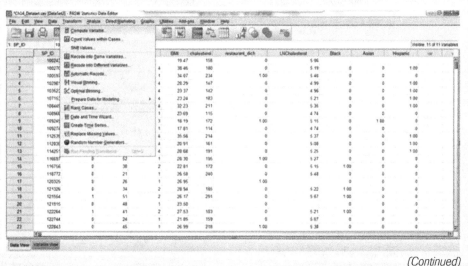

(Continued)

BOX 14-1   USING SPSS TO OBTAIN A MULTIPLE LINEAR REGRESSION MODEL *(Continued)*

Step 1: Go to "Transform," select "Compute Variable."

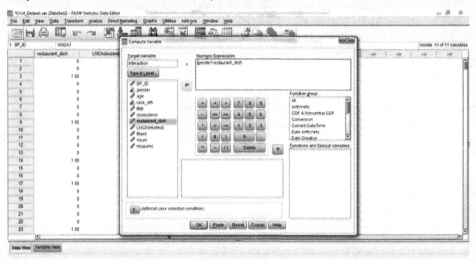

Step 2: In the "Target Variable" box, give the variable a name (perhaps "interaction"), move the "Gender" variable into the "Numeric Expression" window, then type "*" for multiplication, then move the restaurant variable "Restaurant_dicho" into the "Numeric Expression" box. The text should look like "Gender*Restaurant_Dicho."

Step 3: Click on "OK" and the interaction variable is created (you will see it in the Data View window).

V. Assessing assumptions in linear regression

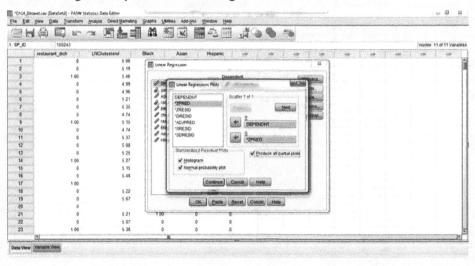

BOX 14-1 USING SPSS TO OBTAIN A MULTIPLE LINEAR REGRESSION MODEL *(Continued)*

Step 1: In the linear regression window (from III above), click on "Plots" and move "Dependent" into the box labeled "Y" and "ZPRED" into the box labeled "X."
Step 2: Check the boxes for "Produce all Partial Plots," "Histogram," and "Normal Probability
Plot" and hit "Continue."

Table 14-2   SPSS OUTPUT FOR MULTIVARIATE LINEAR REGRESSION MODEL REGRESSION VARIABLES ENTERED/REMOVED[a]

Model	Variables Entered	Variables Removed	Method
1	Hispanic, restaurant_dicho, participant gender, age in years, Asian, and Black[b]	.	Enter

[a]Dependent variable: LNCholesterol.
[b]All requested variables entered.

Model Summary

Model	R	R^2	Adjusted R^2	Standard Error of the Estimate
1	.211[a]	.044	.031	.19918

[a]Predictors: (Constant), Hispanic, restaurant_dicho, participant gender, age in years, Asian, and Black.

ANOVA[a]

Model		Sum of Squares	df	Mean Square	F	Significance
1	Regression	.760	6	.127	3.192	.004[b]
	Residual	16.345	412	.040		
	Total	17.105	418			

[a]Dependent variable: LNCholesterol.
[b]Predictors: (Constant), Hispanic, restaurant_dicho, participant gender, age in years, Asian, and Black.

Author Comment The analysis accounted for 3.1% of the variance in the dependent variable.

Author Comment The overall analysis was significant, p = .004.

Table 14-2	SPSS OUTPUT FOR MULTIVARIATE LINEAR REGRESSION MODEL REGRESSION VARIABLES ENTERED/REMOVED[a] *(Continued)*

Coefficients[a]

Model		B	Standard Error	β	T	Significance	Lower Bound	Upper Bound
		Unstandardized Coefficients		Standardized Coefficients			95.0% Confidence Interval for B	
1	(Constant)	5.189	.040		129.516	.000	5.110	5.268
	Participant gender	−.015	.021	−.038	−.750	.453	−.056	.025
	Age in years	.002	.001	.163	3.252	.001	.001	.004
	Restaurant_dicho	.008	.025	.016	.316	.752	−.041	.056
	Black	−.053	.030	−.100	−1.767	.078	−.111	.006
	Asian	.006	.031	.011	.197	.844	−.056	.068
	Hispanic	−.040	.025	−.096	−1.607	.109	−.088	.009

[a]Dependent variable: LNCholesterol.

Author Comment *One of the independent variables (age) is significantly associated with the outcome (p = .001). None of the other variables are significantly related to the outcome.*

The Dependent Variable: Meeting the Assumption of Normality by Using a Linear Transformation

In this example, the dependent variable is total cholesterol (mg/dl). One of the assumptions of multiple linear regression models is that the dependent variable is normally distributed. If we create a histogram of this variable (in SPSS, go to "Graphs," select "Legacy Dialogues," then select "Histogram," and move the variable "Cholesterol" into the "Variable box" and click on "OK"), we can see that cholesterol is slightly skewed. To correct for this, an adjustment called a "linear transformation" of the variable can be made. In this case, the natural log of cholesterol, which is normally distributed, is used in place of the untransformed cholesterol variable (in SPSS, go to "Transform" and select "Compute

Variable." Type the name of the new variable into the "Target Variable" box—perhaps give the variable the name "LNCholesterol." Then, in the "Numeric Expression" box, type "ln" and then put parentheses and move the variable "Cholesterol" over and close the parentheses, so that it reads "ln(Cholesterol)" and click on "OK." This will create a new variable that is the natural log of the original cholesterol variable. Linear transformations are a way to make nonnormally distributed variables take on a more normal distribution. A clear and excellent discussion of different types of linear transformations can be found in the text by Tabachnick and Fidel (2006).

Independent Variables and the Creation of Dummy Variables

In this example, the independent variables (potential predictors) of cholesterol that are examined include gender, age, race/ethnic group, BMI, and frequency of eating out in restaurants (more than five times per week or not). One of the variables, ethnic group, is a nominal variable with four categories: non-Hispanic White, non-Hispanic Black, non-Hispanic Asian, and Hispanic. To use this variable in the linear regression model, a set of dummy variables is needed to represent it.

Regression results, linear, logistic, or of any other form, only have a valid interpretation if the differences in the numerical values of the analysis make sense. Some variables, such as "ethnic group," have multiple categories in which the numerical value of the variable has no meaning. In this example, the difference of three points between "Hispanic" (value = 4) and "non-Hispanic White" (value = 1) has no valid interpretation. However, if dummy variables are created, statements about the differences in total cholesterol that are found in each ethnic group can be made. Using dummy variables is a way to express a nominal variable with multiple categories by a series of dichotomous variables. Creating dummy variables was described in Chapter 13, and here we do an example.

The first step in creating dummy variables is to determine the number of variables that are needed. This will be one less than the number of levels of the variable. Because the variable "race" has four categories, three dummy variables are needed to represent these four categories. The second step is to determine which of the categories will serve as the "reference" category. The choice of reference category is up to the researcher. In this case, "non-Hispanic White" is used as the reference category. Therefore, three dummy variables are created to represent the variable race. In SPSS, we select "Transform," then "Compute Variable." In the "Target Variable" box, put the name of the first dummy variable "Black." In the "Numeric Expression" box, put "1." Click on the "If" button, click on the "If Case Satisfied Condition" button, and then move the variable "Race_Eth" into the box, after which type "=2," so that the text in the box reads "Race_eth=2." Click on "Continue," and then "OK." Then, go back to Transform, Compute Variable, and this time set the new variable "Black" equal to

0 in the "Numeric Expression" box. Click on the "If" button and type "Race_Eth NE 2." NE stands for not equal. When you get a pop-up asking if you want to change the variable, select "Yes." Repeat this procedure to create a dummy variable for Asian and for Hispanic. The three new variables are as follows:

- Black (1 = person is non-Hispanic Black; 0 = person is any other race/ethnicity.)
- Asian (1 = person is non-Hispanic Asian; 0 = person is any other race/ethnicity.)
- Hispanic (1 = person is Hispanic, 0 = person is not Hispanic.)

The final step is to include the dummy variables in place of the original race/ethnicity variable and to then run the linear regression model.

Using SPSS to Obtain a Multiple Linear Regression Model

Box 14-1 illustrates the procedure for obtaining a multiple linear regression model using SPSS. In Step 1, the data set is opened in SPSS. After the data set is open, the menu system is used to obtain the multiple linear regression model by clicking on "Analyze" and then selecting "Regression" and "Linear." In the "Linear Regression" pop-up box, the dependent variable "LNCholesterol" is moved to the "Dependent" slot, and the independent variables ("gender," "age," "restaurant_dicho," "Black," "Asian," and "Hispanic") are moved to the "Independent" slot. Click on "Statistics" and make sure the boxes are checked next to "Estimates," "Model Fit," and "Confidence Intervals" with "Level (%)" set at "95." Click on "Continue" and then the "OK" button. The results appear in the output window.

Interpreting the SPSS Output From a Multiple Linear Regression Model

The output from this multiple linear regression model is shown in Table 14-2. The first box, "Variables Entered/Removed," shows all of the model's variables. The second box, "Model Summary," provides the coefficient of determination (R^2) and the adjusted coefficient of determination (adjusted R^2). In this case, the adjusted coefficient of determination (R^2) is .031. The third box, "ANOVA," provides information about the overall significance of the model; the f-statistic is 3.19 with $p = .004$.

The fourth box, "Coefficients," provides information about the individual predictors (independent variables). This box provides four pieces of information: the value of the regression coefficients (unstandardized B), the confidence interval around B, the adjusted regression coefficients (SPSS calls these "beta"), and the statistical significance of each coefficient. From this box, the overall regression equation can be constructed as follows:

Predicted ln(cholesterol) = 5.189
   – .015(gender) + .002(age) – .053(Black)
   + .006(Asian) – .040(Hispanic)
   + .008(restaurant_dicho)

Looking at the p-values for the regression coefficients, only age is a significant predictor of cholesterol ($p = .001$) and looking at the adjusted regression coefficients (beta), we also see that age is the strongest predictor.

Testing Interactions

As pointed out in Chapter 8, you may be interested in the interaction among independent variables in predicting the dependent variable. Interactions among variables may be examined using regression (linear, logistic, or any other regression form) by creating an interaction term, the product of the two independent variables whose interaction you want to test, and adding it to the model that includes those two independent variables, as well as any other independent variables for which you want to adjust. Suppose you wanted to test the interaction between two categorical variables each with two categories: gender (male or female) and frequency of eating out in restaurants (often vs. not often). You would create a new variable, called the interaction term, which is the product of gender times restaurant (in SPSS, go to "Transform," select "Compute Variable," in the "Target Variable" box, give the variable a name (perhaps "interaction"), move the "Gender" variable into the "Numeric Expression" window, then type "*" for multiplication, and then move the restaurant variable "Restaurant-dicho" into the "Numeric Expression" box. The text should look like "Gender*Restaurant_Dicho." Click on "OK" and the interaction variable is created (you will see it in the Data View window). Then, run the regression model as before (including the independent variables "gender," "age," "restaurant_dicho," "Black," "Asian," and "Hispanic"), but also put the interaction term you created in the Independent(s) window.

From the regression model with the interaction term (see Table 14-3), the only parameter

Putting It All Together

The conclusions can be stated as follows: This model predicts 3.1% of the variance in total cholesterol, and this is statistically significant at $\alpha = .05$. Age is positively associated with total cholesterol such that adjusting for the other variables in the model, for each additional year in age, the natural log (recall that we logged the outcome to make it more normal) of total cholesterol is predicted to increase by .002 units, and this association is statistically significant ($p = .001$). None of the other variables in the model was significantly associated with total cholesterol.

| Table 14-3 | **LINEAR REGRESSION MODEL WITH INTERACTION TERM** |

Variables Entered/Removed[a]

Model	Variables Entered	Variables Removed	Method
1	Interaction, Asian, age in years, Black, participant gender, Hispanic, restaurant_dicho[b]	.	Enter

[a]Dependent variable: LNCholesterol.
[b]All requested variables entered.

Model Summary

Model	R	R²	Adjusted R²	Standard Error of the Estimate
1	.216[a]	.047	.030	.19918

[a]Predictors: (Constant), Interaction, Asian, age in years, Black, participant gender, Hispanic, and restaurant_dicho.

ANOVA[a]

Model		Sum of Squares	df	Mean Square	F	Significance
1	Regression	.799	7	.114	2.878	.006[b]
	Residual	16.306	411	.040		
	Total	17.105	418			

[a]Dependent variable: LNCholesterol.
[b]Predictors: (Constant), Interaction, Asian, age in years, Black, participant gender, Hispanic, and restaurant_dicho.

Coefficients[a]

Model		Unstandardized Coefficients		Standardized Coefficients			95% Confidence Interval for B	
		B	Standard Error	β	t	Significance	Lower Bound	Upper Bound
1	(Constant)	5.185	.040		128.812	.000	5.106	5.264
	Participant gender	−.003	.024	−.008	−.142	.887	−.051	.044
	Age in years	.002	.001	.160	3.171	.002	.001	.003
	Restaurant_dicho	.029	.033	.061	.894	.372	−.035	.094
	Black	−.053	.030	−.100	−1.779	.076	−.111	.006
	Asian	.005	.031	.009	.167	.868	−.057	.067
	Hispanic	−.044	.025	−.106	−1.760	.079	−.094	.005
	Interaction	−.049	.049	−.068	−.995	.320	−.144	.047

[a]Dependent variable: LNCholesterol.

Author Comment *The interaction term is not statistically significant (p = .320).*

you are interested in is the *p*-value associated with the regression coefficient for the interaction term (the last table in the output). The other regression coefficients in this model are not interpretable as measures of association for the sample as a whole, so we ignore them. In our example, we see that the *p*-value for the interaction term is .320, which is greater than .05 and therefore we conclude that there is no significant interaction between gender and frequency of eating in restaurants on the outcome of cholesterol.

APPROACHES TO SELECTING VARIABLES FOR INCLUSION IN MULTIPLE LINEAR REGRESSION MODELS

Because there is so much intercorrelation among variables used in behavioral research, we may want to select a subset of variables that does the best job of predicting a particular outcome. Usually, we want to find the smallest group of variables that will account for the greatest proportion of variance in the dependent variable. Using such information, we can make practical decisions. If two predictors are equally good, we will probably decide to use the one that is easiest to administer, most economical, and so forth. Outlined here are some of the commonly used methods for selecting variables, including standard, stepwise, and hierarchical. In the linear regression menu in SPSS, most of these options can be found in the "Method" drop-down menu.

Standard Approach

All the independent variables are entered at once, which is the method we used in the examples in this chapter. In SPSS, it is called "Enter." All variables are evaluated in relation to the dependent variable and the other independent variables through the use of partial correlation coefficients.

Stepwise Forward and Backward Solutions

In the stepwise forward solution, the independent variable that has the highest correlation with the dependent variable is entered first. The second variable entered is the one that will increase the R^2 the most over and above what the first variable contributed. Say we have four independent variables, and we calculated the correlations between each independent variable and the dependent variable and found the highest correlation to be .50. That independent variable enters the equation and accounts for .50^2 or 25% of the variance. Now we want to know which of the three remaining variables will add the most to the 25% that is already explained. The computer cannot simply select the one with the next-highest correlation with the dependent variable because there is intercorrelation among the independent variables. Therefore, partial correlations are calculated between each of the three remaining independent variables and the dependent variable. Thus, the effect of the first variable is removed from the correlation. The variable that has the highest partial correlation with the dependent variable enters next. Then, the partial correlations between the two remaining independent variables and the dependent variable, taking out the effects of the first two variables in the equation, are calculated. The one with the highest partial correlation is entered next. Various criteria may be set for entry into the regression equation. The .05 level of significance is often used. In that case, a variable has to contribute a significant ($p < .05$) amount of variance to be included in the analysis. Once none of the remaining independent variables can contribute significantly to R^2, the analysis is ended.

In the stepwise backward solution, we start with the overall R^2 generated by putting all of our independent variables in the equation. Then, each variable is deleted one at a time to see whether R^2 drops significantly. If for any of these variables there is a significant drop in R^2, that variable is contributing significantly and will not be removed. If all the variables contribute significantly, the analysis would end with all four variables remaining in the equation. If one is not significant, there would be three variables left in the equation. Then, each of those three variables would be tested to see whether it would contribute significantly if entered last. The analysis continues until all variables in the equation contribute significantly if entered last.

Stepwise Solution

The stepwise solution combines the forward solution with the backward solution and therefore overcomes difficulties associated with each. With the forward solution, once a variable is in the equation, it is not removed. No attempt is made to reassess the contribution of a variable once other variables have been added. The backward solution remedies that problem, but the order of entry is not clear (i.e., which variable enters first and contributes most to the explained variance?). With the stepwise solution, variables are entered in the method outlined for the forward solution and are assessed at each step using the backward method to determine whether their contribution is still significant, given the effect of other variables in the equation.

Hierarchical

The researcher may want to force the order of entry of variables into the equation. Suppose you want to know whether a particular intervention would improve pregnancy outcomes. You already have some givens, such as age, SES, and nutritional status, and you would like to know whether your intervention makes a difference over and above factors that you cannot change. You might then run a linear regression model with just the given variables first and then run another model with both the given variables and the intervention. You could then compare R^2 for the two models to see if the addition of the intervention variables added to the explanatory power of the model.

Summary of Methods of Entry

Selecting a method for entering variables into the equation is an important decision, because the results will differ depending on the method selected. Stepwise methods were in vogue in the 1970s, but they are less popular today. Because the order of entry is based on a statistical rather than a theoretical rationale, the technique is criticized for capitalizing on chance. This is because the entry is based on the correlations among the variables, and these correlations are not stable with time because error is involved in their measurement. This becomes more of a problem when dealing with variables with low reliability.

Nunnally and Bernstein (1994) state that stepwise solutions are particularly problematic when testing hypotheses. The possibility of making a type I error expands dramatically with increased numbers of predictors. They believe that it is preferable to combine stepwise and hierarchical approaches. Variables are not to be "dumped" into an analysis and "large samples are an absolute necessity." They urge a ratio of 50 subjects to 1 variable if you want to use as many as 10 variables. They stress the need to examine the beta weights and R and to cross-validate results.

POWER ANALYSIS

Multiple linear regression is a useful technique, but there are numerous examples of its misuse. A major problem is including too many variables for the number of subjects.

Computer programs provide an adjusted R^2 as well as the actual R^2. The adjusted R^2 is a more conservative estimate given the number of subjects and variables. It also has been called a shrinkage formula, because it predicts how much the R^2 is likely to shrink. There are several formulas for this adjustment; one is given here (Pedhazur & Schmelkin, 1991, p. 446):

$$\text{Adjusted } R^2 = 1 - (1 - R^2)\frac{n-1}{n-k-1}$$

The formula is based on the number in the sample (n) and the number of independent variables (k). The more variables compared to subjects, the greater the shrinkage will be. If you put in the same number of subjects as independent variables, you will get a perfect R^2 (1), no matter which variables you use. (However, the adjusted R^2 will be zero.) Thus, you must always consider the number of subjects and the number of independent variables. Very high and seemingly impressive R^2's may be an artifact of too few subjects. Nunnally and Bernstein (1994, p. 201) state that one should have at least 10 subjects per predictor "in order to even hope for a stable prediction equation."

Cohen (1987) provides a formula for determining sample size, given an effect size index, which he calls L. He defines a small effect as an R^2 of .02, a moderate effect as an R^2 of .13, and a large effect as an R^2 of .30. The formula is as follows:

$$N = \frac{L(1 - R^2)}{R^2} + u + 1,$$

where N is the total sample size, L the effect size index, and u the number of independent variables.

L can be obtained from a table and is defined by Cohen as a function of power and number of independent variables at a given α-level. For our example, we select a power of .80, an α-level of .05, a moderate effect size, and two different numbers of independent variables to determine appropriate sample sizes.

For three independent variables, the value of L is 10.90, and the formula is as follows:

$$N = \frac{10.90(1 - 0.13)}{0.13} + 3 + 1$$

$$N = 77$$

For six independent variables, the value of L is 13.62, and the formula is as follows:

$$N = \frac{13.62(1 - 0.13)}{0.13} + 6 + 1$$

$$N = 98$$

Software programs also can calculate sample size. Sample size must be determined before data collection to ensure an adequate sample to conduct the proposed analyses.

It is possible to increase the accuracy of the prediction by adding predictor variables to the equation. The best additional variables to add are those that are highly correlated with the dependent variable but not highly correlated with the other independent variables. Usually, four or five predictors are enough. Adding more than that may add little to R^2 because of intercorrelations among the predictors.

Because the analysis uses error variance and true variance, the multiple correlation is usually inflated by such error variance. In addition to the shrinkage formula, another way to evaluate R^2 is to calculate it with a second sample. This is called *cross-validation*. A weakness of multiple regression is a tendency to throw variables into the equation. There should be some rationale for each variable included.

TESTING REGRESSION ASSUMPTIONS/REGRESSION DIAGNOSTICS

When multiple linear regression models are being used, it is important to ensure that the data are appropriate to the model. First, we need to check for outliers and be sure that the dependent variable is normally distributed. Next, we should check the bivariate relationships to be sure that they are linear. Scatter diagrams can be used to visualize the relationship between each pair of variables. A problem for behavioral researchers is the interrelatedness of the independent variables. This is called *multicollinearity*.

Multicollinearity

Because variables collected in behavioral research often provide very similar information, they are often highly correlated with each other. Such high interrelatedness makes evaluation of results problematic. Schroeder (1990) and Fox (1997) provide details on diagnosing and dealing with multicollinearity. Indications of the problem include high correlations between variables (>.85), substantial R^2 but statistically insignificant coefficients, unstable regression coefficients (i.e., betas that change dramatically when variables are added or dropped from the equation), unexpected size of coefficients (much larger or smaller than expected), and signs (positive or negative) that are unexpected.

The *tolerance* of a variable is used as a measure of collinearity. It is the proportion of the variance in a variable that is not accounted for by the other independent variables (SPSS, 1999b). To obtain measures of tolerance, each independent variable is treated as a dependent variable and is regressed on the other independent variables. A high multiple correlation indicates that the variable is closely related to the other independent variables. If the R^2 were 1, then the independent variable would be completely related to the others. Tolerance is simply $1 - R^2$; therefore, a tolerance of 0 ($1 - 1 = 0$) indicates perfect collinearity. The variable is a perfect linear combination of the other variables. The *variance inflation factor* is the reciprocal of tolerance (SPSS, 1999b). Therefore, variables with high tolerances have small variance inflation factors, and vice versa.

Testing Assumptions by Analyzing Residuals

Another important tool for checking the assumptions is residual analysis. Verran and Ferketich (1987) present an overview of the use of residual analysis to test linear model assumptions.

The residual is the difference between the actual and the predicted score. If the analysis were perfect, there would be no residuals; they would be zero.

Normal Distribution

If the relationships are linear and the dependent variable is normally distributed for each value of the independent variable, then the distribution of the residuals should be approximately normal (SPSS, 1999b). This can be assessed by using a histogram of the standardized residuals. Figure 14-3 shows this plot for age in our model looking at lnCholesterol as the outcome. The normal curve is interposed on the standardized residuals. It is possible to transform the data mathematically if residual analysis indicates violation of the assumption of normality, as we did by taking the natural log of the outcome.

Homoscedasticity

To check this assumption, the residuals can be plotted against the predicted values and against

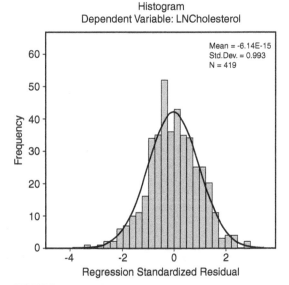

FIGURE 14-3   Histogram of residuals.

the independent variables. When standardized predicted values are plotted against observed values, the data would form a straight line from the lower-left corner to the upper-right corner, if the model fit the data exactly. Although the regression line is not drawn, if you took a ruler and drew a line from the lower-left to the upper-right corner, you would have it. In Figure 14-4, we demonstrate plotting residuals against one of our independent variables, age. Note that the actual scores vary around the prediction line. When the residuals are from a normal distribution, the plotted values fall close to the line in the normal probability plot (SPSS, 1999b). Figure 14-5 is an example from our analysis. Basically, this is a different look at what we saw in the histogram.

Summary of Assessing Assumptions in Regression Analysis

It is important, as always, to check data before it is entered into an analysis for normality, linear relationships, and so forth. In addition, we can request collinearity statistics and analyses of residuals as part of our computer analysis (in the linear regression window, click on "Plots" and move "Dependent" into the box labeled "Y" and "ZPRED" into the box labeled "X"; then check the boxes for "Produce all Partial Plots," "Histogram," and "Normal Probability Plot"; and hit "Continue"). It is very important to check these assumptions; otherwise, the results may be very questionable, and future analyses may show quite different results.

SUMMARY

Multivariate regression may be used for explanation and prediction. It is a flexible technique that allows the use of categorical and continuous variables. Overall, this is one of the most powerful techniques in our field; if used wisely, it can be of great assistance in studying many problems related to human behavior and the health professions.

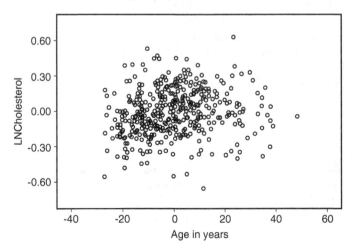

FIGURE 14-4 Plot of residuals against independent variable.

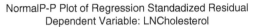

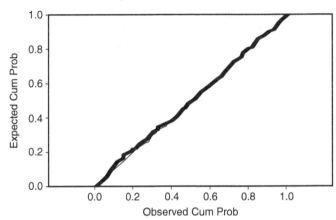

FIGURE 14-5   Normal probability plot.

CHAPTER REVIEW

Multiple-Choice Concept Review

1. Multiple linear regression models are best used with
   a. a dichotomous dependent variable.
   b. any ratio-level variable.
   c. a normally distributed ratio-level variable.
   d. all of the above.

2. The unadjusted regression coefficients (bs) in a multiple linear regression model give information about
   a. the strongest predictor of the dependent variable.
   b. the change in the dependent variable per unit increase in the independent variable.
   c. the adjusted odds of having the condition represented by the dependent variable given that the independent variable is present.
   d. a and b only.

3. The adjusted regression coefficient in a multiple linear regression contains information about
   a. the strongest predictor of the dependent variable.
   b. the change in the dependent variable per unit increase in the independent variable.
   c. the adjusted odds of having the condition represented by the dependent variable given that the independent variable is present.
   d. a and b only.

4. The coefficient of determination in a multiple linear regression contains information about
   a. the strongest predictor of the dependent variable.
   b. the change in the dependent variable per unit increase in the independent variable.
   c. the adjusted odds of having the condition represented by the dependent variable given that the independent variable is present.
   d. the amount of variance in the dependent variable explained by the model.

5. Linear regression models describe
   a. curvilinear relationships only.
   b. linear relationships only.
   c. both a and b.
   d. none of the above.

6. Dummy variables are used to
   a. recode the dependent variable.
   b. represent ratio variables in regression models.
   c. represent ordinal variables in regression models.
   d. represent nominal variables in regression models.

7. Linear regression allows you to test the significance of the following:
   a. The overall model
   b. Each regression coefficient
   c. The risk ratio comparing those with a characteristic to those without
   d. a and b only

8. When the outcome is nominal and dichotomous, which form of regression would be appropriate?
   a. Linear regression
   b. Logistic regression
   c. Multinomial or polytomous regression
   d. All of the above

9. Multivariate regression models, be they linear, logistic, or any other form, allow us to do which of the following?
   a. Simultaneously consider the effects of several independent variables on the dependent variable of interest
   b. Look at the association between two variables of nominal scale
   c. Minimize the risk of obtaining spurious results
   d. a and c

10. Adding an interaction term to the linear regression model allows us to
    a. interpret the adjusted association between each independent variable and the outcome.
    b. assess whether there is significant interaction between the two variables used to create the interaction term.
    c. calculate odds ratios.
    d. all of the above.

Choosing the Best Statistical Test

For each of the following scenarios (1 to 10), choose the most appropriate test (a to l).

a. Independent *t* test
b. Mann-Whitney *U*-test
c. Paired *t* test
d. Wilcoxon matched-pairs test
e. Logistic regression
f. McNemar test
g. Linear regression
h. Repeated-measures ANOVA
i. Friedman's ANOVA by rank
j. Kruskal-Wallis ANOVA
k. Pearson correlation coefficient
l. Spearman correlation coefficient

1. A total of 100 employees were followed for 10 years. Half of the employees were classified as having high-stress jobs, while the other half had low-stress jobs. Which group had a higher probability of having a heart attack over the 10 years of follow-up after adjusting for socioeconomic differences (income, education, and race)?

2. What is the relationship between the number of fruit and vegetables consumed in a week and total cholesterol level after adjusting for age? There are 300 people in the study, and cholesterol level is normally distributed.

3. What is the relationship between score of an exam and staying up all night to study (yes/no)? Exam score is normally distributed.

4. Thirty-five patients underwent a new surgical procedure, while another 35 had the standard procedure. You want to know if the probability of having a postoperative complication differed by procedure type.

5. You want to know if the mean weight of graduate students differs by year of graduate school. Weight is not normally distributed.

6. In order to examine the relationship between pulmonary blood flow and pulmonary blood volume in children with congenital heart disease, 46 such children were randomly sampled and both these variables were measured for each. Both variables are normally distributed.

7. You conduct a study to see if the size of a family's house in rural Bangladesh is associated with the number of family members living in the house and if that association differs by income. You are concerned that for poor families, having a larger family is associated with having a smaller house (a negative association), while larger richer families have larger houses (a positive association).

8. A weight-loss program recruited 30 sibling pairs. One sibling was assigned to an exercise program, while the other was assigned to a nutrition program. The investigator wanted to know which intervention resulted in the most weight lose. Weight lose is normally distributed.

9. A group of researchers is interested in determining if a relationship exists between geographic area (i.e., rural, suburban, and urban) and years of education attained in adults at least 40 years of age. Years of education is not normally distributed.

10. Was there an association between the out-of-pocket charge (dollars paid) to see a physician and rating of the physician visit? Rating is measured on a 10-point scale ranging from very negative to very positive. Neither variable is normally distributed.

Critical Thinking Concept Review

1. Write three multivariate hypotheses that can be tested with multiple linear regression.

2. Locate an article of interest that uses multiple linear regression. Write a brief review of the purpose of the article, the methods, and the findings. Write out the regression equation from information in the Results section. Also, obtain all of the information that you would expect to get from a multiple linear regression model (percent variance explained, unadjusted and adjusted regression coefficients, and statistical significance). Write a brief conclusion based on the information you gleaned from the article.

Computational Problems

1. Consider the following multiple linear regression equation:

$$Y' = 2.75 + 13.42X_1 + .75X_2 - 4.21X_3 + 10.30X_4$$

Find the predicted value of the dependent variable $(\hat{Y})$ given the following situations:
a. The values of all the independent variables are equal to 0.
b. $X_1 = 2; X_2 = 3; X_3 = 1; X_4 = -3$
c. $X_1 = -1; X_2 = 3; X_3 = -1; X_4 = 8$

2. Is BMI associated with eating out in restaurants frequently (more than five times per week on average) after adjusting for gender, age, and race/ethnicity? Use the SPSS data set we used for our example on cholesterol to answer the following questions:
a. First look at a histogram for BMI and decide if you need to log transform the outcome to make it more normal.
b. Next run the linear regression model (make sure to use dummy variables for the race/ethnicity categories) and interpret the results.
c. What is the predicted ln(BMI) of a white woman age 25 who does not eat out often?
d. Is there interaction between gender and eating out often in predicting BMI?

Exploratory Factor Analysis

Jane Karpe Dixon

OBJECTIVES

After studying this chapter, you should be able to:

1. Identify research situations in which factor analysis is appropriate.

2. Describe steps involved in carrying out a factor analysis procedure.

3. Conduct an exploratory factor analysis using the Statistical Package for the Social Sciences (SPSS).

4. Interpret factor analysis results from a computer display or a published study.

OVERVIEW OF FACTOR ANALYSIS

Factor analysis is a statistical tool for analyzing scores on large numbers of variables to determine whether there are any identifiable dimensions that can be used to describe many of the variables under study. Sometimes researchers assume that observed covariation between variables is due to some underlying common factors. The collection of intercorrelations is treated mathematically in such a way that underlying traits are identified.

Factor analysis may be exploratory or confirmatory. Exploratory factor analysis is used to summarize data by grouping together variables that are intercorrelated. Most often, this occurs in the early stages of research. In contrast, confirmatory factor analysis tests hypotheses about the structure of variables. Confirmatory factor analysis may follow an exploratory factor analysis, or it may come directly from theory. Exploratory factor analysis and confirmatory factor analysis are complementary techniques that are often used together in a single study or coordinated program of research. The direct purpose of exploratory factor analysis is to reduce a set of data so that it may be described and used easily. Most often, this occurs in the context of instrument development, although it can also be used in the development of theory.

Researchers in the health care fields often focus their attention on multiple variables. This is a direct result of the nature of the problems under study. In the real world of patient care, problems are complex with many related components. Sometimes, these many components are interrelated parts of a whole. For example, "self-management of chronic disease" is a broad concept that includes a variety of dimensions. Other times, variables may be closely related but still reflect phenomena that are highly distinct and separate. Factor analysis may often serve as an early step in the process of achieving a multivariate perspective on a clinical research problem.

Often, when labeling variables, a single word or phrase is used to represent a phenomenon with multiple parts. Our language may be overly general, blending together the multiple aspects of the phenomenon of interest. Consider, for example, the term *satisfaction with care*. Superficially, it may seem logical to measure this with a single rating. ("Rate your satisfaction with the care you received.") However, such a rating might involve opinions on a variety of matters, such as perceived competence of caregivers, convenience, pleasantness of the environment, and sense of being cared for. (As an exercise, think of at least two other aspects of satisfaction with care.) It is hard to know which of these influences are reflected in a subject's satisfaction rating and what such a rating really means. Instead of a global rating, should the various aspects be measured separately? There are so many potential variables that we may be unable to decide which should be measured and which should not. Factor analysis can help us make such decisions.

The amount of information on which our minds can focus simultaneously is limited. As a convenience, we may concentrate on variables thought to be primary. This will reduce the data burden. In some research endeavors, however, such simplicity of questionnaire may not be necessary, because we have techniques for organizing multivariate data—data on many variables.

Factor analysis can serve the purpose of data reduction by helping us to group a large number of variables into a smaller, more manageable number of "factors." A factor is simply a linear combination of a set of variables. This is analogous to univariate approaches in which a mean, variance, or correlation coefficient is calculated to reduce individual scores on one or two values. In this chapter, the purposes of factor analysis are explained, and the steps used to carry out a factor analysis are introduced. Because factor analysis is a complex technique, and it is carried out by computer, this chapter emphasizes interpretation rather than calculation. The chapter focuses on the most basic form of factor analysis, commonly referred to as exploratory factor analysis.

RESEARCH QUESTIONS

Factor analysis asks the question "how do different sets of variables group together?" We will use a hypothetical example of a factor analysis situation to illustrate this. Suppose we measure six variables within a sample of adult female participants in a health maintenance organization. Three of these variables are aspects of body size: height, arm length, and leg length, and the other three are measures of illness episodes in the past year: number of sore throats, number of headaches, and number of earaches. If we want to see how these variables group—which ones go together and which ones do not and how strongly does each variable go with its group—we can use factor analysis. This technique allows us to explore the many dimensions that are needed to explain relationships among the variables (Nunnally & Bernstein, 1994).

We can begin to explore answers to these questions through careful examination of the patterns of correlations among these variables. In the matrix of correlations for these six

Table 15-1	SIMPLIFIED REPRESENTATION OF A CORRELATION MATRIX					
	Height	**Arm Length**	**Leg Length**	**Number of Sore Throats**	**Number of Headaches**	**Number of Earaches**
Height	—	Hi	Hi	Lo	Lo	Lo
Arm Length		—	Hi	Lo	Lo	Lo
Leg Length			—	Lo	Lo	Lo
Number of Sore Throats				—	Hi	Hi
Number of Headaches					—	Hi
Number of Earaches						—

"Hi" means correlation of high magnitude, regardless of direction (approaching 1.00 or –1.00).
"Lo" means correlation of low magnitude (near zero).

variables (Table 15-1), we see that the three size variables have high intercorrelations and that the three history variables also have high intercorrelations; that is, a woman with longer than average legs also may have longer than average arms. She is also likely to be taller than average. A person reporting frequent sore throats also may report other discomforts. On the other hand, it would be surprising if the size variables and the history variables were highly related.

If we analyze the correlation matrix given in Table 15-1, a factor matrix defining the two groups of variables would be derived, as shown in Table 15-2. Each column in this table reflects one of the variable groupings or factors. The size variables have high values in one column, and the history variables have high values in the other column. This table, indicating the presence of two distinct groups of variables—two factors—summarizes the information contained in the larger correlation matrix. It reduces the data. Thus, we see that much of the information from a 6 × 6 correlation matrix is also conveyed in a 6 × 2 factor matrix.

You may object that the groupings derived were already easily apparent from the correlation table and that an advanced statistical technique is not needed to show what is obvious. This is true, but we have shown a simplified case, created just to be a teaching example. In actual practice, factor analysis does help us know what we would not otherwise know. Suppose that we had a 20 × 20 correlation matrix with widely ranging correlation coefficients, and the groupings among the variables were subtle. The variables would appear in random order, rather than neatly arranged

Table 15-2	ABBREVIATED FACTOR MATRIX DEFINING TWO GROUPS OF VARIABLES	
	Factors	
	I	II
Height	Hi	Lo
Arm length	Hi	Lo
Leg length	Hi	Lo
Number of sore throats	Lo	Hi
Number of headaches	Lo	Hi
Number of earaches	Lo	Hi

"Hi" means above 0.40 or below –0.40 (especially approaching 1.00 or –1.00).
"Lo" means between 0.40 and –0.40 (especially near zero).

according to grouping. Then patterns would not be obvious. Factor analysis is a tool through which we may uncover groupings of variables that are not obvious.

Instrument Development

In the research literature of nursing and other health care professions, factor analysis is most often used as a part of the instrument development process. Factor analysis may be a vital step in the creation of a new measurement tool. It is a method for organizing the items into factors. A factor is a group of items that may be said to belong together. A person who scores high on one item of a particular factor is likely to score above average on other items of the factor and vice versa. Such an item has high correlations with other items of the same factor and not so high correlations with items of different factors. This principle provides the mathematical basis for assignment of items to factors through the statistical technique of factor analysis.

Factor analysis is often used to test the validity of ideas about items in order to decide how items should be grouped together into subscales and which items should be dropped from the instrument entirely. The method helps to provide justification for our use of summated scales (sets of items summed into scale scores). For example, a researcher may start with 18 items and based on factor analysis decide that these should be organized into two subscales: For each subject, two scores will be calculated. It is also common for some items to be dropped from a scale based on factor analysis results. Factor analysis is an important statistical tool for providing validity evidence concerning the internal structure of our instruments. In most cases, this is followed by computation of Cronbach's alpha coefficient, which is a measure of internal consistency reliability. Such reliability is an alternative way of looking at the extent to which items go together, similar to the factor analysis itself; however, in computation

of reliability, only one set of items is dealt with at a time. Also, reliability computations are useful for further identifying weak items that may be omitted in subsequent analysis. In any case, items that form a strong factor in factor analysis generally yield acceptable alpha coefficients when grouped together in a scale, thus providing evidence of internal consistency reliability, as well as supporting beginning evidence of construct validity for a developing scale. Almost all the use of exploratory factor analysis in the health literature is in the context of instrument development and validation.

What are the Factors (Dimensions) of the Environmental Health Engagement Profile?

The author of this chapter, with several colleagues, developed an instrument to measure people's engagement in environmental health (Dixon, Hendrickson, Ercolano, Quackenbush, & Dixon, 2009). We called it the Environmental Health Engagement Profile (EHEP). We developed EHEP through a rigorous, multiphase process. First, we conducted qualitative interviews with 41 urban residents about environmental health (including at least one from each census tract from our area of focus). We used the content of these interviews to inform our process of writing items for the instrument. We wanted the items to reflect what people may think and do about environment and health. For example, a person may come to believe that pollution is a major cause of illness. Likewise, a person may decide to restrict his or her personal use of pesticides in order to avoid toxic exposure (for himself or herself and others). Second, we had experts evaluate these potential items for relevance and clarity to each of three proposed dimensions for EHEP (Concerns, Actions, and Pollution Type). In the third phase, we tested our draft instrument via telephone interviews with 433 residents of the same urban area. We used factor analysis to identify the groupings of items within the instrument. We obtained a five-factor solution, with the proposed dimensions of both Concerns and Actions splitting into two factors, respectively. Based on these results, we then arranged the 44 items of EHEP into five subscales, called Pollution Sensitivity Scale, Pollution-Causes-Illness Scale, Pollution Acceptance Scale, Community Environmental Action Scale, and Personal Action Scale. We were also pleased to see that reliabilities of the subscale were generally adequate.

What are the Factors (Dimensions) of a Self-Report Measure of Self-Management of Diabetes in Adolescents?

The author of this chapter also collaborated in the development of a self-report measure for youth concerning self-management of type 1 diabetes (Schilling et al., 2009). We called the instrument Self-Management of Type 1 Diabetes in Adolescents (SMOD-A). We used state-of-the-art methods of instrument development for this project as well. Development of items was informed first by a previous qualitative descriptive study involving semistructured interviews of youth and their parents (Schilling, Knafl, & Grey, 2006). These potential items for the instrument were then evaluated for item relevance and clarity by experts—including a group of "experiential experts," composed of adolescents deemed to be good self-managers and their parents (Schilling et al., 2007). Then, we conducted a field study with 515 adolescents from two sites to test the instrument, including a look at its underlying structure via factor analysis. Because SMOD-A has two sections, we conducted the factor analysis separately for the sections. We obtained a four-factor solution for Part 1 and a one-factor solution for Part 2. Based on this analysis, we concluded that the SMOD-A has five subscales—Collaboration with Parents, Diabetes Care Activities, Diabetes Problem Solving, Diabetes Communication, and Goals. It was also gratifying to find that subscales' reliabilities were adequate for their separate use.

Theory Building

The building of theory is a principal purpose of research, and factor analysis may support such efforts in a variety of ways: by describing clinical phenomena, exploring relationships, identifying constructs that unite a set of elements, creating units of classification for systems construction, and testing hypotheses. All of these are theory-building functions. Ideally, development of theory and of instruments are closely related endeavors, as researchers build instruments based on theory and then use the findings generated via the instrument to refine the theory. It is in relation to the theory development purpose of factor analysis that the distinction between exploratory and confirmatory goals is of most importance. In a truly exploratory approach, a researcher uses factor analysis to discover a structure that can be meaningfully interpreted. The structure is allowed to unfold from the data, rather than being based on the researcher's preconceptions of what structure will emerge. In a truly confirmatory approach, a hypothesis is developed, and variables relevant to that hypothesis are then identified and (once data are collected) submitted to factor analysis. The researcher asks whether the data fit the hypothesized model better than they fit alternative models. It is not uncommon for exploratory and confirmatory approaches to be combined in a single study, as results obtained through exploratory factor analysis are then refined through confirmatory approaches.

What are the Factors (Dimensions) of the Family Management Measure Concerning the Way That Parents Manage Their Child's Chronic Condition? Do These Fit With the Family Management Style Framework?

The author of this chapter collaborated with Knafl et al., (2009) to develop the Family Management Measure (FaMM) regarding parental perceptions of family management of a child's chronic condition, based on interviews with 579 parents. Items for the FaMM were generated based on dimensions of the Family Management Style Framework (Knafl & Deatrick, 2003). Exploratory factor analysis was used to determine the initial number of factors of the FaMM, and confirmatory analysis techniques were used for refining the factors, including determining item placement. Confirmatory techniques were also used to compare the theory-based model with that of the exploratory analysis. Although the exploratory approach led to stronger scales, still the results are generally consistent with the Family Management Style Framework. Results also suggest areas for further theoretical development to be undertaken.

Using Factor Analysis for Data Reduction

Sometimes factor analysis is used solely for data reduction, simply because such reduction may be needed for subsequent analysis. One goal of scientific inquiry is parsimony or simplicity of explanation; that is, it is preferable to use one variable, rather than many, to explain a phenomenon. Factor analysis provides a means for creating a single composite variable out of many variables. Alternatively, factor analysis may be used to identify several composite variables, which, taken together, summarize the sources of variance contained in all (or most) variables included in a study (or at least of those variables of a particular type). These composite variables are mathematically constructed through a combination of the measured variables. The several composite variables, rather than the larger number of measured variables, are then used in subsequent data analysis. Data reduction of this sort may serve a highly pragmatic function. The researcher may collect a large amount of data, reduce the data through factor analysis, and conduct other analyses (such as regression or analysis of variance) on the reduced data. In these subsequent analyses, the number

of variables relative to the number of subjects is kept within reasonable bounds, reliability is augmented, and provided that the meanings of factors are clearly defined and communicated, interpretation of the analysis may be simplified. Often, this is combined with instrument development or theory development. A special case of this approach occurs in the use of principal components analysis (a closely related technique to factor analysis) in the study of environmental pollution on health.

How Can Environmental Pollutants Best be Measured for Studies of Health Effects?

In research on effects of air pollution on mortality or morbidity, a large number of pollutants may be measured. (In addition to six-criterion air pollutants that can be measured in a variety of ways, the Clean Air Act identifies 187 air toxins, most of which are tracked via national assessment.) Because of potential for high correlations (e.g., collinearity) between pollutants, it is most appropriate statistically to study health effects of combinations of pollutants, rather than attempting to relate health effects to single pollutants. This also fits the reality that humans are exposed to combinations of pollutants (not just to pollutants one at a time)—and effects of combined pollutants may be multiplicative, not just additive. So if combinations are to be employed in investigations of health effects, principal components analysis may be used to identify the relevant combinations. Roberts and Martin (2006) have recently offered a refinement of this approach in which individual variables are included only if they relate to the dependent variable of interest—in their case mortality across nine cities and over time.

TYPE OF DATA REQUIRED

Most often, the factor analysis process begins with a large number of variables gathered from subjects and the calculation of Pearson product–moment correlations between these variables. However, one may also carry out a factor analysis based simply on a correlation matrix, even without access to the raw data by subjects. Whatever the actual starting point, the correlation matrix is the basis for the factor analysis.

You are already familiar with the correlation matrix, the beginnings of many of our statistical treatments. In such a matrix, the two halves are identical; that is, the correlation of X with Y is the same as the correlation of Y with X. We call such a matrix symmetrical. Factor analysis may be performed on any symmetrical matrix of correlations.

In the development of a new instrument, however, it is common for some items to be eliminated from consideration prior to conducting factor analysis. This is based on the univariate and multivariate characteristics of each item. This systematic evaluation of individual items is called *item analysis*. For example, in development of SMOD-A as described above, data were collected from adolescents with diabetes using 86 items, but 13 of the items were eliminated prior to factor analysis, based on the item analysis—usually because the frequency distribution indicated a lack of variability. One of the items eliminated was "My parents encourage me to take care of my diabetes." A large majority of the participants (89%) answered *always* to this item. An item that lacks variability will not show relationships with other items and does not contribute to understanding the concept under study.

Criteria used to select some items for factor analysis and eliminate others vary from one study to another. In addition to indicators of variability, moderate correlation with other items (between .30 and .70) may serve as an additional criterion for screening items. In general, these criteria are largely based on understanding of the assumptions and meaning of correlation and the role of factor analysis in summarizing or reducing a correlation matrix.

ASSUMPTIONS

Factor analysis is based on a matrix of correlations between variables, so all data assumptions applicable to calculation and interpretation of correlations apply to factor analysis as well. Data should be interval level or data that the researcher has specifically decided to treat as interval, as typically occurs with Likert-type self-report data. Data should be approximately normally distributed. It is customary to base factor analysis on variables that are measured on a common metric or response format. Note that a curvilinear relationship between two variables cannot be detected using the Pearson product–moment correlation. Therefore, such a relationship will not be reflected in factor analysis results either.

In general, for meaningful results to be obtained in a factor analysis, correlations between variables should be substantial so that each variable included correlates highly with at least one other variable. It is common to look for correlations with other variables between .30 and .70. Nunnally and Bernstein (1994) recommend inclusion of marker variables with known properties to increase the likelihood of obtaining substantial correlations. Also, all variables included must be reliably measured, and subjects must show some variation in their responses.

SAMPLE SIZE

For statistical tests treated elsewhere in this book, there is a direct relationship between sample size and power of the test to identify statistically significant differences between groups (or relationships between variables), when such differences (or relationships) exist in the population from which the sample is drawn. With a larger sample size, the ability to generalize from the sample to the population is increased. In exploratory models of factor analysis, statistical significance is not tested, and strictly speaking, the concept of "power" does not apply. However, the value of observed sample data in reflecting reality as it exists in the larger population is a major concern in most factor analytic studies, as in most research generally. It is desirable that our results be generalizable beyond the sample from which the data are obtained.

In factor analysis, the number of subjects needed is usually assessed in relation to the number of variables being measured. Although factor analysis is especially appropriate when working with a large amount of data, the number of variables that may be included in a factor analysis procedure is limited. It is tied to sample size. Certainly, the number of cases should always exceed the number of variables. A ratio of at least 10 subjects for each variable is desirable to generalize from the sample to a wider population. With smaller ratios, the influence of relationships based on random patterns within the data becomes more pronounced. However, an alternative perspective on sample size is that a sample size of 100 is fully adequate for exploratory factor analysis for purposes related to measurement (Sapnas & Zeller, 2002), though this alternative perspective has not been widely accepted. Regardless of sample size, the need for replication of factor studies is increasingly apparent. If two different data sets yield similar factor structures, this would greatly increase our confidence that the factor structures obtained may be generalized to other samples not yet studied.

COMPUTING A FACTOR ANALYSIS: SIX MATRICES

The mathematics of factor analysis is complex. It is based on matrix algebra—the branch of mathematics that deals with the manipulation of matrices (i.e., plural of matrix). However, matrix algebra is beyond the scope of this book, and you do not need an understanding of matrix algebra to conduct a factor analysis. Nor should you expect to ever compute a factor analysis by hand or using a calculator—even as a practice

exercise; computations are done through statistical software, such as SPSS, as shown in this chapter. Nevertheless, for undertaking factor analysis or understanding its use in the literature, it is appropriate to have a firm knowledge of what matrices are being manipulated and what information each matrix represents. Conceptually, this process of carrying out a factor analysis may involve as many as six matrices with each matrix derived from a previous one. This section is intended to provide a conceptual and working understanding of these six matrix types.

Raw Data Matrix

These are the data that the researcher collects about the study subjects and enters into the database. In the conceptual form of a raw data matrix, each line contains information about one subject, and each column represents a variable. Such a matrix is the beginning of any data analysis. A raw data matrix to be factor analyzed would contain many variables, with data on each variable from many subjects.

Correlation Matrix

You are also familiar with the correlation matrix. When fully depicted, the correlation matrix is a square, symmetrical matrix in which the number of rows and the number of columns each equals the number of variables. Because the correlation matrix is symmetrical (therefore, containing much duplication), it is often depicted in one of several abbreviated forms. The correlation matrix summarizes information in the raw data matrix. It is smaller, with fewer rows and fewer elements than the raw data matrix. This is the beginning of the data-reduction process. In some situations, the correlation matrix is altered prior to conducting the factor analysis. This alteration concerns the diagonal that extends from the upper-left corner to the lower-right corner—the correlation of each variable with itself. Each variable correlates perfectly with itself, so the conventional correlation matrix contains "1.0" as every element in this diagonal. However, in a correlation matrix to be used for a factor analysis, this may not be maintained. Depending on decisions about the factor analysis model to be used, these 1s are sometimes replaced by a number smaller than 1.0 and selected to be specific for each variable, such as an estimate of the common variance with other variables or the reliability of measurement. This is further explained later in the chapter.

Unrotated Factor Matrix

Based on the correlation matrix, the first of two (or more) factor matrices are calculated. (The unrotated factor matrix is obtained via one of several extraction methods—for more on extraction methods, see the 'Other Options' section on page 393). In an unrotated factor loading matrix, each row represents one variable included in the factor analysis. There are fewer columns, each column representing one factor. In the unrotated factor matrix, the elements within the matrix are the unrotated factor loadings—numbers ranging between –1 and +1, which are like correlations of the variable with the factor. The square of a factor loading represents the proportion of variance that the item and factor have in common; in other words, this is the proportion of item variance explained by the factor. For example, the first variable (1) has a loading of .85 on factor I; approximately 72% of the variance is accounted for by this loading, $(.85)^2 = .7225$. Adding the squared loadings across a row, you arrive at the item communality (h^2). This is the portion of item variance accounted for by the various factors. For variable 1 in Table 15-3, the squared factor loadings are totaled as follows: $.85^2 + .22^2 + .03^2 = .77$. The item communality is .77; that is, 77% of the item variance is "explained" by the three factors.

Likewise, if you add the squared loadings contained in a single column, you will obtain the eigenvalue for the factor. The eigenvalue represents the total amount of variance explained

Table 15-3 FACTOR LOADING MATRIX

Variables		Factors			
		I	II	III	h²
	1	0.85	0.22	0.03	0.77
	2	0.15	•	•	•
	3	0.51	•	•	•
	4	0.83	•	•	•
	5	0.26	•	•	•
Eigenvalues		1.76			
% of variance		0.35			

by a factor. The average of the squared loadings in a column is obtained by dividing the eigenvalue by the number of items in the column (eigenvalue/n). This average represents the percent of interitem variance accounted for by the factor. For the first factor in Table 15-3, the eigenvalue is calculated as follows: $.85^2 + .15^2 + .51^2 + .83^2 + .26^2 = 1.76$. This eigenvalue of 1.76 is divided by 5 (because there are five variables), yielding .352. Thus, approximately 35% of total item variance is accounted for by the first factor. Adding the percent of variance accounted for by each factor tells us how much variance is explained by all the factors.

Factor eigenvalues and variance accounted for are the most important figures contained in the unrotated factor matrix. You may be especially interested in how much variance is accounted for altogether by the important factors; this is simply the sum of variance accounted for by individual factors. Either factor eigenvalues or the variance accounted for by factors may be used to determine the number of potentially interpretable factors contained in the data. Typically, researchers want to interpret the number of factors that each account for at least 5% of variance or the number of factors for which the eigenvalue is 1 or greater. Determination of the appropriate number of factors paves the way for the next matrix of the factor analysis process.

A Note on Extraction Models

For the ambitious reader, further explanation is provided here concerning the choices facing the researcher who is conducting a factor analysis. (If you are a less-ambitious reader, or simply too busy, you may want to skip this section.) The unrotated factor matrix is obtained through the use of an extraction method, and the statistical software packages that are generally used offer a choice of extraction methods. Basically, two general approaches are based on two different assumptions about the data (Ferketich & Muller, 1990).

The distinction has to do with the nature of the variance in the data. One possible assumption is that all measurement error is random. In this case, the mean of deviations (representing the error) is zero. Based on this assumption, a researcher chooses to use the extraction method known as principal components. Using this method of extraction, new variables are exact mathematical transformations of the original data. When this method of extraction is used, all variance in the observed variables contributes to the solution. Because each variable correlates perfectly with itself, the 1s (unities) in the diagonal of the correlation matrix are a part of the variance that is analyzed. Using the principal components method, the goal is to convert a set of variables into a new set of variables that is an exact mathematical transformation of the original data.

The other possible assumption to be made is that measurement error consists of a systematic component and a unique component. The systematic component may reflect common variance due to factors that are not directly measured (Ferketich & Muller, 1990). These are called *latent factors*. Based on this assumption, a researcher chooses to use any of a class of extraction methods categorized as "common factor analysis." This includes methods named *principal axis, alpha, image, generalized least squares*, and *unweighted least squares*. Because the researcher making this assumption wants to focus on the common variance, it is not appropriate to use the full correlation matrix. Instead, the diagonals are altered so that instead of consisting of unities (1s), an estimate of the communalities (h^2) is used. Such modification of a matrix may seem surprising to someone new to factor analysis. In common factor analyses, the matrix analyzed does not reflect the full variance in the data; rather, the covariance is analyzed.

Although some research methodologists place strong emphasis on the distinction between principal components and common factor analysis (Ferketich & Muller, 1990), Nunnally and Bernstein (1994) argue that in a well-designed study involving a sufficient number of subjects, choice of extraction model makes little practical difference in the results obtained. They do note, however, that the principal component method will lead to elements of the matrix being a bit larger. This is because approaches to common factor analysis always involve replacing the "ones" in the diagonal of the correlation matrix with numbers that are less than 1. Thus, the factor loadings that emerge are a bit smaller. We have seen that eigenvalues, variance accounted for by factor, and item communalities are all a direct function of the magnitude of the loadings, so it follows that these are smaller also. Thus, the factor solution may appear to be less good, but this is simply an artifact of the methods decision. Nunnally and Bernstein (1994) also note that the principal components method is more reliable because with this method, you always obtain a factor solution. In common factor analysis, obtaining a solution may not be a sure thing.

Given the potential for differences between extraction methods, some researchers routinely run multiple factor analyses of the same data set with varying methods. This enables the researcher to gauge the importance of these distinctions and other decision points in the factor analytic process as these affect the specific data under study.

Factor Matrix, Rotated

The unrotated factors are created so that the amount of variance accounted for by each successive factor is maximized. This means that variables may be associated with more than one factor. It is usually difficult to give a meaningful interpretation to unrotated factors. However, just as you may alter an algebraic equation by performing the same operation on both sides, you may transform or "rotate" a factor matrix into any one of an infinite number of mathematically equivalent matrices. If factor rotation is conducted according to the criterion of simple structure as described by Thurstone (1947), the result is a set of factors that are distinct from one another and that, in most situations, can be meaningfully and creatively interpreted by the researcher.

In simple structures, factors are set to maximize the number of loadings of great magnitude (near –1 and + 1) and loadings of small magnitude (near 0.00) for each factor; that is, a distinct pattern emerges in the factor matrix so that each factor has certain variables that go with it, while other variables do not. Likewise, as a simple structure is approached, each variable is identified with only one factor. According to Thurstone (1947), the following occurs in a rotated factor matrix:

1. Each row should have at least one loading close to zero.
2. Each column should have at least as many variables with near-zero loadings as there are factors.
3. For pairs of columns (factors), several variables should load on one and not on the other.

The essence of interpreting factor analytic results is the process of identifying, from the rotated factor matrix, which variables go with a factor and then naming the factor based on whatever meanings these variables with substantive loadings have in common. The criterion for considering a loading substantive varies from study to study. Most studies use a cutoff of .35 or higher; however, some studies will employ cutoff points as low as .20 (Parshall, 2002; Schilling et al., 2009), especially when the analysis also involves other processes through which individual items may be dropped from composite score calculation.

When naming and describing factors, the researcher uses not only knowledge of the statistical technique and how it works but also an understanding of the subject matter under study, especially an ability to construct new understandings of that subject matter. By facilitating the organization of individual variables into variable groupings, factor analysis opens the door to new conceptualizations and new ways of thinking, provided that the researcher is ready to discover these in the data. More than any other statistical technique, factor analysis requires the full exercise of creative potential.

Factor Score Matrix

Based on the rotated factor matrix, a score for each subject on each factor may be computed. To calculate such factor scores, an individual's score on each variable included in a factor is multiplied by the factor loading for the particular variable. The sum of these products is the individual's factor score. Factor scores can be calculated automatically within factor analysis procedures in statistical software such as SPSS. Consider an individual included in the data who received scores as follows:

Variable	Scores
1	2
2	4
3	1
4	5
5	2

This person's factor score on factor 1 would be calculated as follows:

$$(.85)(2)+(.15)(4)+(.51)(1)+(.83)(5)+(.26)(2)$$
$$=1.7+.6+.51+4.15+.52 = 7.48$$

This factor score, based on the strength of the loading of each variable on the factor, could be used instead of the individual's unweighted (i.e., summative) score on the factor. The factor score is based on the relative "importance" of each variable to the factor as indicated by the item loadings on the factor. It is conventional among researchers to use factor scores when conducting further analysis on the same data set. This operationalizes the data reduction purpose of factor analysis.

In contrast, when factor analysis is used primarily for the purpose of instrument development (as is often the case), it is conventional to derive an approach for the creation of unweighted scores from the factor results obtained. These are the summative scales (often referred to as subscales) that become a part of the protocol for how the instrument is to be scored and interpreted in future usage. This individual's unweighted score would be simply the sum of the scores on the three variables with substantial loadings on the factor $(2 + 1 + 5 = 8)$. This is a much more user-friendly approach for other researchers who will utilize the instrument in future studies. The factor score matrix has as many rows as subjects, with each column representing one factor. It is smaller than the raw data matrix because there are fewer factors than variables. The data have been reduced in Table 15-4.

Factor Correlation Matrix

Factor rotation is often orthogonal, with resulting factors uncorrelated with each other. This is usually desirable for instrument development, in which the researcher seeks to create subscales that are independent of one another.

Table 15-4	FACTOR SCORE MATRIX			
		Factors		
		I	II	•	•
Subjects	1	7.48	•	•	•
	2	•			
	•	•			
	•	•			
	•	•			
	N	•			

Alternatively, factor rotation also may be oblique, with factors that are not totally unrelated to each other. Advocates of oblique rotation assert that in the real world, important factors are likely to be correlated; thus, searching for unrelated factors is unrealistic. Novice factor analysts should probably plan to use an orthogonal, rather than oblique, rotation because it is easier to interpret. The Varimax (variance-maximized) method is available on widely used computer packages. This tends to produce factors that have low loadings with some variables and high loadings with other variables. Other alternatives are Quartimax, which is likely to yield a first, very general factor with many high loadings, and Equamax, which combines characteristics of Quartimax and Varimax, balancing the advantages and disadvantages of each.

With orthogonal rotation, one factor-loading matrix is produced. It represents both regression weights (called a *pattern matrix*) and correlation coefficients (called a *structure matrix*). Because the solution is orthogonal, the regression weights are equal to the correlation coefficients. The loadings are interpreted as were those in the unrotated factor matrix. A squared loading represents the variance accounted for in a variable by a particular factor. The squared loadings may be added across a row to determine the total variance accounted for in a variable by all the factors and so on.

Because with oblique rotation there is a correlation among the factors, the factor pattern matrix (the regression weights) and the factor structure matrix (containing correlation coefficients) are not the same. The two matrices are produced and interpreted differently. The pattern matrix is generally considered preferable as a basis for interpreting the meanings of factors. The square of a loading in a factor pattern matrix represents the variance accounted for by a particular variable, but because other factors may share some of this variance (due to intercorrelation among factors in an oblique solution), the total variance in an item accounted

Table 15-5	FACTOR CORRELATION MATRIX		
	Factor 1	Factor 2	Factor 3
Factor 1	1.00	0.65	0.30
Factor 2		1.00	0.45
Factor 3			1.00

for by all the factors cannot be determined by adding the squared loadings in a row (h^2).

In oblique rotation, a matrix displaying the correlation of each factor with every other factor is displayed in a factor correlation matrix. The structure of such a matrix is shown in Table 15-5.

STEPS OF A FACTOR ANALYTIC STUDY

The steps of a factor analytic study are as follows:

1. Formulate a research question or hypothesis. If factor analysis is the appropriate statistical technique for answering research questions or testing the hypothesis, proceed with the following steps.
2. Collect data of interest.
3. Calculate and examine univariate data on a variable-by-variable basis, identifying variables that should not be included in the factor analysis because of failure to meet initial assumptions or criteria.
4. Calculate and examine bivariate relationship data—again with an eye toward identifying variables and relationships that should not be included in the factor analysis.
5. Conduct the factor analysis. Unless you have a good reason to do otherwise, use an orthogonal rotation. If you have predicted certain factors, specify how many factors you expect; otherwise, let the computer determine the number of factors in the course of the factor analysis, based on eigenvalues in the unrotated factor matrix. Note the total proportion of interitem variance accounted for by the factor solution and the number of factors involved. Arriving at the most appropriate number of factors is one of the key elements of arriving at a factor solution that best reflects the data.

6. Name and interpret factors from the rotated factor loading matrix. (Sometimes researchers experiment with several factor solutions to choose the one that can be most meaningfully interpreted.)
7. If subsequent analyses are planned, use factor analysis results to decide how to combine variables; calculate these new or combined variables for each subject. (Usually, factor scores can be easily calculated within the statistical software for factor analysis.) Consider the reliabilities of the derived scores. Then conduct the subsequent analyses.
8. Relate findings to the existing literature, and disseminate results through presentation and publication. If appropriate, repeat the analysis with other available populations.

Note that factor analysis is often used as an early stage of a multistage analysis, as indicated by steps 7 and 8. Subsequent analyses may be conducted as part of an instrument development and validation process or because of substantive interest. For example, after Lenoci, Telfair, Cecil, and Edwards (2002) identified three factors of their Chronic Illness Assessment Interview for Sickle Cell Disease and determined internal consistency of these as subscales (as well as test–retest reliability), they assessed construct validity by performing a multiple regression analysis using the factors scores to predict self-care behaviors. Scores on *Personal Satisfaction and Perceived Control* factor and *Feeling Concerned and Worried* factor were both positive predictors of self-care behaviors. In another analysis, scores on the *Feeling Supported* factor were related to satisfaction with services received from staff and physicians.

The authors note that these findings are consistent with prior studies and with their expectations. These data were taken as evidence of the potential usefulness of the new instrument for adults with sickle cell disease. Such findings may have important substantive and instrument development implications. Generally, factor analysis tends to be most useful when combined with other analyses within a single study.

COMPUTING A FACTOR ANALYSIS USING SPSS

As an example, we now illustrate computation of a factor analysis (via principal components extraction) using SPSS. The data to be analyzed are from the Inventory of Personal Attitudes (IPA), which was used as a part of a survey with students at Boston College School of Nursing and provided by Barbara Hazard Munro, PhD, FAAN. These data were collected to provide a sample data set for statistics learning. The data set includes 30 IPA items. Full data on each of the variables were provided by 661 subjects. Thus, there are 22 subjects per variable—well above the 10 to 1 ratio that is often recommended.

To compute a factor analysis using SPSS, the menu system may be used (Box 15-1). We will analyze these data by principal components extraction method with Varimax rotation. First, we click on "Analyze," then select "Dimension reduction," and then "Factor." We then follow the instructions as shown in Box 15-1. Note that if item analysis has not previously been conducted, there is an opportunity to do it now via selection of "Univariate statistics" under "Statistics," and also we may select "coefficients" and "significance levels" under correlation matrix, but these procedures are not our focus here.

The result of the analysis is shown in Figure 15-1. The first part of the printout shows two measures that are used to examine the strength of the relationships among the variables as a part of deciding whether factor analysis is appropriate (Norusis, 2003). The Kaiser-Meyer-Olkin (KMO) measure is based on the principle that if variables share common factors, then partial correlations between pairs of variables should be small when the effects of other variables are controlled. The KMO measure provides an approach to comparing the zero-order correlations to the partial correlations. The KMO measure may vary between zero and one with larger numbers indicating a greater difference between the zero-order correlations and the partial correlations. If a KMO measure in the .80s or higher is achieved, this supports the use of factor analysis for the data. In this analysis, the KMO measure of sampling adequacy is .964.

Bartlett's test of sphericity is used to evaluate whether a correlation matrix is suitable for factor analysis by testing the hypothesis that the matrix is an identity matrix—a matrix in which all coefficients not in the diagonal are zeroes. If a low probability is obtained and the hypothesis of an identity matrix is rejected, this supports the use of factor analysis as an appropriate procedure. In this analysis, the p-value (probability) is .000. These calculations provide support for proceeding with the analysis.

The next table shows communalities for each of the items. The column labeled "initial" presents 1.000 for each of the 30 variables. This simply indicates that the number 1.000 was kept in the diagonal of the correlation matrix that was analyzed—always the case when using the extraction method of principal components. In the column labeled "extraction," there is a listing of communalities as calculated for each item, based on the four-factor solution (as explained below). The communality for the first item may be rounded to .49, indicating that $.49^2$ or 24% of the variance in that item is accounted for by the four factors.

The next table contains information needed relative to general characteristics of the factors, both before and after rotation. SPSS uses the term components because we chose principal components analysis as the extraction method. Nevertheless, we will continue to use the term factors, as the components of principal components analysis and the factors of other forms of factor analysis are so closely analogous. Note that

BOX 15-1 USING SPSS TO COMPUTE A FACTOR ANALYSIS

Step 1: Enter data into SPSS. Click on "Analyze," then select "Dimension reduction," and then "Factor."

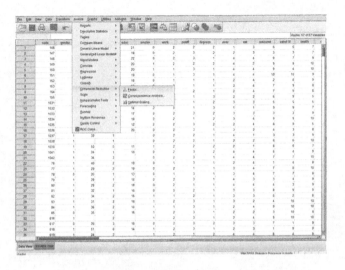

Step 2: In the pop-up box, we move the variables to be included into the box labeled "variables."

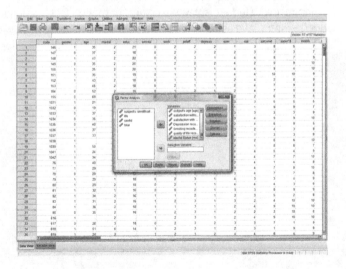

(Continued)

BOX 15-1   USING SPSS TO COMPUTE A FACTOR ANALYSIS *(Continued)*

Step 3: In "Descriptives" under "Statistics," we select "initial solution," and under "Correlation matrix" we select "KMO and Bartlett's test of sphericity."

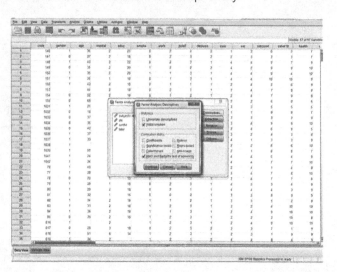

Step 4: Next, in the "extraction" box, we keep selection of "principal components," which is also the default method of extraction. Also, under "analyze," we select "correlation matrix." Under display, we select "unrotated factor solution" and "scree plot." Under "extract," we select "Based on eigenvalue" and we stick with the default value "Eigenvalue greater than 1." We also stick with the number 25, for "maximum iterations for convergence."

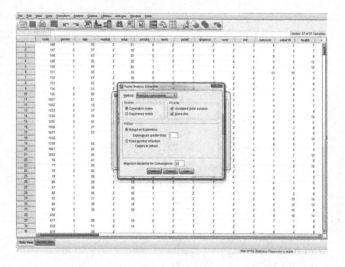

BOX 15-1   USING SPSS TO COMPUTE A FACTOR ANALYSIS *(Continued)*

Step 5: Next, in the "rotation" box, under "method," we select "Varimax." Under "display," we select "rotated solution." Again for "maximum iterations for convergence," we stick with the number "25."

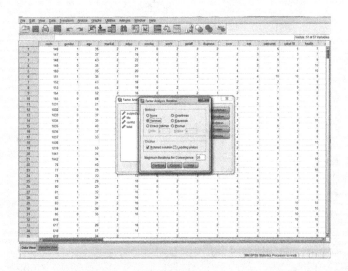

Step 6: Next, in the box for "options," under "missing values," we select "exclude cases listwise." Under "coefficient display format," we select "sorted by size" and "suppress small coefficients" with "absolute value below" kept at the default value of .10.

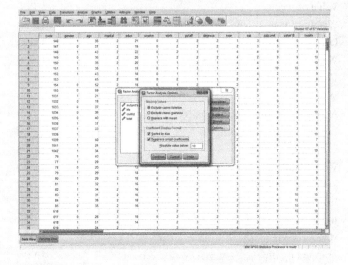

Kaiser-Meyer-Olkin and Bartlett's Test

Kaiser-Meyer-Olkin (KMO) measure of sampling adequacy		.964
Bartlett's test of sphericity	Approximate chi-square	10,608.051
	df	435
	Significance	.000

Author Comment *In this section, KMO measure of sampling adequacy and Bartlett's test of sphericity are shown. These results meet criteria and support the use of factor analysis for this data.*

Communalities

	Initial	Extraction
Energy level	1.000	.492
Reaction to pressure	1.000	.651
Characterization of life as a whole	1.000	.617
Daily activities	1.000	.553
Experience anxiety	1.000	.630
Expectations of every day	1.000	.566
Fearful	1.000	.581
Think deeply about life	1.000	.508
Productivity of life	1.000	.585
Making mistakes	1.000	.525
Value of work	1.000	.516
Wishing I was different	1.000	.645
Defined goals for life	1.000	.517
Worrying that bad things will happen	1.000	.622
Concentration during stress	1.000	.649
Standing up for myself	1.000	.492
Adequacy in most situations	1.000	.556
Frustration to problems	1.000	.548
Sad things	1.000	.514
Worthwhile life	1.000	.646
Satisfaction of present life	1.000	.629
Respond positively in difficult situations	1.000	.595
Joy in heart	1.000	.623
When relaxing	1.000	.492
Trapped by life	1.000	.615
Panic in frightening situations	1.000	.672
Thinking about past	1.000	.427

FIGURE 15-1 Computer printout of a principal component analysis.

Communalities

	Initial	Extraction
Feeling loved	1.000	.612
Worry about future	1.000	.474
Thinking about problems	1.000	.596

Extraction method: Principal component analysis.

Author Comment *This table shows initial "communalities" of correlation matrix as well as communalities derived through the analysis.*

Total Variance Explained

Component	Initial Eigenvalues			Extraction Sums of Squared Loadings			Rotation Sums of Squared Loadings		
	Total	% of Variance	Cumulative %	Total	% of Variance	Cumulative %	Total	% of Variance	Cumulative %
1	12.633	42.110	42.110	12.633	42.110	42.110	5.874	19.579	19.579
2	2.107	7.023	49.133	2.107	7.023	49.133	4.422	14.740	34.319
3	1.233	4.111	53.243	1.233	4.111	53.243	3.469	11.563	45.883
4	1.176	3.921	57.164	1.176	3.921	57.164	3.384	11.281	57.164
5	.947	3.158	60.322						
6	.843	2.811	63.134						
7	.777	2.592	65.725						
8	.714	2.379	68.104						
9	.674	2.246	70.350						
10	.648	2.159	72.509						
11	.630	2.101	74.610						
12	.573	1.909	76.519						
13	.536	1.788	78.307						
14	.534	1.780	80.086						
15	.513	1.710	81.796						
16	.475	1.582	83.378						
17	.450	1.500	84.878						
18	.446	1.486	86.364						
19	.425	1.417	87.781						
20	.406	1.354	89.134						
21	.396	1.321	90.456						
22	.376	1.254	91.709						
23	.373	1.242	92.952						
24	.342	1.142	94.093						
25	.335	1.116	95.210						

FIGURE 15-1   (*Continued*)

Total Variance Explained

Component	Initial Eigenvalues			Extraction Sums of Squared Loadings			Rotation Sums of Squared Loadings		
	Total	% of Variance	Cumulative %	Total	% of Variance	Cumulative %	Total	% of Variance	Cumulative %
26	.323	1.077	96.287						
27	.295	.982	97.269						
28	.293	.977	98.246						
29	.273	.909	99.155						
30	.254	.845	100.000						

Extraction method: Principal component analysis.

Author Comment In this table, variance accounted for by factors before rotation and after rotation is shown. "Total" refers to total variance accounted for by the factor. This is the eigenvalue. Four factors have eigenvalues greater than one. Only these factors are rotated. "Cumulative %" refers to the percent of variance accounted for cumulatively by previous factors plus this factor. Thus, the first four factors account for 57.164% of the variance—rounded to 57.2%. After rotation, the cumulative % of the four-factor solution remains the same at 57.2%. However, after rotation, variance is more evenly distributed between factors. Display of this table on screen shows all 10 columns as a single table, but depending on printer settings, it may print as two separate tables.

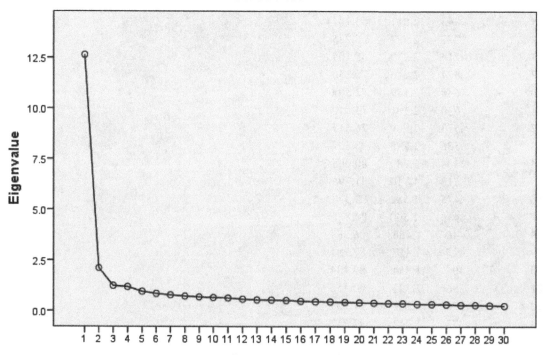

Scree Plot

FIGURE 15-1 (*Continued*)

Component Matrix[a]

	Component			
	1	2	3	4
Thinking about problems	.764			
Joy in heart	.752	−.211		−.118
Respond positively in difficult situations	.737			.227
Satisfaction of present life	.734	−.280		
Worthwhile life	.732	−.265	−.177	
Trapped by life	.722	−.178		−.233
Wishing I was different	.720		−.327	−.129
Characterization of life as a whole	.709	−.240	.235	
Sad things	.693	.172		
Feeling loved	.690	−.238	−.227	−.165
Frustration to problems	.663	.301		.133
Productivity of life	.662	−.304	−.206	.113
When relaxing	.659		.136	−.171
Adequacy in most situations	.655	.154	−.316	
Value of work	.646	−.303		
Defined goals for life	.637	−.304		.137
Think deeply about life	.634	−.314		
Daily activities	.622	−.287	.285	
Thinking about past	.613		−.154	−.165
Fearful	.611	.338	.116	−.284
Panic in frightening situations	.610	.471		.279
Experience anxiety	.609	.390	.174	−.279
Concentration during stress	.607	.380		.368
Making mistakes	.602	.228	−.329	
Energy level	.593		.305	.214
Standing up for myself	.573	.203	−.348	
Worry about future	.549	.112	.197	−.349
Reaction to pressure	.524	.450		.404
Expectations of every day	.522	−.214	.470	.164
Worrying that bad things will happen	.512	.406	.245	−.368

Extraction method: Principal component analysis.
[a]Four components extracted.

Author Comment *This is the unrotated matrix. You do not use this to interpret the meanings of the factors. Loadings that are near zero are not printed. This helps to make the matrix easier to read.*

FIGURE 15-1   *(Continued)*

Rotated Component Matrix[a]

	Component			
	1	2	3	4
Daily activities	.695	.111	.124	.205
Characterization of life as a whole	.694	.198	.173	.256
Expectations of every day	.688	−.121	.209	.186
Satisfaction of present life	.647	.363		.268
Defined goals for life	.611	.341	.160	
Value of work	.592	.381	.123	
Think deeply about life	.590	.379	.115	
Joy in heart	.575	.434		.309
Worthwhile life	.561	.541	.186	
Energy level	.560		.374	.195
Trapped by life	.548	.366		.424
Productivity of life	.534	.528	.145	
Respond positively in difficult situations	.507	.328	.453	.159
Wishing I was different	.309	.678	.164	.251
Feeling loved	.446	.604		.218
Adequacy in most situations	.159	.602	.316	.262
Making mistakes		.576	.344	.263
Standing up for myself		.562	.376	.168
Thinking about problems	.468	.483	.260	.275
Thinking about past	.274	.480	.139	.319
Reaction to pressure	.156		.769	.168
Concentration during stress	.216	.194	.731	.172
Panic in frightening situations	.114	.255	.728	.252
Frustration to problems	.239	.302	.548	.315
Sad things	.330	.335	.432	.326
Worrying that bad things will happen			.234	.742
Experience anxiety	.144	.191	.319	.686
Fearful	.153	.246	.281	.646
Worry about future	.280	.180		.598
When relaxing	.368	.258	.223	.490

Extraction method: Principal component analysis. Rotation method: Varimax with Kaiser normalization.
[a]Rotation converged in 13 iterations.

Author Comment *This is the rotated matrix. Use this one to interpret meanings of the factors.*

FIGURE 15-1 *(Continued)*

some information ("initial eigenvalues") is provided for 30 potential factors. This is because the number of unrotated factors obtainable equals the number of variables included in a principal components analysis. The purpose of this part of the analysis is, however, to determine how many of the 30 potential factors should be rotated for conceptual interpretation. Three types of information are given about each potential factor: This includes the total eigenvalue, percent of variance accounted for by this factor, and the cumulative percent of variance accounted for by all factors so far (indicated as "Cumulative %").

The first four factors each have an eigenvalue greater than one. The variance accounted by these factors (as rounded) is 42%, 7%, 4%, and 4%, respectively. Together, these factors account for 57.2% of the overall variance between items. Based on the criterion that the minimum eigenvalue (for rotated factors) is one, the first four factors are rotated. The second set of three columns simply repeats information already provided for these first four factors. The third set of three columns (under the heading "Rotation Sums of Squared Loadings") provides equivalent information for the factors after rotation. Note that numbers listed under "total" are now considerably closer to each other in value than were the original eigenvalues of the unrotated factors, indicating that the variance is now more equally distributed between the factors. However, both sets account for 57.2% of the variance. The total variance accounted for by the four factors has not changed.

In this display, a plot of eigenvalues was requested. This is called the scree plot. It provides a graphic representation of the relative values of eigenvalues. Because eigenvalues often are the key criteria for determining the number of factors to be rotated, this can be useful because it provides a basis for identifying a logical breaking point between eigenvalues. This visual representation of eigenvalues may help the researcher to determine the number of factors in the data.

The next table, labeled "Component Matrix," is analogous to the unrotated factor matrix.

This table presents loadings for the four factors extracted. As usual, the first factor is a generalized factor on which all variables load. The other factors have only a few loadings in the moderate range and none above .5. Typically, no attempt is made to derive conceptual interpretations of these unrotated factors.

The last portion of the printout, titled "Rotated Component Matrix," is the most important, as it contains the rotated solution that we will interpret. In this portion, the four factors with eigenvalues greater than 1 are rotated, and the final solution is displayed. These rotated factors are to be conceptually interpreted. Note that the items are listed by the strength of loading, not by the order in which they were entered. In SPSS, this is done by checking "sorted by size" under "Options."

After inspecting the items that load on a factor and their respective loadings, the investigator gives each factor an appropriate name as a way of capturing its meaning. Note that, in contrast to the unrotated matrix previously displayed, this analysis results in a distribution of highest loadings among the four factors. In the naming process, the researcher gives most emphasis to the three or four variables with the highest loadings. Keep in mind that items with negative wordings were reversed as they were coded. In this analysis, the factors may be named Life Satisfaction, Self-Love, Reactivity, and Pessimistic Worry. The researcher should not expect that all items loading on a factor will seem to fit conceptually or that factor names selected will perfectly reflect the meanings of all items. In any case, one could calculate a score for each subject on each factor, and these could be used for further analysis.

Other Options

A factor analysis may be considerably more complicated than the one shown here. Rather than principal components analysis, any of a variety of extraction methods representing common factor analysis may be used. Principal axis extraction method is often selected (Henson & Roberts, 2006). Principal axis differs from principal components mainly in that the correlation matrix diagonals are squared multiple correlations, rather than 1s, in the first step. Following this initial step, communalities are estimated from the factor matrix, and factoring is repeated with these communalities in the diagonal. Each such step is one iteration. This is repeated until the estimated communalities and calculated communalities are approximately the same.

Another important method of extraction within the class of common factor analysis is alpha factoring, which is designed to maximize the internal consistency reliability (e.g., Cronbach's alpha) of the factors. It is assumed that the particular variables measured are a sample of the universe of variables represented by the factor. You want to generalize not to the population of cases from which research subjects were drawn, but to the universe of variables from which the measured variables were sampled. Ferketich and Muller (1990) point out that this method is highly appropriate for instrument development efforts, particularly the early stages. Schilling et al. (2009) used the alpha extraction method in identifying subscales of SMOD-A, as described earlier in the chapter.

Other extraction methods available in the common statistical packages are image factoring, unweighted least squares, and generalized least squares. However, these may be less important to the sort of applications discussed here. Finally, the maximum likelihood method of extraction is an available option. This method provides a form of confirmatory factor analysis.

CONCEPTUAL UNDERSTANDING: AN EXAMPLE FROM THE LITERATURE

For many readers of this chapter, it will be most important to have a conceptual understanding of factor analysis, so that you may make

sense of articles with factor analysis that you encounter in your area of interest. Toward this end, we will take a close look at a published article that employed factor analysis in developing an instrument to measure sensory qualities of dyspnea among persons with exacerbated chronic obstructive pulmonary disease (COPD) (Parshall, 2002). The researcher notes that dyspnea is the most common symptom of COPD patients in the emergency department (ED).

In this study, 104 patients who presented to the ED with exacerbated COPD were asked to rate the intensity of the 16 dyspnea sensory quality descriptors, as experienced at two points in time—when the person made the decision to come to the ED and 1 week earlier. Intensity ratings could vary from 0 to 10. Factor analysis was reported in detail for the data describing the time point of the decision to come to the ED.

One item ("I felt that I was breathing more.") was eliminated prior to the analysis. The researcher reported that this item was confusing to subjects, and the frequency of use by subjects was low. The remaining 15 items were included in an exploratory factor analysis using principal axis factor analysis with Varimax rotation. With 104 subjects and 15 items, there is a ratio of 6.9 subjects per item. Another item was then omitted based on the initial factor analysis results. The item ("My breath did not go all the way in.") had weak loadings on multiple factors, rather than being strongly associated with a single factor. Thus, the item did not meet the threshold loading used in this study, nor was the item consistent with simple structure.

After this item was eliminated, multiple runs of factor analysis were conducted, varying the number of factors. The researcher found that the five-factor solution was best at yielding a clear pattern of loadings. This solution accounted for almost 63% of the total variance between items. This factor solution from the article is reproduced here in Table 15-6. In a footnote, Parshall indicates the names that he assigned to the four factors—*Work/Effort,*

Table 15-6	ROTATED FACTOR MATRIX FOR "DESCRIPTIVE" SOLUTION (14 DESCRIPTORS) AT DECISION (*N* = 98)					
	Factor[a]					
Descriptor	1	2	3	4	5	h[2b]
Effort	.79		.29	.25		.81
Work	.70	.29	.30			.72
Out of breath	.54	.33			.26	.52
Suffocating	.22	.87		.27		.94
Smothering	.22	.63	.40		.30	.72
Couldn't breathe	.39	.53			.25	.52
Hunger for air	.44	.48	.30		.28	.62
Heavy	.28	.21	.61			.52
Not out all the way			.59			.40
Rapid	.22	.33	.46			.41
Constricted	.40			.83		.89
Tight		.37		.58		.52
Not enough	.41	.22			.71	.73
Shallow			.26		.58	.46
Initial eigenvalues[c]	6.56	1.14	1.03	0.98	0.88	
Rotation sums of squares	2.32	2.27	1.54	1.35	1.30	
Percentage of variance explained	16.6	16.2	11.0	9.6	9.3	
Cronbach's α[d]	.84	.87	.67	.74	.67	

Bold type indicates primary factor loading for each item.
[a]Factor 1 = Work/Effort; Factor 2 = Suffocating/Smothering; Factor 3 = Heavy/Rapid; Factor 4 = Tight/Constricted; Factor 5 = Shallow/Not enough. Factor loadings <.20 not shown.
[b]h^2 = extraction (final) communalities (row sums of squared loadings).
[c]Eigenvalues = prerotation column sums of squared loadings.
[d]Cronbach's α reported for primary loadings (bold type).
Source: Data from Parshall, M. B. (2002). Psychometric characteristics of dyspnea descriptor ratings in emergency department patients with exacerbated chronic obstructive pulmonary disease. *Research in Nursing and Health,* 25, 339.

Suffocating/Smothering, Heavy/Rapid, Tight/Constricted, and *Shallow/Not Enough.*

Note that this table is constructed such that the loadings above .45 are indicated in bold type, other loadings of magnitude greater than .2 are indicated in type that is not bold, and lower loadings are simply omitted, leaving some blank spaces in the published table. This approach to presenting a factor table in publication is reader-friendly in that it emphasizes the information that is most important and it omits information of lesser importance. The connection between item wordings and factors names is, thus, made clear, even to readers who may not be familiar with the details of factor analysis but who may be very interested in the content of the research. The table also includes supplementary information about item and factors. Item communalities are shown in a column to the right of the factors. For each factor, information is provided concerning the initial eigenvalues (before rotation), variance accounted for after rotation (rotation sum of squares), percentage of variance explained (also after rotation), and internal consistency reliability as indicated by Cronbach's alpha of the items loading on the factor.

Parshall (2002) notes that two of the five factors had low internal consistency reliability, as indicated by Cronbach's alpha below .70. He suggests that this argues "against retention" of these factors. The researcher proceeded to eliminate items one at a time, rerunning the analysis at each step. The optimal solution consisted of seven items and three factors. Factors were named as follows: *Smothering/Suffocating/Hunger for air, Effort/Work,* and *Tight/Constricted.* This reduced factor solution from the article is shown in Table 15-7. This solution accounted for almost 74% of the variance between items. Parshall (2002) observed that the item referring to *Hunger for air* had a clearer primary loading in the reduced analysis. Further, the explained variance of factor *Tight/Constricted* was twice as high in the reduced analysis (from 9.6% to 18.1%). These results were consistent

Table 15-7	ROTATED FACTOR MATRIX FOR REDUCED SOLUTION AT DECISION (*N* = 98)			
	Factor[a]			
Descriptor	1	2	3	h[2b]
Smothering	.82	.26	.21	.79
Suffocating	.79	.22	.34	.79
Hunger for air	.61	.48		.63
Effort	.24	.90	.20	.91
Work	.38	.71		.68
Tight	.32		.77	.71
Constricted		.47	.64	.65
Initial eigenvalues[c]	4.16	.90	.87	
Rotation sums of squares	2.00	1.89	1.27	
Percentage of variance explained	28.5	27.0	18.1	
Cronbach's α[d]	.87	.87	.74	

Bold type indicates primary factor loading for each item.
[a]Factor 1: Smothering/Suffocating/Hunger for air; Factor 2: Effort/Work; Factor 3: Tight/Constricted Loadings <.20 not shown.
[b]h 2¼ extraction (final) communalities (row sums of squared loadings).
[c]Eigenvalues ¼ prerotation column sums of squared loadings.
[d]Cronbach's a reported for primary loadings (bold type).
Source: Data from Parshall, M. B. (2002). Psychometric characteristics of dyspnea descriptor ratings in emergency department patients with exacerbated chronic obstructive pulmonary disease. *Research in Nursing and Health, 25,* 339.

with qualitative data that were also collected. Ratings describing the 1-week earlier time point did not follow the same pattern. It is concluded that this shorter list of items can be used to reliably measure the dyspneic sensations of COPD patients presenting in the ED.

SUMMARY

The factor analysis techniques presented in this chapter are distinct from many other statistical techniques in the tremendous potential for researcher creativity to shape the understanding of the results obtained. Through application of statistical techniques of factor analysis, the researcher arrives at numbers that indicate groupings of variables in the data. These groups must then be named or described by the researcher, a creative process in which clinical wisdom, knowledge of the literature, and research sophistication must be integrated. This creative process is the key element on which the value of the factor analysis must rest. A factor analysis solution is well suited to inform the creative process. However, factor loadings and eigenvalues are only as valuable as the interpretation of the factors is insightful.

CHAPTER REVIEW

Multiple-Choice Concept Review

1. Factor analysis can best be described as
   a. a step in the process of achieving a multivariate perspective on a research problem.
   b. a technique done by computer.
   c. an approach to organizing individual variables into groups of related variables.
   d. all of the above.

2. Which of the following is true about exploratory factor analysis?
   a. It tests the means of multiple variables.
   b. It is used as the last step in research.
   c. It is often used as a part of instrument development.
   d. None of the above.

3. Factor analysis can be used
   a. to determine the internal structure of a new instrument.
   b. to reduce the number of variables in preparation for subsequent analysis.
   c. to support the development of theory.
   d. for all of the above.

4. When conducting factor analysis, data usually are
   a. determined to have a curvilinear relationship.
   b. tested for statistical significance.
   c. interval level of measurement (or treatable as interval).
   d. unreliable.

5. Which of the following is not a step in factor analysis?
   a. Run it using orthogonal rotation.
   b. Collect data.
   c. Create a research question.
   d. Include only a small number of variables.

6. When there are multiple variables that might explain a health condition, the researcher should (check all that apply)
   a. always analyze each one separately.
   b. determine which mean is different from the others.
   c. determine if there is a bivariate relationship.
   d. determine if there is a pattern of correlation between the variables.

7. The test used to establish correlations between variables is
   a. Pearson.
   b. ANOVA.
   c. *t* test.
   d. *z*-score.

8. In factor analysis, the matrix that is used for naming factors and interpreting their meaning is the
   a. raw data matrix.
   b. correlation matrix.
   c. unrotated factor matrix.
   d. rotated factor matrix.

9. To determine the number of factors for rotation, a researcher might consider
   a. proportion of variance accounted for by each factor.
   b. eigenvalues of each factor.
   c. graphic representation of eigenvalues in scree plot.
   d. all of the above.

10. Exploratory factor analysis
    a. tests for statistical significance.
    b. can never be generalized.
    c. is only used when the sample size is large.
    d. none of the above.

Critical Thinking Concept Review

1. Develop three research questions for which factor analysis would be appropriate.

2. For each of the research questions you develop for review problem 1, determine whether you would take an exploratory or a confirmatory approach and why.

3. Take another look at the rotated component matrix in Figure 15-1. Naming factors based on a rotated matrix is potentially a creative process. Different researchers looking at the same results may assign names with subtle differences. Each factor name should reflect what the items with high loadings on the factor have in common—with most emphasis on the top three items. Consider the names given—Life Satisfaction, Self-love, Reactivity, and Pessimistic Worry. What would you name these factors? (Once you have decided on names, discuss with classmates and try to come to agreement regarding the very best names.)

Computational Problems

There are many decisions to be made in any factor analysis, and it is common to run factor analysis more than one way in order to see how results compare. Using the data (available on the Web site that accompanies this book), perform another factor analysis of the 30 items in the IPA scale. According to the developers of the scale, LIFE consists of the following 17 questions: items 1, 3, 4, 6, 8, 9, 11, 12, 13, 19, 20, 21, 23, 25, 27, 28, 30. CONFIDENCE consists of 13 questions: items 2, 5, 7, 10, 14, 15, 16, 17, 18, 22, 24, 26, 29. This suggests that you might restrict rotation to two factors in order to see how results compare.

Path Analysis

CHAPTER

16

Anne E. Norris

OBJECTIVES

After studying this chapter, you should be able to:

1. State the three conditions necessary for causality.

2. Draw a recursive path model.

3. Identify which independent variables are theorized to have indirect effects in addition to direct effects on the dependent variable.

4. Identify the appropriate regression analyses needed to calculate the path coefficients in a model.

5. Calculate the direct and indirect effects of an independent variable in a model.

OVERVIEW OF PATH ANALYSIS

Path analysis is used to answer questions regarding the relationships between a set of independent variables and a dependent variable. Path analysis is based on simple regression techniques, but it moves beyond the traditional regression analysis discussed in Chapter 14 to examining relationships among and between the variables. Asher (1983) argues that by taking this step beyond regression analysis, we achieve a richer understanding of our phenomena. Path models are considered a type of causal model, and path analysis is referred to as a causal modeling technique. Path models depict theorized, directional relationships among a set of variables.

Path analysis is literally an analysis of the paths or lines in a model that represent the influence of one variable on another. It is used to answer research questions about the effect of a given independent (X_1) variable on the dependent variable (Y) in the model. As you learn in this chapter, independent variables may have both direct ($X_1 \rightarrow Y$) and indirect effects. Indirect effects arise when the independent variable is theorized to influence other independent variables in the model. In Robinson's (1995) path model, social support, income and education, and spiritual beliefs influence coping, which, in turn, influences the widow's grief response. Thus, the diagram indicates that these variables have indirect effects on the dependent variable (grief response) through their influence on coping. The direct lines between these three variables and the dependent variable, grief response, indicate that these variables have direct effects on the dependent variable as well.

By analyzing the paths, path analysis provides information about the consistency between data and a theorized path model. If the data do not fit the theorized relationships in the model, this suggests that the model (and the theory that generated it) may warrant revision. However, data that are consistent with the model are supportive but not definitive; such data merely indicate that the model (and the theory) was not disconfirmed.

Ideally, the path model should be drawn before the data are collected. However, in secondary data analysis, the model is drawn after the data are collected but before the analysis is conducted. In both primary and secondary data analysis, the model may also be drawn after completing a regression analysis because the researcher wishes to examine the relationships between the independent variables. In either case, Asher (1983) recommends working with a model based on an a priori theoretical or substantive understanding of the relationships between variables in the model. Although it is important to modify a model in response to statistical results, the path analysis should not become a mindless attempt to find a model that best fits the data. Such attempts result in models that may not replicate and may have questionable theoretical value.

RESEARCH QUESTIONS FOR PATH ANALYSIS

In general, the research questions for path analysis relate to the testing of relationships that are hypothesized to exist between and within a dependent variable and a set of predictor variables. In general, path analysis helps us address the following questions:

1. Are the paths in the model supported by the data?
2. What is the total effect (direct plus indirect) of a predictor variable?
3. Does one of the independent variables mediate the effect of another variable on the dependent variable?

What Are the Effects of Self-Efficacy Regarding Illness Self-Management and Self-Management Behavior on a Kidney Transplant Patient's Quality of Life?

Weng, Dai, Huang, and Chiang (2010) surveyed 150 adults living in Taiwan who had undergone a kidney transplant anywhere from 6 months to 10 years prior to study participation. These adults completed a self-administered questionnaire at two different points in time with a 6-month interval between the two data collections. Their measure of self-efficacy assessed a variety of areas (e.g., diet, exercise, blood pressure monitoring) as a single unitary concept. In contrast, self-management (problem solving, patient–provider partnership, and self-care behavior) and health-related quality of life (physical, mental) had multiple components. This meant that the authors had two separate dependent variables (physical quality of life and mental quality of life). The authors used linear regression and path analysis to test the hypotheses listed below (see Fig. 16-1).

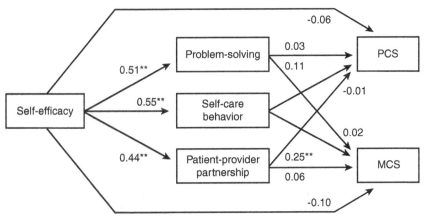

FIGURE 16-1   Robinson's (1995) path model. Model from Weng et al. (2010) depicting effects of self-efficacy on self-management (problem solving, self-care behavior, patient–provider relationship), and physical (PCS) and mental (MCS) quality of life.

1. Self-efficacy at time 1 is positively and significantly related to time 2 problem solving, patient–provider partnership, and self-care behavior
2. Self-efficacy at time 1 is positively and significantly related to time 2 physical and mental quality of life
3. Time 2 problem solving, patient–provider partnership, and self-care behavior are positively and significantly related to time 2 physical and mental quality of life.

Weng et al. (2010) found support for paths between self-efficacy and the three self-management components (β values ranged from .44 to .51), but no support for the paths between self-efficacy and physical and mental quality of life ($\beta < |.10|$). However, using path analysis, the authors found that self-efficacy had an indirect effect on mental quality of life through its effect on self-care behavior. Meanwhile, only the path between self-care behavior and mental quality of life was supported in the analyses addressing hypothesis 3 ($\beta = .25$). These findings argue for revising the path model or revisiting sampling and other aspects of the study design. Weng et al. point

out that relationships in their model might be different for the sample of people who were in their first 6 months postkidney transplant or if the interval between time 1 and time 2 had been longer. Nevertheless, the finding of an indirect effect for self-efficacy on mental quality of life is an important finding and it would have been missed if path analysis had not been used.

Does Prayer Mediate the Effect of Caregiving Burden on Resiliency? An Example of Using Path Analysis to Test for Mediation

This cross-sectional study examined the relationships between prayer, caregiving burden, and resiliency in a sample of 304 Alzheimer's caregivers using self-administered questionnaires (Wilks & Vonk, 2008). The authors used path analysis to test for mediation, with prayer being identified as the mediator variable. Mediation occurs when the relationship (or path) between an independent and a dependent variable is decreased by the addition of a third "mediator" variable. Following Baron and Kenny's (1986) procedures for testing for mediation, Wilks and

Vonk conducted a series of regression analyses to determine

1. The effect of burden on prayer (mediator)
2. The effect of burden on resiliency (dependent variable)
3. The effect of burden on resiliency when prayer is included in the analysis

Baron and Kenny (1986) assert that mediation is present when the regression coefficient observed in step 2 decreases in magnitude and/or becomes nonsignificant when the mediator variable (e.g., prayer) is entered into the analysis (step 3). Wilks and Vonk (2008) found that the regression coefficient for burden decreased from −.53 to −.41 (see Table 3, page 124 of the Wilks and Vonk [2008] article) when prayer was added. This substantive change in the magnitude of the coefficient argues for mediation.

TYPE OF DATA REQUIRED

Path analysis requires the same type of data as linear multiple regression. In other words, you need a dependent variable that is continuous and normally distributed. Ideally, the independent variables are also continuous. Some researchers use the coding techniques (dummy, effect, and orthogonal) discussed in Chapter 13 to include categorical variables, but by doing so, they violate a statistical assumption underlying path analysis (see later discussion of assumptions) and jeopardize the validity of their findings. In addition, the researcher should strive to have a large enough data set to follow Nunnally and Bernstein's (1994) recommendation of 30 subjects per independent variable in the model to increase the likelihood that findings can be replicated and are not mere artifact. Although path analysis is considered a causal modeling technique, it can be performed with either cross-sectional

or longitudinal data. For example, Robinson's data were cross-sectional.

ASSUMPTIONS

There are two types of assumptions that must be considered with path analysis: theoretical and statistical.

Theoretical Assumptions

In the strictest sense, causation is investigated with experimental designs in which the independent variable is manipulated, the subsequent effects of this are measured, and variables that could confound or influence the effect of the independent variable are controlled for (e.g., subjects are randomized by condition). However, path analysis typically involves testing a causal or path model with data that do not result from an experimental design. For example, path analysis can be done with survey data, data produced by a review of medical records, and so forth. Given this, many researchers have reservations about using such models to imply causation (Pedhazur, 1997). Hence, although the notion of causation is implicit, careful terminology is used. For example, independent variables may be referred to as predictor variables but are described as influencing rather than causing the dependent variable.

Causation

Theoretical assumptions of causation are implicit in path analysis, and such assumptions are strengthened when three conditions of causation are met (Kenny, 1979). First, there must be an observed and measurable relationship between X_1 and Y. In other words, X_1 and Y must be correlated. Second, X_1 should precede Y in time; that is, it must be possible to temporally order X_1 and Y such that X_1 occurred first in time. This condition may seem easy to meet, but it can be quite complicated. Consider a cross-sectional data set concerning a health behavior such as engaging in regular exercise, and predictors of this behavior, such as education and beliefs about exercise. For education, the matter is straightforward. It is safe to assume that education temporally precedes current exercise. For beliefs, it is less clear. Do we assume that beliefs about exercise were present first? This would be consistent with hypothesizing that these beliefs lead to engaging in regular exercise. However, could the exercise have occurred before the beliefs developed or were fully formed? This would be consistent with hypothesizing that engaging in regular exercise changes or alters beliefs about exercise. Unfortunately, the researcher must take a stand on the hypothesized causal direction; otherwise, the model would be nonrecursive, and nonrecursive path models cannot be tested with cross-sectional data.

This example illustrates the problem with using causal modeling techniques to imply causation. It also underscores the importance of theory: We can use theory to resolve the dilemma of whether the belief or the behavior came first. For example, Pender's (1987) Health Promotion Theory and Fishbein and Ajzen's (1975) Theory of Reasoned Action both specify that beliefs guide behavior. Therefore, we can use these theories to guide us in assigning a direction between beliefs and behaviors such that beliefs are theorized to influence engaging in exercise (Fig. 16-2).

Nonspurious Relationships

It is assumed that X_1 and Y have a nonspurious relationship. This means that the observed, measurable, and temporally ordered relationship between X_1 and Y will not disappear when the effects of other variables on this relationship are controlled. For example, suppose in our predictors of exercise analysis, we found that the relationship between beliefs and engaging in exercise disappeared when the effects of intention to exercise were controlled for statistically (i.e., we entered intention into a regression analysis predicting exercise behavior first, with belief entered on the second step, and found that the beta for belief was no longer significant). This would mean that the earlier relationship between belief and exercise was spurious—it only appeared to exist because both belief and exercise were correlated with intention. Another way to say this is that the relationship was confounded by intention. If we found this, we would modify the diagram of our causal model from the one in Figure 16-2 to the one in Figure 16-3.

We can use regression to test whether the data meet this assumption, but the problem is that we can do this only if we have measured the right confounding variable. It is difficult (perhaps impossible) to identify and rule out all the variables that could confound the observed relationship between X_1 and Y. The solution is to use theory, existing literature, and discussions with colleagues to identify the variables that seem clearly likely to confound the relationships in the model, and then include measures of such variables in the analysis (Asher, 1983). Unfortunately,

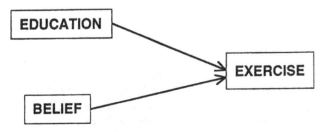

FIGURE 16-2   Education influences exercise. Belief influences exercise.

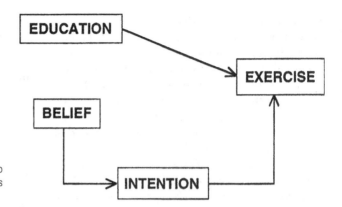

FIGURE 16-3   Intention confounds the relationship between belief and exercise because belief influences intention, which, in turn, influences exercise.

in secondary data analysis, the researcher works with an existing data set and can include only the variables that are contained in the data set. Thus, such researchers may need to recognize this as a limitation of their results.

Statistical Assumptions

The statistical assumptions in path analysis are of two types. The first you are already familiar with: the assumptions of normal distributions, homoscedasticity, and linear relationships that have been discussed in previous chapters. These assumptions arise because path analysis consists of a series of regression equations and shares the same assumptions as multiple linear regression (Chapter 14).

The second type of assumptions is unique to path analysis. These assumptions are necessary if we want to use path analysis to calculate the direct and indirect effects of variables in the path model. There are four such assumptions (Pedhazur, 1997):

1. When two independent variables are correlated with one another and diagrammed as having no other variables influencing them, their relationship cannot be analyzed, and it is assumed that the magnitude of this relationship is represented by the correlation coefficient.

2. It is assumed that the flow of causation in the model is unidirectional. The model is recursive: If we start with any independent variable in a model and move our fingers along the straight lines in the direction of the arrows from one variable to the next, we will not come back to the independent variable we started with; we will not find ourselves moving in a circle.

3. It is assumed that the variables in the model are measured on an interval scale. However, Asher (1983) argues that this assumption can be somewhat relaxed with ordinal variables, particularly as the number of categories in the ordinal variable increases.

4. All variables in the model are measured without error; measurement error is assumed to be zero. This last assumption underscores the importance of having reliable measures of variables in the path model.

POWER

Power analyses in path analysis are the same as those discussed in Chapter 14 for multiple regression and so are not discussed in detail here. As you will see later in the examples in this chapter, path analysis involves more than one regression analysis. Hence, the power analysis should be calculated for the regression equation that involves the smallest effect size (or requires the largest number of subjects because it contains the most variables). This will ensure that you have enough power to detect the significance of important paths in the model.

KEY TERMS

Path analysis brings with it a set of terms that are common to causal models in general. We have already discussed recursive and nonrecursive models and direct and indirect effects. In this next section, we will discuss these terms in more detail and then introduce some additional ones.

Recursive and Nonrecursive Models

As discussed earlier in this chapter, an assumption in path analysis is that the model is recursive; that is, there is a one-way flow of causation in the model. Another way of thinking about this is that in a recursive model, all the paths between variables are one-way roads. The only exception is when theory and previous research is insufficient to support a direction being assigned to the "road." In this case, a correlational rather than a directional relationship

is assumed, indicated by a curved line with an arrow at each end. In a nonrecursive model, at least one of the paths between two variables is a two-way road, or there is a set of paths in the model that are circular. These models do not meet the assumptions necessary for standard path analysis. There is a way to use longitudinal data to translate some theoretical models that are inherently nonrecursive into a recursive form that can then be tested with path analysis (see Asher, 1983, and Pedhazur, 1997, for examples of this and other ways to approach recursive models).

Indirect and Direct Effects

A given independent variable in a model can be diagrammed as having one of three kinds of effects on the dependent variable, depending on its relationships with other variables in the model: only direct, only indirect, or both direct and indirect. Let us return to a path model of factors influencing engaging in regular exercise. In Figure 16-4, intention has only a direct effect on the dependent variable. This effect is reflected in the direct line between intention and exercise that points toward exercise. In this same figure, age and education also have direct effects on exercise, and age and education are correlated.

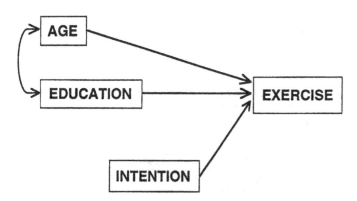

FIGURE 16-4   Age, education, and intention have direct effects.

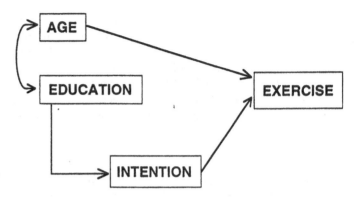

FIGURE 16-5   Education has an indirect effect. Age and intentions have direct effects.

In Figure 16-5, education has only an indirect effect on exercise through its relationship with intention. There is no direct line between education and exercise, as there was in Figure 16-4. However, there is a direct line between education and intention that points toward intention, and between intention and the dependent variable. In Figure 16-6, education has both direct and indirect effects on the dependent variable. As in Figures 16-4 and 16-5, intention has only a direct effect.

Endogenous and Exogenous Variables

All variables in a path model can be described as either endogenous or exogenous. This is an important distinction, because to do path analysis we need to perform a regression analysis for every endogenous variable in the model. Endogenous variables are variables that are diagrammed as being influenced by other variables in the model. The variables diagrammed as independent of any influence are the exogenous variables (Bollen, 1989).

Dependent variables are always endogenous, but some independent (or predictor) variables can be endogenous if they are themselves being influenced by other independent variables in the model. Thus, in Figure 16-6, intention is both an independent variable and an endogenous variable. This means that to analyze the path model depicted in Figure 16-6, we need two regression analyses—one with exercise regressed onto age, education, and intention and one with intention regressed onto education. This second regression only involves one independent variable. Hence the path coefficient is simply the correlation between intention and education. Age is not included in this second regression because

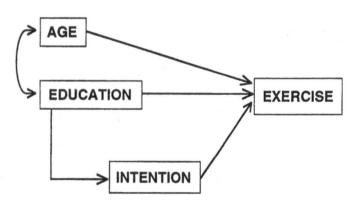

FIGURE 16-6   Education has direct and indirect effects.

it has no direct or indirect effect on this intention. Note that for any given endogenous variable, all variables that are exogenous to it (i.e., any that have direct or indirect effects) need to be entered into the regression equation for that specific endogenous variable.

In the diagrams you have seen in this chapter, both endogenous and exogenous variables are indicated with a square drawn around them. This square is used to indicate that these variables correspond to a subject's response or score in a particular data set. Variables demarcated with a square are referred to as measured variables or indicators of specific theoretical constructs. As you will learn in Chapter 17, circles are used to indicate that a variable is an unmeasured, theoretical construct.

Path Coefficients

Path coefficients are produced by the various regression analyses used in the path analysis. They represent the magnitude of the influence of one variable on another in the path model. The subscripts used in the notation for path coefficients are ordered such that the letter or abbreviation representing the variable being influenced is always listed first and the one for the variable doing the influencing is listed second. Thus, in Figure 16-6, the path coefficient for the path between intention and exercise is $p_{e,i}$.

Either the standardized (β) or the nonstandardized (b) regression coefficient can be used as the value for the path coefficient, but use of the former is more common. Use of the standardized

coefficient allows comparison of the magnitude of one path in the model with that of other paths in the model. Thus, use of the standardized coefficient makes it possible for the reader to determine which independent variable has the greatest direct effect on the dependent variable. In contrast, use of the nonstandardized coefficient makes it possible to evaluate how the magnitude of a particular path varies in different sample subgroups or study populations. Pedhazur (1997) recommends that both coefficients should be reported; if only standardized coefficients are reported, then the standard deviations of all the variables should be reported as well, so that interested readers can calculate the nonstandardized value. Use of standardized path coefficients may be more common because these coefficients are needed to determine the direct, indirect, and total effect of an independent variable. The determination of these effects is discussed later (see the sections on determining direct and indirect effects, and conducting a path analysis).

Identification

Causal models can be overidentified, just identified, or underidentified. Visually, just identified models are easy to recognize because all the variables in the model are interconnected with each other by a path (Pedhazur, 1997). Such models can become overidentified through the process of "theory trimming" or the deletion of nonsignificant paths in the model (Heise, 1969). Note how the overidentified model in Figure 16-7 becomes the just identified model in Figure 16-8 with the

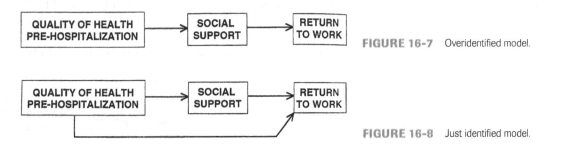

FIGURE 16-7   Overidentified model.

FIGURE 16-8   Just identified model.

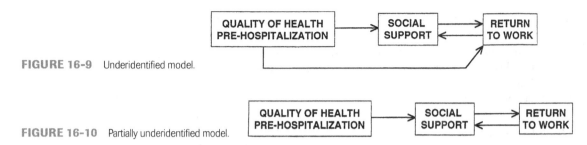

FIGURE 16-9   Underidentified model.

FIGURE 16-10   Partially underidentified model.

addition of the direct path between quality of health prehospitalization and return to work ($p_{r,q}$). The just identified model becomes underidentified in Figure 16-9 when the path $p_{s,r}$ is added and the model becomes nonrecursive. In Figure 16-10, the addition of this same path to the overidentified model in Figure 16-7 results in a nonrecursive model that is partially underidentified.

An advantage of overidentified models is that unlike just identified or underidentified models, the model as a whole can be statistically evaluated for its fit to the data. The results of this statistical test can be used to support the validity of the path model, although this is not commonly done in the published literature. A discussion of this statistic is beyond the scope of this chapter, but if readers are interested in learning more about it, Pedhazur (1997) is an excellent resource.

INTERPRETING PATH MODELS: DETERMINING DIRECT AND INDIRECT EFFECTS

Being able to determine the direct and indirect effects of an independent variable is an important advantage of path analysis (Asher, 1983). It allows you to know the total effect of an independent variable, which could be important in deciding which independent variables you

might want to target in an intervention. Being able to determine these effects also allows you to compare them. For example, an independent variable can have an indirect effect that is greater than its direct effect, or vice versa. It is also possible that the two effects may cancel each other out, in the sense that they could be similar in magnitude but opposite in direction (one positive, the other negative).

Pedhazur (1997) presents a method for using matrix algebra to ease the calculation of direct and indirect effects for more complex models (i.e., models with many variables and many paths). However, for simplicity an alternative method developed by Wright (1934) is presented in this chapter that does not require a knowledge of matrix algebra. Using Wright's method, you can work directly from the diagram of the path model and identify the simple (direct effect) and compound (more than one path is involved) paths relevant to a particular variable. These compound effects can either be meaningful (indirect) or nonmeaningful (noncausal).

According to Wright, the value of any one compound path is equal to the product of the simple paths that make it up. Thus, in the hypothetical model shown in Figure 16-11, the compound path from quality of health prehospitalization to return to work through social support is equal to $p_{s,q}$ multiplied by $p_{r,s}$. In the

FIGURE 16-11   Model with one compound path from quality of health prehospitalization to return to work through social support.

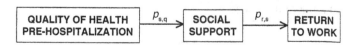

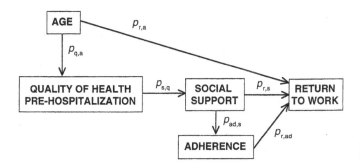

FIGURE 16-12   Model with two meaningful and one nonmeaningful compound paths from quality of health pre-hospitalization to return to work.

hypothetical model shown in Figure 16-12, there are two possible meaningful compound paths between quality of health prehospitalization and return to work, $(p_{s,q})(p_{r,s})$, and a new one that takes us from quality of health prehospitalization to return to work through social support and adherence. The value of this new compound path is $(p_{s,q})(p_{ad,s})(p_{r,ad})$. There is also a nonmeaningful compound (or noncausal) path between quality of health prehospitalization and return to work through age: This compound path is equal to $(p_{r,a})(p_{q,a})$. This compound path ignores the direction of the relationships specified by the path model. This is why it is noncausal and is considered nonmeaningful. However, it is an important component of the correlation between quality of health prehospitalization and return to work.

Wright (1934) found that when a path model is correctly specified, the correlation between two variables is equal to the sum of the simple (direct effect) and all possible compound paths (indirect effect and noncausal) between these two variables. Measurement error may enter in and cause the correlation to be approximately, rather than exactly, equal to the sum of the direct effect, indirect effect, and noncausal component. However, incorrect specification of the model could cause the sum of the direct and indirect effects and noncausal component to be noticeably less than the correlation. This noticeable difference between the sum and the correlation is an indication that the model may need revision (Asher, 1983).

Thus, in Figure 16-12, we could describe the correlation between quality of health prehospitalization and return to work with the following equation:

$$r = (p_{s,q})(p_{r,s}) + (p_{s,q})(p_{ad,s})(p_{r,ad}) + (p_{r,a})(p_{q,a})$$

In this equation, there is no direct effect, $(p_{s,q})(p_{r,s}) + (p_{s,q})(p_{ad,s})(p_{r,ad})$ is the sum of the total indirect effect of the variable, and $(p_{r,a})(p_{q,a})$ is the noncausal component of the correlation.

It is important to identify all the compound paths in a model that are relevant to the correlation between two variables. Otherwise, one might, through error, conclude incorrectly that a path model needs respecification. Fortunately, Wright has provided three rules that, if followed, result in the identification of all possible compound paths between two particular variables. These rules guide the researcher in looking at a diagram of a path model and tracing the possible compound paths. The goal is for the researcher to identify compound paths that are meaningful (indirect effects) and not meaningful (noncausal), because both are part of the correlation.

Wright's three rules for identifying all compound paths are as follows:

1. No compound path involves going through the same variable more than once.
2. No compound path involves going forward with the direction of an arrow through a variable and then backward

against the direction of a second arrow through a second variable (although it is perfectly acceptable to go backward first and then forward).

3. No compound path involves going through a curved, double-headed arrow line (i.e., a diagrammed relationship between two variables that has been left as a correlation) more than once.

The second rule sounds complicated, but we have already been applying it to identify the nonmeaningful compound path shown in Figure 16-12 for the variables quality of health prehospitalization and return to work. Look back over the diagram in Figure 16-12 and trace this path once more. The third rule hints at the problem with including a correlation in a path model, namely, that the correlation may get in the way of determining the indirect effect of an independent variable. For this reason, researchers should assign a direction to hypothesized relationships between variables whenever possible, but not at the expense of theory or logic and reason.

CONDUCTING A PATH ANALYSIS

Conducting a path analysis involves preparation, analysis, and a consideration of the analysis' limitations. In this section we go through the steps needed to conduct a path analysis, an example of a study of factors influencing individuals' perceptions of their overall state of health using data collected for earlier editions of this book. This study illustrates how researchers can use path analysis to move a step beyond traditional regression analysis. Here, the researchers start the path analysis after completing a regression analysis in which the factors that influence an individual's perception of health have been identified.

The independent variables in this example are satisfaction with current weight, frequency of exercise, and scores on an inventory of personal attitudes about self, life, and work. Age and education were tested for inclusion as independent variables but were not significant in this final regression model and were dropped. The sample size is 659, and the independent variables are continuous and fairly normally distributed. We are comfortable in continuing with the analysis because we know that multiple regression is somewhat robust to (i.e., able to tolerate) mild to moderate violations of normality, particularly as the sample size increases. The only information we have about measurement error is that the Cronbach's alpha for the inventory of personal attitudes is .95.

Step 1: Draw the Model

The first step is to draw the model to be tested with path analysis. This path model is drawn after having used regression analysis to identify which variables from a theoretical framework are significantly related to the dependent variable of interest. The results of this regression analysis are depicted in Table 16-1. To draw the model we will also need a table of correlations among the variables in the regression (Table 16-2); familiarity with the research findings and theory pertinent to this topic; logic and reason to assign, where possible, a temporal order to the independent variables that are correlated with one another and for which research findings and theory are not available; and awareness of the need to maintain a one-way flow of causation to meet the assumptions necessary for path analysis.

An examination of the correlations listed in Table 16-2 reveals that all the independent variables are correlated with one another. This means that we must now attempt to assign a direction to these relationships. Theories about health behavior hold that attitudes guide behavior (Norris & Ford, 1995). Therefore, we can assign a direction to the relationship between

Table 16-1	**REGRESSION RESULTS USED TO CREATE PATH MODEL IN COMPUTER EXAMPLE**

Model Summary

Model	R	R^2	Adjusted R^2	Standard Error of the Estimate
1	.580[a]	.336	.333	1.143

ANOVA[b]

Model		Sum of Squares	df	Mean Square	F	Significance
1	Regression	663.461	3	221.154	110.725	.000[a]
	Residual	1308.247	655	1.997		
	Total	1971.709	658			

Coefficients[b]

Model		Unstandardized Coefficients		Standardized Coefficients	t	Significance
		B	Standard Error	β		
1	(Constant)	2.690	0.312		8.634	.000
	Exercise	0.375	0.059	.220	6.314	.000
	Personal attitudes	0.023	0.002	.370	10.990	.000
	Satisfaction with current weight	0.124	0.022	.193	5.546	.000

[a]Predictors: (Constant), satisfaction with current weight, personal attitudes, and exercise.
[b]Dependent variable: overall state of health.

Table 16-2	**CORRELATIONS AMONG VARIABLES IN COMPUTER EXAMPLE**

		Overall State of Health	**Exercise**	**Satisfaction With Current Weight**	**Total**
Pearson correlation	Overall state of health	1.000	.394	.369	.482
	Exercise	.394	1.000	.363	.281
	Satisfaction with current weight	.369	.363	1.000	.260
	Personal attitudes	.482	.281	.260	1.000

personal attitudes and frequency of exercise and draw a path $(p_{f,p})$ to represent this (Fig. 16-13). Research on exercise suggests that people who exercise moderately and regularly may be more satisfied with their weight (Tucker & Maxwell, 1992), and there is no evidence that those in our sample exercise excessively. Consequently, we draw a path $(p_{s,f})$ in Figure 16-13 to represent the influence of frequency of exercise on satisfaction with current weight. Research and theory are not available for assigning a direction to the relationship between personal attitudes and satisfaction with current weight, so here we use logic and reason and awareness of the need to maintain a one-way flow of causation. It seems reasonable to hypothesize that a general set of attitudes should influence satisfaction with something specific such as current weight. So we assign a direction to the path between these two variables $(p_{s,p})$ to represent this. There is in fact only one direction that can be assigned to this relationship that will ensure that the model meets the necessary assumption of a one-way flow of causation. If we instead hypothesized that satisfaction with current weight influenced personal attitudes, the model would have a component that is circular or nonrecursive. You can see this if you redraw the model in Figure 16-13 such that it contains the path $p_{p,s}$ in place of $p_{s,p}$.

Step 2: Identify the Regression Analyses Needed to Calculate and Test the Path Coefficients

Look at the model in Figure 16-13 and count the number of endogenous variables to determine the number of regression analyses needed. You should come up with three endogenous variables: the dependent variable, overall state of health; frequency of exercise, which is endogenous to personal attitudes; and satisfaction with current weight, which is endogenous to frequency of exercise and personal attitudes. Checking to be sure that we have identified all the variables that have direct or indirect effects on a specific endogenous variable, we identify the three regression analyses needed for this model as follows:

1. Overall state of health (o) regressed on satisfaction with current weight (s), frequency of exercise (f), and personal attitudes (p)
2. Frequency of exercise regressed on personal attitudes
3. Satisfaction with current weight regressed on frequency of exercise and personal attitudes

The second regression analysis is nothing more than the correlation between frequency

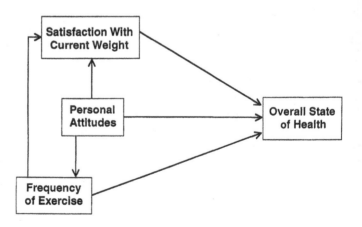

FIGURE 16-13 Diagram of initial path model.

of exercise and personal attitudes. It is always the case that the path between an endogenous and an exogenous variable is equal to the correlation between these two variables whenever (1) there is an endogenous variable with only one variable exogenous to it, and (2) the exogenous variable is fully exogenous and has no other variables influencing it.

Step 3: Calculate the Path Coefficients

Calculating the path coefficients is easy! We actually know what many of these coefficients are from our prior work. Figure 16-14 shows what we know using information from Tables 16-1 and 16-2. We are using the betas or the standardized coefficients for our diagram because we are not looking at group differences.

To calculate the remaining coefficients, we run the third regression analysis we identified in step 2—the one with satisfaction with current weight as the dependent variable. The results of this third regression analysis are shown in Table 16-3.

Step 3: Assess Need to Modify or Respecify the Path Model

At this point in the analysis it is time to identify what paths are and are not significant in the model. If there are paths that are not significant, they can be dropped from the model.

At this point, power and effect size should be considered. In an analysis that is underpowered, the researcher may want to retain a nonsignificant path in the model, if the size of the path coefficient is substantive. The significance test of the path coefficient is biased by sample size. Thus, it is important to consider the given variables in the analysis, and the likelihood that measurement error may contribute to a small effect size. What is considered meaningful will vary with the nature of the phenomenon being studied (Cohen, 1988), but if in doubt Cohen's effect sizes of small ($|.10|$), medium ($|.30|$), and large ($|.50|$) may be used as a guide (Cohen, Cohen, West, & Aiken, 2003).

Returning to our example, we see from the results in Table 16-3 that the remaining paths $(p_{s,p}, p_{s,f})$ are statistically significant ($p < .001$). Hence, there is no need to modify our model, and we can proceed to calculating the direct and indirect effects of the independent variables. Figure 16-15 depicts our final path model. We will need to refer to this model to complete this second step of the analysis.

Step 4: Determine the Direct, Indirect, and Total Effects of the Independent Variables

To accomplish step 4, we need to construct Table 16-4 to help us use Wright's (1934)

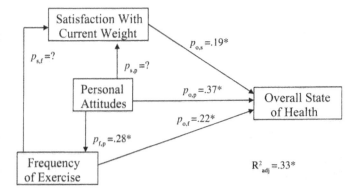

FIGURE 16-14 Diagram of model prior to running third regression analysis to test paths to endogenous variables. (*Path coefficient is significant at $p < .001$.)

Table 16-3	**REGRESSION RESULTS FOR PATHS TO ENDOGENOUS INDEPENDENT VARIABLES IN COMPUTER EXAMPLE**

Model Summary

Model	R	R^2	Adjusted R^2	Standard Error of the Estimate
1	.399[a]	.159	.157	2.459

ANOVA[b]

Model		Sum of Squares	df	Mean Square	F	Significance
1	Regression	751.371	2	375.686	62.116	.000[a]
	Residual	3967.591	656	6.048		
	Total	4718.962	658			

Coefficients[b]

Model		Unstandardized Coefficients		Standardized Coefficients		
		B	Standard Error	β	t	Significance
1	(Constant)	1.423	.539		2.638	.009
	Exercise	.830	.098	.315	8.455	.000
	Personal attitudes	.016	.004	.172	4.598	.000

[a]Predictors: (Constant), personal attitudes, and exercise.
[b]Dependent variable: satisfaction with current weight.

work about the components of a correlation. Next, we fill in Table 16-4 using the correlation values from Table 16-2 for the left column and the beta weights from Table 16-1 for the simple paths column. These beta weights are the direct effects of the independent variable on the overall state of health.

Figure 16-15 is used to identify the paths that need to be multiplied to determine the values for the compound paths. Wright's rules are used

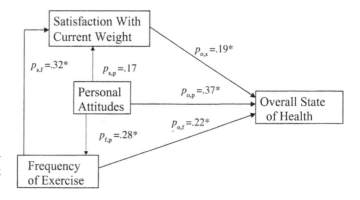

FIGURE 16-15   Final path analysis results for computer example. (*Path coefficient is significant at $p \leq .001$.)

Table 16-4	**TABLE USED TO DETERMINE DIRECT AND INDIRECT EFFECTS OF INDEPENDENT VARIABLES IN FIGURE 16.15**				
$r =$ Direct	+	(Indirect)		+	(Noncausal)
$r =$ Simple	+	Compound + $\cdots$ + Compound		+	Compound + ... + Compound
$r_{f,o} = p_{o,f}$	+	$(p_{s,f})(p_{o,s})$		+	$(p_{f,p})(p_{o,p}) + (p_{f,p})(p_{s,p})(p_{o,s})$
.39 = .22	+	(.32)(.19)		+	(.28)(.37) + (.28)(.17)(.19)
$r_{p,o} = p_{o,p}$	+	$(p_{f,p})(p_{o,f}) + (p_{f,p})(p_{s,f})(p_{o,s}) + (p_{s,p})(p_{o,s})$		+	None
.48 = .37	+	(.28)(.22) + (.28)(.32)(.19) + (.17)(.19)		+	0
$r_{s,o} = p_{o,s}$	+	None		+	$(p_{s,f})(p_{o,f}) + (p_{s,p})(p_{o,p}) + (p_{s,p})(p_{f,p})$ $(p_{o,f}) + (p_{s,f})(p_{f,p})(p_{o,p})$
.37 = .19	+	0		+	(.32)(.22) + (.17)(.37) + (.17) (.28)(.22) + (.32)(.28)(.37)

to trace the paths needed to calculate these compound paths. For example, the second rule tells us that the coefficients for $p_{f,p}$ and $p_{o,p}$ should be multiplied to determine the noncausal component of $r_{f,o}$. Note that the compound paths are sorted into (1) indirect effects, which are the sums of products for meaningful compound paths, and (2) noncausal components, which are the sums of products for compound paths that are meaningless.

Table 16-5 contains the value of the direct and indirect effects as determined by using Wright's formula for the components of a correlation coefficient and his rules for calculating compound paths. Personal attitudes appear to have the greatest effect (0.48) on the overall state of health. Also, all but one of the sums

of the total effect and noncausal components match the magnitude of the respective correlation coefficient. The one sum that does not (satisfaction with current weight) is very close (within .01).

Step 6: Considering the Analysis' Limitations

Now that we have a final path model, it is important to review the assumptions underlying path analysis to be aware of the limitations of the analysis we have just conducted. First, we need to consider whether any of the relationships in the model may be spurious (i.e., violate the third condition of causation). Are there potentially confounding variables that we should have

Table 16-5	**TABLE OF DIRECT EFFECTS, INDIRECT EFFECTS, AND NONCAUSAL COMPONENTS ASSOCIATED WITH EACH INDEPENDENT VARIABLE IN FIGURE 16.15**				
	Direct	**+**	**Indirect**	**Total Effect**	**Total Effect + Noncausal**
Frequency of exercise ($r = .39$)	.22	+	.06	.28	.39
Personal attitudes ($r = .48$)	.37	+	.11	.48	.48
Satisfaction with current weight ($r = .37$)	.19	+	0	.19	.36

included? Second, can we assume that there is no measurement error in our measures? What evidence do we have to support the reliability of our measures? Finally, we should also remind ourselves of the need to replicate this model with longitudinal data. In this example, we were forced to make assumptions regarding the directions between the variables in our model because we were working with cross-sectional data. For example, it may be the case that having a positive perception of their overall state of health causes individuals to exercise more, but we have no way of knowing this. Path analysis does not allow us to evaluate the correctness of the directions we have assigned. Rather, we have assumed that these are the correct directions. Path analysis can only tell us that given our assumptions, this particular path is or is not statistically significant.

SUMMARY

Path analysis is a data analysis technique that can be used to inform our understanding of phenomena. It is useful because, at the very least, it challenges us to think of the effects of independent variables in more complex ways (Asher, 1983). Although on the surface it may appear complex, path analysis is a relatively simple data analysis technique. It is nothing more than a series of regression analyses and some hand calculations. The difficulty is in thinking through the relationships among a set of variables, and correctly specifying the regression equations to be tested. Path analysis, like any statistic, is just a tool in the hands of the researcher. The validity of the model testing and theory building it produces depends on the quality of the data and the thinking that accompanies the use of the statistic.

CHAPTER REVIEW

Multiple-Choice Concept Review

1. Path analysis is useful when
   a. spurious relationships exist within a set of variables.
   b. linear relationships exist within a set of variables.
   c. the size of the sample is small.
   d. none of the above.

2. The dependent variable in path analysis
   a. should be continuous and normally distributed.
   b. should be measured at two points in time.
   c. should be categorical.
   d. none of the above.

3. Endogenous variables are
   a. always influenced by other variables in the model.
   b. never influenced by other variables in the model.
   c. always independent variables.
   d. usually ordinal.

4. Path analysis
   a. is based on regression techniques.
   b. is considered a type of causal model.

   c. examines relationships between variables.
   d. all of the above.

5. Variables in a path model
   a. are either endogenous or exogenous.
   b. demonstrate a one-way flow of causation.
   c. have a U-shaped distribution.
   d. both a and b.

6. Causation can be implied in path analysis when
   a. there is no correlation between the independent and dependent variables.
   b. there is a correlation between the independent and dependent variables.
   c. Y precedes X in time.
   d. causation can never be implied.

7. Effects in path analysis
   a. have little impact on the study.
   b. can be used to determine which variable to target in an intervention.
   c. can be direct or indirect.
   d. both b and c.

8. Indirect effects
   a. involve an exogenous variable and an endogenous variable that is exogenous to Y, the dependent variable.
   b. occur because an independent variable is theorized to influence other independent variables.
   c. arise when the dependent variable is theorized to influence other independent variables.
   d. exacerbate underlying problems with measurement error and multicollinearity.

9. Which of the following is not a limitation of the path model?
   a. Relationships are spurious.
   b. There is measurement error.
   c. It only works with cross-sectional data.
   d. There are confounding variables that could have been included.

10. Which of the following is a statistical assumption in path analysis?
   a. Measurement error is equal to ± 1.
   b. The flow of causation is unidirectional.
   c. Correlational paths can be fully analyzed.
   d. All variables are measured at the ordinal level.

Critical Thinking Concept Review

1. Develop a research question for which path analysis would be appropriate. Specify your variables and determine whether they are endogenous or exogenous. Identify how many regression analyses you would have to conduct.

2. Using the research question you developed for problem 1, identify the steps you would take to conduct a path analysis assuming that you have used regression

analysis to identify which variables from a theoretical framework are significantly related to the dependent variable of interest. As you do not have actual results of this regression analysis, use hypothetical values.

3. How might you evaluate whether your path model is correctly specified? How might measurement error affect your correlation?

Structural Equation Modeling

Anne E. Norris

CHAPTER

17

OBJECTIVES

After studying this chapter, you should be able to:

1. Describe at least three types of research questions that can be addressed with structural equation modeling (SEM).

2. Identify three data set requirements for conducting SEM.

3. Describe the relationship between the measurement model and the theoretical model in SEM.

4. Describe the role of theory in the SEM process.

5. Critique an SEM analysis on the basis of the model fit statistics and description of the modeling process.

OVERVIEW OF STRUCTURAL EQUATION MODELING

This chapter is intended as an introduction to structural equation modeling (SEM) and assumes an understanding of the concepts and issues discussed in Chapter 16 with respect to path analysis. The purpose of this chapter is to acquaint readers with the possibilities SEM offers and aid them in interpreting SEM results

published in the literature. Readers who are interested in gaining a more in-depth knowledge of SEM are encouraged to read one or more of the following sources—Bollen (1989), Byrne (2006), Hayduk (1996), or Schumacker and Lomax (2004)—and to consult the *Journal of Structural Equation Modeling*.

Like path analysis, SEM is used to test theoretical models depicting relationships between concepts. Over the years, SEM has been referred to as covariance structure modeling, because covariances are analyzed in SEM; latent variable analysis, because SEM analyzes relationships between latent (i.e., abstract or unmeasured) variables; and a LISREL analysis, because LISREL was the name of the first software available for conducting SEM.

SEM challenges us to think about how we measure theoretical constructs. In fact, it allows us to use multiple measures of theoretical constructs. For example, researchers do not have to settle for one measure of health. They can use psychological, performance, and physiological measures, and the response options for these measures can vary with the measure. Alternatively, they can use a health attitudes questionnaire, but instead of totaling item responses into one lump sum, each item can be treated as a separate measure of health.

The measurement of theoretical constructs is critical in SEM. SEM tests two models simultaneously: a measurement model and a theoretical model. Together these two models are referred to as the full model. The measurement model is a model of how theoretical constructs are measured. The theoretical model is a model of the hypothesized relationships between the theoretical constructs. Valid tests of the theoretical model are dependent on a good fit of the measurement model to the data. The statistics produced in SEM help the researcher determine how good this fit is.

RESEARCH QUESTION

SEM allows us to ask old questions in new and more powerful ways, and new questions that could not have been addressed without the technology and thinking that underlie SEM. The latter sort of questions is only just beginning to be identified and pursued.

We can break the research questions addressed by SEM into four categories. The first category is testing theoretical models. Like path analysis, SEM can be used to test a causal model. However, unlike path analysis, measurement error is estimated and removed from the relationships between theoretical constructs. Thus, it is possible to get a more precise test of theories. In addition, SEM can be used to analyze nonrecursive models (i.e., models with two-way paths).

A second category relates to measurement issues. SEM provides a new way to examine the factor structure of an instrument because it allows assigning items to specific factors, identifying which items "load" on more than one factor, and specifying which factors are or are not correlated with one another. Model fit statistics can then be used to determine how well this factor structure fits the data. The fit of alternative factor structures can be compared, making it possible to statistically identify which factor structure provides a better fit to the data. With respect to reliability, a whole new level of sophistication is possible when the consistency in both factor loadings and measurement error can be examined over time. Additionally, SEM can be used to accurately estimate reliability in large-sample studies of well-constructed scales where the factor model is correctly specified (Yang & Green, 2010).

Third, SEM provides new ways to look at group differences. For example, the fit of a factor structure in different groups of people can be compared to determine whether the factor structure is the same in the various groups. We can compare the magnitude of the factor "loadings" (path coefficients in the measurement model) or the factor correlations as well as test the assumption that these values are equivalent in the groups. Determining whether the factor structures are the same with this level of specificity allows us to identify when group differences at the factor-score level are real and not an artifact of measurement differences.

With SEM, it is also possible to determine whether the same theoretical model works equally well for explaining the data in different sample subgroups. SEM can be used to examine whether individual paths in the model differ in magnitude across the two groups. Individual differences (e.g., ethnic, gender, diagnostic group differences) can be explored, as well as moderator effects.

Finally, SEM opens the door to new questions. For example, with SEM, it is possible first to assume that different levels of measurement error are present in data and then to test the effect of these different levels on the theoretical relationships specified in the model. Thus, conclusions could be made about the robustness of these relationships to problems such as subjects' poor memories, tendency to alter responses to make a better impression, misreading the question, and so forth.

Do Attitudes and Norms Predict Changes in Sexual Risk Behavior Over Time or Does Sexual Risk Behavior Predict Changes in Attitudes and Norms Over Time? An Example of a Theory Testing SEM Analysis

This longitudinal study examined attitudes and norms related to sexual risk behavior and sexual risk behaviors in gay and bisexual men (n = 1,465) at two different points in time, separated by approximately 18 months (Huebner, Neilands, Rebchook, & Kegeles, 2011). The authors used a single SEM to simultaneously test three alternative hypotheses:

1. Attitudes and perceived norms will be related to sexual risk behavior when measured at a single point in time (i.e., cross-sectionally).
2. Attitudes and perceived norms will predict changes in sexual risk behavior over time, consistent with health behavior theories.
3. Sexual risk behavior will predict changes in attitudes and perceived norms over time, consistent with self-perception and/or cognitive dissonance theories (Huebner et al., 2011, p. 112).

SEM analysis provided significance tests for the different paths associated with these three hypotheses. In addition, it provided information regarding the magnitude of these paths and how well the theoretical model that contained these different paths explained observed relationships (i.e., covariances in the time 1 and time 2 data sets). The authors found that norms and attitudes were related to unprotected anal sex in the cross-sectional data set for both time points. However, attitudes and norms at time 1 did not predict unprotected anal sex at time 2 after controlling for the effect of time 1 behavior on the time 2 measure of behavior. This suggests that behavior at time 1 mediates (is responsible for) the relationship between time 1 attitudes and norms and time 2 behavior. Moreover, they found that, contrary to health behavior theories (e.g., Fishbein & Ajzen's [1975] Theory of Reasoned Action), behavior at time 1 predicted time 2 attitudes and norms. Their work has critical implications for theory about health behaviors and the development of more effective health promotion interventions.

What Factor Structure Best Explains Responses to the Scales for Diagnosing Attention Deficit Hyperactivity Disorder (SDADHD)? An Example of Using SEM to Conduct a Confirmatory Factor Analysis

The SDADHD contains 39 items and is based on the *Diagnostic and Statistical Manual of Mental Disorders, Fourth Edition* (*DSM-IV-TR*) (APA, 2000) criteria for attention deficit hyperactivity disorder (ADHD). These *DSM-IV-TR* criteria identify three different symptom dimensions: inattention, hyperactivity, and impulsivity. However, for diagnostic purposes, an individual must meet symptom criteria for inattention and either hyperactivity or impulsivity, raising the issue of whether the SDADHD items form a two- or three-factor scale. On the other hand, it is possible that the symptom criteria specified by the *DSM-IV-TR* do not represent two or three distinct dimensions, but instead indicate that ADHD is a single-dimensional construct. Comparing results for a single-, two-, and three-factor structure would resolve this issue and address an important gap in the clinical literature with respect to ADHD.

The SDADHD is available in two forms, a version to be completed by parents, the Home Rating Scale (HRS), and a version to be completed by teachers, the School Rating Scale (SRS). Ryser, Campbell, and Miller (2010) used both versions in their analysis of normative data collected for a nationally representative sample of children between the ages of 5 and 18 who were not diagnosed with ADHD. In essence, their study asked three questions:

1. What factor structure fits best: a single-, two-, or three-factor structure?
2. Is the factor structure the same for the HRS and the SRS versions?
3. What is the evidence for the internal consistency of the two versions?

Using SEM and data from both HRS ($n = 803$) and SRS ($n = 1,263$) samples, Ryser et al. (2010) were able to compare statistical results for three different factor structures, separately for each sample. They compared the model fit statistics produced in the analysis and determined that a two-factor structure fit as well as a three-factor structure in both samples and that both structures had better model fit statistics than a single-factor structure. They chose not to test for statistically significant differences in the fit of their factor models and instead argued for the two-factor structure on the basis of parsimony.

Ryser et al. (2010) then computed factor reliability (internal consistency) using path coefficients in the factor model (analogous to factor loadings in traditional factor analysis) obtained in HRS and SRS samples. Reliabilities were excellent: .91 for inattention and .92 for hyperactivity/

impulsivity in the HRS sample and .97 for inattention and .96 for hyperactivity/impulsivity in the SRS sample.

How Do Pathways From Academic Competence, Negative Life Events, and Peer User Affiliations to Level of Substance Use and From Level of Substance Use to Behavior Problems Differ in High–School Students as a Function of High and Low Self-Regulation? An Example of a Multiple-Group SEM

This cross-sectional study of 1,116 public high-school students in the New York metropolitan area used a set of psychological and behavioral measures with acceptable to good internal consistency (alpha values ranged from .69 to .96) as single indicators of their theoretical constructs (Wills, Pokhrel, Morehouse, & Fenster, 2011). The authors used a multiple-group analysis to compare the path coefficients obtained for a model of students who were high in self-regulation ($n = 524$) with those obtained for a model of students who were low in self-regulation ($n = 545$). Their use of single indicators prevented them from estimating measurement error in their analysis and removing its effect from the paths they were interested in studying. However, they were more interested in establishing the presence of moderators than estimating the effect size of the paths in their model. Moderation was hypothesized to occur at two places in the theoretical model:

1. Self-regulation would moderate paths from life events and peer deviance to level of substance use.
2. Self-regulation would alter the paths from level of substance use to behavior and emotional problems.

Using SEM, Wills et al. (2011) tested their theoretical model in each subgroup. They were able to obtain significance tests for specific paths in the model for each self-regulation group as well as determine that the paths from negative life events to level of substance abuse (hypothesis 1; *p* < .01) and from level of substance abuse to behavior problems were significantly different in the high and low self-regulation groups (hypothesis 2; *p* < .001). These results supported their moderation hypotheses with respect to high and low behavioral self-regulation but not high and low emotional self-regulation.

KEY TERMS

Before talking about the type of data and assumptions required for SEM, we must discuss some of the terms used in SEM. Frequently, different names have evolved to refer to the same term. These different names result from differences in the software used for SEM and in the orientation to SEM. Currently, the most commonly used software programs are M*plus*, LISREL, AMOS, and EQS. In this section, names for terms that are unique to these programs are noted. M*plus* and AMOS use a minimum of terms, relying more on the names of the variables or in the case of AMOS, a diagram of the model, to drive the analysis.

Indicators, Measured Variables, Proxies, and Manifest Variables

Indicators, measured variables, proxies, and manifest variables are different terms used in SEM to refer to the same thing: measures of a theoretical construct. For simplicity, *indicator* will be used in the remainder of this chapter to refer to these measures. Indicators are directly measured by the researcher: They correspond to a specific response on a questionnaire or piece of data in a data set. In LISREL, the letters X and Y are used to refer to indicators for theoretical constructs that are exogenous and endogenous, respectively. (As you may recall from Chapter 16, endogenous variables are

influenced by other variables in the model, whereas exogenous variables are independent of such influences.) In EQS, the letter V is used for all indicators. A universal way of designating a variable as an indicator is to enclose it in a square in the SEM diagram. Hence, we could say that the construct health in Figure 17-1 has six indicators: well-being, happiness, Karnofsky's Performance Status, percentage of activities of daily living (ADLs), treadmill performance, and resting heart rate.

Residuals and Measurement Error

Residuals and measurement error represent the imprecision inherent to some extent in any research measure, whether it is an item on a questionnaire or the results of an HIV viral load test. For simplicity, *measurement error* is used in the remainder of this chapter to refer to this inherent imprecision. Measurement error may be theorized to be correlated if some systematic (i.e., nonrandom) error is expected in the data. This might occur if certain items in a questionnaire elicit social desirability concerns, or when the same measure is used at different points in time.

Although measurement error is sometimes left out of SEM diagrams, it is always estimated in SEM analyses unless an indicator is assumed

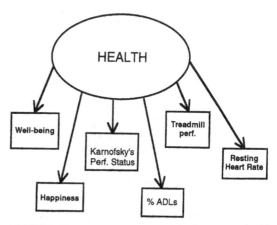

FIGURE 17-1   Measurement model for the construct health.

to have no measurement error. An indicator is assumed to have no measurement error if it is the only indicator used to measure a theoretical construct. This often occurs when a theoretical construct is low in abstraction (e.g., age or height) or when multiple measures of the construct are not available.

In *Mplus*, measurement error is referred to as the residual variance for a particular indicator variable. In LISREL, measurement error is represented by the lowercase Greek letter δ (delta) if the theoretical construct is exogenous and ∈ (epsilon) if the construct is endogenous. In Amos, the letter d is used, and in EQS, the letter E is used for the measurement error associated with both types of theoretical constructs.

Measurement Model

The measurement model is a model of how theoretical constructs are measured. For example, Figure 17-1 is a measurement model for the construct health. The model, as diagrammed, indicates that we are hypothesizing that well-being, happiness, Karnofsky's Performance Status, percentage of activities of daily living self-completed, treadmill performance, and resting heart rate are all indicators for the construct health. Some measurement error is expected for each of these six indicators, but this has not been included in the diagram.

Sometimes the focus of the SEM is on the measurement model, as when SEM is used for confirmatory factor analysis to examine an instrument's construct validity. Other times the measurement model receives little attention because the researcher is focused on examining relationships between theoretical constructs. However, the validity of any theory testing that SEM provides is dependent on the fit of the measurement model to the data. If the measurement model does not fit the data well, we cannot determine whether a failure to find a hypothesized relationship is due to a problem with the theory or a problem with the measurement.

Theoretical Constructs, Unmeasured Variables, and Latent Variables

In SEM, theoretical constructs are often called unmeasured or latent variables because they are not measured directly by the researcher. To minimize confusion, theoretical constructs will be referred to as latent variables for the remainder of the chapter. Latent variables are free of the random or systematic measurement error inherent in indicator variables (Bollen, 1989). A universal way of identifying a theoretical construct as a latent variable is to demarcate it with a circle in a diagram of an SEM model. Thus, it can be said that the model in Figure 17-1 has one latent variable—health.

In LISREL, latent variables are designated as ξ (xi) or η (eta), depending on whether the latent variable is exogenous or endogenous. In EQS, all latent variables are designated with an F for factor. Let us revisit our measurement model for health. Figure 17-1 represents health as a single latent variable with psychological, performance, and physiological indicators. Alternatively, we could hypothesize that health is a multidimensional construct with psychological, performance, and physiological indicators measuring its different dimensions. This hypothesis would be consistent with a model for health such as that shown in Figure 17-2. The advantage of SEM is that we can test both models (or hypotheses about how to measure Health) and see which one fits the data better before going on to test a larger theoretical model about factors that influence health. (Measurement error would be estimated for both models, although it is only included in the diagram for Fig. 17-2.)

Disturbance

The disturbance is the error in the prediction of an endogenous latent variable by other latent variables in the model. It is analogous to the error variance (i.e., residual) in linear regression

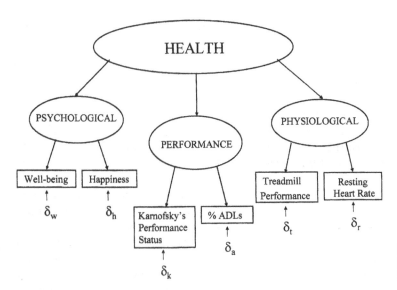

FIGURE 17-2 Measurement model for the construct health as a second-order factor with error terms included.

analysis. The disturbance is often left out of SEM diagrams. If present, it is designated by a *short arrow* pointing at the endogenous latent variable. In M*plus*, the disturbance is referred to as the residual. In LISREL, ζ (zeta) is used to refer to the disturbance, whereas EQS uses the letter D.

Theoretical Model

The theoretical model is a model of the hypothesized relationships between latent variables. For example, in Figure 17-3, we are hypothesizing

that health is influenced by age, health attitudes, and health behaviors. Health attitudes are diagrammed as having only an indirect effect on health. Within the theoretical model, variables are designated as endogenous or exogenous, just as they are in path analysis. Thus, in Figure 17-3, health behaviors and health are endogenous variables. In LISREL, Greek letters are used: ξ (xi) for endogenous and η (eta) for exogenous latent variables. M*plus*, AMOS, and EQS do not make this distinction. In EQS, endogenous and exogenous latent variables are referred to as factors (e.g., F1, F2, F3).

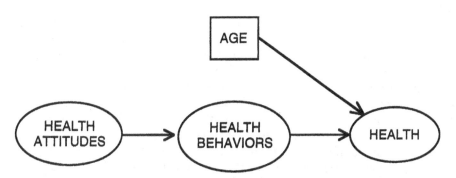

FIGURE 17-3   Hypothetical model predicting health as a function of age, health attitudes, and health behaviors.

Coefficients, Parameters, and Parameter Estimates

Researchers refer to path coefficients in the measurement and theoretical model as coefficients, parameters, or parameter estimates. These words are often used interchangeably because they mean the same thing, but for the sake of clarity, the word *parameter* will be used for the rest of the chapter. Unlike *Mplus*, AMOS, or EQS, which uses no special notation to denote parameters, the LISREL software uses a system of Greek letters to categorize parameters according to the paths they define. Consequently, researchers (regardless of the software they use) may talk about lambda parameters (λ) when referring to paths in the measurement model, beta parameters (β) when referring to paths between endogenous variables, or gamma parameters (γ) when referring to paths between two exogenous variables or one exogenous and one endogenous variable. Researchers further define these parameters by using the same subscript notation discussed in Chapter 16 (e.g., $\gamma_{1,2}$).

Parameters are often referred to as fixed or free. A fixed parameter is not estimated in the SEM analysis; instead, the researcher assigns it a particular value. For example, researchers typically fix a parameter in the measurement model to 1.0. This allows a measurement scale (e.g., 0 to 10 or 1 to 4) to be determined for the latent variable. Other parameters are fixed to 0 to represent the absence of a path between two latent variables or between an indicator and a latent variable.

A free parameter has no value assigned to it. Free parameters are estimated in the SEM analysis: The computer calculates the value as part of the analysis using the covariances of the various indicators. Both standardized and nonstandardized parameters (i.e., path coefficients) are estimated in SEM. SEM computer programs provide significance tests of these parameters as part of the analysis. It is possible to use the standardized parameter estimated and Wright's (1934) method to compute the indirect and total effects of latent variables, just as you would in path analysis (see Chapter 16).

Model Fit Statistics

SEM software programs produce a variety of statistics pertaining to the fit of the model. Unfortunately, the major statistical packages, including *Mplus*, LISREL, EQS, and AMOS, automatically include in their default options indices that are known to have undesirable properties (Marsh, Balla, & Hau, 1996). We try to restrict our discussion here to those indices that are most commonly used in the literature and review any undesirable properties that have been identified. There is currently no consensus on which indices are best, and research on the properties of these indices is ongoing.

Two indices commonly reported in the literature are the goodness-of-fit index (GFI) and the comparative fit index (CFI). Both the GFI and the CFI can range from 0 to 1.0. Historically, a good-fitting model is one that has a GFI or a CFI greater than .90 (Bentler & Bonnett, 1980). However, some work suggests that even this cutoff may not be high enough in all cases given certain sample sizes, estimation methods, and distributions (Hu & Bentler, 1995). Values equal to or greater than .95 may be more desirable because they decrease the chance of making a type II error. Type II error is a concern in SEM because the fit statistics are being used to make the case that there is no difference between the covariance matrices expected based on the analysis specifications and the covariance matrices observed in the data.

Some researchers recommend the CFI over the GFI because Monte Carlo simulation studies suggest that it is less influenced by sample size (Tanguma, 2001; Wang, Fan, & Willson, 1996). However, neither of these indices takes into account how many parameters are included in the model, and model fit can be enhanced (i.e., made closer to 1.0) by merely adding additional parameters (Bollen & Long, 1993). Unfortunately, many indices developed to reward parsimony (e.g., Incremental Fit Index (IFI), Parsimony Goodness of Fit Index (PGFI), and Akaike's Information Criterion [AIC]) have not proved satisfactory for a variety of reasons and are not recommended for general use (Marsh et al., 1996). Two indices that reward parsimony and appear to have some promise, based on recent work with Monte Carlo simulations, are the non-normed fit index and the normed Tucker Lewis index (Marsh et al., 1996). These indices range, like the CFI and the GFI, between 0 and 1.0, with values greater than .90 indicating a good fit. For sample sizes greater than 250, the TLI is less sensitive to sample size and consistently performs well even when models deviate from multivariate normality assumptions (Hu & Bentler, 1998).

The root mean squared residual (RMR) and the standardized root mean squared residual (SRMR) are absolute misfit indices that differ from many other fit indices (e.g., GFI, NFI) in that they are not based on the chi-square. Both indices are solely based on the residual matrix and unlike the GFI and NFI, they decrease as the fit improves, with 0 indicating a perfect fit. However, the scaling (and magnitude) of the RMR is influenced by the scaling of the indicators in the analysis. The SRMR overcomes this problem because it is standardized (Bentler, 1995). The SRMR should be less than .05 for a good fit (Hu & Bentler, 1995), with values smaller than .10 considered acceptable (Schermelleh-Engel, Moosbrugger, & Muller, 2003). In contrast, a value greater than .10 argues for the model being rejected due to a poor fit to the data (Bachand & Beard, 1995).

Generally, a good SRMR value is found when chi-square–based fit indices such as the CFI or the GFI are greater than .95. However, on occasion, the SRMR may suggest that the model fits very well, but the CFI or the GFI may indicate a poor model fit (Browne et al., 2002). This occurs when measurement is very precise, making error variance low—a rare phenomenon in health behavior research, but more common in physiological research. In such cases, one should conclude that the model being tested does provide a good fit to the data despite the discrepancy between the SRMR and the chi-square–based fit indices (Browne et al., 2002).

The root mean square error of approximation (RMSEA) is also a misfit index. Like the RMR, values close to 0 indicate a good fit, with values less than .05 indicating a very good fit (Hu & Bentler, 1995) and those below .10 indicating a reasonable fit (Fan, Thompson, & Wang, 1999). The RMSEA is a little different from the RMR in that it attempts to correct for the number of parameters in the model being tested, and is based on the chi-square. There is good support for using the RMSEA given moderate to large sample sizes (i.e., $n > 200$), but the statistic is likely to be biased at smaller sample sizes (Curran, Bollen, Paxton, Kirby, & Chen, 2002). Other strengths of the RMSEA are that it does not appear overly influenced by the choice of estimation method used for the analysis (Fan et al., 1999), and is sensitive to model misspecification under conditions where indicator reliability and/or the number of parameters vary (Jackson, 2007).

All SEM programs produce a model chi-square. This chi-square assesses the difference between observed data and a restricted structure resulting from the full (i.e., measurement and theoretical) model (Byrne, 2006). This means that in SEM, the researcher wants the chi-square test to be nonsignificant: the researcher seeks to confirm the null hypothesis (i.e., there is no difference between the data and the model).

A limitation of the model chi-square is that it is greatly influenced by sample size and violations of multivariate normality (Jöreskog & Sörbom, 1988). In fact, Bollen and Long (1993) say that any work that uses only the model chi-square to draw conclusions about model fit should be greeted with skepticism.

Two hand-calculated statistics are also used to assess model fit. One of these, Carmines and McIver's (1983) relative chi-square (ratio of chi-square to degrees of freedom) is calculated by dividing the model chi-square by its degrees of freedom. There is no consensus on what value constitutes a good fit (Bollen, 1989), but Carmines and McIver recommend that relative chi-squares be less than 3.

A second type of hand-calculated statistics, the nested chi-square, is used to determine which of two competing models fits the data significantly better. This is the test we would use to determine which measurement model of health, Figure 17-1 or Figure 17-2, is better. A nested chi-square is calculated by subtracting the chi-square and degrees of freedom for one model from those associated with another competitive model. The significance level associated with this nested chi-square is used to determine whether the fit of one model differs significantly from that of the other. Table 17-1 contains an example of how to calculate the nested chi-square to determine if one measurement model for health fits the data significantly better than the other. Note that the chi-square for Figure 17-2 (second-order factor model) is smaller than the one for Figure 17-1. This suggests that the second-order factor model fits the data better (remember, in SEM, we want the chi-square to be nonsignificant). The significance level associated with the nested chi-square confirms this: $\chi^2 = |15.21|$, df = 2, $p < .001$.

The AIC and the Bayesian Information Criterion (BIC) are two alternative statistics used to compare competing models, involving the same number of indicator variables and the same data set (Akaike, 1987; Raftery, 1995; Schermellah-Engel, Moosbrugger, & Muller, 2003). Neither criteria is a test of significance and neither is normed, so they cannot be interpreted in isolation. Instead, the model with the lowest AIC or BIC of a set of models computed for the same data set is argued to be the superior model, and other fit statistics are used to support selection of this model. A difference in BIC values for two models of 5 points or more argues for the models being different, with differences of 10 points or more indicating more certainty in this difference, and the best model being the one with the lowest BIC (Raftery, 1993). Both criteria correct for the number of parameters in the model being estimated but do so in different ways. The AIC corrects by a factor of 2 for each parameter estimated. The BIC is a stronger correction with the magnitude of the correction increasing as the sample size increases.

In general, a variety of fit statistics should be used to evaluate model fit (Gonzalez & Griffin, 2001; Hu & Bentler, 1999; Jackson, 2007). For example, a researcher may choose to report the CFI, chi-square test, RMSEA, and relative chi-square ratio. A model may be interpreted as fitting the data even when the chi-square is statistically significant if the CFI or GFI is greater than .90 and the relative chi-square is less than 3. Certain fit statistics are less influenced by reliability of the indicators, while others are less influenced by sample size or the number of parameters being tested (Jackson, 2007).

Table 17-1	EXAMPLE OF HOW TO CALCULATE A NESTED CHI-SQUARE	
Chi-square statistic for model of health depicted in Figure 17-1:		2,006.37, df = 1,202
Chi-square statistic for model of health depicted in Figure 17-2:		2,021.58, df = 1,200
Nested chi-square[a]:		−15.21, df = 2

[a]Sign (negative or positive) of the nested chi-square does not matter.

Hence, a combination of fit and misfit statistics is recommended.

Identification

Identification of both the measurement model and the theoretical model is critical to the estimation of parameters and testing of model fit that occurs in SEM. Just as in path analysis, these models can be overidentified (e.g., when the number of covariances or known information exceeds the number of parameters being estimated), just identified (e.g., when the number of covariances or known information is equal to the number of parameters being estimated), or underidentified (e.g., when the number of parameters being estimated exceeds the number of covariances or known information). In SEM, the measurement and theoretical models being tested must be overidentified. The computer program cannot generate model fit statistics if the model is just identified; if the model is underidentified, the program either will not run or will run only after the software chooses specific parameters in the model to constrain to be equal to 0.

Unfortunately, identification (i.e., delineating a model that is overidentified) is not an easy or straightforward task. For example, it is possible for a model to be overidentified on paper but empirically underidentified on the computer due to the statistical properties of the indicators (e.g., problems with normality, high intercorrelations). Templin and Peters (2002) provide a simple method to make sure that a model is at least overidentified on paper based on calculation of the model's degrees of freedom. According to this method, it is only when the model's degrees of freedom are positive that the model is overidentified. The model's degrees of freedom are equal to the unadjusted degrees of freedom minus the number of parameters in the model (i.e., all variances, disturbances, free paths in both measurement and theoretical model, free covariances [specified correlations]).

The unadjusted degrees of freedom are equal to the number of distinct variances and covariances in the model to be tested or

$$P \times \frac{(p+1)}{2} \qquad (1)$$

where p is equal to the number of manifest variables.

Thus, the formula for calculating a model's degrees of freedom can be written as follows:

$$\text{Model df} = \left[P \times \frac{(p+1)}{2} \right] - k \qquad (2)$$

where k is the number of parameters that will be estimated when the model is analyzed in SEM.

Modification Indices

In addition to model fit statistics and parameter estimates, SEM programs provide statistics predicting the potential change in model fit (change in chi-square) associated with adding or deleting parameters. Researchers may use these statistics to guide them in making changes in their model. Two specific types of modification indices produced by EQS are the Lagrange multiplier test (for adding parameters) and Wald test (for deleting nonsignificant parameters). The modification indices produced by LISREL are simply referred to as modification indices or MI and indicate only whether specific parameters should be added.

Multiple-Group Analysis

Multiple-group analysis is a type of analysis in which group differences in measurement and theoretical models are tested. A researcher could use this type of analysis to determine whether the factor structure of an instrument is the same in different sample subgroups (e.g., different age, gender, or ethnic groups). Group differences in theoretical models are explored when the measurement model is equivalent or at least partially invariant across groups (Byrne, 2006). An equivalent measurement model means that the free parameters are not significantly different across groups. A partially invariant measurement model has at least one free parameter that is equivalent across groups (i.e., the difference is not statistically significant). It is important to establish that the measurement model is equivalent or partially invariant to avoid having group differences in the theoretical model confounded by measurement differences.

TYPE OF DATA REQUIRED

SEM requires data to have three characteristics. First, the data should be continuous and normally distributed. However, new techniques are being developed for categorical data (Maydeu-Olivares, 2006; Muthén, 2001; West, Finch, & Curran, 1995). Special estimation methods and scaled statistics are available that are robust to violations of normality (Byrne, 2006; Hu & Bentler, 1995), but the best approach currently available is to use *Mplus,* which has special estimation procedures (e.g., weighted least squares) and model fit statistics (e.g., weighted root mean residual) that allow fitting of measurement models that contain categorical and continuous indicator variables.

Second, the data should contain multiple indicators of latent variables. At least three indicators of a latent variable are needed for its measurement model to be just identified. Fixing the parameter for one of the three indicators to be equal to 1.0 makes the model overidentified. As noted earlier, this is a common practice because it also allows a measurement scale to be determined for the latent variable. Measurement models with less than three indicators can become overidentified if the researcher makes certain assumptions (i.e., fixes certain parameters), such as assuming a measure has no measurement error. It is important that these multiple indicators capture different aspects or characteristics of a latent variable. Indicators cannot be so redundant (i.e., highly correlated) that one can be used to predict another perfectly or nearly perfectly. This type of redundancy is called linear dependency. It prevents the model from being empirically identified (Chou & Bentler, 1995). This means that although the model as diagrammed looks identified, high intercorrelations in the data render it empirically underidentified.

Third, the data should be numerous: SEM requires a large sample size. Assuming the most common method for estimating the parameters in SEM (maximum likelihood [ML]), a past recommendation has been a minimum of 100 to 200 subjects (100 to 200 per group in a multiple-group analysis). However, there are at least five reasons why this recommended sample size minimum should be revised to 500 or more. First, Fan and Wang's (1998) work with computer simulations of a simple, three-factor model suggests that sample sizes of 100 and 200 are more likely to lead to improper solutions (i.e., those with statistically impossible values such as negative variances). Sample sizes of 500 did not produce these same improper solutions. Second, Curran et al. (2002) found that even models with only small to moderate misspecification had biased mean and variance estimates when the sample size was 200 or less. Third, model fit statistics are influenced by unreliability of the indicator variables (average magnitude of path between the indicator and the latent variable) when sample size was less than 400 (Jackson, 2007). Fourth, larger sample sizes decrease the effects of nonnormality on model fit statistics and parameter estimates (West et al., 1995), and nonnormality frequently occurs in nursing and health-related research data sets. Fifth, a parameter's standard error (used to compute parameter significance tests) varies across equivalent models when sample sizes are less than 500 (Gonzalez & Griffin, 2001). This means that different conclusions about a parameter's significance may be arbitrarily reached when testing equivalent or competing models. It is disturbing to realize that much of the research demonstrating problems when sample sizes dip below 500 was conducted using simple models. It is unclear whether similar problems would arise for sample sizes of 500 or more when models are more complex (i.e., have more theoretical variables and hence more parameters to be estimated)! We do know that as theoretical models become more complex, a larger sample size is needed. And as discussed later in this chapter, one approach to power analysis suggests that power is likely to be inadequate when models are tested in sample sizes of 200 or less. Therefore, until additional research is conducted, a minimum sample size of 500, even for fairly simple models, seems advisable, particularly when data are not normally distributed.

Although SEM is considered a causal modeling technique, it can be performed with either cross-sectional or longitudinal data. For example, the data used by Wills et al. (2011) in their multiple-group analysis are from a survey and are cross-sectional. Thus, it is important to be aware of theoretical assumptions pertaining to causation in SEM.

ASSUMPTIONS

There are three types of assumptions that must be considered with SEM: theoretical, general statistical, and estimation method-specific.

Theoretical Assumptions

In SEM, the importance of using theory to guide your work cannot be emphasized enough. As in path analysis, theoretical (or causal) assumptions are made in the process of identifying a model to be tested. However, with SEM, assumptions of causation are made regarding both measurement of latent variables (e.g., this indicator measures this construct) and relationships between latent variables (e.g., attitudes influence behavior). Assumptions are made when paths are drawn (i.e., parameter does not

equal 0) and not drawn (i.e., parameter equals 0). For example, in Figure 17-2, there are no paths connecting well-being, happiness, treadmill performance, and resting heart rate with the performance construct; thus, it is assumed that the parameters between these indicators and the performance construct are equal to 0.

As in path analysis, it is important to consider the three conditions of causation: the presence of an observed and measurable relationship between variables, temporal ordering, and nonspuriousness (see Chapter 16 for a discussion of these three conditions). Bollen (1989) and others writing specifically about SEM use the terms *association, direction of influence,* and *isolation* to refer to these three conditions of causation. Bollen talks about meeting a condition of pseudoisolation to emphasize the researcher's inability to be certain that a relationship between two latent variables is nonspurious. Further, he emphasizes the need to recognize the tentativeness of any claims made through SEM about causality, and argues for replication as an important check on whether the conditions of association and isolation have been met.

General Statistical Assumptions

There are three types of general statistical assumptions in SEM. Violating these assumptions makes it difficult to identify a model that fits the data well and typically results in poorer fit indices.

The first type of assumption should already be familiar to you. These are the assumptions of normal distributions, homoscedasticity, and linear relationships discussed in Chapter 14 for regression analysis. These assumptions arise because, like path analysis, SEM also involves solving a series of regression equations. Although SEM is somewhat robust to violations of normality, including categorical variables can bias significance tests of parameters and the model chi-square test by increasing the likelihood that they will be significant (West et al., 1995) unless special estimation procedures are used such as those provided in M*plus*. Unless these procedures are used, the effect of categorical variables is contingent on their correlation with other variables in the measurement model and must be examined on a case-by-case basis (Bollen, 1989). Variables should be transformed so that their relationships are linear, and a multiple-group analysis should be conducted when interactions are predicted. For example, Norris and Ford (1995) used a multiple-group analysis to show that different models of condom use were needed for each gender or ethnic subgroup in their sample. Their findings confirmed the effect of a gender-by-ethnicity interaction on condom use.

Second, there are assumptions regarding the error terms in SEM. These assumptions are similar to those made in regression regarding the residuals and are typically met in the course of meeting other SEM assumptions. (Specifically, it is assumed that error terms in the model are not correlated with any latent variables, are independent of one another, and are normally distributed; Fox, 1984.) Although these assumptions are violated when the data are not multivariate normal, they are robust when the sample size is large (Chou & Bentler, 1995).

The third type of assumption pertains to sample size. It is assumed that the sample is asymptotic—so large as to approach infinity (Bollen, 1989). Smaller sample sizes (e.g., less than 100 for a simple model when ML is used to estimate parameters) increase the probability of rejecting a true model (one that fits the data) (West et al., 1995).

Estimation of Method-Specific Statistical Assumptions

In addition to general statistical assumptions, there are distributional assumptions associated with the method used to estimate the parameters in SEM. This discussion is limited to ML because it is the most commonly used estimation method (Chou & Bentler, 1995) and performs, on average, better than most other estimation methods, even when its assumptions are violated (Schermelleh-Engel, Moosbrugger, & Muller, 2003). See Bollen (1989) and West et al. (1995) for a discussion of other estimation methods and their robustness. An exception are adjusted or corrected ML estimation methods (see Satorra & Bentler, 1994) that outperform ML when indicator variables extremely nonnormally distributed (Chou & Bentler, 1995) require relatively large sample sizes (e.g., $n \geq 2,000$; Yang-Wallentin & Joreskog, 2001).

ML assumes that no single variable or group of variables perfectly explains another in the data set (Bollen, 1989) and that indicators have a distribution that is multivariate normal (West et al., 1995). This first assumption is why indicators cannot be redundant (i.e., highly intercorrelated). ML is not very robust to violations of this first assumption: models with variables that correlate at or above .90 cannot be estimated.

Although the multivariate normal assumption is difficult to meet, ML is fortunately fairly robust to violation of this assumption (Chou & Bentler, 1995). However, there are two exceptions: when the sample size is small and the model is complex, and when categorical or dichotomous variables are used. Special techniques and estimation methods for models with categorical variables are available, although the sample size requirement can become so large as to be impractical (see Maydeu-Olivares, 2006; Muthén, 2001; Yang & Dunson, 2010 for a discussion of these techniques and estimation methods). In addition, it often makes more theoretical (as well as statistical) sense to perform a multiple-group analysis when dichotomous variables represent group differences such as gender or employment status.

Power

Power is an important issue in SEM in two respects. First, given the same model, a larger sample is more likely to generate a significant model chi-square and hence rejection of the model regardless of its truth (Bollen, 1989; Kaplan, 1995) unless multiple measures of fit are used (Gonzalez & Griffin, 2001). Even models that fit the data well have small specification errors because it is difficult, if not impossible, to specify a model perfectly. Large sample sizes magnify the effects of these small specification errors, leading to a significant chi-square (i.e., chi-square test is overpowered). Conversely, a small sample size will mask the effect of large specification errors, generating a nonsignificant chi-square and acceptance of a model when it should be rejected.

Second, the probability of committing a type II error (i.e., accepting a model that should be rejected—accepting the null hypothesis) increases as models are respecified and tested (Kaplan, 1995). However, as is demonstrated later in this chapter in the computer examples, respecifying and retesting models is an inherent part of conducting an SEM analysis. Undue inflation of type II error can be avoided when the SEM analysis is guided by theory, and modifications are selected in model specification that result in the greatest change in model fit (i.e., have the most power). In addition, Chou and Bentler (1995) recommend splitting a data set in half (when the sample size allows this) and developing a model with one half. The final model can then be retested with the remaining half of the data.

Although power is an important consideration in SEM, evaluating how much power is available in a given SEM analysis is not a simple or straightforward matter. Power is influenced by both sample size and misspecification errors (Kaplan, 1995), but misspecification errors are not typically known to the researcher. Different methods of power analysis have been proposed, but a discussion of these and their various shortcomings is beyond the scope of this chapter. Interested readers are encouraged to consult Kaplan (1995) and Saris and Satorra (1993)

for a discussion of specific methods of power analysis, or MacCallum, Browne, and Suawara (1996) and Hancock and Freeman (2001) for a new approach that allows calculation of minimum sample sizes. Note, Hancock and Freeman (2001) provide select sample size and power tables for models with varying degrees of freedom (calculation described previously in the identification section) based on the MacCallum et al. (1996) method. A review of these tables indicates that even using least-conservative assumptions, power is less than .80 for models with less than 70 degrees of freedom and a sample size of 200 or less. Moreover, a sample size of 100 only yields a power of .80 when the model has 225 or more degrees of freedom. These tables provide further support for raising the SEM minimum sample size well beyond 200.

CONDUCTING SEM

Like path analysis, SEM involves preparation (model specification), analysis (model estimation and testing), and a consideration of the analysis's limitations. Preparation involves drawing a full model (i.e., delineating the measurement model for each latent variable as well as the hypothesized relationships between these constructs) and fixing parameters to either zero or a nonzero value (e.g., .5, 1.0) for identification purposes. Once the full model has been specified (and the data have been collected), a computer program estimates the parameters and tests the fit of the model to the data. The measurement model is evaluated first, and once the researcher determines that the measurement model fits the data, the theoretical model can be tested.

Fitting the model to the data is rarely accomplished in a single analysis. More often, the computer output suggests that certain parameters are not statistically significant and could be dropped, or additional respecification of the model is needed (i.e., GFI or CFI is less than .90). For example, modification indices (in EQS, the Lagrange multiplier test) may suggest adding parameters to the model. If this makes good theoretical sense, the researcher makes the change, and then the fit of this respecified model is tested. Although it may make for more model testing, the addition of parameters (i.e., paths) should be made incrementally to observe whether the parameter contributes substantively to the fit of the model (Kaplan & Wenger, 1993).

In the end, the limitations of the SEM analysis are considered to help put the results in the proper context. For example, the researcher might consider whether certain assumptions about measurement may have influenced the results in some way. Concern about the validity of the final model can also arise if many models were tested in the process of finding one that fit the data well.

In the remainder of this section, a computer example of SEM is discussed. The computer example provides a flavor of the SEM analysis process.

Example of a Multiple-Group SEM Using EQS

This example uses SEM to test a theoretical model of condom use for African American men with a partner they know well. Specifically, we use SEM to determine which parameters are significant and whether the model as a whole provides a good fit to the data. If additional parameters are added to the model, we need to be able to justify this on theoretical grounds.

The data and model testing results reported here are part of a larger multiple-group analysis published by Norris and Ford (1995) in the *Journal of Applied Social Psychology*. The sample size is 203, and the data are cross-sectional. The SEM software is EQS (Bentler, 1995), and the method of estimation is ML. Variables are excluded from the analysis if they have skew or kurtosis of |1.5| or more.

The theoretical model being tested is depicted in Figure 17-4. This model is an integration of three different health behavior models: Health Belief Model (Janz & Becker, 1984), Theory of Reasoned Action (Fishbein & Ajzen, 1975), and Construct Accessibility Model (Norris & Devine, 1992). The effects of talking about AIDS, age, and alcohol use are also included in response to findings in the literature.

As can be seen in Figure 17-4, the theoretical model contains eight latent variables. Interpersonal consequences, embarrassing, and pleasure are three different types of condom beliefs (i.e., three condom-belief factors). Condom predisposition is a new latent variable that combines concepts from the Theory of Reasoned Action (condom attitude, partner norm) and Construct Accessibility Model (state of information in memory). Other latent variables include AIDS communication, AIDS concern (AIDS susceptibility), alcohol use, and condom use. Age is also included: It is demarcated with a square because it has only one indicator and is assumed to be measured without error. This theoretical model is overidentified using criteria described elsewhere (Bollen, 1989; Hayduk, 1987).

The measurement model for the latent variables fit the data well. Separate measurement models were tested for each latent variable: The CFIs for these were .91 or more, and the relative chi-squares ranged from .20 to 1.80.

Although the model shown in Figure 17-4 is overidentified on paper, the computer found that the model was empirically underidentified when it estimated and tested the model. The computer made the model overidentified by constraining the error associated with condom predisposition to be equal to 0. This is indicated by the warning in Table 17-2 that test results may not be appropriate due to condition code and that the parameter D10,D10 (the error term for condom predisposition) is constrained at lower bound.

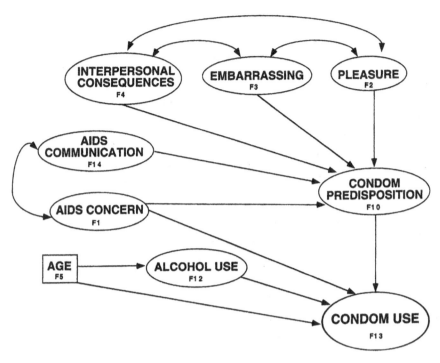

FIGURE 17-4   Initial theoretical model for computer example.

The computer's constraining of the error term associated with condom predisposition (D10,D10) gives us some direction as to how to respecify the model to improve the likelihood that it can be empirically overidentified. The computer's choice of this particular constraint suggests there are too many latent variables diagrammed as influencing condom

Table 17-2	MODEL FIT STATISTICS FOR INITIAL THEORETICAL MODEL IN COMPUTER EXAMPLE
Parameter	Condition code
D10,D10	Constrained at lower bound
Goodness-of-fit summary	
Chi-square = 371.158 based on 242 degrees of freedom	
Probability value for the chi-square statistic is less than .001	
The normal theory RLS chi-square for this ML solution is 338.987	
Bentler-Bonnett normed	Fit index = .7.55
Bentler-Bonnett nonnormed	Fit index = .881
Comparative fit index	= .896

WARNING Test results may not be appropriate due to condition code.

Note: Bentler (1992) recommends the comparative fit index over the other fit indices provided above.
ML, maximum likelihood.

predisposition. But how do we know which parameters to drop? The answer is in the Wald test results presented in the top half of Table 17-3. The Wald test predicts whether dropping a particular parameter would significantly worsen the fit of the model. The Wald predicts that three parameters in the model that involve condom predisposition (F10) could be dropped without worsening the fit of the model: F10,F4; F10,F3; and F10,F1. None of these parameters are associated with a significant change in the

chi-square (i.e., probability associated with the change is ≥.46). Dropping the paths represented by these three parameters results in the respecified model shown in Figure 17-5 and should have no effect on the overall fit of the model. Note, we ignore results for the Lagrange multiplier test in the bottom half of Table 17-3 because the constraint imposed by the computer on D10,D10 may affect their validity. We also do not make any further changes in the model because our goal is to create a

Table 17-3	RESULTS OF WALD AND LAGRANGE MULTIPLIER TESTS FOR INITIAL THEORETICAL MODEL IN COMPUTER EXAMPLE			
Step	Parameter	Chi-Square	df	Probability
Wald test (for dropping parameters)				
1	F13,F5	0.036	1	.850
2	F10,F4	0.382	2	.944
3	F10,F3	0.658	3	.956
4	D13,D13	1.449	4	.919
5	F13,F12	2.871	5	.825
6	F13,F1	4.861	6	.677
7	F10,F1	7.712	7	.462
Multivariate Lagrange multiplier test by simultaneous process in stage 1				
1	V11,F13	14.847	1	.000
2	V22,F1	28.271	2	.000
3	V23,F13	36.500	3	.000
4	V34,F5	43.684	4	.000
5	V7,F4	50.027	5	.000
6	V30,F12	55.977	6	.000
7	V26,F13	60.882	7	.000
8	V13,F5	65.656	8	.000
9	V9,F13	70.214	9	.000
10	V8,F12	74.643	10	.000
11	F14,F4	79.050	11	.000
12	V9,F5	83.102	12	.000
13	V1,F3	86.974	13	.000

WARNING Test results may not be appropriate due to condition code multivariate Wald test by simultaneous process.

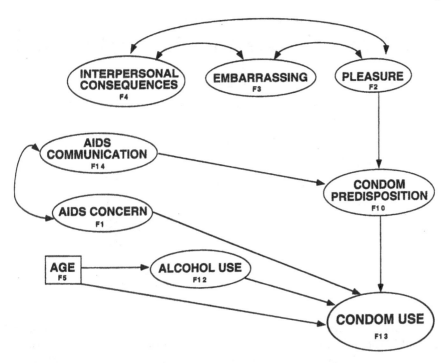

FIGURE 17-5   First respecified model for computer example.

model that is statistically overidentified without needing to constrain any variance terms to 0 before we make any additional changes. At this point in the analysis, we only know that there are identification problems with respect to the regression equation predicting the condom predisposition variable in the theoretical model.

We proceed directly to testing the respecified model shown in Figure 17-5. The Lagrange multiplier test for this next analysis will tell us whether any of the parameters we have dropped should be added back to the model. Although the Wald test in Table 17-3 argues against these parameters being in the model, it is good to review the Lagrange multiplier test for the respecified model to confirm the decisions we made earlier. It is important to confirm these decisions because the statistics that guided them (i.e., those in Table 17-3) were created only after constraining the disturbance term or error

in the regression equation predicting condom predisposition. This term needs to be estimated if we want to remove error variance from our estimates of the path coefficients for the latent variables we hypothesize to influence condom predisposition. Once we have estimated and have a good sense of the value of the disturbance term, we could choose to constrain it. However, constraining this term when we do not know its value is questionable and hence the statistics produced in the previous SEM may not be reliable.

Model fit statistics for the respecified model (Fig. 17-5) are provided in Table 17-4. Note that there is no warning about a condition code: Fortunately, we solved the identification problem. Also, the fit of this new model is acceptable. The model chi-square is significant, but the CFI equals .90. The relative chi-square (375.296/246) is 1.53. This also argues for the fit of the model because it is less than 3.0. Given acceptable model fit statistics, we want to know

Table 17-4	MODEL FIT STATISTICS FOR FIRST RESPECIFIED THEORETICAL MODEL IN COMPUTER EXAMPLE	

Goodness-of-Fit Summary

Independence model chi-square = 1,517.312 on 276 degrees of freedom

Independence AIC =	965.31161	Independence CAIC =	–200.99448
Model AIC =	–116.70398	Model CAIC =	–1,156.23766

Chi-square = 375.296 based on 246 degrees of freedom

Probability value for the chi-square statistic is less than .001

The normal theory RLS chi-square for this ML solution is 342.759

Bentler-Bonett normed	Fit index =		.753
Bentler-Bonett nonnormed	Fit index =		.883
Comparative fit index		=	.896

Note: Bentler (1992) recommends the comparative fit index over the other fit indices provided above.
ML, maximum likelihood; AIC, Akaike's Information Criterion; CAIC, Consistent Akaika Information Criterion; RLS, Recursive Least Squares.

whether all the paths in this respecified theoretical model are necessary. Would dropping any of the parameters representing these paths significantly affect the fit of the model? We want to minimize the probability of our making a type II error here, so it is important to review the rest of the output.

The Wald test results in Table 17-5 indicate that there are three parameters that could be dropped: F13,F5; F13,F12; and F13,F1. These represent the paths from age (F5), alcohol use (F12), and AIDS concern (F1) to condom use (F13). Dropping them results in a second respecified model, depicted in Figure 17-6.

Now we turn to the Lagrange multiplier test results in Table 17-5 and ask ourselves, should any parameters be added to the model? The answer to this question is "no." None of the parameters listed involve two latent variables (i.e., there are no pairs of Fs). Instead they refer to potential changes in our measurement model that cannot be justified on theoretical grounds and therefore should not be made. Moreover, the measurement model has already been determined to fit the data well and is not the focus of analysis at this point.

The results of the Lagrange multiplier test in Table 17-5 support our earlier decision to drop the three parameters representing the influence of interpersonal consequences, embarrassing, and AIDS concern on condom use. The pattern of findings from this model testing and estimation argue for assuming that these latent variables have no influence on condom predisposition (i.e., the parameters are equal to 0). As can be seen in Table 17-6, the fit statistics for the second respecified model (see Fig. 17-6) differ little from those for the first respecified model in Table 17-4. This is good: We have simplified our model without sacrificing model fit. In Table 17-7, the Wald test does not suggest dropping any additional paths between the latent variables, and the Lagrange multiplier test does not suggest adding any such paths. Together with the model fit statistics, these two tests argue against any further respecification of the model. Also, the Lagrange multiplier test results in the context of these model fit statistics support assuming that the paths from age, alcohol use, and AIDS concern to condom use are equal to 0.

The SEM test of the theoretical model is concluded at this point. We now consider three

Table 17-5	**RESULTS OF WALD AND LAGRANGE MULTIPLIER TESTS FOR FIRST RESPECIFIED MODEL IN COMPUTER EXAMPLE**			
		Cumulative Multivariate Statistics		
Step	Parameter	Chi-Square	df	Probability
Wald test (for dropping parameters):Multivariate Wald test by simultaneous process				
1	F13,F5	0.040	1	.841
2	D13,D13	0.790	2	.674
3	F13,F12	2.141	3	.544
4	F13,F1	4.599	4	.331
Multivariate Lagrange multiplier test by simultaneous process in stage 1				
1	V11,F13	12.514	1	.000
2	V23,F13	23.205	2	.000
3	V22,F14	32.068	3	.000
4	V7,F4	39.285	4	.000
5	V34,F5	46.470	5	.000
6	V29,F12	52.430	6	.000
7	V26,F13	58.037	7	.000
8	V9,F13	62.870	8	.000
9	V1,F10	67.682	9	.000
10	V13,F5	72.444	10	.000
11	V9,F5	76.782	11	.000
12	V8,F12	80.774	12	.000

limitations of the analysis. First, due to sample size constraints, we did not randomly split the data set in half, develop our model with one half, and then retest it with the remaining half of the data. Thus, it is possible that our findings could result from a type II error. However, only three models were specified and tested. This limited number of models argues against our findings being the result of a type II error. On the other hand, a second and more serious issue, sample size, makes a stronger argument for type II errors remaining a concern. None of our groups had a sample size of 500 or more. This argues for the need to replicate these findings before using them to guide practice or revise theory.

Finally, these data are cross-sectional, but our model implies causal relationships (e.g., talking about AIDS makes people more predisposed to use condoms). These theoretical relationships need to be validated with longitudinal data.

SUMMARY

SEM is a valuable data analysis tool in many respects. For example, SEM affords us greater precision in testing theories and in evaluating construct validity. However, SEM is still just a tool: SEM in and of itself cannot be used to imply causation or ensure construct validity. The use of theory to guide the analysis is essential, but

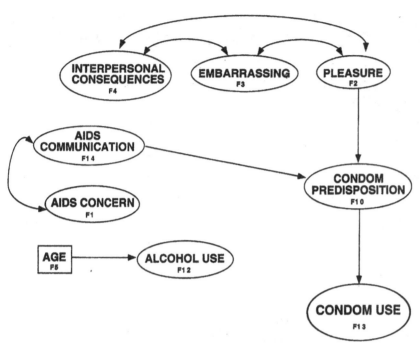

FIGURE 17-6 Second respecified model for computer example.

the validity of the result is also influenced by the data and how SEM is used. A beautiful theory can be contradicted by the data, such as when the CFI or the GFI is less than .90. Alternatively, the theory can be unnecessarily distorted as a result of type II error when too many models are run, and problematic data can also make the use of SEM unfeasible.

Table 17-6	MODEL FIT STATISTICS FOR SECOND RESPECIFIED THEORETICAL MODEL IN COMPUTER EXAMPLE		

Goodness-of-Fit Summary

Independence model chi-square = 1,517.312 on 276 degrees of freedom

Independence AIC =	965.31161	Independence CAIC =	−200.99448
Model AIC =	−118.75645	Model CAIC =	−1,170.96737

Chi-square = 379.244 based on 249 degrees of freedom

Probability value for the chi-square statistic is less than .001

The normal theory RLS chi-square for this ML solution is 349.732

Bentler-Bonett normed	Fit index =		.750
Bentler-Bonett nonnormed	Fit index =		.884
	=		.895

Note: Bentler (1992) recommends the comparative fit index over the other fit indices provided above.
ML, maximum likelihood; AIC, Akaike's Information Criterion; CAIC, ; RLS.

Table 17-7	RESULTS OF WALD AND LAGRANGE MULTIPLIER TESTS FOR SECOND RESPECIFIED MODEL IN COMPUTER EXAMPLE			
		Cumulative Multivariate Statistics		
Step	Parameter	Chi-Square	df	Probability
Wald test (for dropping parameters): Multivariate Wald test by simultaneous process				
1	D13,D13	1.365	1	.243
Multivariate Lagrange multiplier test by simultaneous process in stage 1				
1	V11,F13	12.213	1	.000
2	V22,F14	23.845	2	.000
3	V23,F13	32.416	3	.000
4	V7,F4	39.514	4	.000
5	V34,F5	46.056	5	.000
6	V30,F12	52.014	6	.000
7	V1,F13	57.443	7	.000
8	V13,F5	62.278	8	.000
9	V9,F12	66.804	9	.000
10	V9,F13	71.246	10	.000
11	V3,F12	75.267	11	.000

CHAPTER REVIEW

Multiple Choice Concept Review

1. SEM can be used to address all of the following research issues except
   a. modeling delay in occurrence of a particular event.
   b. reliability of measures.
   c. validity of measures.
   d. group differences.

2. SEM is different from traditional path analysis because
   a. identification is less problematic (more straightforward) in SEM.
   b. the reliability with which variables are measured does not matter.
   c. measurement error can be estimated for model concepts (latent variables).
   d. path coefficients are defined with exogenous variable listed first, then endogenous variables.

3. In SEM, a parameter is another name for
   a. an observed variable.
   b. a path coefficient.
   c. model fit statistic.
   d. a latent variable.

4. Model fit is best evaluated using
   a. a model chi-square test.
   b. parameter significance tests.
   c. Akaike's Information Criterion.
   d. a combination of fit statistics (e.g., CFI, RMSEA, SRMR).

5. Which of the following is true about model fit indices?
   a. The model chi-square test is not influenced by sample size.
   b. Research argues that an SRMR less than .05 indicates good model fit.
   c. The RMSEA does not correct for the number of parameters being estimated.
   d. Research argues that a relative chi-square value of 5.0 indicates good model fit.

6. All of the following are assumptions for SEM except
   a. independent variables must be made up of mutually exclusive groups.
   b. relationships between latent variables are nonspurious.
   c. error terms are normally distributed.
   d. the sample size is asymptotic.

7. Data concerns in SEM include all of the following except
   a. distribution of indicator variables.
   b. distribution of latent variables.
   c. reliability of measures.
   d. large sample size.

8. In SEM analysis, it is best to
   a. retain a model if the GFI or CFI is less than .05.
   b. begin without any a priori ideas about the paths in a model.
   c. use a combination of theory, fit statistics, and modification indices to guide model respecification.
   d. test multiple models, systematically adding parameters until fit statistics and modification indices indicate that the model is saturated.

9. Which of the following is important to do in the early stages of an SEM analysis?
   a. Identify a good-fitting measurement model.
   b. Identify a limited number of theoretical models for testing.
   c. Randomly select a small sample ($n = 100$) for preliminary analyses.
   d. Both a and b.

10. Which of the following is true about multiple-group analysis?
    a. A nested chi-square test can be used to evaluate full or partial measurement invariance.
    b. Measurement model invariance is less important than theoretical model invariance.
    c. The analysis can only proceed if each group uses an identical set of parameters.
    d. The study sample size needs to be 500 or more (minimum of 100 in each group).

Critical Thinking Concept Review and Computational Problems

Review the fit information listed in Exercise Figures 17-1 and 17-2. Which model provides a better fit to these data? Do any additional models need to be run? Does the model with the best fit still need to be respecified and reanalyzed?

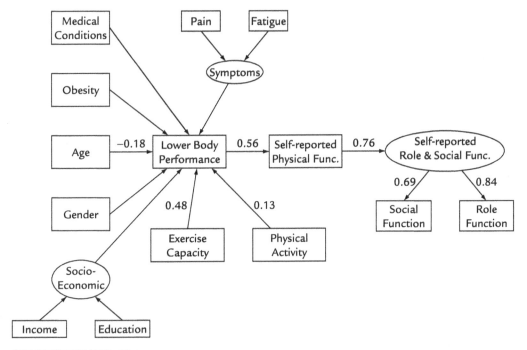

EXERCISE FIGURE 17-1

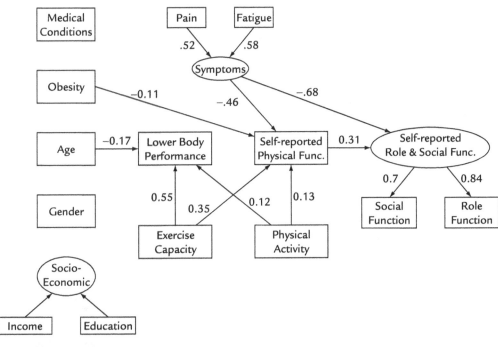

EXERCISE FIGURE 17-2

Writing and Presenting for Publication

Laurel S. Garzon Shepherd
• Stacey B. Plichta

CHAPTER

18

OBJECTIVES

After studying this chapter, you should be able to:

1. Explain the importance of publishing your results.
2. Articulate the structure of academic papers, presentations, and posters.
3. Draft a presentation to share your study results with others.
4. Create a poster to share your study results with others.
5. Discuss the problems and issues with redundant publications.

INTRODUCTION

Research is not useful unless the results are shared with the practice and professional community. It is also important to share your results with the people who participated in your research. This can be accomplished through local grand rounds, talks given at public health departments, and talks given at local community centers, regional conferences, and newsletters. A higher level of dissemination occurs when a paper or poster is presented in peer-reviewed arenas such as state and national conferences. Publishing in a peer-reviewed journal that is indexed in a national index (e.g., CINAHL or MEDLINE) provides the best way to widely disperse the results of a study.

Health care professionals publish research findings for many reasons. The first and most obvious reason is to pass on new findings or to reinforce existing practices through research. This allows health care providers to provide evidence-based care to their patients and enables policymakers to craft good policies based on scientific evidence. Writing for publication not only increases scientific knowledge, but it may also advance a researcher's career as well as improve the reputation of the institution where the research took place (Cetin & Hackam, 2005; McGhee & Gilhotra, 2005; Rosenfeldt, Dowling, Pepe, & Fullerton, 2000; Teijlingen & Hundley, 2002).

Getting your paper into print, however, can be a complicated and stressful task because writing for publication involves much more than reporting research results. You must consider the journal and its requirements for publishing works, the target audience of the journal, and the space allocated in a journal for publishing research. Perhaps most importantly, you must find the right journal for the research conducted. This last consideration can be daunting because the researcher may want to publish in a certain journal, only to be told by the committee reviewing the manuscript that it is not relevant for the journal's readers (Teijlingen & Hundley, 2002). Almost all professional journals publish guidelines so that there is a clear understanding of what is expected in manuscripts that are received for review (Boushey, Harris, Bruemmer, Archer, & Van Horn, 2006; Gilhotra & McGhee, 2006).

ANATOMY OF A SCIENTIFIC PAPER

Scientific journals generally all use the same format, which includes the following: title, abstract, introduction, methods, results, discussion, conclusion, and references (Box 18-1). There may also be supplementary sections such as acknowledgments, figures, and tables (Cetin & Hackam, 2005; Rosenfeldt et al., 2000). The length of a manuscript is generally between 3,000 and 5,000 words, not including references.

Title

The title is the first part of the article that is retrieved electronically, and it may be the basis on which readers decide that the article is applicable to their area of interest. A good title should inform readers as well as pique their interest in the article. It may be appropriate to decide on the title once the article is written, so that the title conveys a clear statement concerning the content. The title should inform readers if the research was conducted on humans or animals or if it was benched based, and it should be neither too long nor too short but should clearly describe the research (McGhee & Gilhotra, 2005).

Abstract

The abstract may also be the only portion of the article that appears in electronic print; therefore, it is crucial that the abstract provides a good first impression of the research. Usually 250 to 350 words in length, the abstract deals primarily with the methods and key results of the work (Kurmis, 2003; McGhee & Gilhotra, 2005). The abstract should be written after the final manuscript has been written, and it should be written to attract readers to the article itself (Kurmis, 2003).

Introduction

The purpose of the introduction is to explain the reason or justification for the study. This section should tell readers what is already known about the subject, what is not known, and what the researcher is trying to find out (hypothesis). A complete literature review of the area of study, including the identification of gaps of knowledge, helps to explain the motivation for the study (Cetin & Hackam, 2005; Kurmis, 2003).

If the author used any specific tools, techniques, or approaches that are not commonly used or are considered experimental, they should be introduced here; however, it is not necessary to provide lengthy explanations because they will be covered in the "Methods" section (Kurmis, 2003). Finally, the introduction should end

BOX 18-1   SECTIONS OF A RESEARCH PAPER

I. Abstract

State the problem, the methods (including number of subjects), and the main conclusions. The abstract is usually limited to 150 to 350 words.

II. Introduction

Provide the context and rationale for the study. State the purpose of the study, provide a review of the literature, point out deficiencies in the current body of research, and state how the study hopes to address one or more of these deficiencies.

III. Methods

Provide the "map" or "recipe" for conducting the study and be sure it is written so that any investigator can repeat the study. This section usually includes the following:

- A description of how the data were collected
- A description of the sample (including the sample size and demographics)
- The response rate
- Methods for assignment into treatment and control groups (if applicable)
- Variable definitions, including recoding and modification of variables
- A discussion of the statistical methods used and any special challenges or adjustments made

IV. Results

Only actual findings are presented. Descriptive statistics about the outcome variables of interest are usually presented first. The results of both bivariate and multivariate analyses are presented in this section. Note that important findings are presented in both tables and the text; less-important or less-interesting findings can be discussed in one or the other. Interpretation of the findings should not appear in the "Results" section.

V. Discussion

Study limitations and strengths appear in this section. The implications of the findings are discussed here. This section usually includes a comparison of findings with those of earlier studies, a discussion of the implications of the findings for clinical practice and health policy, and the need for future research.

---

with a clear statement of the specific problem or hypotheses that will lead to the aim of the research findings (Cetin & Hackam, 2005; Kurmis, 2003).

Methods

This section should include the details of how the research was conducted so that readers can repeat the experiment if they wish. In other words, this section should include details of the study design, the time frame, the description and number of participants involved in the study, and the technical and statistical methods used. This section may also be divided into subsections with key information in each section (Cetin & Hackam, 2005; Gilhotra & McGhee, 2006; Kurmis, 2003).

Reviewers critically evaluate the experimental design presented in the "Methods" section. Thus, it is imperative that researchers provide clear explanations of statistical methods used and analysis of the results to assess the validity of the study (Rosenfeldt et al., 2000).

If a researcher has an outside funding source, it should be acknowledged with a statement in the "Methods" sections if the funding source had any involvement in the design of the study. Studies often receive funding from drug companies, biomedical equipment companies, and other private firms, which may influence a study design and increase the potential for bias (Gilhotra & McGhee, 2006).

Results

The "Results" section should contain only the results of the study, including all data that support or refute the hypothesis. The researcher should not interpret the data in this section, and background findings should not be presented here. Instead, this material should be presented in the introduction or discussion sections (Cetin & Hackam, 2005; Rosenfeldt et al., 2000). Sentences in this section should be concise and easy to understand; the past tense may be used to state the findings. It is also helpful to readers if the results are presented in the same sequence in which the experiment was listed in the "Methods" section (Gilhotra & McGhee, 2006). Gilhotra and McGhee (2006) provide a list of simple rules for authors to follow when presenting results:

- Provide data relevant to the research.
- Present the data in a clear and simple way.
- Show absolute numbers as well as percentages.
- State the statistical analyses applied, not simply p-values.
- Report p-values up to three decimal places.
- Present findings in a logical sequence with the most important findings first.

- Use graphs, tables, figures, or illustrations to present data.
- Do not repeat data in the text that are presented in graphs, tables, or figures.
- Include an analysis of data by variables such as age, gender, or ethnicity, if appropriate.

When reporting p-values, explicitly state the p-value and not just $p < .05$, so that the readers can draw their own conclusions and the significance of the results (Kurmis, 2003). Statistics are a key element of all research, and authors should be careful not to misrepresent statistical data (Gilhotra & McGhee, 2006).

Discussion

The author may begin the "Discussion" section with a brief review of the original research results and the important aspects of the study. This allows the author to make a statement describing the significance of his or her work (Cetin & Hackam, 2005; Gilhotra & McGhee, 2006). Cetin and Hackam (2005) state, "Subsequent paragraphs are devoted to expanding on themes that the authors feel are important for the reader to understand the significance of the work." In the "Discussion" section, it is appropriate to use the present tense and active voice.

Key results should be discussed in order of their importance. These ideas are usually stated in the "Introduction" section so that readers are not introduced to them for the first time in the "Discussion" section. Authors should compare and contrast findings with comparable studies and discuss how their findings add to, support, or change the current body of scientific knowledge (Gilhotra & McGhee, 2006; Kurmis, 2003; Rosenfeldt et al., 2000).

The limitations of a study should also be discussed in this section. Doing so shows that the authors have remained unbiased (Kurmis, 2003). Furthermore, by citing the limitations, the authors can avoid seeing the limitations pointed out in letters to the editor after the manuscript has been published (Gilhotra & McGhee, 2006).

Conclusions

A "Conclusions" section may be included within the "Discussion" section, or it may be presented separately. This section should be brief (no more than a couple of paragraphs), and it should not reiterate the discussion (Gilhotra & McGhee, 2006; Kurmis, 2003). It is important not to state any conclusions that are not supported by the results in the study. No new information should be introduced at this point. Authors may make recommendations for interpretation or application of the findings in the "Conclusions" section (Kurmis, 2003).

References

The "References" section should list all works referenced in the manuscript. How the references are cited in the manuscript depends on the journal to which the paper is submitted. All journals have their own style for reference citations. The author can find details for the presentation of citations in the "Instruction to Authors" section found in each journal (Kurmis, 2003). Authors should carefully cite all references; original resources should be used whenever possible (Gilhotra & McGhee, 2005).

ANATOMY OF CONFERENCE PRESENTATONS AND POSTERS

In addition to published papers, many researchers present their work at peer-reviewed conferences, such as the annual meeting of the American Public Health Association. These presentations are an excellent way for new researchers to learn how to communicate their findings. The presentations are typically in the form of either a poster or a talk (with PowerPoint slides). While these presentations have the same format as peer-reviewed journal articles (title, abstract; introduction, methods, results, discussion, conclusion, and references), they are much shorter. For both posters and presentations, you should focus on a single key result in a short talk or poster, rather than trying to cover the entire scope of the research.

Posters

Poster presentations are a great way for new researchers to present their work to professional colleagues. Most national and state-level health-related professional conferences have poster sections, and local organizations may sponsor these as well. Many schools also hold a "poster day" to highlight the research of their students. In a typical poster session, presenters will stand by their boards for an hour or two while people come by to view the poster and talk about the results. These sessions allow the researchers to have more personal interactions with the audience than do a talk or paper and can reach people who might not be in their specific field of research.

The most important thing to remember about a poster is that it is a visual representation of your work. It should be easy to read and pleasing to the eye. An excellent (and amusing) overview of how to construct a poster is provided by Colin Purrington (2011) on his Web site. Additional information can also be found in an older but still quite relevant article by Block (1996).

In general, the first thing you will need to know is the size of the poster. Most conferences will provide you with guidelines. It is important to adhere to these, because if you arrive with a poster that is too large, it may not fit on the board that was assigned to you. Today, almost all posters are printed using a professional large-format printer—many schools have in-house capacity and there are also a number of low-cost vendors that you can find online to use. Most vendors will provide you with a "template" to complete; many of these employ PowerPoint

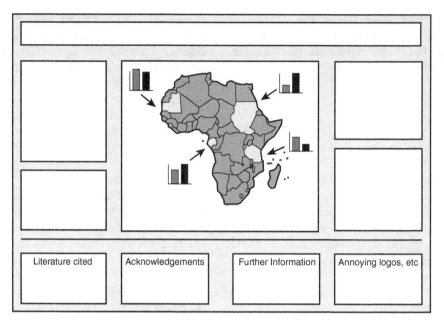

Literature cited | Acknowledgements | Further Information | Annoying logos, etc

FIGURE 18-1 An example of a poster layout. Adapted from Purrington, C. B. (2011). *Advice on designing scientific posters.* Retrieved March 2011 from http://www.swarthmore.edu/NatSci/cpurrin1/posteradvice.htm

software. Figure 18-1 shows a "typical" poster layout. As noted by Purrington (2011), "unless you possess artistic ability, you should not attempt to build a poster by cutting and pasting content onto panels of colored matte board, the default method for the most of the last century."

The key to making a great poster is to make it readable. Table 18-1 presents some general tips on creating posters that are adapted from Purrington's Web site with his permission (note his Web site has great visuals and is much more amusing to read than our abstraction of his comments). Your poster should contain the following sections:

- *Title:* Should convey the issue succinctly. Maximum length of one line.
- *Abstract:* Do not include an abstract on a poster! Your poster is essentially an expanded abstract.
- *Introduction:* This should be short and to the point. State your main hypothesis.

- *Methods:* Briefly describe your methods, but not with the detail used for a manuscript: use figures, flowcharts, and tables where possible.
- *Results:* First, state your main finding and descriptive results. In the second paragraph, present the data analysis that specifically addresses the hypothesis. Make use of tables, charts, and figures here. Provide figure legends that are self-explanatory.
- *Conclusions:* State whether your hypothesis was supported. Discuss why your results are conclusive and interesting. Note the relevance to policy, practice, and future research.
- *Literature cited* Follow standard format (e.g., American Psychological Association). Maximum length: approximately 10 citations. This can be in one of the smaller fonts in a less-central part of the poster.

Table 18-1	**TIPS FOR MAKING GOOD POSTERS**

- Keep your poster to about 800 words. The number one mistake is to make your poster too long.
- Use a large font throughout (at least 20 point) and organize the text so that the reader can easily read all the information in 4–5 min from a distance of 6–8 feet or so.
- Use a nonserif font (e.g., Helvetica) for title and headings and a serif font (e.g., Palatino) for body text (serif-style fonts are much easier to read at smaller font sizes).
- Do not "bullet" or otherwise punctuate section headers. The use of a larger font size for headers, coupled with a simple "bolded" format, is sufficient for demarcating sections.
- The width of text boxes should be approximately 40 characters (on average: 11 words per line). Lines that are shorter or longer are harder to read quickly.
- Avoid blocks of text longer than 10 sentences.
- Whenever possible, use lists of sentences rather than blocks of text.
- Use italics instead of underlining.

Source: Adapted from Purrington, C. B. (2011). *Advice on designing scientific posters*. Retrieved March 2011 from http://www.swarthmore.edu/NatSci/cpurrin1/posteradvice.htm

- *Acknowledgments:* Thank individuals for specific contributions to the project and include in this section explicit disclosures of any conflicts of interest and conflicts of commitment.
- *Further information:* Use this section to provide your e-mail address, your Web site address, and perhaps a URL where they can download a PDF version of the poster.

Presentations

Professional presentations are usually given at the annual conferences of professional organizations such as the American Public Health Association. These are typically talks of about 15 minutes or so, given as part of a larger panel on a single topic. Keep in mind that a talk has both a visual component (usually PowerPoint slides) and an oral (talking) component. In order to keep the interest of your audience, you will need to provide both interesting visuals and keep your voice energetic and enthusiastic. You should plan on about 20 to 28 slides for a 15-minute talk. Table 18-2 provides some general tips for creating slideshows that are visually appealing. An excellent guide to producing an academic presentation is de Szendeffy's (2005) book *A Practical Guide to Using Computers in Language Teaching*.

In general, academic presentations all follow the same format, as outlined below.

- *Title:* Should convey the issue succinctly. You should also put your coauthors and your institutional affiliations on this slide. If your acknowledgments are not too lengthy, you can also put them on this slide (one slide).

Table 18-2	**TIPS FOR MAKING GOOD SLIDESHOWS**

- Keep your slideshow to about 22–30 slides for a 15-min talk.
- Use a large font throughout (at least 20 point for footnotes, 30 point for main text, and 44 point for titles). Make sure that the slide is readable from the back of a large room.
- Use a consistent background (Master slide) and font—changes can be distracting to the reader.
- Keep slides simple. Busy slides are hard to read.
- Do not read your slides. Highlight facts in the slides and then speak using the slides as a visual aid.
- Use visual aids (e.g., pictures, charts, graphics) where appropriate.

- *Abstract:* Do not include an abstract in a presentation. It is appropriate to have a one-page synopsis of your work to hand out to interested listeners.
- *Introduction:* State the research problem you are addressing first. Then, in a few slides, give a brief review of the literature (three to four slides).
- *Methods:* Briefly describe your methods, but not with the detail used for a manuscript: use figures, flowcharts, and tables where possible. Keep the slides uncluttered. You can talk your audience through your methods (five to six slides).
- *Results:* In the first slide, state your main finding. In subsequent slides, you can show tables (not too busy) and graphs. You can explain each of these to your audience as you go through your presentation (five to eight slides).
- *Conclusions:* In the first slide, state whether your hypothesis was supported. Discuss why your results are conclusive and interesting. Note the relevance to policy, practice, and future research (five to eight slides).
- *Acknowledgments:* Thank individuals for specific contributions to the project and include in this section explicit disclosures of any conflicts of interest and conflicts of commitment (if not done on the first slide).
- *Closing slide:* End with this slide. Provide your e-mail address, your Web site address, and other contact information.
- *Literature cited:* This should be last. You would not present this slide, but it might be useful to later viewers to have a slide with the references on it.

WHAT AUTHORS NEED TO KNOW ABOUT REDUNDANT PUBLICATION

How does redundant or duplicate publication occur? Redundant publications occur when authors publish an article that is very similar to one that they have already published, either electronically or in print. Also referred to as "self-plagiarism," this can be a violation of publishing ethics and copyright laws (Hegyvary, 2005). To avoid duplicate publication, authors should become aware of what it is, how to avoid it, what happens when it occurs, and what penalties there may be for the author.

The International Committee of Medical Journal Editors has published guidelines regarding duplicate or redundant publications, and all authors should visit the ICMJE's Web site if they are considering publishing in more than one journal and read the section titled "Redundant Publication" (Hegyvary, 2005; International Committee of Medical Journal Editors, 2005).

Duplicate publishing can present many problems. As previously stated, it can be a violation of copyright laws, and it may cause other authors to double count the results of a study if they are using it in a meta-analysis or literature review (DeAngelis, 2004). Duplicate publishing also consumes an editor's time investigating the possibility of duplicate publishing. If the duplicate article is in print, then it may prevent or delay the publication of other articles (Hegyvary, 2005). If duplication is caught before publication, then the manuscript is rejected. If it is not caught until after publication, then notices are published in both journals, the author's employer is notified, and indexes such as PubMed are notified. The author of the duplication may also be asked to provide a written statement to accompany the notice of duplicate publication. In some cases, the redundant article may be retracted after publication (Hegyvary, 2005).

Hegyvary (2005) notes that authors can take certain steps to avoid redundant or duplicate publication:

- Cite all related papers, including those submitted but not yet accepted.
- Be clear in submitting a manuscript what new information it contains.

- Understand what conditions all authors listed on a manuscript endorse in giving permission to publish a manuscript.
- Give preference to publishing a potentially "classic" and comprehensive article instead of dissecting results into minimally publishable pieces.
- Challenge criteria for promotion that indicate greater emphasis on quantity than quality of publications.

SUMMARY

Research is not useful unless the results are shared with the practice and professional community, and, when possible, the study participants. Research results can be shared via talks at local venues, posters presented at school events and professional conferences, and publication in both lay and peer-reviewed venues. Each of these forums requires a different approach in order to communicate clearly to your audience.

CHAPTER REVIEW

Critical Thinking Concept Review

1. Choose three peer-reviewed research articles and write a short review of each of them that includes the following:
   a. Write the problem statement.
   b. Name the theoretical model used or briefly describe the overall conceptual model.
   c. Write out the main research questions. What is the rationale for the question?
   d. List the main hypotheses that the study seems to be testing.
   e. Define the dependent variable and the main independent variables.
   f. Briefly describe the research design.
   g. Describe the sample (e.g., size, sociodemographic characteristics) and how it was obtained.
   h. List the statistics used to test the hypotheses.
   i. Identify the main assumptions and limitations.

a: Intercept constant. The point at which the regression line intercepts the Y-axis.

Absolute value: The positive numeric value of a number (the minus sign in front of the number is disregarded).

Abstract: A short description of a completed research project. Typically, it is between 150 and 300 words and contains information on the purpose, methods, results, and conclusions of the study.

Adjusted group mean: Group mean scores that have been adjusted for the effect of the covariate on the dependent variable.

Adjusted R^2: R^2 adjusted for the number of subjects and variables.

Alpha: The probability of making a type I error.

Alpha level (α-level): The *p*-value defined by the researcher as being statistically significant. It is the chance that the researcher is willing to take of committing a type I error. The most commonly used α-levels are .05, .01, and .10.

Alternative hypothesis (H$_a$): The hypothesis that states a statistically significant relationship exists between the variables. It is the hypothesis opposite to the null hypothesis. It is also referred to as the "acting" hypothesis or the research hypothesis.

Analysis of covariance (ANCOVA): A combination of regression and analysis of variance techniques that allows comparison of group means after adjustment for the effect of the covariate.

Analysis of variance (ANOVA): A parametric statistical technique used to compare the means of three or more groups as defined by one or more factors.

A priori contrasts: Planned comparisons based on orthogonal hypotheses.

b: Regression coefficient. In linear regression, it is the rate of change in Y with a one-unit change in X, and it is used to calculate predicted scores. In logistic regression, it is used to calculate probabilities.

Bar graph: A graph used for nominal or ordinal data. A space separates the bars.

Bartlett's test: A chi-square statistic used to test the significance of lambda.

Baseline: Measures taken at the start of a study before any interventions; sometimes referred to as the pretest.

Bell shaped: A graphical shape, typical of the normal distribution.

Beta coefficients: In a regression equation, the weight associated with standardized scores on the variables; a partial correlation coefficient.

Beta (β-level): The probability of making a type II error.

Between-group variance: A measure of the deviation of group means from the grand mean.

Biserial correlation: A technique used when one variable is dichotomized and the other is continuous to estimate what the correlation between the two variables would be if the dichotomized variable were continuous.

Blinding: Keeping subjects and observers unaware of treatment assignments.

Bonferroni *t* test: A *post hoc* test used in ANOVA to help determine which of the means are significantly different from each other after an ANOVA has been found to be statistically significant. It is a type of *t* test that adjusts the α-level for multiple comparisons that are being made.

Box plots: A graphic display that uses descriptive statistics based on percentiles.

Box's M/Box's test of equality of covariance matrices: A test of the assumption that the variance–covariance matrices are equal across all levels of the between-subjects factor in a repeated-measures analysis of variance.

Canonical coefficient: Equivalent to a *b*-weight in regression; can be used to calculate predicted scores based on actual scores.

Canonical correlation: A measure of the relationship between a set of independent variables and a set of dependent variables.

Canonical variate: A weighted composite of the variables in a set.

Canonical weights: Standard score weights generated in a canonical correlation; like betas in regression; used more for explanation than prediction.

Causal relationship: A relationship in which one or more variables are presumed to cause changes in another variable.

Central limit theorem: When many samples are drawn from a population, the means of these samples tend to be normally distributed.

Centroid: The mean of the discriminant scores for a given group.

Chi-square: A nonparametric test used to assess whether a statistically significant association exists between the rows and columns in a cross-tabulation (contingency) table. The chi-square test statistic is used to compare the proportion of participants having a given characteristic among different groups.

Coefficient of determination: The correlation coefficient squared (r^2); a measure of the variance shared by the two variables; a measure of the "meaningfulness" of the relationship.

Coefficient of variation: Measures the spread of a set of data as a proportion of its mean; usually expressed as a percentage.

Common factor analysis: Based on the assumption that there is systematic and random error in measurement. Analysis is based on common variance only.

Communality: The portion of item variance accounted for by the factors.

Compound symmetry: An assumption made when conducting a repeated-measures ANOVA. It means that the correlations and variances across the measurements are equivalent.

Conditional probability: The likelihood that an event will occur given the knowledge that another event has already occurred.

Confidence interval: A range within which the population parameter is estimated to fall based on the statistic and the standard error.

Confirmatory factor analysis (CFA): A special application of structural equation modeling and a theory-driven method for testing an instrument's factor structure.

Contingency coefficient: A nonparametric technique to measure the relationship between two nominal-level variables.

Continuity correction (Yates correction): Used in chi-square analysis when the expected frequency in cells in 2 × 2 tables is less than 5.

Continuous variable: A variable that can take on any possible value within a range. For example, weight is a continuous variable because a weight of 152.5 lb makes sense. In contrast, number of children is a discrete variable because it can take on only certain values (0, 1, 2, and so on). A value of 1.2 for children does not make any conceptual sense.

Control group: The group that is used for comparison in an experimental or quasi-experimental study.

Correlated t test (paired t test): A parametric test to compare two pairs of scores.

Correlation coefficient: A measure of the extent to which the variation in one variable is related to the variation in another variable. Values range from −1 to +1.

Correlation matrix: A square symmetric matrix containing correlations between pairs of variables.

Covariate: A continuous variable used to adjust the mean scores of groups; a method for control of extraneous variation.

Cramer's V: Modified phi, used to assess the relationship between categorical variables; used with tables larger than 2 × 2.

Critical value: The value or values that determine the rejection region or threshold for a specific computed statistic to be defined as statistically significant (eg, that will result in the researcher's rejecting the null hypothesis). The critical value of each statistic is based on the distribution of that particular statistic. Depending on the particular statistical test, the computed value must either exceed or be less than the critical value for the test to be defined as statistically significant.

Cronbach's alpha: A measure of internal consistency reliability.

Cross-tabulation: A way of presenting the relationship between two variables in a table format; the rows and columns of the table are labeled with the values of the variables.

Cross-validation: Checking the validity of R^2 by calculating it in a second sample.

Data set: Collection of different values of all the variables used to measure the characteristics of the sample or population.

Degrees of freedom: The freedom of a variable's values to vary given what is already known about the other values and the sum of the values.

Dependent variable: The variable that measures the effect of some other variable (eg, the variable whose values are expected to be predicted by the independent variable). Also referred to as the outcome variable or the response variable.

Descriptive statistics: Statistics used to summarize and describe data.

Deviance: In logistic regression, the comparison between the predicted probability of being in the correct group based on the model to the perfect prediction. Large values indicate poor model fit.

Deviation coding (effect coding): A method of coding nominal-level variables using 1s, –1s, and 0s; reflects the comparison of each group mean with the grand mean.

Dichotomous variable: A nominal variable having only two categories.

Directional hypothesis: States a relationship between the variables being studied or a difference between experimental treatments that the researcher expects to emerge.

Discriminant function: The mathematical function that combines information from predictor variables to obtain the maximum discrimination among groups.

Discriminant function analysis: A statistical technique that provides a prediction of group membership based on predictor variables.

Dummy coding (indicator coding): A method of coding nominal-level variables using 1s and 0s; reflects a comparison of the control group mean with other group means.

Effect coding (deviation coding): A method of coding nominal-level variables using 1s, –1s, and 0s; reflects the comparison of each group mean with the grand mean.

Effect size: The impact made by the independent variable on the dependent variable.

Efficiency: The degree to which the test result and the diagnosis agree, that is, the overall accuracy of a test in measuring true findings; expressed as a percentage.

Eigenvalue: The amount of variance explained by a factor or discriminant function.

Empirical study: Study based on observation or experience.

Endogenous variables: Variables influenced by other variables in a model.

Epsilon: A correction used in repeated-measures analysis of variance when the assumption of compound symmetry has not been met. Epsilon is multiplied by the degrees of freedom for the within-subjects factor(s), making them smaller, and thus making the test more conservative.

Equamax rotation: Combines the characteristics of Quartimax and Varimax rotation.

Estimation: The procedure for testing a model whereby a sample of observed data is used to make estimations of population parameters.

Eta: Sometimes called the correlation ratio. It can be used to measure a nonlinear relationship. The range of values is from 0 to 1.

Exogenous variables: Variables that are not influenced by other variables in a model.

Exp(*B*): The exponent of *b* or the odds ratio.

Experiment: A research study with the following characteristics: an intervention that the investigator controls and that only some groups receive, random selection of participants into the study, and random assignment of participants to intervention and control groups.

External validity: The extent to which the results of a study can be generalized to other populations or settings than the sample that was studied.

Extraneous variable: A variable that confounds the relationship between the dependent variable and the independent variable.

F: A measure of the ratio of between to within variance produced by analysis of variance.

Factor(s): In an ANOVA model, the variable(s) that defines the groups whose means are being compared.

Factor analysis: A statistical tool for analyzing scores on large numbers of variables to determine whether any identifiable dimensions can be used to describe many of the variables under study. Intercorrelations are treated mathematically in such a way that underlying traits are identified.

Factor loadings: Correlations of variables with a factor.

Factor matrix: Each row represents one variable; each column represents a factor.

Factor pattern matrix: A matrix produced by oblique rotation in factor analysis. It contains regression weights. It is generally preferable to the structure matrix for interpretation.

Factor scores: Actual scores weighted by factor loadings.

Factor structure matrix: A matrix produced by oblique rotation in factor analysis. It contains correlation coefficients.

Fisher's exact test: An alternative to chi-square for 2 × 2 tables when sample size and expected frequencies are small.

Fisher's Z: Transformation of correlation coefficients into Fisher's Z to create a normal distribution.

Frequency distribution: A systematic array of data together with a count of the raw frequency that each value occurs, the relative frequency with which it occurs, and the cumulative frequency with which it occurs.

Friedman's ANOVA by rank: A nonparametric analogue to the repeated-measures ANOVA. It is often used to compare rankings and preferences.

Friedman matched samples: A nonparametric analogue of repeated-measures analysis of variance.

F-statistic: A statistic computed by measuring the ratio of two variances to each other.

Generalizability: The extent to which the research findings can be applied to situations beyond those of the immediate group that was studied. The extent to which the findings can be used to make inferences about the population that the sample came from.

Goodness-of-fit statistic: A measure of how well the data fit the model; compares the observed probabilities to those predicted by the model.

Graphs: The visual representations of frequency distributions.

Greenhouse-Geisser: A conservative epsilon value used to alter the degrees of freedom for the within-subjects factor(s) in repeated-measures analysis of variance when the assumption of compound symmetry has not been met.

Heteroscedasticity: Refers to situations in which the variability of the dependent variable is not equivalent across the values of the independent variable.

Hierarchical regression: The researcher determines the order of entry of the variables into the equation. Variables may be entered one at a time or in subsets.

Histogram: A way of graphically displaying ordinal-, interval-, and ratio-level data. It shows the shape of the distribution.

Homogeneity of regression: The direction and strength of the relationship between the covariate and the dependent variable must be similar in each group.

Homogeneity of variance: When there are no significant differences in the variance of the values of the dependent variable within two or more groups that are being compared with each other. It is also called homoscedasticity.

Hotelling-Lawley trace: The sum of the ratio of the between and within sum of squares for each of the discriminant variables.

Huynh-Feldt: A value for the epsilon correction factor in repeated-measures analysis of variance that is less conservative than Greenhouse-Geisser.

Hypothesis: Formal statement of the expected relationships between variables or differences between groups.

Identification: A necessary condition for conducting confirmatory factor analysis and structural equation modeling, where the amount of information or known values in the data exceed the information being estimated or unknown values.

Improvement: In logistic regression, the change in −2LL between successive steps of building a model.

Imputation: Estimation of missing values in a data set based on prior knowledge, mean or median substitution, or regression techniques.

Independent random sample: A sample in which the value of the variables for each subject is not related to the value of the variables for the other subjects and in which each and every subject has an equal chance of being selected to be in the study.

Independent samples: Groups or samples in which the measurements of the members of one sample have no preexisting relationship to the measurements of members of the other sample(s).

Independent *t* test: A parametric test used to determine whether the means of two independent groups are significantly different from each other.

Independent variable: The variable that is seen as having an effect on the dependent variable. In experimental designs, the treatment is manipulated.

Indicator: A measured variable in structural equation models; may also be called a manifest variable.

Indicator coding (dummy coding): A method of coding nominal-level variables using 1s and 0s. Reflects a comparison of the control group mean with other group means.

Inference: A conclusion about a population drawn from results based on a sample of data from that population.

Institutional review board (IRB): An established body of individuals that convenes to review proposed and ongoing studies to protect the welfare of human subjects recruited to participate in biomedical or behavioral research. IRBs are typically located on college campuses, at medical facilities, and in governmental institutions.

Intercept constant (a): The point at which the regression line intercepts the *Y*-axis.

Internal validity: The extent to which the findings of a study truly and accurately represent the relationship between the independent variable(s) and the dependent variable.

Interquartile range: The range of values extending from the 25th to the 50th percentile.

Interval-level measurement: A rank-order scale with equal intervals between units but no true zero. IQ scores, SAT scores, and GRE scores are all examples of interval-level data.

Just identified model: All variables in the model are interconnected with each other by a path.

Kendall's tau: A nonparametric measure of relationship between two ordinal variables.

Kruskal-Wallis *H*-test: A nonparametric alternative to ANOVA. It is used to determine the difference in the medians between three or more groups.

Kurtosis: A measure of whether the curve is normal, flat, or peaked.

Lambda: Wilks' lambda varies from 0 to 1 and represents the error variance. $1 - \text{lambda} = R^2$.

Latency effect: Interaction between treatments in repeated-measures designs.

Latent variable: A theoretical construct in structural equation models that is not directly measured but represented by measured variables.

Least significant difference test: A *post hoc* test that is a modified version of multiple *t* tests.

Levene's test: A test for homogeneity of variance that tests the null hypothesis that the variances of two or more distributions are equal. It is less sensitive to departures from normality than are other tests of this type.

Likelihood: The probability of the observed results given the parameter estimates.

Likert scale: A measurement scale that asks respondents to register the level to which they agree or disagree with a set of statements. There are typically five to seven response categories that range from strongly disagree to strongly agree. Other descriptors, such as level of satisfaction, may be used instead of level of agreement.

Line chart: The preferred type of chart to show many changes over time for many periods of time, or to place emphasis on a particular factor.

Listwise deletion: Cases (subjects) are dropped from analysis if they have any missing data.

Logistic regression: A technique designed to determine which variables affect the probability of an event.

Lower-bound epsilon: The most conservative approach to "correcting" the degrees of freedom in repeated-measures analysis of variance when the assumption of compound symmetry has not been met.

Mann-Whitney *U*-test: The nonparametric analogue of the independent *t* test. It is used to determine the statistical significance of the difference in the medians of two independent groups.

Matched-pairs design: Test design in which study participants are matched based on characteristics that might influence their treatment reactions.

Mauchly's test of sphericity: A test of the assumption of compound symmetry in repeated-measures analysis of variance.

Maximum likelihood (ML) method: A method of estimation used in CFA and structural equation modeling.

McNemar: A nonparametric measure of difference between two paired dichotomous measures; used to measure change.

Mean: A measure of central tendency. It is the arithmetic average of a set of data.

Meaningfulness: The clinical or substantive meaning of the results of statistical analysis.

Mean replacement: Substitution of the mean of the distribution for missing values on a specific variable.

Measurement: The assignment of numerals to objects or events, according to a set of rules (Stevens, 1946).

Median: The middle value or subject in a set of ordered numbers.

Median replacement: Substitution of the median of the distribution for missing values on a specific variable. Often used if the variable distribution is skewed.

Missing values: Values that are missing from a variable for some participants. These values may be missing because the participant refused to answer certain questions or because certain questions do not apply to the participant (eg, the question, "Are you pregnant?" would be missing for male study participants).

Mixed design: A study that includes between- and within-group factors.

Mode: The most frequently occurring number or category.

Model chi-square: In logistic regression, the difference between –2 log likelihood (–2LL) for the model with only a constant and –2LL for the complete model; tests the null hypothesis that the coefficients for all the independent variables equal zero.

Model modification: Respecifying an initially hypothesized model in confirmatory factor analysis and structural equation modeling to test the newly proposed model for improved data–model fit.

Multicollinearity: Interrelatedness of independent variables.

Multiple correlation: The relationship between one dependent variable and a weighted composite of independent variables.

Multiple group comparisons: The two most common are a priori (before the fact) and *post hoc* (after the fact) comparisons of group means.

Multivariate analysis of variance: An analysis of variance with more than one dependent variable.

Mutually exclusive and exhaustive categories: Each participant (eg, item, event) can fit into one and only one category, and each participant (eg, item, event) fits into a category.

N: The total number of participants in a study across all groups.

n: The number of participants in specific subgroups.

Negatively skewed distribution: Asymmetric distribution that has a disproportionate number of cases with high values and a tail that points to the left. Also called a left-skewed distribution.

Negative predictive value: The proportion of people who do not have the disease who tested negative for the disease, that is, "true negatives"; expressed as a percentage.

Negative relationship: As the value of one variable increases, the value of the other decreases. Also called an inverse relationship.

Nominal: The lowest level of measurement; consists of organizing data into discrete units.

Nominal measure: A measurement scale in which the numbers have no intrinsic meaning but are merely used to label different categories. Ethnic identity, religion, and health insurance status (eg, none, Medicaid, Medicare, private) are all examples of nominal-level data.

Nondirectional hypothesis: A specific statement that a difference exists between groups or a relationship exists between variables, with no specification of the direction of the difference or relationship.

Nonparametric tests: Statistical tests designed to be used when the data fail to meet one or more of the assumptions required of parametric tests. These tests are "distribution free" but usually have less power than parametric tests.

Nonrecursive model: A model in which causal flow is not unidirectional.

Normal curve: A theoretically perfect frequency polygon in which the mean, median, and mode all coincide in the center, and which takes the form of a symmetrical bell-shaped curve.

Normal distribution: A theoretical probability distribution in which the horizontal axis represents all possible values of a variable and the vertical axis represents the probability that these values will occur. Normal distributions are unimodal (mean, median, and mode are the same), symmetrical about the mean, and have a shape commonly described as a bell-shaped curve.

Null hypothesis: The hypothesis that states that two or more variables being compared will not be related to each other (ie, no significant relationship between the variables will be found).

Oblique rotation: The resulting factors are correlated with each other.

Observed variables: The indicators for the latent variable or the items on a research instrument.

Odds ratio: The probability of occurrence over the probability of nonoccurrence.

One-tailed test of significance: A test used with a directional hypothesis that proposes extreme values are in one tail of the distribution.

One-way analysis of variance: Analysis of variance with one factor (independent variable).

Ordinal scale: A measurement scale that ranks participants on some variable. The interval between the ranks does not necessarily have to be equal. Examples of ordinal variables are scale items that measure any subjective state (eg, happiness: very happy, somewhat happy, somewhat unhappy, very unhappy; attitude: strongly agree, somewhat agree, somewhat disagree, strongly disagree; and military rank: general, colonel, sergeant, private).

Orthogonal: Independent of each other.

Orthogonal coding: A method of coding orthogonal contrasts between groups. A priori contrasts can be tested through this method of coding.

Orthogonal rotation (Varimax): The resulting factors are not correlated with each other.

Outliers: Extreme values of a variable that are at the tail end of the distribution of the data. Sometimes outliers are defined as being greater than ±3.0 standard deviations from the mean.

Overidentified model: A model that contains at least one less path than a just identified model.

Paired *t* test: A parametric test to compare two pairs of scores.

Pairwise deletion: In correlational analyses, cases (subjects) are excluded when they are missing one of the two variables being correlated.

Parameters: Characteristics of the population.

Parametric tests: Statistical tests based on assumptions that the sample is representative of the population and that the scores are normally distributed.

Partial correlation: A measure of the relationship between two variables after statistically controlling for the influence of some other variable(s) on both of the variables being correlated.

Path analysis: A causal model analytic technique using least squares regression.

Path coefficients: The magnitude of the influence of one variable on another in the path model.

Path model: A causal model.

Pearson correlation coefficient: A parametric test used to determine if a linear association exists between two measures of interval or ratio measurement scale. The variables need to be normally distributed.

Percentile: Describes the relative position of a score.

Phi: A shortcut method of calculating Pearson correlation coefficient when both variables are dichotomous.

Pie chart: A circle that is partitioned into percentage distributions of qualitative variables.

Pillai-Bartlett trace: Represents the sum of the explained variances.

Point-Biserial coefficient: A shortcut method of calculating *r* when there is one dichotomous and one continuous variable.

Point estimate: A single number that serves as the estimate of the population parameter.

Polygon: A graph for interval- or ratio-level variables that is the equivalent of the histogram but appears smoother. It is constructed by joining the midpoints of the top of each bar.

Population: The entire group having some characteristic (eg, all people with depression, all residents of the United States). Often a sample is taken of the population and then the results are generalized to that population.

Positive predictive value: The proportion of people with the disease who tested positive for the disease, that is, "true positives"; expressed as a percentage.

Positive relationship: Also called a "direct" relationship. The values of *x* and *y* increase or decrease together. As *x* increases, *y* also increases.

Positively skewed distribution: An asymmetric distribution with a disproportionate number of cases with a low value. The tail of this distribution points to the right. Also known as a right-skewed distribution.

***Post hoc* tests:** Tests of paired comparisons made when an overall test, such as an ANOVA, is statistically significant. *Post hoc* tests are used to control for the problems caused by multiple comparisons. Many *post hoc* tests, including the Scheffe test, Tukey's honestly significant difference test, and Bonferroni *post hoc* test, are available.

Power: The probability that the null hypothesis will be correctly accepted by the test. It is denoted by β.

Principal components analysis: A type of analysis that is based on the assumption that all measurement error is random and includes 1s in the diagonal of the correlation matrix that is analyzed.

Probability: A quantitative description of the likely occurrence of a particular event, conventionally expressed on a scale from 0 to 1.

Probability value (*p*-value): In a statistical hypothesis test, the likelihood of getting the value of the statistic by chance alone.

p-value: The actual probability of getting the obtained results or results even more extreme. The smaller the *p*-value, the more statistically significant (ie, the less likely the result is due to chance).

Quartile: The four "quarters" of the data distribution. The first quartile is the 25th percentile, the second quartile is the 50th percentile, the third quartile is the 75th percentile, and the fourth quartile is the 100th percentile.

Quartimax rotation: A method of rotation in factor analysis that tends to produce a first, very general, factor with high loadings.

R: Multiple correlation.

R^2: Squared multiple correlation; the amount of variance accounted for in the dependent variable by a combination of independent variables.

Randomization: Assignment of individuals to groups by chance (ie, every subject has an equal chance of being assigned to a particular group).

Range: The difference between the maximum and minimum values in a distribution.

Ratio-level measurement: The highest level of measurement. In addition to equal intervals between data points, there is an absolute zero.

Ratio scale: A measurement scale in which there are both equal intervals between units and a true zero. Most biologic measures (eg, weight, pulse rate) are ratio-level variables.

Raw data matrix: A matrix containing raw scores for each subject on each variable. The rows represent subjects, and the columns represent variables.

Receiver operator characteristic (ROC) curve: Graphic representation of the trade-off between false-positive and false-negative rates for every possible cutoff value. The graph plots the false-positive rate on the *x*-axis and the true-positive rate (1 − the false-negative rate) on the *y*-axis. The area under the curve is of primary interest as it measures the correlation between the category predicted by the test and the true category into which the case falls.

Recursive model: The flow of causation in the model is unidirectional.

Redundancy: In canonical correlation, the percentage of variance the canonical variates from the independent variables extract from the dependent variables and vice versa.

Reflect a variable: A form of recording a variable so that scores are reversed, that is, the highest score becomes the lowest, and so forth.

Regression: A statistical method that makes use of the correlation between two variables and the notion of a straight line to develop a prediction equation.

Regression coefficient (*b*): The rate of change in *Y* with a one-unit change in *X*.

Regression line: The line of best fit formed by the mathematical technique called the method of least squares.

Regression sum of squares: The variance that is accounted for by the variables in the equation.

Rejection region: The region of a statistical distribution not under the null hypothesis. The null hypothesis is rejected if the computed value of the sample statistic falls into the rejection region. These regions are typically located at the extreme tail(s) of a sampling distribution.

Relative risk: The risk given one condition versus the risk given another condition.

Reliability: The degree of consistency with which an instrument measures what it purports to measure. Reliability can be broken down into test–retest reliability, interrater reliability, and internal consistency.

Repeated-measures analysis of variance: A method of analyzing within-cell designs in which subjects are measured more than once on the same variable or where subjects are exposed to all treatments, thus serving as their own controls.

Research problems: Questions that can be answered by collecting facts.

Residual: The difference between the actual and predicted scores; the variance that is not shared by the variables in the correlation; the unexplained or error variance.

Risk: The number of occurrences out of the total.

Roy's greatest characteristic root: An outcome statistic generated by multivariate analysis of variance and based on the first discriminate variate.

R statistic: In logistic regression, the partial correlation.

Sample: A group selected from the population in the hope that the smaller group will be representative of the entire population.

Sample size: Number of subjects included in the study.

Scatter diagram: A diagram that graphically represents the relationship of two ordinal-, interval-, or ratio-level variables to each other. The diagram is typically presented with correlation coefficients.

Scheffé test: A conservative *post hoc* test; may be used with groups of equal or unequal size.

Scree test: A plot of eigenvalues.

Semipartial correlation: The correlation between two variables with the effect of another variable(s) removed from one of the variables being correlated.

Sensitivity: The proportion of people with disease who have a positive test result.

Shrinkage formula: An equation that provides an estimate of how much the multiple correlation coefficient is likely to shrink.

Significance level: Specifies the risk of rejecting the null hypothesis when it is true.

Significance test: A statistical calculation that assigns a probability to a statistical estimate; a small probability implies a significant result.

Simple structure: A criterion for factor rotation that seeks to maximize high and low loadings to reduce ambiguity.

Skewness: A measure of the shape of an asymmetrical distribution.

Spearman rho: A shortcut formula for *r* when there are two sets of ranks.

Specification: The process of specifying or delineating the structural relationships among the component parts of a model.

Specificity: The proportion of people without the disease who have a negative test result.

Standard deviation: A measure of dispersion of scores around the mean. It is the square root of the variance.

Standardized canonical correlations: Similar to beta weights in regression. They are based on the standard scores of the variables and indicate the relative importance of each variable.

Standard regression: All the independent variables are entered together.

Standard scores: *z*-scores; represent the deviation of scores around the mean in a distribution with a mean of "0" and a standard deviation of "1."

Statistics: The field of study that is concerned with obtaining, describing, and interpreting data; the characteristics of samples.

Stepwise regression: Variables are entered into the equation based on their measured relationship to the dependent variable. Methods include forward entry, backward removal, and a combination of forward and backward called stepwise.

Structural equation modeling: A method of testing theoretical models that analyzes covariances. It tests a measurement model and a theoretical model made up of measured and latent variables.

Structure coefficients: The correlations between the dependent and canonical variates. They are generally used for interpretation of results. Values of .30 or greater are considered meaningful.

Student-Newman-Keuls: A *post hoc* test that is similar to Tukey's honestly signifant difference (HSD) test, but the critical values do not remain constant.

Subjective probability: An individual's personal judgment of the likelihood of a particular event occurring.

Sum of squares: The sum of the squared deviations of each of the scores around a respective mean.

Tables: When data are organized into values or categories and then described with titles and captions, the result is a statistical table.

Tetrachoric: A coefficient that estimates r from the relationship between two dichotomized variables.

Theoretical model: A model of the hypothesized relationship between two latent variables.

Theory: A well-tested and systematic explanation about the relationships that make up a phenomenon.

Tolerance: A measure of collinearity. The proportion of the variance in a variable that is not accounted for by the other independent variables $(1 - R^2)$.

Transformation to normality: Altering data values in a skewed distribution to produce a normal or nearly normal distribution.

Trimmed mean: A statistical average calculated after removal of a certain percentage of extreme values from both ends of the distribution.

t test: A parametric statistical test for comparing the means of two independent groups.

Tukey's honestly significant difference (HSD): The most conservative *post hoc* test.

Tukey's wholly significant difference: A *post hoc* test that is intermediate in conservatism between Newman-Keuls and Tukey's HSD.

Two-tailed test of significance: A test used with a nondirectional hypothesis, in which extreme values are assumed to occur in either tail of the distribution.

Type I error: Rejecting the null hypothesis when it is true.

Type II error: Accepting the null hypothesis when it is false.

Underidentified model: A nonrecursive model. It contains paths that are not undirectional.

Validity: The extent to which an instrument measures what it intends to measure; the extent to which the measurements are "true."

Valid percent: The percentage with missing data excluded.

Variable: A measured characteristic that can take on different values.

Variance: A measure of the dispersion of scores around the mean. It is equal to the standard deviation squared.

Variance inflation factor: The reciprocal of tolerance.

Varimax rotation: Orthogonal rotation resulting in factors that are not correlated with each other.

Wald statistic: A value tested for significance in logistic regression.

Wilcoxon matched-pairs signed rank test: A nonparametric technique analogous to the paired t test. Used to compare paired measures.

Winsorized mean: A statistical average calculated after replacing the highest and lowest extreme values with the next-highest and next-lowest value.

Wilks' lambda: Represents the unexplained or error variance.

Within-groups variance: Variation of scores within the respective groups; represents the error term in analysis of variance.

Within-sample independence: Observations within the sample are independent of each other.

Within-subjects designs: Subjects serve as their own controls. Subjects are measured more than once on the same variable, or subjects are exposed to more than one treatment.

Y': The predicted score in a regression equation.

Zero-order correlation: The measured relationship between two variables.

z-scores: Standardized scores calculated by subtracting the mean from an individual score and dividing the result by the standard deviation; represents the deviation from the mean in a normal distribution.

CHAPTER ONE

Critical Thinking Concept Review

1. A peer-reviewed article may not explicitly state the different steps (e.g., problem statement and hypotheses). However, you should be able to identify each of these items through a careful reading of the article.

2. Any study that affected either clinical practice or health policy is acceptable.

3. The important thing in this exercise is to follow the 10-step plan.

CHAPTER TWO

Multiple-Choice Concept Review

1 (a), 2 (c), 3 (d), 4 (d), 5 (a), 6 (b), 7 (d), 8 (b), 9 (a), 10 (d)

Choosing the Correct Measurement Scale

1 (a), 2 (c), 3 (d), 4 (d), 5 (d), 6 (b), 7 (a), 8 (a), 9 (d), 10 (b), 11 (b), 12 (a), 13 (c), 14 (a), 15 (b), 16 (d), 17 (a), 18 (d), 19 (b), 20 (d)

Computational Problems

1.

Statistic	Data Set 1: Number of Hospitals in 25 Selected Counties in Yunan, China	Data Set 2: Cholesterol (in mg/dL) Levels in 32 Health Fair Participants
Mean	31.68	199.38
Standard deviation	17.797	16.974
Median	28.0	196.50
Interquartile range	17.00–46.00 hospitals	188.00–202.25
Mode	13, 30 (2 modes)	200
Range	8–79	178–259

2.

Characteristic	Value
Percentage married	64.7
Mean age (standard deviation)	38.82 (8.974)
Number older than age 30 years	12

(Continued)

2.	Characteristic	Value
	Percentage older than age 30 years	70.6
	Percentage male	17.6
	Mean number of years of work experience (standard deviation)	15.59 (9.063)
	Percentage with a BS degree	52.9

3.	Statistic	Department A	Department B
	Mean	42.11	44.31
	Standard deviation	10.839	15.377
	Median	40.00	42.50
	Interquartile range	37.00–49.50	34.75–53.00
	Mode	40	41
	Range	18–78	18–84

Interpretation

The age distribution in the two departments is similar, but the range of ages in Department B appears to be slightly wider. In both cases, the mean is slightly larger than the median, indicating the distributions are slightly positively skewed.

4.	Statistic	Group A	Group B
	Mean	167.29	198.38
	Standard deviation	42.589	39.586
	Median	155.00	199.00
	Interquartile range	130.50–200.00	168.75–225.00
	Mode	130	145, 165, 200, 225, 260 (multiple modes)
	Range	100–270	115–280

Interpretation

Group B appears to weigh more, as a group, than group A. However, the mean in group A is much larger than the median, indicating the data are positively skewed, whereas the mean and median are very similar in group B, suggesting a more bell-shaped distribution.

CHAPTER THREE

Multiple-Choice Concept Review
1 (b), 2 (d), 3 (c), 4 (b), 5 (a), 6 (d), 7 (c), 8 (a), 9 (b), 10 (c)

Conceptual Questions

1. In a positively skewed distribution, the tail is to the **right** or **higher** scores of the distribution.

2. A standard score distribution has a **mean of** 0 and an **SD of 1**.

Computational Problems

3. Marginal Probabilities

p (did not achieve goal weight)
$$\frac{120}{200} = .60$$

p (achieved goal weight)
$$\frac{80}{200} = .40$$

p (used diet alone)
$$\frac{100}{200} = .50$$

p (used diet and exercise)
$$\frac{100}{200} = .50$$

Joint Probabilities

p (did not achieve goal weight with diet alone)
$$\frac{80}{200} = 0.8$$

p (did not achieve goal weight with diet and exercise)
$$\frac{40}{200} = .20$$

p (achieved goal weight with diet alone)
$$\frac{20}{200} = .10$$

p (achieved goal weight with diet and exercise)
$$\frac{60}{200} = .30$$

Conditional Probabilities

p (did not achieve goal weight given diet alone)
$$\frac{80}{100} = 0.8$$

p (did not achieve goal weight given diet and exercise)
$$\frac{40}{100} = 0.4$$

(Continued)

---

p (achieved goal weight given diet alone)

$$\frac{20}{100} = 0.2$$

p (achieved goal weight given diet and exercise)

$$\frac{60}{100} = 0.6$$

---

2. **Marginal Probabilities**

p (less than high school diploma)

$$\frac{325}{2519} = .129$$

p (high school diploma or GED)

$$\frac{855}{2519} = .3394$$

p (2-year college degree)

$$\frac{708}{2519} = .2811$$

p (4-year college degree)

$$\frac{441}{2519} = .1751$$

p (postgraduate degree)

$$\frac{190}{2519} = .0754$$

p (does not smoke)

$$\frac{1960}{2519} = .7780$$

p (smokes)

$$\frac{559}{2519} = .2219$$

Joint Probabilities

p (less than high school diploma and does not smoke)

$$\frac{250}{2519} = .0992$$

p (less than high school diploma and smokes)

$$\frac{75}{2519} = .0298$$

p (high school diploma or GED and does not smoke)

$$\frac{620}{2519} = .2461$$

p (high school diploma or GED and smokes)

$$\frac{235}{2519} = .0933$$

p (2-year college degree and does not smoke)

$$\frac{554}{2519} = .2199$$

p (2-year college degree and smokes)	$\dfrac{154}{2519} = .0611$
p (4-year college degree and does not smoke)	$\dfrac{369}{2519} = .1465$
p (4-year college degree and smokes)	$\dfrac{72}{2519} = .0286$
p (postgraduate degree and does not smoke)	$\dfrac{167}{2519} = .0663$
p (postgraduate degree and smokes)	$\dfrac{23}{2519} = .0091$

Conditional Probabilities

p (does not smoke given less than high school diploma)	$\dfrac{250}{325} = .7692$
p (smokes given less than high school diploma)	$\dfrac{75}{325} = .2308$
p (does not smoke given high school diploma or GED)	$\dfrac{620}{855} = .7252$
p (smokes given high school diploma or GED)	$\dfrac{235}{855} = .2749$
p (does not smoke given 2-year college degree)	$\dfrac{554}{708} = .7825$
p (smokes given 2-year college degree)	$\dfrac{154}{708} = .2175$
p (does not smoke given 4-year college degree)	$\dfrac{369}{441} = .8367$
p (smokes given 4-year college degree)	$\dfrac{72}{441} = .1633$
p (does not smoke given postgraduate degree)	$\dfrac{167}{190} = .8789$
p (smokes given postgraduate degree)	$\dfrac{23}{190} = .1211$

3. A. $z = \dfrac{78 - 82}{6.58} = -0.6079$ round to -0.61, take the absolute value, and look up

$z = 0.61$ to get $p(0 \leq z \leq 0.61) = 22.97$. So, 22.97% of scores fall between the

mean, which is zero, and 0.61 on the standard normal distribution and therefore 22.97% of scores of the normally distributed exam fall between the mean of 82 and 78. Percentile rank = 50 − 22.92 = 27.08. This means that 27.08% of students score below 78%.

B. $z = \dfrac{82 - 82}{6.58} = 0$; $p(z = 0) = 0$: $p(0 \leq z \leq 0) = 0$. Percentile rank = 50 + 0 = 50,

so 50% of exam scores are below 82.

C. $z = \dfrac{88 - 82}{6.58} = .9119$ round to 0.91: $p(0 \leq z \leq 0.91) = 31.86$. Percentile rank =

50 + 31.86 = 81.86, so 81.86% of scores are below 88.

D. $z = \dfrac{95 - 82}{6.58} = 1.976$ round to 1.98: $p(0 \leq z \leq 1.98) = 47.61$. Percentile rank =

50 + 47.61 = 97.61, so 97.61% of scores are below 95.

4. With a mean of 70 and an SD of 15:
   a. 68% of scores = ±1SD; therefore, 68% fall between 55 and 85.
   b. 96% of scores = ± 2SD; therefore, 96% fall between 40 and 100.

5. z-scores $\mu = 70$ and $\sigma = 5$.

Raw Score	Standard Score $z = \dfrac{x - \mu}{\sigma}$	Absolute Value
58	$z = (58 - 70)/5 = -2.4$	2.4
65	$z = (65 - 70)/5 = -1.0$	1.0
73	$z = (73 - 70)/5 = 0.6$	0.6
82	$z = (82 - 70)/5 = 2.4$	2.4

b. Percentiles: Areas between mean and z-score (Appendix B)

Raw Score	|z-Score|	p ($\mu \leq z \leq$ |z-score|)	Tabled Value Percentiles
58	2.4	49.18	50 − 49.18 = 0.82
65	1.0	34.13	50 − 34.13 = 15.87
73	0.6	22.57	50 + 22.57 = 72.57
82	2.4	49.18	50 + 49.18 = 99.18

6. 364/1,500 = .243, or (0.243 × 100) = 24.3%.

7. a. Sensitivity is calculated as follows:
   $$Sn = (TP/[TP + FN]) \times 100$$
   $$= (731/[731 + 78]) \times 100$$
   $$= [731/809] \times 100$$
   $$= 90.4\%$$
   Specificity is calculated as follows:
   $$Sp = (TN/[TN + FP]) \times 100$$
   $$= (1500/[1500 + 270]) \times 100$$
   $$= [1500/1770] \times 100$$
   $$= 84.7\%$$
   Positive predictive value is calculated as follows:
   $$PPV = (TP/[TP + FP]) \times 100$$
   $$= (731/[731 + 270]) \times 100$$
   $$= [731/1001] \times 100$$
   $$= 73.0\%$$
   Negative predictive value is calculated as follows:
   $$NPV = (TN/[TN + FN]) \times 100$$
   $$= (1500/[1500 + 78]) \times 100$$
   $$= [1500/1578] \times 100$$
   $$= 95.1\%$$
   Efficiency is calculated as follows:
   $$Eff = ([TP + TN]/[TP + TN + FP + FN]) \times 100$$
   $$= ([731 + 1500]/[731 + 1500 + 270 + 78]) \times 100$$
   $$= [2231/2579] \times 100$$
   $$= 86.5\%$$

   b. These results indicate that 90.4% of patients with iron deficiency anemia have a positive serum ferritin level test result (Sn), and 85% of patients who do not have the disorder test negative (Sp). Seventy three percent of those who receive a positive serum ferritin level test actually have iron deficiency anemia (PPV), while only 27 out of every 100 (100–73=27%) patients who tested positive actually do not have iron deficiency anemia (1-PPV). Meanwhile, of those who test negative on the serum ferritin level test, 95.1% truly do not have iron deficiency anemia (NPV), while (100–95.1=4.9%) of those testing negative actually do have the deficiency (1-NPV). The serum ferritin level test is 86% accurate (EFF) in diagnosing patients with iron deficiency anemia.

CHAPTER FOUR

Multiple-Choice Concept Review

        1 (b), 2 (c), 3 (b), 4 (d), 5 (b), 6 (a), 7 (d), 8 (b), 9 (c), 10 (c)

Critical Thinking Concept Review

1. Any five hypotheses that are similar to these are fine:

   $H1_0$: Infant birth weight will not differ by polychlorinated biphenyl (PCB) exposure.
   $H1_A$: Infants born in zip codes with documented PCBs will have lower birth weights than infants born in zip codes without PCBs who were not exposed.
   $H2_0$: Maternal smoking will not be associated with infant birth weight.
   $H2_A$: Infants born to women who smoke will have lower birth weights than will infants born to women who do not smoke.
   $H3_0$: Ethnicity will not be associated with infant birth weight.
   $H3_A$: Infants born to African American women will have lower birth weights than infants born to women of other ethnicities.
   $H4_0$: The mother's marital status will not be associated with infant birth weight.
   $H4_A$: Infants born to single mothers will have lower birth weights than will infants born to married women.
   $H5_0$: Income will not be associated with infant birth weight.
   $H5_A$: Infants born to families with a per capita income of less than $15,000 a year will have lower birth weights than will infants born to families with a per capita income of $15,000 or more a year.

2. Any five hypotheses that contain one dependent variable and one independent variable are fine. The hypotheses should all relate to the central research question of the article.

3. The write-up should follow the 10-step plan detailed in Chapter 1. Make sure that the purpose is stated clearly, that there are at least two research questions related to that purpose, and that there are at least two hypotheses for each research question.

Computational Problems

1. a. $z = \dfrac{31.3 - 26.8}{4.6/\sqrt{25}} = \dfrac{4.5}{4.6/5} = \dfrac{4.5}{.92} = 4.89$; not on the chart, but it is known that

   $p < .0001$: significant.

   b. $z = \dfrac{47 - 45.2}{17.5/\sqrt{36}} = \dfrac{1.8}{17.5/6} = \dfrac{4.5}{2.92} = 1.54$; $pz \geq 1.54 = .0618$: not significant.

   c. $z = \dfrac{38.2 - 40.0}{8.2/\sqrt{49}} = \dfrac{-1.8}{8.2/7} = \dfrac{-1.8}{1.17} = -.0855$; $pz \leq -.0855 = .1977$: not

   significant.

2. a. Find the standard error of the mean.

$$se_{\overline{X}} = \frac{6}{\sqrt{120}} = .5477$$

b. Set up the 95% confidence interval for the mean.

95%CI $= 75 \pm (1.96 \times .5477)$

95%CI $= 75 \pm (1.073)$

95%CI $= (73.927, 76.073)$

c. Set up the 99% confidence interval for the mean.

99%CI $= 75 \pm (2.58 \times .5477)$

99%CI $= 75 \pm (1.413)$

99%CI $= (73.587, 76.413)$

CHAPTER FIVE

Multiple-Choice Concept Review

1 (b), 2 (a), 3 (b), 4 (c), 5 (d), 6 (a), 7 (b), 8 (b), 9 (b), 10 (a), 11 (c), 12 (a), 13 (d), 14 (d), 15 (d), 16 (a), 17 (d), 18 (b), 19 (b), 20 (a)

Critical Thinking Concept Review

1. Any hypothesis in which the grouping variable has two categories and the other variable is at least ordinal in measurement is acceptable.

2. (a) 2.08, (b) 2.704, (c) 1.658, (d) 2.110, (e) 1.671, (f) 3.055

3. (a) 34, (b) 11, (c) 139, (d) 1, (e) 27, (f) 16

Computational Problems

1. **Independent t test:** The group that took the placebo had an average of 4.4 hours of sleep a night (standard deviation, 1.44), and the group that took the herbal formula had an average of 4.9 hours of sleep a night (standard deviation, 0.87). The f-test was not significant (the computed value of 2.74 did not exceed the critical value of 4.95). Because the f-test was not statistically significant, homogeneity of variance is assumed, and independent t test formula is used for pooled samples. Also, in SPSS, the Levene's test p-value is .381, which is not significant. The computed independent t test statistic is .741, and the critical value is 2.201. Because the computed value does not exceed the critical value, it can be concluded that no statistically significant difference exists between the two groups. Also, in SPSS, the p-value for the t test is .474. Thus, the conclusion is that people who took the herbal formula did not sleep any more or less, on average, than people who took the placebo.

Mann-Whitney U-test: The sum of the ranks assigned to the placebo group is 42.5, and the sum of the ranks of the formula group is 48.5. The independent t test statistic is 14.5. The critical value ($n = 7$; $m = 6$) at a .05 level (two-tailed) is 7. Because 14.5 > 7, the null hypothesis cannot be rejected. Using SPSS, the p-value for the Mann-Whitney U-test is .352, which is not less than $\alpha = .05$. Therefore, it is concluded that there is no significant difference between the two groups. Thus, the conclusion is that the people who took the herbal formula did not sleep any more or less than the people who took the placebo.

2. **Independent t test:** The group of children at home had an average of 2.86 (standard deviation, 1.35) aggressive acts in a 4-hour period, and the group in the day-care center had an average of 2.33 (standard deviation, 1.63) aggressive acts in a 4-hour period. The f-test was not significant (the computed value of 1.46 did not exceed the critical value of 4.39). Also, in SPSS, the Levene's test p-value is .471, which is greater than the cutoff of .05. Therefore, homogeneity of variance is assumed, and the independent t test formula for pooled samples is used. The computed independent t test statistic is 0.635, and the critical value is 2.201. Because the computed value does not exceed the critical value, it can be concluded that no statistically significant difference exists between the two groups. In SPSS, the p-value for the t test is .538, which is greater than .05. Thus, the conclusion is that children who are in day-care settings do not engage more frequently in aggressive acts than those in home settings.

   Mann-Whitney U-test: The sum of the ranks assigned to the in-home group is 52.5, and the sum of the ranks of the day-care group is 38.5. The Mann-Whitney U-test statistic is 17.5. The critical value ($n = 7$; $m = 6$) at a .05 level (two-tailed) is 7. Because 17.5 > 7, the null hypothesis cannot be rejected. In SPSS, the p-value is .611. It can be concluded that there is no significant difference between the two groups. Thus, the conclusion is that children who are in day-care settings do not engage in aggressive acts any more frequently than children who are in home settings.

3. **Independent t test:** The uninsured group had an average of 1.73 (standard deviation, 1.46) visits to the primary care physician per year, and the insured group had an average of 2.77 (standard deviation, 1.54) visits per year. The f-test was not significant (the computed value of 1.11 did not exceed the critical value of 1.85). In SPSS, the Levene's test p-value is .883. Therefore, homogeneity of variance is assumed, and the independent t test formula for pooled samples is used. The computed independent t test statistic is –2.704, and the critical value is ≈2.000. Because the absolute value of the computed independent t test exceeds the critical value, it is concluded that a statistically significant difference exists. In SPSS, the p-value is .009 and is less than .05. Thus, the conclusion is that women with health insurance make significantly more outpatient physician visits per year than women without health insurance.

   Mann-Whitney U-test: The sum of the ranks assigned to the no-insurance group is 748, and the sum of the ranks of the insurance group is 1,143. The test statistic is 283. Because both n and m are greater than 20, the Mann-Whitney U-statistics table cannot be used to obtain the critical value. In this case, it is necessary to compute a z-score, $z = (t - mn/2)/[nm\ (n + m + 1)/12]$ and compare the result, for the significance, with critical values of the standard normal distribution. In this case, $z = -2.674$ has a p-value of .008 (two-tailed), so the null hypothesis can be rejected at the .05 level. In SPSS, $p = .008$. It can be concluded that a significant difference exists between the two groups. Thus, the conclusion is that women with health insurance make significantly more visits to their primary care physician in a year than women without health insurance.

4. **Independent t test:** The group living in poverty had an average depression score of 6.45 (standard deviation, 3.33), and the group living above the poverty line had an average depression score of 4.86 (standard deviation, 2.27). The f-test was significant (the computed value of 2.15 exceeded the critical value of 1.80). The Levene's test p-value is .037. Therefore, heterogeneity of variance cannot be assumed. Using SPSS, we can find the independent samples' t test for separate variances. Under equal variances not assumed, the value of the test statistic in SPSS is 2.250 and p is .029. Because the p-value is less than .05, it can be concluded that a statistically significant difference exists. Thus, the conclusion is that people living at or below the poverty line score significantly higher on the depression scale than those living above the poverty line.

   Mann-Whitney U-test: The sum of the ranks assigned to the below-poverty group is 1,230, and the sum of the ranks of the above-poverty group is 1,048. The test statistic is 382. Because both n and m are greater than 20, the Mann-Whitney U-test table cannot be used to obtain the critical value. In this case, it is necessary to compute a z-score, $z = (t - mn/2)/[nm\ (n + m + 1)/12]$ and compare the result, for the significance, with the critical values of the standard normal distribution. In this case, $z = -2.229$ has a p-value of .026 (two-tailed). In SPSS, $p = .026$. Therefore, the null hypothesis is rejected at the $\alpha = .05$ level. It can be concluded that a significant difference exists between the two groups. Thus, the conclusion is that people living at or below the poverty line score significantly higher on the depression scale than those living above the poverty line.

5. **Independent t test:** The dental hygienists who did not read journal articles in their field were in practice for an average of 11.83 years (standard deviation, 7.67), and the dental hygienists who did read journal articles regularly were in practice for an average of 15.71 years (standard deviation, 8.84). The f-test was not significant (the computed value of 1.33 did not exceed the critical value of 1.39). Therefore, homogeneity of variance is assumed, and the independent t test for pooled variances is used. The computed t-statistic is 3.540, and the critical value is 1.96. Because the computed value exceeds the critical value, it can be concluded that a statistically significant difference exists between the two groups. Thus, the conclusion is that dental hygienists who read journal articles on a regular basis have been in practice for a significantly longer time than dental hygienists who do not read journal articles.

CHAPTER SIX

Multiple-Choice Concept Review
> 1 (b), 2 (d), 3 (c), 4 (d), 5 (c), 6 (d), 7 (b), 8 (d), 9 (d), 10 (a)

Choosing the Best Statistical Test
> 1 (a), 2 (d), 3 (b), 4 (a), 5 (b), 6 (a), 7 (a), 8 (d), 9 (b), 10 (c)

Critical Thinking Concept Review

> 1. These should be any five hypotheses that compare two different measures of the same variable in either a pretest/posttest design or a case and a matched-control design. The characteristic of interest should be at least ordinal in measurement scale.

> 2. Critical value of the Wilcoxon matched pairs:
>   a. 3
>   b. 0
>   c. 100
>   d. 5
>   e. 35

> 3. A study with a case and a matched control compares the measure of the dependent variable in the case group (which received some type of intervention) with the measure of the dependent variable in the control group (which does not receive any intervention). A study that has each person act as his or her own control compares two measures (pretest and posttest) on the same person: one before the intervention takes place and one after the intervention takes place. This is a weaker design.

Computational Problems

> 1. Paired t test: The participants have a mean fun score of 4.90 (standard deviation, 0.88) when wearing the blond wig and a mean fun score of 2.90 (standard deviation, 1.29) with their own brown hair. The computed t test statistic is -3.873, and the critical value is 2.262 (α-level = .05; two-tailed test; degrees of freedom, 9). The p-value from SPSS is .004. Because the absolute value of the computed value exceeds the critical value and the p-value is less than .05, it can be concluded that a statistically significant difference exists between the two hair colors. The conclusion is that blonds do have more fun.

> Wilcoxon matched-pairs test: The participants have a median fun score of 5.0 when wearing the blond wig and a median fun score of 3.0 with their own brown hair. The sum of positive ranks is 53, and the sum of the negative ranks is 2. The result that is smaller is compared with a table of Wilcoxon's signed-rank probabilities to check for significance. When the number of pairs is 10, a value of 8 or less is significant at .05. The p-value from SPSS is .008. Because the result of 2 is

smaller than 10 and the *p*-value is less than .05, it can be concluded that a statistically significant difference exists.

2. Paired *t* test: The participants leave an average of 8.40 oz (standard deviation, 4.70) of salad A and an average of 11.30 oz (standard deviation, 3.30) of salad B. The computed *t* test statistic is –2.240, and the critical value is 2.262 (α-level = .05; two-tailed test; degrees of freedom, 9). The *p*-value from SPSS is .052. Because the absolute value of the computed value does not exceed the critical value and because the *p*-value is not less than .05, it can be concluded that no statistically significant difference exists between the two salads in terms of their popularity using the paired *t* test. However, the result does come close to significance (*p* = .052) and would be worth pursing further.

   Wilcoxon matched-pairs test: The participants leave a median of 8.0 oz of salad A and a median of 11.5 oz of salad B. The sum of negative ranks is 5, and the sum of positive ranks is 40. The result that is smaller is compared with a table of Wilcoxon's signed-rank probabilities to check for significance. When the number of pairs is 10, a value of 8 or less is significant at .05 level using a two-tailed test. Because the result of 5 is smaller than 8, it can be concluded that a statistically significant difference exists. In SPSS, the *p*-value is .036, which is less than .05. Using the Wilcoxon matched-pairs test, it is concluded that salad A is more popular than salad B.

   The results obtained by using the paired *t* test and Wilcoxon do not agree. In this case, it should be noted that the data do not really meet the assumptions for the paired *t* test and that the Wilcoxon matched-pairs test is actually the better test to use.

3. Paired *t* test: The mean pretest knowledge score is 5.76 (standard deviation, 1.86), and the mean posttest knowledge score is 5.82 (1.74). The computed paired *t*-statistic is –.194, and the exact *p*-value from the SPSS printout is .848. Therefore, it can be concluded that the intervention did not increase knowledge about domestic violence in nurse practitioner students.

   Wilcoxon matched-pairs test: The median pretest knowledge score is 6.0, and the median posttest knowledge score is 6.0. The sum of the negative ranks is 30, and the sum of the positive ranks is 25. The exact *p*-value from the SPSS printout is .782. Therefore, it can be concluded that the intervention does not significantly increase knowledge about domestic violence in nurse practitioner students.

4. Paired *t* test: The participants smoked an average of 14.43 cigarettes daily (standard deviation, 3.39) before participating in the program and an average of 7.71 cigarettes daily (standard deviation, 1.67) after participating in the program. The computed *t* test statistic is 12.22 with an exact *p*-value from the SPSS printout of less than .000. It can be concluded that the participants smoke significantly less daily after participating in the smoking cessation program.

   Wilcoxon matched-pairs test: The participants smoked a median of 14 cigarettes daily before participating in the program and a median of 8 cigarettes daily after participating in the program. The sum of the positive ranks is 0, with an exact *p*-value from the SPSS printout of less than .000. It can be concluded that the participants smoke significantly less daily after participating in the smoking cessation program.

CHAPTER SEVEN

Multiple-Choice Concept Review
1 (c), 2 (b), 3 (c), 4 (b), 5 (b), 6 (a), 7 (b), 8 (b), 9 (d), 10 (a)

Choosing the Best Statistical Test
1 (f), 2 (a), 3 (c), 4 (d), 5 (e), 6 (b), 7 (e), 8 (f), 9 (a), 10 (e)

Critical Thinking Concept Review
1. Any hypotheses that ask to test for differences in the means of three or more groups (as defined by a single variable).

2. The following table lists the critical values.

α-Value	Degrees of Freedom (Numerator)	Degrees of Freedom (Denominator)	One-Way ANOVA
.01	2	30	5.39
.05	2	30	3.32
.01	3	25	4.68
.05	3	25	2.99

3. The following table is the completed ANOVA table.

Source of Variance	Sum of Squares	Degrees of Freedom	Mean Square	F-Ratio	p-Value
Between groups	97.4	2	48.7	245.46	<.01
Within groups	12.3	62	0.1984		
Total	109.7				

Computational Problems
1. One-way ANOVA: The mean reading speeds in words per minute and standard deviations are as follows: Group 1: 15.6 (standard deviation, 6.50), Group 2: 16.25 (standard deviation, 3.59), and Group 3: 10.0 (standard deviation, 1.83). Because the Levene's test was not significant ($p = .159$), there is homogeneity of variance. The computed f-test is 2.225, with an associated p-value of .159 (not significant). Thus, the conclusion is that no significant difference exists in the mean reading speed of people in the three groups.

Kruskal-Wallis H-test: The computed Kruskal-Wallis H-statistic p-value is .099 (not significant at $\alpha = .05$). Thus, the conclusion is that no significant difference exists in the distribution of reading speed of people in the three groups.

2. One-way ANOVA: The mean number of traffic accidents and standard deviations are as follows: City A: 15.0 (standard deviation, 4.0), City B: 9.71 (standard deviation, 4.72), and City C: 7.71 (standard deviation, 5.02). Because the Levene's test was not significant ($p = .876$), homogeneity of variance is present. The computed f-test is 4.688 with an associated p-value of .023 (significant). Thus, the conclusion is that a significant difference exists in the mean number of traffic accidents in the three cities. The Bonferroni *post hoc* test reveals that City A and City C ($p = .025$) are significantly different from each other and that no other differences exist.

   Kruskal-Wallis H-test: The computed Kruskal-Wallis H-statistic p-value is .030. Thus, the conclusion is that a significant difference exists in the number of traffic accidents in the three cities.

3. One-way ANOVA: The mean self-esteem scores and standard deviations are as follows: less than a high school diploma: 17.8 (standard deviation, 3.55), high school only: 23.3 (standard deviation, 3.30), some college: 25.7 (standard deviation, 1.89), and 4-year college or higher: 30.5 (3.03). Because the Levene's test was not significant ($p = .379$), homogeneity of variance is present. The computed f-test is 30.762 with an associated p-value of .000 (significant). Thus, the conclusion is that a significant difference exists in the mean self-esteem of women in the different educational groups. The Bonferroni *post hoc* tests reveal that women with less than a high school education had significantly lower self-esteem than women in the other three groups and that women with a 4-year college degree had significantly higher self-esteem than women in all the other groups. No significant difference was present in the self-esteem of women with high school education and women with some college.

   Kruskal-Wallis H-test: The computed Kruskal-Wallis H-statistic p-value is .000. Thus, the conclusion is that a significant difference exists in the self-esteem of women in the four groups.

4. One-way ANOVA: The mean monthly salaries and standard deviations are as follows: University A: \$1,861.0 (standard deviation, \$337.81), University B: \$4,740.38 (standard deviation, \$379.29), University C: \$2,595.11 (standard deviation, \$355.97), University D: \$3,492.25 (standard deviation, \$306.71), and University E: \$5,812.75 (standard deviation, \$257.94). Because the Levene's test was not significant ($p = .746$), homogeneity of variance is present. The computed f-test is 202.639 with an associated p-value of .000 (significant). Thus, the conclusion is that a significant difference exists in the mean salaries of assistant professors at the five universities. The *post hoc* tests reveal that all the salaries were significantly different from each other.

   Kruskal-Wallis H-test: The computed Kruskal-Wallis H-statistic p-value is .000. Thus, the conclusion is that a significant difference exists in the distribution of salaries of at least one of the four groups.

5. One-way ANOVA: The mean cholesterol levels and standard deviation are as follows: Tract A: 186.19 (standard deviation, 35.09), Tract B: 178.28 (standard deviation, 38.38), Tract C: 207.68 (standard deviation, 46.06), and Tract D: 185.36 (standard deviation, 45.44). Because the Levene's test was not significant ($p = .660$), homogeneity of variance is present. The computed f-test is 3.079 with an associated p-value of .030 (significant). Thus, the conclusion is that a significant difference exists between at least two of the mean cholesterol levels of patients from the four different census tracts. The Bonferroni *post hoc* tests reveal that only Tract B and Tract C differ from each other significantly ($p = .038$).

Kruskal-Wallis H-test: The computed Kruskal-Wallis H-statistic p-value is .054. Thus, the conclusion is that a significant difference does not exist in the distribution of cholesterol levels of the four census tracts (assuming an α-level of .05). The one-way ANOVA and Kruskal-Wallis tests disagree, likely because the data violate one or more of the assumptions required for the one-way ANOVA test.

CHAPTER EIGHT

Multiple-Choice Concept Review

1 (b), 2 (d), 3 (d), 4 (b), 5 (a), 6 (b), 7 (a), 8 (c), 9 (d), 10 (a)

Choosing the Best Statistical Test

1 (c), 2 (d), 3 (g), 4 (a), 5 (f), 6 (g), 7 (f), 8 (b), 9 (g), 10 (h)

Critical Thinking Concept Review

1. Any hypotheses that ask to test for differences in the means of four or more groups (as defined by two factors/independent variables).

2. Any hypotheses that ask to test for the differences in the means of two dependent variables among three or more groups as defined by one or more factors/independent variables.

3. The following table is the completed ANOVA table.

Two-Way ANOVA Table (n = 66)

Source of Variation	Sum of Squares	Degrees of freedom (df_x)	Mean Square	F (Variance Ratio)	Significant at $\alpha = .05$?
Factor A	11.6	2	11.6/2 = 5.8	5.8/2.5 = 2.32	F_{crit} = 3.14, so $p > .05$
Factor B	98.9	1	98.9/1 = 98.9	98.9/2.5 = 39.56	F_{crit} = 3.99, so $p < .05$
Interaction (AB)	1,948.7– (11.6 + 98.9 + 1,746.8) = 91.4	2 × 1 = 2	91.4/2 = 45.7	45.7/2.5 = 18.28	F_{crit} = 3.14, so $p > .05$

Treatments			
Residual (error)	1,746.8	688	1,746.8/688 = 2.5
Total	**1,948.7**		

Computational Problems

1. The SPSS results are below. Briefly, because the Levine's test is not significant ($p = .395$), we can conduct a three-way ANOVA. From the Tests of Between-Subjects Effects, we see that maternal race/ethnicity is significantly associated with birth weight. From the Bonferroni *post hoc* test, we see that Black/African Americans have a significantly lower mean birth weight (2,440.25 g) compared to Whites/Caucasians (3,485.87 g) and Hispanics (3,399.33 g). In addition, we found significant interaction between maternal age and smoking ($p = .007$).

		Notes	
Output created		16-Mar-2011 15:30:37	
Comments			
Input	Data	C:\Documents and Settings\ekelvin\Desktop\ Kelvine\Stat book editing\chapter 8 low birth weight problems.sav	
	Active Data set	DataSet2	
	Filter	<none>	
	Weight	<none>	
	Split File	<none>	
	No. of Rows in Working Data File	60	
Missing value handling	Definition of Missing	User-defined missing values are treated as missing.	
	Cases Used	Statistics are based on all cases with valid data for all variables in the model.	
Syntax		UNIANOVA Birth weight BY RaceEth Mat_Age MatSmoking	
		/METHOD=SSTYPE(3)	
		/INTERCEPT=INCLUDE	
		/POSTHOC=RaceEth Mat_Age(BONFERRONI)	
		/PRINT=HOMOGENEITY DESCRIPTIVE	
		/CRITERIA=ALPHA(.05)	

(Continued)

		Notes *(Continued)*
		/DESIGN=RaceEth Mat_Age MatSmoking RaceEth*Mat_Age RaceEth*MatSmoking Mat_Age*MatSmoking RaceEth*Mat_Age*MatSmoking.
Resources	Processor Time	00:00:00.016
	Elapsed Time	00:00:00.016

[Data Set2] C:\Documents and Settings\ekelvin\Desktop\Kelvine\Stat book editing\chapter 8 low birthweight problems.sav

Between-Subjects Factors

		Value Label	N
Maternal primary race/ethnicity	1	Black/African American	20
	2	White/Caucasian	20
	3	Hispanic	20
Maternal age category during pregnancy	1	Under 18 years	19
	2	18–34 years	21
	3	35 years and older	20
Maternal history of smoking	0	Never smoked	35
	1	Smoker	25

Descriptive Statistics
Dependent Variable: Birth Weight of Infant in Grams

Maternal Primary Race/Ethnicity	Maternal Age Category During Pregnancy	Maternal History of Smoking	Mean	Standard Deviation	N
Black/African American	Under 18 years	Never smoked	2,457.28	644.431	5
		Smoker	2,137.58	262.117	3
		Total	2,337.39	533.212	8
	18–34 years	Never smoked	2,916.95	752.713	5
		Smoker	1,390.38	344.029	3
		Total	2,344.48	990.857	8
	35 years and older	Never smoked	2,709.81	300.962	2
		Smoker	2,965.19	662.117	2
		Total	2,837.50	445.044	4
	Total	Never smoked	2,690.90	642.945	12
		Smoker	2,064.28	738.179	8
		Total	2,440.25	734.353	20
White/Caucasian	Under 18 years	Never smoked	3,395.54	766.370	6

		Smoker	3,433.38	.	1
		Total	3,400.95	699.743	7
	18–34 years	Never smoked	4,341.38	.	1
		Smoker	3,353.93	672.493	5
		Total	3,518.50	724.091	6
	35 years and older	Never smoked	3,227.66	847.894	4
		Smoker	3,963.04	216.718	3
		Total	3,542.82	727.756	7
	Total	Never smoked	3,420.48	780.634	11
		Smoker	3,565.79	572.092	9
		Total	3,485.87	681.204	20
Hispanic	Under 18 years	Never smoked	3,575.25	.	1
		Smoker	3,499.58	32.765	3
		Total	3,518.50	46.336	4
	18–34 years	Never smoked	3,575.25	418.311	7
		Total	3,575.25	418.311	7
	35 years and older	Never smoked	3,107.06	508.908	4
		Smoker	3,291.50	478.605	5
		Total	3,209.53	470.213	9
	Total	Never smoked	3,419.19	468.207	12
		Smoker	3,369.53	377.885	8
		Total	3,399.33	424.439	20
Total	Under 18 years	Never smoked	3,019.57	816.621	12
		Smoker	2,906.41	735.538	7
		Total	2,977.88	768.775	19
	18–34 years	Never smoked	3,380.99	681.871	13
		Smoker	2,617.59	1,151.075	8
		Total	3,090.17	941.815	21
	35 years and older	Never smoked	3,075.85	613.583	10
		Smoker	3,427.70	560.649	10
		Total	3,251.77	599.837	20
	Total	Never smoked	3,169.89	712.126	35
		Smoker	3,022.51	875.539	25
		Total	3,108.48	780.663	60

Levene's Test of Equality of Error Variances[a]
Dependent Variable: Birth Weight of Infant in Grams

F	df1	df2	Significance
1.088	16	43	.395

Tests the null hypothesis that the error variance of the dependent variable is equal across groups.

[a]Design: Intercept + RaceEth + Mat_Age + MatSmoking + RaceEth* Mat_Age + RaceEth* MatSmoking + Mat_Age* MatSmoking + RaceEth* Mat_Age* MatSmoking.

Tests of Between-Subjects Effects
Dependent Variable: Birth Weight of Infant in Grams

Source	Type III Sum of Squares	df	Mean Square	F	Significance
Corrected model	2.138E7	16	1,336,531.760	3.944	.000
Intercept	4.548E8	1	4.548E8	1,341.942	.000
RaceEth	1.173E7	2	5,864,510.451	17.305	.000
Mat_Age	219,017.396	2	109,508.698	.323	.726
MatSmoking	750,643.562	1	750,643.562	2.215	.144
RaceEth* Mat_Age	1,704,590.617	4	426,147.654	1.257	.301
RaceEth* MatSmoking	395,703.503	2	197,851.752	.584	.562
Mat_Age* MatSmoking	3,725,744.928	2	1,862,872.464	5.497	.007
RaceEth* Mat_Age *MatSmoking	60,418.063	3	20,139.354	.059	.981
Error	1.457E7	43	338,887.122		
Total	6.157E8	60			
Corrected total	3.596E7	59			

[a]$R^2 = .595$ (adjusted $R^2 = .444$).

POST HOC TESTS

Maternal Primary Race/Ethnicity

Multiple Comparisons

Birth Weight of Infant in Grams Bonferroni

(I) Maternal Primary Race/ Ethnicity	(J) Maternal Primary Race/ Ethnicity	Mean Difference I − J	Standard Error	Significance	95% Confidence Interval Lower Bound	Upper Bound
Black/African American	White/ Caucasian	−1,045.62[a]	184.089	.000	−1,504.23	−587.01
	Hispanic	−959.07[a]	184.089	.000	−1,417.69	−500.46
White/ Caucasian	Black/African American	1,045.62[a]	184.089	.000	587.01	1,504.23
	Hispanic	86.54	184.089	1.000	−372.07	545.16
Hispanic	Black/African American	959.07[a]	184.089	.000	500.46	1,417.69
	White/ Caucasian	−86.54	184.089	1.000	−545.16	372.07

Based on observed means.
The error term is Mean Square (Error) = 338,887.122.
[a]The mean difference is significant at the .05 level.

HOMOGENEOUS SUBSETS

Maternal Age Category During Pregnancy

Multiple Comparisons

Birth Weight of Infant in Grams Bonferroni

(I) Maternal Age Category During Pregnancy	(J) Maternal Age Category During Pregnancy	Mean Difference I − J	Standard Error	Significance	95% Confidence Interval Lower Bound	Upper Bound
Under 18 years	18–34 years	−112.29	184.319	1.000	−571.48	346.90
	35 years and older	−273.89	186.495	.448	−738.50	190.72
18–34 years	Under 18 years	112.29	184.319	1.000	−346.90	571.48
	35 years and older	−161.60	181.884	1.000	−614.72	291.52
35 years and older	Under 18 years	273.89	186.495	.448	−190.72	738.50
	18–34 years	161.60	181.884	1.000	−291.52	614.72

Based on observed means.
The error term is Mean Square (Error) = 338,887.122.

2. Because the Box's test of equality of variances (p = .295) and the Levine's test (p = .451 and p = .474) are not significant, we can do a MANOVA test. We find that the dietary intervention has a significant impact on weight loss (p = .007) and cholesterol level (p = .000), and the exercise intervention has a significant impact on cholesterol level (p = .006). In addition, there is significant interaction between diet and exercise on weight loss (p = .000).

General Linear Model

Notes		
Output created		16-Mar-2011 15:48:54
Comments		
Input	Data	C:\Documents and Settings\ ekelvin\Desktop\Kelvine\Stat book editing\chapter 8 exercise and diet.sav
	Active Data set	DataSet3
	Filter	<none>
	Weight	<none>
	Split File	<none>
	No. of Rows in Working Data File	60
Missing value handling	Definition of Missing	User-defined missing values are treated as missing
	Cases Used	Statistics are based on all cases with valid data for all variables in the model
Syntax		GLM LbsLost Cholesterol BY Diet Exercise
		/METHOD=SSTYPE(3)
		/INTERCEPT=INCLUDE
		/PRINT=DESCRIPTIVE HOMOGENEITY
		/CRITERIA=ALPHA(.05)
		/DESIGN= Diet Exercise Diet*Exercise.
Resources	Processor Time	00:00:00.000
	Elapsed Time	00:00:00.032

[Data Set3] C:\Documents and Settings\ekelvin\Desktop\Kelvine\Stat book editing\chapter 8 exercise and diet.sav

Between-Subjects Factors

		Value Label	N
Diet: Changed or not	0	No change	30
	1	Experimental diet	30
Exercise: Changed or not	0	No change in exercise routine	30
	1	Experimental exercise routine	30

Descriptive Statistics

	Diet: Changed or not	Exercise: Changed or not	Mean	Standard Deviation	N
Number of pounds lost during experiment period	No change	No change in exercise routine	3.53	1.642	15
		Experimental exercise routine	6.87	1.767	15
		Total	5.20	2.384	30
	Experimental diet	No change in exercise routine	7.40	2.098	15
		Experimental exercise routine	5.53	1.356	15
		Total	6.47	1.978	30
	Total	No change in exercise routine	5.47	2.700	30
		Experimental exercise routine	6.20	1.690	30
		Total	5.83	2.264	60
Total cholesterol at end of experiment	No change	No change in exercise routine	183.47	34.525	15
		Experimental exercise routine	208.73	25.429	15
		Total	196.10	32.446	30
	Experimental diet	No change in exercise routine	151.07	26.111	15
		Experimental exercise routine	165.73	20.927	15
		Total	158.40	24.417	30
	Total	No change in exercise routine	167.27	34.294	30
		Experimental exercise routine	187.23	31.651	30
		Total	177.25	34.232	60

Box's Test of Equality of Covariance Matrices[a]	
Box's M	11.468
F	1.192
df1	9
df2	35,937.955
Significance	.295

Tests the null hypothesis that the observed covariance matrices of the dependent variables are equal across groups.

[a]Design: Intercept + Diet + Exercise + Diet* Exercise.

	Multivariate Tests[a]					
Effect		Value	F	Hypothesis df	Error df	Significance
Intercept	Pillai's trace	.982	1,490.594[b]	2.000	55.000	.000
	Wilks' lambda	.018	1,490.594[b]	2.000	55.000	.000
	Hotelling's trace	54.203	1,490.594[b]	2.000	55.000	.000
	Roy's largest root	54.203	1,490.594[b]	2.000	55.000	.000
Diet	Pillai's trace	.414	19.392[b]	2.000	55.000	.000
	Wilks' lambda	.586	19.392[b]	2.000	55.000	.000
	Hotelling's trace	.705	19.392[b]	2.000	55.000	.000
	Roy's largest root	.705	19.392[b]	2.000	55.000	.000
Exercise	Pillai's trace	.153	4.951[b]	2.000	55.000	.011
	Wilks' lambda	.847	4.951[b]	2.000	55.000	.011
	Hotelling's trace	.180	4.951[b]	2.000	55.000	.011
	Roy's largest root	.180	4.951[b]	2.000	55.000	.011
Diet* Exercise	Pillai's trace	.376	16.561[b]	2.000	55.000	.000
	Wilks' lambda	.624	16.561[b]	2.000	55.000	.000
	Hotelling's trace	.602	16.561[b]	2.000	55.000	.000
	Roy's largest root	.602	16.561[b]	2.000	55.000	.000

[a]Design: Intercept + Diet + Exercise + Diet* Exercise.
[b]Exact statistic.

Levene's Test of Equality of Error Variances[a]

	F	df1	df2	Significance
Number of pounds lost during the experiment period	.891	3	56	.451
Total cholesterol at the end of the experiment	.847	3	56	.474

Tests the null hypothesis that the error variance of the dependent variable is equal across groups.
[a]Design: Intercept + Diet + Exercise + Diet* Exercise.

Tests of Between-Subjects Effects

Source	Dependent Variable	Type III Sum of Squares	df	Mean Square	F	Significance
Corrected model	Number of pounds lost during the experiment period	133.533[a]	3	44.511	14.767	.000
	Total cholesterol at the end of the experiment	27,720.717[b]	3	9,240.239	12.494	.000
Intercept	Number of pounds lost during the experiment period	2,041.667	1	2,041.667	677.330	.000
	Total cholesterol at the end of the experiment	1,885,053.750	1	1,885,053.750	2,548.813	.000
Diet	Number of pounds lost during the experiment period	24.067	1	24.067	7.984	.007
	Total cholesterol at the end of the experiment	21,319.350	1	21,319.350	28.826	.000
Exercise	Number of pounds lost during the experiment period	8.067	1	8.067	2.676	.107
	Total cholesterol at the end of the experiment	5,980.017	1	5,980.017	8.086	.006
Diet* Exercise	Number of pounds lost during the experiment period	101.400	1	101.400	33.640	.000

(*Continued*)

Tests of Between-Subjects Effects (*Continued*)

Source	Dependent Variable	Type III Sum of Squares	df	Mean Square	F	Significance
	Total cholesterol at the end of the experiment	421.350	1	421.350	.570	.454
Error	Number of pounds lost during the experiment period	168.800	56	3.014		
	Total cholesterol at the end of the experiment	41,416.533	56	739.581		
Total	Number of pounds lost during the experiment period	2,344.000	60			
	Total cholesterol at the end of the experiment	1,954,191.000	60			
Corrected total	Number of pounds lost during the experiment period	302.333	59			
	Total cholesterol at the end of the experiment	69,137.250	59			

[a]$R^2 = .442$ (Adjusted $R^2 = .412$).
[b]$R^2 = .401$ (Adjusted $R^2 = .369$).

CHAPTER NINE

Multiple-Choice Concept Review
    1 (c), 2 (d), 3 (c), 4 (b), 5 (a), 6 (d), 7 (d), 8 (c), 9 (b), 10 (a)

Choosing the Best Statistical Test
    1 (h), 2 (b), 3 (a), 4 (e), 5 (h), 6 (b), 7 (g), 8 (d), 9 (g), 10 (c)

Critical Thinking Concept Review

    1. Any hypothesis that compares three or more repeated measures is acceptable.

    2. a. Any study that repeats a measure (eg, blood pressure) on the same person at three or more different points in time.
       b. Any study that has three or more related measures (eg, test anxiety, generalized anxiety, and performance anxiety) taken on the same person at one point in time.

c. Any quasiexperimental or experimental study that uses one case and at least two matched controls.

3. The following table is the completed ANOVA table.

Source of Variation	Sum of Squares	Degrees of Freedom	Mean Square	Variance Ratio (*f*-Test)	*p*-Value
Treatments	8.2	2	4.1		
Blocks	2.5	58			
Error	3.5				
Total	14.2				

Computational Problems

1. **Repeated-measures ANOVA:** The mean anxiety levels (standard deviation) during trials 1 to 4 are as follows: Trial 1: 16.50 (standard deviation, 2.07), Trial 2: 11.50 (standard deviation, 2.43), Trial 3: 7.75 (standard deviation, 2.42), and Trial 4: 4.25 (standard deviation, 2.86). The repeated-measures ANOVA-computed *f*-test is 127.56 with an associated *p*-value of ≤.00. The Bonferroni *post hoc* tests indicate that all four means are significantly different from each other.

    Friedman's ANOVA by rank: The median anxiety levels (interquartile range) during trials 1 to 4 are as follows: Trial 1: 16.00 (interquartile range, 2.00), Trial 2: 12.00 (interquartile range, 3.50), Trial 3: 8.00 (interquartile range, 4.00), and Trial 4: 4.00 (interquartile range, 5.50). The Friedman's ANOVA by rank chi-square is 35.72 with an associated *p*-value of ≤.00.

2. **Repeated-measures ANOVA:** The mean pulse rates (standard deviation) using each machine, equip 1 to equip 3, are as follows: Equip 1: 86.50 (standard deviation, 16.73), Equip 2: 133.11 (standard deviation, 21.75), and Equip 3: 188.56 (standard deviation, 27.75). The repeated-measures ANOVA-computed *f*-test is 633.46 with an associated *p*-value of <.00. The Bonferroni *post hoc* tests indicate that all three means are significantly different from each other.

    Friedman's ANOVA by rank: The median pulse rates (interquartile range) using each machine, Equip 1 to Equip 3, are as follows: Equip 1: 85.50 (interquartile range, 17.75), Equip 2: 131.50 (interquartile range, 34.00), and Equip 3: 185.00 (interquartile range, 39.50). The Friedman's ANOVA by rank chi-square is 36.00 with an associated *p*-value of <.00.

3. **Repeated-measures ANOVA:** The mean scores (standard deviation) after each course are as follows: baseline: 75.7 (standard deviation, 11.03), basic: 78.6 (standard deviation, 10.05), and advanced: 80.23 (standard deviation, 10.20). The repeated-measures ANOVA-computed *f*-test is 83.60 with an associated *p*-value of ≤.00. The Bonferroni *post hoc* tests indicate that all three means are significantly different from each other.

Friedman's ANOVA by rank: The median scores (interquartile range) after each course are as follows: baseline: 76.00 (interquartile range, 14.25), basic: 79.00 (interquartile range, 14.50), and advanced: 81.00 (interquartile range, 14.00). The Friedman's ANOVA by rank chi-square is 52.56 with an associated p-value of $\leq .00$.

4. **Repeated-measures ANOVA:** The mean temperatures (standard deviation) at each time are as follows: baseline: 30.26 (standard deviation, 4.91), Hour 1: 30.27 (standard deviation, 4.90), Hour 2: 30.31 (standard deviation, 4.91), Hour 3: 30.82 (standard deviation, 4.81), and Hour 4: 35.10 (standard deviation, 5.27). The repeated-measures ANOVA-computed f-test is 306.35 with an associated p-value of $\leq .00$. The Bonferroni *post hoc* tests indicate that the baseline, first-hour, and second-hour means are not significantly different from each other but that the third- and fourth-hour means are significantly different from each other and from all the other means.

   Friedman's ANOVA by rank: The median temperatures (interquartile range) at each time are as follows: baseline: 30.00 (interquartile range, 4.70), Hour 1: 29.95 (interquartile range, 4.725), Hour 2: 29.95 (interquartile range, 4.65), Hour 3: 30.50 (interquartile range, 4.325), and Hour 4: 34.30 (interquartile range, 5.20). The Friedman's ANOVA by rank chi-square is 69.14 with an associated p-value of $\leq .00$.

5. **Repeated-measures ANOVA:** The mean 6-second pulse rates (standard deviation) at 5-minute intervals over the course of the operation are as follows: Minute 0: 8.33 (standard deviation, 0.95), Minute 5: 8.70 (standard deviation, 0.90), Minute 10: 7.96 (standard deviation, 0.86), Minute 15: 8.75 (standard deviation, 0.82), Minute 20: 7.97 (standard deviation, 0.68), Minute 25: 8.66 (standard deviation, 1.09), Minute 30: 7.96 (standard deviation, 0.98), and Minute 35: 8.27 (standard deviation, 1.10). The repeated-measures ANOVA computed f-test is 32.47 with an associated p-value of $\leq .000$. The Bonferroni *post hoc* tests indicate that the mean pulse at Minute 0 and Minute 35 are not different from each other; that the mean pulse at Minute 5, Minute 15, and Minute 25 are not significantly different from each other; and that the mean pulse at Minute 10, Minute 20, and Minute 30 are not significantly different from each other. All other means are significantly different from each other.

   Friedman's ANOVA by rank: The median 6-second pulse rates (interquartile range) at 5-minute intervals over the course of the operation are as follows: Minute 0: 8.4 (interquartile range, 1.6), Minute 5: 8.85 (interquartile range, 0.825), Minute 10: 7.20 (interquartile range, 0.825), Minute 15: 8.05 (interquartile range, 0.45), Minute 20: 7.30 (interquartile range, 0.725), Minute 25: 8.80 (interquartile range, 2.10), Minute 30: 7.65 (interquartile range, 1.65), and Minute 35: 7.85 (interquartile range, 2.175). The Friedman's ANOVA by rank chi-square is 122.11 with an associated p-value of $\leq .00$.

CHAPTER TEN

Multiple-Choice Concept Review

1 (c), 2 (d), 3 (a), 4 (d), 5 (b), 6 (d), 7 (a), 8 (a), 9 (d), 10 (d)

Choosing the Best Statistical Test

1 (h), 2 (g), 3 (d), 4 (a), 5 (b), 6 (a), 7 (f), 8 (i)

Computational Problems

1. a. Maternal BMI and birth weight are significantly negatively correlated ($r =$ $-.20$, $p = .013$).
   b. There is no significant interaction between maternal BMI and smoking history in predicting birth weight ($p = .584$).
   c. The Levene's test for homogeneity of variance is not statistically significant ($p = .968$) and therefore ANCOVA can be used. After adjusting for maternal BMI, there is a significant difference in the mean birth weight by smoking status ($p = .028$). Looking at the pairwise comparisons, we can see that current smokers (mean birth weight = 2,802.84 g) have a significantly lower birth weight compared to both past smokers (mean = 3,183.95, $p = .037$) and never smokers (mean = 32,36.91, $p = .011$) while there was no significant difference between never smokers and past smokers ($p = .752$).

2. Age and HITS score are significantly correlated with each other ($r = .20$, $p = .043$); there is no significant interaction between age and history of intimate partner violence ($p = .859$) or age and drug use ($p = .332$); and the Levene's test is not significant ($p = .343$); therefore, ANCOVA can be used. From the ANCOVA results, we see that there is a significant main effect of history of intimate partner violence ($p = .000$) such that those who have experiences partner violence in the past have a higher mean HITS score (12.99) compared to those who have not (11.78) after adjusting for age. Furthermore, the difference in mean HITS score by history of intimate partner violence is larger among drug users compared to nondrug users (interaction between drug use and history of intimate partner violence; $p = .035$).

CHAPTER ELEVEN

Multiple-Choice Concept Review

1 (b), 2 (a), 3 (c), 4 (c), 5 (d), 6 (b), 7 (d), 8 (a), 9 (c), 10 (d)

Choosing the Best Statistical Test

1 (b), 2 (a), 3 (c), 4 (e), 5 (k), 6 (j), 7 (b), 8 (f), 9 (i), 10 (k)

Critical Thinking Concept Review

1. Any hypothesis in which both variables are at least ordinal in measurement scale.

2. a (.468), b (.393), c (.164), d (.367), e (.622)

Computational Problems

1. The mean self-rated health is 3.33 (standard deviation, 1.23), and the mean number of physician visits in the past year is 3.5 (standard deviation, 1.31). The Pearson correlation coefficient (r) is –.67, and the r^2 is .45; the associated p-value is .016. The Spearman correlation coefficient is –.76, and the r^2 is .58; the associated p-value is .004. Although technically the Spearman test of correlation is more appropriate than the Pearson test in this case because the two variables are not normally distributed, the results from the two tests give us the same overall conclusion. The conclusion is that a statistically significant and strong inverse correlation exists between self-rated health and the number of physician visits a person makes in a year. In other words, the number of physician visits a year increases as self-rated health decreases.

2. The mean age is 38.52 years (standard deviation, 14.81), and the mean number of poor mental health days in the past month is 8.33 (standard deviation, 10.14). The Pearson correlation coefficient (r) is .15, and the r^2 is .02; the associated p-value is .520. The Spearman correlation coefficient is .31, and the r^2 is .10; the associated p-value is .168. The Spearman test of correlation is more appropriate than the Pearson test in this case because number of poor mental health days (a count variable) is not precisely normally distributed; however, the results from the two tests give us the same overall conclusion. The conclusion is that no statistically significant relationship exists between age and number of poor mental health days in the past month in this sample of cancer patients.

3. The mean number of physician visits in the past year is 4.13 (standard deviation, 3.0), and the mean satisfaction score is 1.90 (standard deviation, .98), where a higher score means greater satisfaction. The Pearson correlation coefficient (r) is –.12, and the r^2 is .01; the associated p-value is .518. The Spearman correlation coefficient is –.04, and the r^2 is .00; the associated p-value is .827. The difference between the Pearson and Spearman tests is because the assumption of normality is likely violated (number of physician visits and satisfaction score are not normally distributed variables), but this violation does not impact the final conclusion of the two tests. The conclusion is that no statistically significant relationship exists between the number of physician visits in the past year and satisfaction with the physician among women attending the health care center.

4. The mean communication score is 9.08 (standard deviation, 3.35), and the mean satisfaction level is 3.08 (standard deviation, 1.30). The Pearson correlation coefficient (r) is .73, and r^2 is .53; the associated p-value is .000. The Spearman correlation coefficient is .74, and r^2 is 55; the associated p-value is .000. Again, the variables are not precisely normal, but the conclusion from the Pearson and Spearman tests are the same despite the violation of this assumption. The conclusion is that a strong and statistically significant positive relationship exists between communication with the physician and patient satisfaction with the physician.

CHAPTER TWELVE

Multiple-Choice Concept Review
>   1 (c), 2 (d), 3 (d), 4 (b), 5 (c), 6 (d), 7 (c), 8 (d), 9 (a), 10 (b)

Choosing the Best Statistical Test
>   1 (k), 2 (j), 3 (c), 4 (l), 5 (e), 6 (b), 7 (k), 8 (d), 9 (k), 10 (l)

Critical Thinking Concept Review
>   1. a. 2.71
>   b. 3.84
>   c. 6.64
>   d. 5.99
>   e. 13.28

>   2. Any three hypotheses that are testing two nominal variables that are theoretically independent of each other are acceptable here.

>   3. Any three hypotheses that are testing two nominal variables that have a known preexisting relationship (eg, pretest–posttest or matched case–control) are acceptable here.

>   4. The answer will vary by article chosen.

>   5. The answer will vary by article chosen.

Computational Problems
>   1. A total of 44.44% of those who do not use steroid cream have flare-ups compared with 85.7% of those who do use steroid cream. The computed chi-square statistic is 5.723 with a *p*-value of .017. This is statistically significant.

>   2. A total of 88.6% of the rabbits receiving the drug through injection contracted nasal cancer compared with 73.2% of the rabbits who received the drug through oral means. The computed chi-square statistic is 3.90 with an associated *p*-value of .048. This is statistically significant.

>   3. A total of 37.8% of the senior citizens with regular Medicare had an annual examination in the past year compared with 44.9% of the senior citizens with HMO Medicare. The computed chi-square statistic is 4.065 with an associated *p*-value of .044. This is statistically significant.

>   4. A total of 36.1% of people with less than a high school education reported getting regular exercise compared with 33.6% of people with a high school education only and 35.9% of people with at least some college. The computed chi-square statistic is 0.234 with an associated *p*-value of .890. This is not statistically significant.

>   5. Among the 21- to 30-year-old age group, 34.6% report being always happy in the winter, 27.2% report being sometimes happy, and 38.3% report being rarely happy. Among the 31- to 40-year-old age group, 27.4% report being always happy, 32.3%

report being sometimes happy, and 40.3% report being rarely happy. Among the 41- to 50-year-old age group, 27.1% report being always happy, 22.9% report being sometimes happy, and 50.0% report rarely being happy. The computed chi-square statistic is 3.284 with an associated *p*-value of .511. This is not statistically significant.

6. a. A total of 70.6% of those living above 200% of the poverty level have a medical home compared with 61.5% of those living at or below poverty. Because one expected cell count is less than 5, the appropriate Fisher's exact test, with a two-sided *p* = .705, is the appropriate test. The association between being 200% above the poverty level and having a medical home is not statistically significant.

Cross-Tab

| | | | Participant Has a Home for Medical Needs | | |
			No	Yes	Total
Poverty level	Above 200% of poverty level	Count	5	12	17
		Percentage within poverty level	29.4	70.6	100.0
	At or below 200% of poverty level	Count	5	8	13
		Percentage within poverty level	38.5	61.5	100.0
Total		Count	10	20	30
		Percentage within poverty level	33.3	66.7	100.0

Chi-Square Tests

	Value	df	Asymptotic Significance (Two-Sided)	Exact Significance (Two-Sided)	Exact Significance (One-Sided)
Pearson chi-square	.271[a]	1	.602		
Continuity correction[b]	.017	1	.896		
Likelihood ratio	.270	1	.603		
Fisher's exact test				.705	.446
Linear-by-linear Association	.262	1	.608		
Number of valid cases	30				

[a] 1 cell (25.0%) has expected count less than 5. The minimum expected count is 4.33.
[b] Computed only for a 2 × 2 table.

b. A total of 23.5% of those living above 200% poverty level had an unmet need for care in the past year compared with 61.5% of those living at or below 200% of the poverty level. The computed chi-square statistic is 4.434 with an associated *p*-value of .035. This association is statistically significant.

Cross-Tab

			Participant Has Unmet Medical Needs		
			No	Yes	Total
Poverty level	Above 200% of poverty level	Count	13	4	17
		Percentage within poverty level	76.5	23.5	100.0
	At or below 200% of poverty level	Count	5	8	13
		Percentage within poverty level	38.5	61.5	100.0
Total		Count	18	12	30
		Percentage within poverty level	60.0	40.0	100.0

Chi-Square Tests

	Value	df	Asymptotic Significance (Two-Sided)	Exact Significance (Two-Sided)	Exact Significance (One-Sided)
Pearson chi-square	4.434[a]	1	.035		
Continuity correction[b]	2.992	1	.084		
Likelihood ratio	4.507	1	.034		
Fisher's exact test				.061	.042
Linear-by-linear Association	4.287	1	.038		
Number of valid cases	30				

[a]1 cells (.0%) have expected count less than 5. The minimum expected count is 5.20.
[b]Computed only for a 2 × 2 table.

7. Overall, 70.6% of the nurses rated the exam as complete, compared to 47.1% of the "patients." The *p*-value for the McNemar test is .219. The difference in ratings is not statistically significant.
Nurse/patient agreement:

Case Processing Summary

	Cases					
	Valid		Missing		Total	
	N	Percent	*N*	Percent	*N*	Percent
Student nurse assessment of exam completion* Patient assessment of exam completion	17	100.0	0	.0	17	100.0

CHAPTER THIRTEEN

Multiple-Choice Concept Review

1 (d), 2 (a), 3 (c), 4 (b), 5 (a), 6 (b), 7 (c), 8 (c), 9 (d), 10 (b)

Choosing the Best Statistical Test

1 (a), 2 (l), 3 (e), 4 (c), 5 (g), 6 (e), 7 (e), 8 (l), 9 (d), 10 (i)

Critical Thinking Concept Review

1. Any three hypotheses that have a dichotomous dependent variable are acceptable.

2. Any article that uses logistic regression is acceptable.

Computational Problems

1. On a Sports Team	Smokes		Row Totals
	Yes	No	
No	270	500	770
Yes	50	430	480
Total	320	930	1,250

Probabilities:

Of smoking when not on team	270/770 = 0.35
Of not smoking when not on team	500/770 = 0.65
Of smoking when on team	50/480 = 0.10
Of not smoking when on team	430/480 = 0.90

Odds:

Of smoking when not on team	0.35/0.65 = 0.54
Of smoking when on team	0.10/0.90 = 0.11
Odds ratio:	0.54/0.11 = 4.91

Risks:

Of smoking when not on team	270/770 = 0.35
Of smoking when on team	50/480 = 0.10
Relative risk:	0.35/0.10 = 3.5

The odds of smoking among those not on a team are 4.91 times higher than that of those on a team. The risk of smoking among those not on a team is 3.5 times higher than that of those on a sports team.

2. a. The odds of trying to lose weight in the past year for women are 2.06 times that of men after adjusting for BMI. This difference in odds is statistically significant ($p = .000$).

   b. For each unit increase in BMI, the odds of trying to lose weight in the past year increases by 1.14 times. This difference in odds is statistically significant ($p = .000$).

   c. For the Hosmer and Lemeshow test, $p = .055$. This is not significant at the $\alpha = .05$ level, and, therefore, we do not reject the null hypothesis that our model is a good fit (although the p-value is borderline).

CHAPTER FOURTEEN

Multiple-Choice Concept Review

1 (c), 2 (b), 3 (a), 4 (d), 5 (b), 6 (d), 7 (d), 8 (b), 9 (d), 10 (b)

Choosing the Best Statistical Test

1 (e), 2 (g), 3 (a or g), 4 (e), 5 (b), 6 (g or k), 7 (g), 8 (c), 9 (j), 10 (l)

Critical Thinking Concept Review

1. Any three hypotheses that have a ratio-level dependent variable and more than one independent variable are acceptable.

Computational Problems

1. a. 2.75
   b. −3.27
   c. 78.19

2. a. BMI is somewhat right skewed. After taking the natural log, it seems more normal, so we will use the log-transformed BMI as the outcome in the linear regression model.

b. The model explains 9.0% of the variance of BMI and this is statistically significant ($p = .000$). Eating out in restaurants frequently is not significantly associated with BMI ($p = .512$). However, gender, age, and black race (compared to white) are all significantly positively associated with BMI.

c. Predicted $\ln(\text{BMI}) = 3.136 - .015(0) + .016(1) + .003(25) + .087(0) - .062(0) + .058(0) = 3.136 + .016 + .075 = 3.227$; predicted BMI $= e^{3.227} = 25.2$.

CHAPTER FIFTEEN

Multiple-Choice Concept Review

1 (d), 2 (c), 3 (d), 4 (c), 5 (d), 6 (a, c, d),7 (a), 8 (d), 9 (d), 10 (c)

Computational Problem

We reran the principal components factor analysis with Varimax rotation, again using SPSS, but this time we forced the number of factors to 2. We do this by selecting "Fixed number of factors" under "Extract" in the Extraction pop-up box. "Factors to extract" is 2. Results of our analysis are contained in Exercise Figure 15-1. You can compare your results with ours. You may have selected different rotation and extraction methods, or your display may look different from ours if you selected different options for presentation or if you used different statistical software. To save space, we show here only Communalities, Total Variance Explained, and Rotated Component Matrix. The KMO and Bartlett's test and the scree plot would be the same as shown in Exercise Figure 15-1.

We see that first two factors together account for 49.1% of the variance between items. Variances explained by the two rotated factors are 8.2 and 6.5, respectively. The first factor contains 16 of the 17 questions associated with the life purpose and satisfaction scale. Only one item from the self-confidence scale (item 22—"*respond*

Communalities

	Initial	Extraction
energy level	1.000	.353
reaction to pressure	1.000	.477
characterization of life as a whole	1.000	.561
daily activities	1.000	.469
experience anxiety	1.000	.523
expectations of every day	1.000	.318
fearful	1.000	.487
think deeply about life	1.000	.500
productivity of life	1.000	.530
making mistakes	1.000	.415
value of work	1.000	.510

EXERCISE FIGURE 15-1 Factors analysis of IPA items. (*Continued*)

Communalities

	Initial	Extraction
wishing I was different	1.000	.521
defined goals for life	1.000	.498
worrying that bad things will happen	1.000	.426
concentration during stress	1.000	.512
standing up for myself	1.000	.369
adequacy in most situations	1.000	.453
frustration to problems	1.000	.530
sad things	1.000	.510
worthwhile life	1.000	.606
satisfaction of present life	1.000	.618
respond positively in difficult situations	1.000	.543
joy in heart	1.000	.610
when relaxing	1.000	.444
trapped by life	1.000	.553
panic in frightening situations	1.000	.593
thinking about past	1.000	.376
feeling loved	1.000	.533
worry about future	1.000	.314
thinking about problems	1.000	.588

Extraction Method: Principal component analysis.

Total Variance Explained

Component	Initial Eigenvalues			Extraction Sums of Squared Loadings			Rotation Sums of Squared Loadings		
	Total	% of Variance	Cumulative %	Total	% of Variance	Cumulative %	Total	% of Variance	Cumulative %
1	12.633	42.110	42.110	12.633	42.110	42.110	8.235	27.451	27.451
2	2.107	7.023	49.133	2.107	7.023	49.133	6.504	21.681	49.133
3	1.233	4.111	53.243						
4	1.176	3.921	57.164						
5	.947	3.158	60.322						
6	.843	2.811	63.134						
7	.777	2.592	65.725						

EXERCISE FIGURE 15-1 (Continued)

Total Variance Explained

Component	Initial Eigenvalues			Extraction Sums of Squared Loadings			Rotation Sums of Squared Loadings		
	Total	% of Variance	Cumulative %	Total	% of Variance	Cumulative %	Total	% of Variance	Cumulative %
8	.714	2.379	68.104						
9	.674	2.246	70.350						
10	.648	2.159	72.509						
11	.630	2.101	74.610						
12	.573	1.909	76.519						
13	.536	1.788	78.307						
14	.534	1.780	80.086						
15	.513	1.710	81.796						
16	.475	1.582	83.378						
17	.450	1.500	84.878						
18	.446	1.486	86.364						
19	.425	1.417	87.781						
20	.406	1.354	89.134						
21	.396	1.321	90.456						
22	.376	1.254	91.709						
23	.373	1.242	92.952						
24	.342	1.142	94.093						
25	.335	1.116	95.210						
26	.323	1.077	96.287						
27	.295	.982	97.269						
28	.293	.977	98.246						
29	.273	.909	99.155						
30	.254	.845	100.000						

Extraction Method: Principal component analysis.

Rotated Component Matrix[a]

	Component	
	1	2
satisfaction of present life	.741	.261
worthwhile life	.730	.271
joy in heart	.710	.325

EXERCISE FIGURE 15-1   *(Continued)*

Rotated Component Matrix[a]

	Component	
	1	2
productivity of life	.701	.196
characterization of life as a whole	.696	.275
value of work	.689	.187
think deeply about life	.687	.170
defined goals for life	.682	.180
feeling loved	.680	.265
trapped by life	.666	.331
daily activities	.660	.183
thinking about problems	.622	.448
wishing I was different	.581	.428
respond positively in difficult situations	.562	.476
expectations of every day	.536	.174
energy level	.478	.353
thinking about past	.464	.400
panic in frightening situations	.161	.753
experience anxiety	.213	.691
reaction to pressure	.109	.682
concentration during stress	.218	.682
frustration to problems	.312	.658
fearful	.248	.652
worrying that bad things will happen	.128	.640
sad things	.418	.579
making mistakes	.312	.563
adequacy in most situations	.400	.541
standing up for myself	.305	.525
when relaxing	.442	.498
worry about future	.346	.441

Extraction Method: Principal component analysis. Rotation Method: Varimax with Kaiser Normalization.
[a] Rotation converged in 3 iterations.

positively in most situations") also loaded on this scale. This item also had a slightly smaller but still substantial loading (.48) on Factor 2. The second factor contains 12 of the 13 self-confidence items plus one item from the life purpose and satisfaction scale (item 19—*"sad things"*). This item also had a substantial loading (.42) on Factor 1. Thus, this analysis generally supported the structure proposed by the authors of the scale. The scree plot also suggests a potential for a two-factor solution, although some might argue that the high eigenvalue of the first factor, as well as multiple loadings of some items, indicates a unidimensional scale. Conceptually, does the two-factor solution make good sense to you? Which provides a better conceptual fit—this two factor solution or the four-factor solution presented previously? Helping us to see how the items of an instrument fit together is among the most important purposes of this statistical technique.

CHAPTER SIXTEEN

Multiple-Choice Concept Review

1 (b), 2(a), 3(a), 4(d), 5(d), 6(b), 7(d), 8(b), 9(c), 10 (b)

Critical Thinking Concept Review

1. Remember that endogenous variables have at least one arrow coming into them, whereas exogenous variables (or fully exogenous variables) have no arrows coming into them. You will need one regression analysis for each endogenous variable. This endogenous variable will be the dependent variable in the regression analysis needed to estimate the paths that have an arrow coming into this endogenous variable.

2. Using the research question you developed for Problem 1, identify the steps you would take to conduct a path analysis assuming that you have used regression analysis to identify which variables from a theoretical framework are significantly related to the dependent variable of interest. As you do not have actual results of this regression analysis, use hypothetical values.

3. To investigate whether your model may be a misspecified model, you would need to use Wright's (1934) formula for the components of the correlation between a particular independent variable and the dependent variable being equal to the sum of the direct, indirect, and noncausal components. If the magnitude of the sum of the components is greater than the correlation, this argues that the model is misspecified. Keep in mind that rounding error may lead to small differences between the sum and the actual correlation (eg, one hundredth of a point). Misspecification would be associated with larger differences and is easy to detect if you calculate direct, indirect, and noncausal components for a model in which paths that are small in magnitude are retained instead of being dropped (eg, $p_{y.x} < |.10|$). Measurement error would make your correlation and path coefficients smaller—it would underestimate the relationship between X and Y.

CHAPTER SEVENTEEN

Multiple-Choice Concept Review
1 (a), 2 (c), 3 (b), 4 (d), 5(b), 6 (a), 7 (b), 8 (c), 9 (d), 10 (a)

Critical Thinking Concept Review and Computational Problem

The model fit statistics for the model in Exercise Figure 17-1 are not acceptable. The goodness-of-fit index is equal to .89 and the comparative fit index is equal to .76. Note also that the root mean square error of approximation (RMSEA) is greater than .10. These results argue for this model being respecified. The authors did this and after testing three more models, they arrived at the model in Exercise Figure 17-2. The fit statistics for this model argue that it is a very good fit to the data. Thus, these statistics argue against the model needing to be respecified and reanalyzed. However, look at the variables in the model. Do you see any variables that are categorical? There is one variable that is. Given this and the lack of effect this variable has on other variables in the model, it makes sense to rerun the analyses without this variable. The fit statistics should not change, but by meeting the statistical assumptions, you will get better estimates of the parameters in the model.

	Degrees of Freedom	Chi-Square (χ^2)	p-Value	Goodness of Fit	Nonnormed Fit	Comparative Fit	RMSEA
Full model fit	32	272.99	<.01	.89	.33	.76	.18

Exercise Figure 17-1. From Bennett, J. A., Stewart, A. L., Kayser-Jones, J., & Glaser, D. (2002). The mediating effect of pain and fatigue on level of functioning in older adults. *Nursing Research, 51*(4), 259.

	Degrees of Freedom	Chi-Square (χ^2)	p-Value	Goodness of Fit	Nonnormed Fit	Comparative Fit	RMSEA
Full model fit	27	30.25	.30	.98	.99	.99	.02

EXERCISE FIGURE 17-2. From Bennett, J. A., Stewart, A. L., Kayser-Jones, J., & Glaser, D. (2002). The mediating effect of pain and fatigue on level of functioning in older adults. *Nursing Research, 51*(4), 262.

Entering Data into SPSS

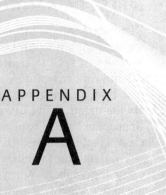

APPENDIX

A

Emily Greene

OBJECTIVES

After studying this appendix, you should be able to:

1. Create an SPSS database, or spreadsheet, into which data can be entered.
2. Enter data directly into SPSS completely and correctly.
3. Import data sets into SPSS from Excel and SAS files.

USING SPSS

Throughout this text, we use data and data analysis to answer various health-related questions. Statistical analysis can be a helpful and powerful tool, but before any analysis, even simple frequencies can be run, data must first be entered into a database. In this text, we use a software package called IBM SPSS. SPSS stands for "Statistical Program for the Social Sciences," and it was acquired by IBM in 2009. You can learn more about IBM SPSS at http://www.spss.com/.

When you open SPSS, there are three "windows": the syntax window, the output window,

and the data editor window. In this tutorial, we focus on the data editor window. This is the place where you open or create the database, in the form of a spreadsheet, which SPSS will use to access the data. Once you have entered your data into SPSS or opened an already created database, be it an SPSS database or a database created using some other software, you are ready to start analyzing your data in SPSS.

What follows is a brief introduction to database design and data entry in SPSS. There are two routes of data entry into SPSS: (1) direct data entry and (2) importing from other programs.

DIRECT DATA ENTRY

Direct data entry is the most basic way of entering data into SPSS. In order to enter the data, we will first need to create a database with one column for each variable and one row for each case that we are going to enter. After we create the database, we can enter the data into it. Remember to save your work often, even when creating and labeling your variables.

The data editor window is the place where we create the database. When we first open SPSS, we are in this window. This window has two tabs at the bottom of the screen: data view and variable view. In order to create the database and define its format (e.g., specify the names, format, and labels of variables), we must be in the variable view (as shown in Fig. A-1). The first step in creating the database is to define each variable.

Defining Variables in the Variable View

There are several columns to fill in to define each variable for SPSS. Figure A-2 shows an example with the variable "Gender" defined.

1. **Name:** This column is for the name of the variable that SPSS will use. It should be short and descriptive. A few pointers on variable names:

- *Keep variable names short and straightforward.*
  If the data come from a survey, create names that correspond to the survey questions. For example, if the survey question number is 15, then naming the variable Q15 makes sense. Alternately, short descriptive variable names work too (e.g., "gender" and "age").
- *Confine your variable name to a single word.*
  SPSS does not allow blank spaces or hyphens in variable names. If the variable name must contain multiple words, each word must be separated by an underscore (i.e., _). For example, if you are inputting depression scores, the best variable name would be depression, but you could also name the variable "depression_score."
- *Variable names must begin with a letter.*
  SPSS does not allow you to begin a variable name with a number or

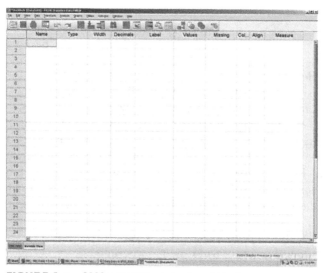

FIGURE A-1 SPSS data editor window in variable view.

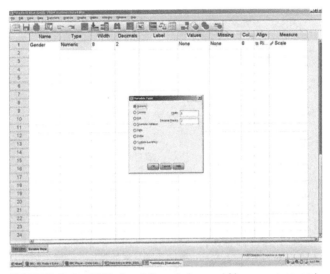

FIGURE A-2 SPSS data editor window—variable name, type, and width.

symbol. Therefore, if you are naming the variables based on question number in a survey, you have to put a letter before the question number (e.g., "Q15" rather than just "15").

2. **Type:** Variable type tells SPSS what kind of data we will enter for the variable (Fig. A-2). Variable types include numeric, which can be a number such as age, or the numeric codes assigned to represent categories of a categorical variables (e.g., 0 = male and 1 = female), date, which can be in various formats (e.g., mm/dd/yyyy or dd/mm/yyyy), or string, which means text. While this may seem trivial, it is not. Statistical tests can only be performed on numbers; therefore, we often assign numeric codes to represent nonnumeric data (e.g., gender) so that we can use statistical tests to analyze these data. Unless you have some compelling reason to do otherwise, it is best to use all numbers for all coded responses and to define the type as "numeric."

3. **Width:** Here is where we set the maximum number of spaces allocated to the variable (Fig. A-2). For example, a gender variable (0 = male and 1 = female) needs only a width of 1, while an age variable may need a width up to 3 to cover an age range of 0 to 100 years. If any possible values include negative numbers, remember that the negative sign will require a space, so –1 would need a width of 2.

4. **Decimal:** Similar to width above, this allows us to set the maximum number of decimal places SPSS will allow us to enter (Fig. A-2). The default value for a numeric variable is 2, but it is upwardly/downwardly adjustable. Some variables will not need any decimals (e.g., gender). Remember when setting the width that the decimal point will need a space too.

5. **Label:** Variable labels are used to describe the variable (Fig. A-3). The labels are for the convenience of the researcher and are not used by the program to refer to the variable. For example, if survey question for Q15 is annual income, the variable label for Q15 could be "Annual Income." Labels can help the researcher to remember what each question is about. SPSS has an

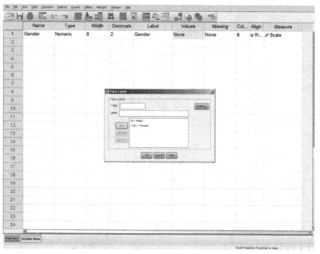

FIGURE A-3 SPSS data editor window—value labels.

option that allows you to have the labels and values (below) appear on the printout.

6. **Values:** This column allows us to provide text labels for specific numeric values that represent categories of a variable (Fig. A-3). For example, if gender is coded 0 and 1, we can label these values as 0 = male and 1 = female. For variables in which the data are an actual number (e.g., age), we do not need to enter anything under values. This is also an aid to the researcher and will appear on the printout.

7. **Missing:** This is largely a more advanced function, so for most purposes, just make sure it says "none." If, however, your survey allows for user-defined missing data ("don't know" or "refuse to answer," etc.), the missing dialogue allows you to tell SPSS which values to code as missing. Commonly used missing codes in surveys are –99, 998, 999, but this is not an exhaustive list. If, in the income variable (Q15), there is a refuse to answer option that you code as –99, you can specify –99 as a discrete missing value in the missing dialogue box (Fig. A-4).

8. **Columns:** This tells us how many columns the variable will appear across when we look at it. The default, 8, is fine to leave as is.

9. **Align:** This is just alignment of the variable and whatever the default setting is can be left. Changing this will have no effect of data entry or analysis.

10. **Measure:** Throughout the text, we have referred to data by measure type: scale, nominal, ordinal, etc. SPSS allows us to set the variable type, but it can make things unnecessarily complicated. As long as the variable type is *numeric*, it is fine to leave the measure at the default setting.

11. **Role:** Again, we leave this at the default of input.

Entering Data Into the Database

Once you have set up your database in the variable view of the data editor, it is time to start entering data. Click on the Data view tab to move from the variable window to the data window and begin adding data. Simply click in a cell and enter

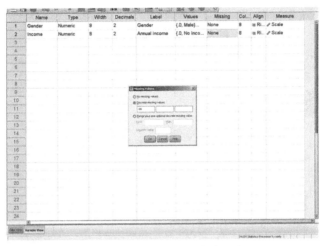

FIGURE A-4   SPSS data editor window—missing values.

the appropriate data in that cell before moving to the next. Note that each row in the spreadsheet represents a different study participant while each column represents a different variable. Figure A-5 shows data entry for the gender and income variables for 20 participants in a study.

Entering data by hand can be time-consuming and prone to error. Just set up your database and take your time entering data. Be sure to check over your data before you begin any analysis. Once your data are entered, you can view them either as the numeric data themselves, in which case all coded categorical variables will show the numeric code, or by label, in which case you will see the categories assigned to any numeric codes that you defined under Value Labels. If you would like to change the view, click on View from the upper left-hand side of the menu and then select Value Labels (Fig. A-6).

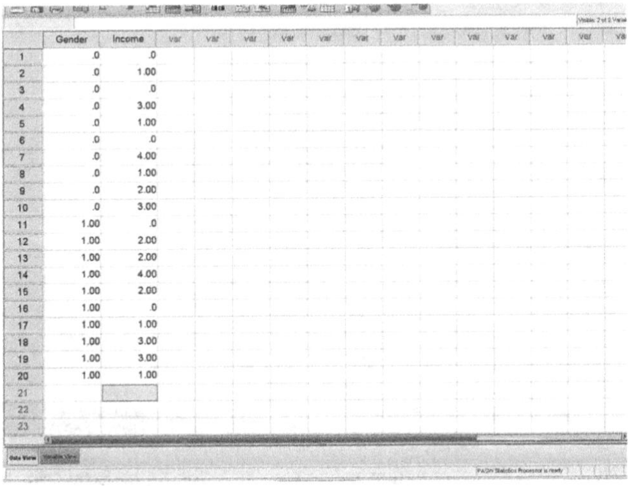

FIGURE A-5   Data entry example.

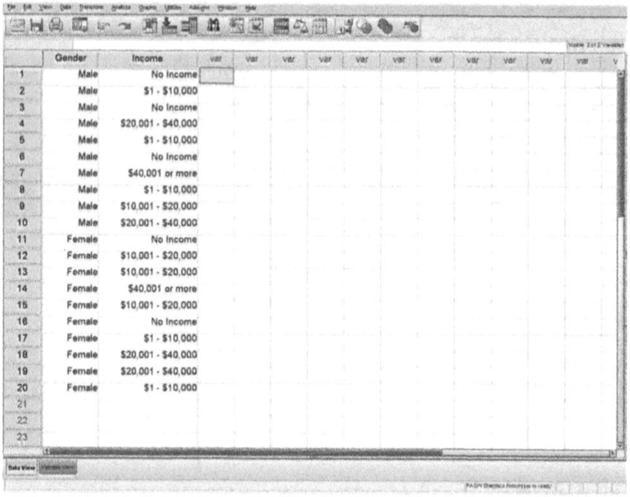

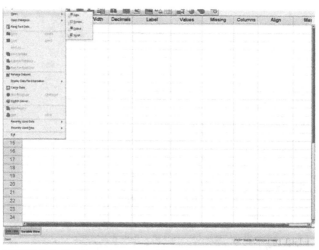

FIGURE A-6 Viewing data with value labels.

IMPORTING DATA

Data already entered into a database created in different software (e.g., Excel, SAS, STATA) can also be used by SPSS. While this saves time because data do not need to be entered manually, there are a few things that must be considered. The first thing is to open the data set of interest using SPSS.

In many cases, we can open the database in the same way you would open an SPSS database. The difference is that we need to follow the SPSS prompts to pull the data into SPSS from its original format. If we are opening an Excel database, we would follow the procedure as in Figs. A-7 to A-11.

FIGURE A-7 Step 1 in opening Excel files in SPSS (the Excel data file is called survey01.xls).

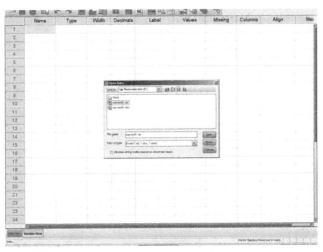

FIGURE A-8   Step 2 in opening Excel files in SPSS.

Select the data file you wish to open and click "Open." This will open a dialogue box with options for importing the Excel file.

Make sure that "read variable names from the first row of data" is checked if the Excel file contains variable names in the first row. Further, if the Excel file has multiple worksheets, select the one you want to open. Then click "ok."

Once the SPSS data editor is open, you will notice that the variable names are present, but much of the information discussed above (e.g., label, values) are empty. You will need to fill in this information just as you would with direct data entry. Once you have completed this, be sure to name your file and save it as an SPSS data set (go to File and select "Save As").

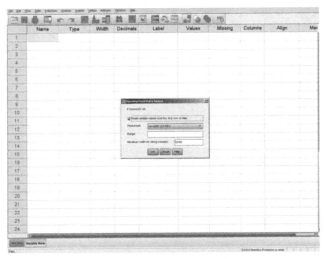

FIGURE A-9   Step 3 in opening Excel files in SPSS.

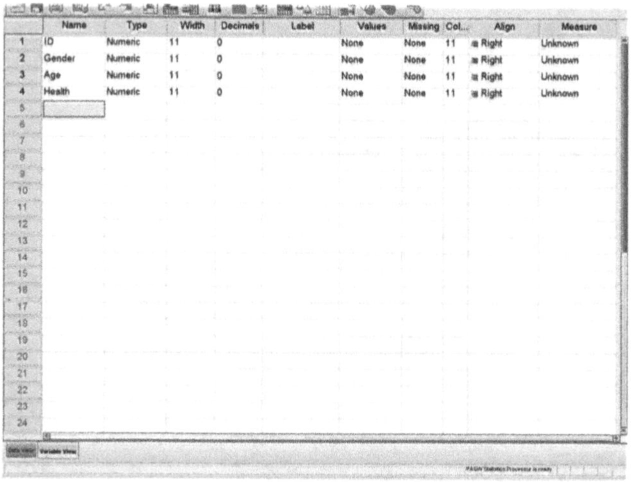

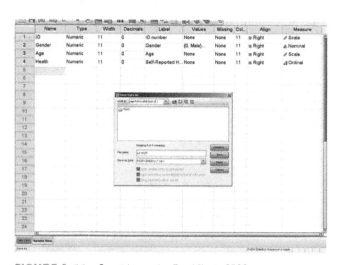

FIGURE A-10 Step 4 in opening Excel files in SPSS.

If we are opening an SAS data file, we would follow basically the same procedure as above, except that we would select SAS as the File Type. For example, the same survey data above have been saved as an SAS file with the .sas-7bdat file extension (note SAS files can also be identified as an .xpt file type).

FIGURE A-11 Step 5 in opening Excel files in SPSS.

Percent of Total Area of Normal Curve Between a z-Score and the Mean

z	0.00	0.01	0.02	0.03	0.04	0.05	0.06	0.07	0.08	0.09
0.0	00.00	00.40	00.80	01.20	01.60	01.99	02.39	02.79	03.19	03.59
0.1	03.98	04.38	04.78	05.17	05.57	05.96	06.36	06.75	07.14	07.53
0.2	07.93	08.32	08.71	09.10	09.48	09.87	10.26	10.64	11.03	11.41
0.3	11.79	12.17	12.55	12.93	13.31	13.68	14.06	14.43	14.80	15.17
0.4	15.54	15.91	16.28	16.64	17.00	17.36	17.72	18.08	18.44	18.79
0.5	19.15	19.50	19.85	20.19	20.54	20.88	21.23	21.57	21.90	22.24
0.6	22.57	22.91	23.24	23.57	23.89	24.22	24.54	24.86	25.17	25.49
0.7	25.80	26.11	26.42	26.73	27.04	27.34	27.64	27.94	28.23	28.52
0.8	28.81	29.10	29.39	29.67	29.95	30.23	30.51	30.78	31.06	31.33
0.9	31.59	31.86	32.12	32.38	32.64	32.90	33.15	33.40	33.65	33.89
1.0	34.13	34.38	34.61	34.85	35.08	35.31	35.54	35.77	35.99	36.21
1.1	36.43	36.65	36.86	37.08	37.29	37.49	37.70	37.90	38.10	38.30
1.2	38.49	38.69	38.88	39.07	39.25	39.44	39.62	39.80	39.97	40.15
1.3	40.32	40.49	40.66	40.82	40.99	41.15	41.31	41.47	41.62	41.77
1.4	41.92	42.07	42.22	42.36	42.51	42.65	42.79	42.92	43.06	43.19
1.5	43.32	43.45	43.57	43.70	43.83	43.94	44.06	44.18	44.29	44.41
1.6	44.52	44.63	44.74	44.84	44.95	45.05	45.15	45.25	45.35	45.45
1.7	45.54	45.64	45.73	45.82	45.91	45.99	46.08	46.16	46.25	46.33
1.8	46.41	46.49	46.56	46.64	46.71	46.78	46.86	46.93	46.99	47.06
1.9	47.13	47.19	47.26	47.32	47.38	47.44	47.50	47.56	47.61	47.67
2.0	47.72	47.78	47.83	47.88	47.93	47.98	48.03	48.08	48.12	48.17

(Continued)

z	0.00	0.01	0.02	0.03	0.04	0.05	0.06	0.07	0.08	0.09
2.1	48.21	48.26	48.30	48.34	48.38	48.42	48.46	48.50	48.54	48.57
2.2	48.61	48.64	48.68	48.71	48.75	48.78	48.81	48.84	48.87	48.90
2.3	48.93	48.96	48.98	49.01	49.04	49.06	49.09	49.11	49.13	49.16
2.4	49.18	49.20	49.22	49.25	49.27	49.29	49.31	49.32	49.34	49.36
2.5	49.38	49.40	49.41	49.43	49.45	49.46	49.48	49.49	49.51	49.52
2.6	49.53	49.55	49.56	49.57	49.59	49.60	49.61	49.62	49.63	49.64
2.7	49.65	49.66	49.67	49.68	49.69	49.70	49.71	49.72	49.73	49.74
2.8	49.74	49.75	49.76	49.77	49.77	49.78	49.79	49.79	49.80	49.81
2.9	49.81	49.82	49.82	49.83	49.84	49.84	49.85	49.85	49.86	49.86
3.0	49.87									
3.5	49.98									
4.0	49.997									
5.0	49.99997									

From Hald, A. (1952). *Statistical tables and formulas*. New York, NY: John Wiley & Sons. (Table 1).

Distribution of *t*

	Level of Significance for One-Tailed Test					
	0.10	0.05	0.025	0.01	0.005	0.0005
	Level of Significance for Two-Tailed Test					
df	0.20	0.10	0.05	0.02	0.01	0.001
1	3.078	6.314	12.706	31.821	63.657	636.619
2	1.886	2.920	4.303	6.965	9.925	31.598
3	1.638	2.353	3.182	4.541	5.841	12.941
4	1.533	2.132	2.776	3.747	4.604	8.610
5	1.476	2.015	2.571	3.365	4.032	6.859
6	1.440	1.943	2.447	3.143	3.707	5.959
7	1.415	1.895	2.365	2.998	3.499	5.405
8	1.397	1.860	2.306	2.896	3.355	5.041
9	1.383	1.833	2.262	2.821	3.250	4.781
10	1.372	1.812	2.228	2.764	3.169	4.587
11	1.363	1.796	2.201	2.718	3.106	4.437
12	1.356	1.782	2.179	2.681	3.055	4.318
13	1.350	1.771	2.160	2.650	3.012	4.221
14	1.345	1.761	2.145	2.624	2.977	4.140
15	1.341	1.753	2.131	2.602	2.947	4.073
16	1.337	1.746	2.120	2.583	2.921	4.015
17	1.333	1.740	2.110	2.567	2.898	3.965
18	1.330	1.734	2.101	2.552	2.878	3.922

(Continued)

	Level of Significance for One-Tailed Test					
	0.10	0.05	0.025	0.01	0.005	0.0005
	Level of Significance for Two-Tailed Test					
df	0.20	0.10	0.05	0.02	0.01	0.001
19	1.328	1.729	2.093	2.539	2.861	3.883
20	1.325	1.725	2.086	2.528	2.845	3.850
21	1.323	1.721	2.080	2.518	2.831	3.819
22	1.321	1.717	2.074	2.508	2.819	3.792
23	1.319	1.714	2.069	2.500	2.807	3.767
24	1.318	1.711	2.064	2.492	2.797	3.745
25	1.316	1.708	2.060	3.485	2.787	3.725
26	1.315	1.706	2.056	2.479	2.779	3.707
27	1.314	1.703	2.052	2.473	2.771	3.690
28	1.313	1.701	2.048	2.467	2.763	3.674
29	1.311	1.699	2.045	2.462	2.756	3.659
30	1.310	1.697	2.042	2.457	2.750	3.646
40	1.303	1.684	2.021	2.423	2.704	3.551
60	1.296	1.671	2.000	2.390	2.660	3.460
120	1.289	1.658	1.980	2.358	2.617	3.373
∞	1.282	1.645	1.960	2.326	2.576	3.291

From Fisher, R. A. (1970). *Statistical methods for research workers* (14th ed.). Darien, CT: Hafner Publishing. (Table IV, p. 176).

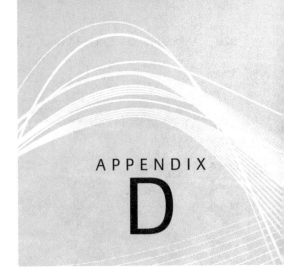

Critical Values of the U-Statistic

Probability of obtaining a U smaller than that tabulated in comparing two samples of size n and m

	Level of Significance for the One-Tailed Test ≤				
	.10	.05	.025	.01	.005
	Level of Significance for the Two-Tailed Test ≤				
n = # in sample #1	.20	.10	.05	.02	.01
m = # in sample 2					
n = 3					
m = 2	0	—	—	—	—
m = 3	1	0	—	—	—
n = 4					
m = 2	0	—	—	—	—
m = 3	1	0	—	—	—
m = 4	3	1	0	—	—
n = 5					
m = 2	1	0	—	—	—
m = 3	2	1	0	—	—
m = 4	4	2	1	0	—
m = 5	5	4	2	1	0
n = 6					
m = 2	1	0	—	—	—
m = 3	3	2	1	—	—

(Continued)

	Level of Significance for the One-Tailed Test $\leq$				
	.10	.05	.025	.01	.005
	Level of Significance for the Two-Tailed Test $\leq$				
n = # in sample #1	.20	.10	.05	.02	.01
m = # in sample 2					
m = 4	5	3	2	1	0
m = 5	7	5	3	2	1
m = 6	9	7	5	3	2
n = 7	.10	.05	.025	.01	.005
m = 2	1	0	—	—	—
m = 3	4	2	1	0	—
m = 4	6	4	3	1	0
m = 5	8	6	5	3	2
m = 6	11	8	6	4	3
m = 7	13	11	8	6	4
n = 8					
m = 2	2	1	0	—	—
m = 3	5	3	2	0	—
m = 4	7	5	4	2	1
m = 5	10	8	6	4	3
m = 6	13	10	8	6	4
m = 7	16	13	10	8	6
m = 8	19	15	13	10	8

Adapted from Mann, H. B., & Whitney, D. R. (1947). On a test of whether one of two random variables is stochastically larger than the other. *The Annals of Mathematical Statistics, 18*(1), 50–60.

Critical Values of the Wilcoxon Signed-Rank Statistic

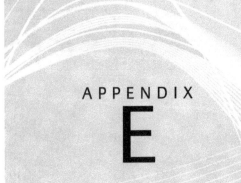

Where T *is the largest integer value such that* $Pr[T \, |N] \leq \alpha_t$

	Level of Significance for the One-Tailed Test				
	.10	.05	.025	.01	.005
	Level of Significance for the Two-Tailed Test				
n	.20	.10	.05	.02	.01
5	2	0	—	—	—
6	3	2	0	—	—
7	5	3	2	0	—
8	8	5	3	1	0
9	10	8	5	3	1
10	14	10	8	5	3
11	17	13	10	7	5
12	21	17	13	9	7
13	26	21	17	12	9
14	31	25	21	15	12
15	36	30	25	19	15
16	42	35	29	23	19
17	48	41	34	27	23
18	55	47	40	32	27
19	62	53	46	37	32
20	69	60	52	43	37

(Continued)

	Level of Significance for the One-Tailed Test				
	.10	.05	.025	.01	.005
	Level of Significance for the Two-Tailed Test				
n	.20	.10	.05	.02	.01
21	77	67	58	49	42
22	81	75	65	55	48
23	94	83	73	62	54
24	104	91	81	69	61
25	113	100	89	76	68
26	124	110	98	84	75
27	134	119	107	92	83
28	145	130	116	101	91
29	157	140	126	110	100
30	169	151	137	120	109

Critical values for $\alpha \leq .10$ (one-tailed) have been obtained from Daniel W. W. (2005). *Biostatistics*. Hoboken, NJ: Wiley & Sons. Adapted from McCornack, R. L. (1965). Extended tables of the Wilcoxon matched pair signed rank statistic. *Journal of the American Statistical Association, 60*(311), 864–871.

The 5% and 1% Points for the Distribution of F

n₁ Degrees of Freedom (For Greater Mean Square)ᵃ

n_2^b	1	2	3	4	5	6	7	8	9	10	11	12
1	161	200	216	225	230	234	237	239	241	242	243	244
	4,052	4,999	5,403	5,625	5,764	5,859	5,928	5,981	6,022	6,056	6,082	6,106
2	18.51	19.00	19.16	19.25	19.30	19.33	19.36	19.37	19.38	19.39	19.40	19.41
	98.49	99.00	99.17	99.25	99.30	99.33	99.34	99.36	99.38	99.40	99.41	99.42
3	10.13	9.55	9.38	9.12	9.01	8.94	8.88	8.84	8.81	8.78	8.76	8.74
	34.12	30.82	29.46	28.71	28.47	27.91	27.67	27.49	27.34	27.23	27.13	27.05
4	7.71	6.94	6.59	6.39	6.26	6.16	6.09	6.04	6.00	5.96	5.93	5.91
	21.20	18.00	16.69	15.98	15.52	15.21	14.98	14.80	14.66	14.54	14.45	14.37
5	6.61	5.79	5.41	5.19	5.05	4.95	4.88	4.82	4.78	4.74	4.70	4.68
	16.26	13.27	12.06	11.39	10.97	10.67	10.45	10.27	10.15	10.05	9.96	9.89
6	5.99	5.14	4.76	4.53	4.39	4.28	4.21	4.15	4.10	4.06	4.03	4.00
	13.74	10.92	9.78	9.15	8.75	8.47	8.26	8.10	7.98	7.87	7.79	7.72
7	5.59	4.74	4.35	4.12	3.97	3.87	3.79	3.73	3.68	3.63	3.60	3.57
	12.25	9.55	8.45	7.85	7.46	7.19	7.00	6.84	6.71	6.62	6.54	6.47
8	5.32	4.46	4.07	3.84	3.69	3.58	3.50	3.44	3.39	3.34	3.31	3.28
	11.26	8.65	7.59	7.01	6.63	6.37	6.19	6.03	5.91	5.82	5.74	5.67
9	5.12	4.26	3.86	3.63	3.48	3.37	3.29	3.23	3.18	3.13	3.10	3.07
	10.56	8.02	6.99	6.42	6.06	5.80	5.62	5.47	5.35	5.26	5.18	5.11
10	4.96	4.10	3.71	3.48	3.33	3.22	3.14	3.07	3.02	2.97	2.94	2.91
	10.04	7.56	6.55	5.99	5.64	5.39	5.21	5.06	4.95	4.85	4.78	4.71
11	4.84	3.98	3.59	3.36	3.20	3.09	3.01	2.95	2.90	2.86	2.82	2.79
	9.65	7.20	6.22	5.67	5.32	5.07	4.88	4.74	4.63	4.54	4.46	4.40
12	4.75	3.88	3.49	3.26	3.11	3.00	2.92	2.85	2.80	2.76	2.72	2.69
	9.33	6.93	5.95	5.41	5.06	4.82	4.65	4.50	4.39	4.30	4.22	4.16
13	4.67	3.80	3.41	3.18	3.02	2.92	2.84	2.77	2.72	2.67	2.63	2.60
	9.07	6.70	5.74	5.20	4.86	4.62	4.44	4.30	4.19	4.10	4.02	3.96
14	4.60	3.74	3.34	3.11	2.96	2.85	2.77	2.70	2.65	2.60	2.56	2.53
	8.86	6.51	5.56	5.03	4.69	4.46	4.28	4.14	4.03	3.94	3.86	3.80
15	4.54	3.68	3.29	3.06	2.90	2.79	2.70	2.64	2.59	2.55	2.51	2.48
	8.68	6.36	5.42	4.89	4.56	4.32	4.14	4.00	3.89	3.80	3.73	3.67
16	4.49	3.63	3.24	3.01	2.85	2.74	2.66	2.59	2.54	2.49	2.45	2.42
	8.53	6.23	5.29	4.77	4.44	4.20	4.03	3.89	3.78	3.69	3.61	3.55
17	4.45	3.59	3.20	2.96	2.81	2.70	2.62	2.55	2.50	2.45	2.41	2.38
	8.40	6.11	5.18	4.67	4.34	4.10	3.93	3.79	3.68	3.59	3.52	3.45
18	4.41	3.55	3.16	2.93	2.77	2.66	2.58	2.51	2.46	2.41	2.37	2.34
	8.28	6.01	5.09	4.58	4.25	4.01	3.85	3.71	3.60	3.51	3.44	3.37

14	16	20	24	30	40	50	75	100	200	500	∞
245	246	248	249	250	251	252	253	253	254	254	254
6,142	6,169	6,208	6,234	6,258	6,286	6,302	6,323	6,334	6,352	6,361	6,366
19.42	19.43	19.44	19.45	19.46	19.47	19.47	19.48	19.49	19.49	19.50	19.50
99.43	99.44	99.45	99.46	99.47	99.48	99.48	99.49	99.49	99.49	99.50	99.50
8.71	8.69	8.66	8.64	8.62	8.60	8.58	8.57	8.56	8.54	8.54	8.53
26.92	26.83	26.69	26.60	26.50	26.41	26.35	26.27	26.23	26.18	26.14	26.12
5.87	5.84	5.80	5.77	5.74	5.71	5.70	5.68	5.66	5.65	5.64	5.63
14.24	14.15	14.02	13.93	13.83	13.74	13.69	13.61	13.57	13.52	13.48	13.46
4.64	4.60	4.56	4.53	4.50	4.46	4.44	4.42	4.40	4.38	4.37	4.36
9.77	9.68	9.55	9.47	9.38	9.29	9.24	9.17	9.13	9.07	9.04	9.02
3.96	3.92	3.87	3.84	3.81	3.77	3.75	3.72	3.71	3.69	3.68	3.67
7.60	7.52	7.39	7.31	7.23	7.14	7.09	7.02	6.99	6.94	6.90	6.88
3.52	3.49	3.44	3.41	3.38	3.34	3.32	3.29	3.28	3.25	3.24	3.23
6.35	6.27	6.15	6.07	5.98	5.90	5.85	5.78	5.75	5.70	5.65	5.65
3.23	3.20	3.15	3.12	3.08	3.05	3.03	3.00	2.98	2.96	2.94	2.93
5.56	5.48	5.36	5.28	5.20	5.11	5.06	5.00	4.96	4.91	4.88	4.86
3.02	2.98	2.93	2.90	2.86	2.82	2.80	2.77	2.76	2.73	2.72	2.71
5.00	4.92	4.80	4.73	4.64	4.56	4.51	4.45	4.41	4.36	4.33	4.31
2.86	2.82	2.77	2.74	2.70	2.67	2.64	2.61	2.59	2.56	2.55	2.54
4.60	4.52	4.41	4.33	4.25	4.17	4.12	4.05	4.01	3.96	3.93	3.91
2.74	2.70	2.65	2.61	2.57	2.53	2.50	2.47	2.45	2.42	2.41	2.40
4.29	4.21	4.10	4.02	3.94	3.86	3.80	3.74	3.70	3.66	3.62	3.60
2.64	2.60	2.54	2.50	2.46	2.42	2.40	2.36	2.35	2.32	2.31	2.30
4.05	3.98	3.86	3.78	3.70	3.61	3.56	3.49	3.46	3.41	3.38	3.36
2.55	2.51	2.46	2.42	2.38	2.34	2.32	2.28	2.26	2.24	2.22	2.21
3.85	3.78	3.67	3.59	3.51	3.42	3.37	3.30	3.27	3.21	3.18	3.16
2.48	2.44	2.39	2.35	2.31	2.27	2.24	2.21	2.19	2.16	2.14	2.13
3.70	3.62	3.51	3.43	3.34	3.26	3.21	3.14	3.11	3.06	3.02	3.00
2.43	2.39	2.33	2.29	2.25	2.21	2.18	2.15	2.12	2.10	2.08	2.07
3.56	3.48	3.36	3.29	3.20	3.12	3.07	3.00	2.97	2.92	2.89	2.87
2.37	2.33	2.28	2.24	2.20	2.16	2.13	2.09	2.07	2.04	2.02	2.01
3.45	3.37	3.25	3.18	3.10	3.01	2.96	2.89	2.86	2.80	2.77	2.75
2.33	2.29	2.23	2.19	2.15	2.11	2.08	2.04	2.02	1.99	1.97	1.96
3.35	3.27	3.16	3.08	3.00	2.92	2.86	2.79	2.76	2.70	2.67	2.65
2.29	2.25	2.19	2.15	2.11	2.07	2.04	2.00	1.98	1.95	1.93	1.92
3.27	3.19	3.07	3.00	2.91	2.83	2.78	2.71	2.68	2.62	2.59	2.57

n_1 Degrees of Freedom (For Greater Mean Square)[a]

n_2[b]	1	2	3	4	5	6	7	8	9	10	11	12
19	4.38	3.52	3.13	2.90	2.74	2.63	2.55	2.48	2.43	2.38	2.34	2.31
	8.18	5.93	5.01	4.50	4.17	3.94	3.77	3.63	3.52	3.43	3.36	3.30
20	4.35	3.49	3.10	2.87	2.71	2.60	2.52	2.45	2.40	2.35	2.31	2.28
	8.10	5.85	4.94	4.43	4.10	3.87	3.71	3.56	3.45	3.37	3.30	3.23
21	4.32	3.47	3.07	2.84	2.68	2.57	2.49	2.42	2.37	2.32	2.28	2.25
	8.02	5.78	4.87	4.37	4.04	3.81	3.65	3.51	3.40	3.31	3.24	3.17
22	4.30	3.44	3.05	2.82	2.66	2.55	2.47	2.40	2.35	2.30	2.26	2.23
	7.94	5.72	4.82	4.31	3.99	3.76	3.59	3.45	3.35	3.26	3.18	3.12
23	4.28	3.42	3.03	2.80	2.64	2.53	2.45	2.38	2.32	2.28	2.24	2.20
	7.88	5.66	4.76	4.26	3.94	3.71	3.54	3.41	3.30	3.21	3.14	3.07
24	4.26	3.40	3.01	2.78	2.62	2.51	2.43	2.36	2.30	2.26	2.22	2.18
	7.82	5.61	4.72	4.22	3.90	3.67	3.50	3.36	3.25	3.17	3.09	3.03
25	4.24	3.38	2.99	2.76	2.60	2.49	2.41	2.34	2.28	2.24	2.20	2.16
	7.77	5.57	4.68	4.18	3.86	3.63	3.46	3.32	3.21	3.13	3.05	2.99
26	4.22	3.37	2.98	2.74	2.59	2.47	2.39	2.32	2.27	2.22	2.18	2.15
	7.72	5.53	4.64	4.14	3.82	3.59	3.42	3.29	3.17	3.09	3.02	2.96
27	4.21	3.35	2.96	2.73	2.57	2.46	2.37	2.30	2.25	2.20	2.16	2.13
	7.68	5.49	4.60	4.11	3.79	3.56	3.39	3.26	3.14	3.06	2.98	2.93
28	4.20	3.34	2.95	2.71	2.56	2.44	2.36	2.29	2.24	2.19	2.15	2.12
	7.64	5.45	4.57	4.07	3.76	3.53	3.36	3.23	3.11	3.03	2.95	2.90
29	4.18	3.33	2.93	2.70	2.54	2.43	2.35	2.28	2.22	2.18	2.14	2.10
	7.60	5.42	4.54	4.04	3.73	3.50	3.33	3.20	3.08	3.00	2.92	2.87
30	4.17	3.32	2.92	2.69	2.53	2.42	2.34	2.27	2.21	2.16	2.12	2.09
	7.56	5.39	4.51	4.02	3.70	3.47	3.30	3.17	3.06	2.98	2.90	2.84
32	4.15	3.30	2.90	2.67	2.51	2.40	2.32	2.25	2.19	2.14	2.10	2.07
	7.50	5.34	4.46	3.97	3.66	3.42	3.25	3.12	3.01	2.94	2.86	2.80
34	4.13	3.28	2.88	2.65	2.49	2.38	2.30	2.23	2.17	2.12	2.08	2.05
	7.44	5.29	4.42	3.93	3.61	3.38	3.21	3.08	2.97	2.89	2.82	2.76
36	4.11	3.26	2.86	2.63	2.48	2.36	2.28	2.21	2.15	2.10	2.06	2.03
	7.39	5.25	4.38	3.89	3.58	3.35	3.18	3.04	2.94	2.86	2.78	2.72
38	4.10	3.25	2.85	2.62	2.46	2.35	2.26	2.19	2.14	2.09	2.05	2.02
	7.35	5.21	4.34	3.86	3.54	3.32	3.15	3.02	2.91	2.82	2.75	2.69
40	4.08	3.23	2.84	2.61	2.45	2.34	2.25	2.18	2.12	2.07	2.04	2.00
	7.31	5.18	4.31	3.83	3.51	3.29	3.12	2.99	2.88	2.80	2.73	2.66
42	4.07	3.22	2.83	2.59	2.44	2.32	2.24	2.17	2.11	2.06	2.02	1.99
	7.27	5.15	4.29	3.80	3.49	3.26	3.10	2.96	2.86	2.77	2.70	2.64
44	4.06	3.21	2.82	2.58	2.43	2.31	2.23	2.16	2.10	2.05	2.01	1.98
	7.24	5.12	4.26	3.78	3.46	3.24	3.07	2.94	2.84	2.75	2.68	2.62

14	16	20	24	30	40	50	75	100	200	500	∞
2.26	2.21	2.15	2.11	2.07	2.02	2.00	1.96	1.94	1.91	1.90	1.88
3.19	3.12	3.00	2.92	2.84	2.76	2.70	2.63	2.60	2.54	2.51	2.49
2.23	2.18	2.12	2.08	2.04	1.99	1.96	1.92	1.90	1.87	1.85	1.84
3.13	3.05	2.94	2.86	2.77	2.69	2.63	2.56	2.53	2.47	2.44	2.42
2.20	2.15	2.09	2.05	2.00	1.96	1.93	1.89	1.87	1.84	1.82	1.81
3.07	2.99	2.88	2.80	2.72	2.63	2.58	2.51	2.47	2.42	2.38	2.36
2.18	2.13	2.07	2.03	1.98	1.93	1.91	1.87	1.84	1.81	1.80	1.78
3.02	2.94	2.83	2.75	2.67	2.58	2.53	2.46	2.42	2.37	2.33	2.31
2.14	2.10	2.04	2.00	1.96	1.91	1.88	1.84	1.82	1.79	1.77	1.76
2.97	2.89	2.78	2.70	2.62	2.53	2.48	2.41	2.37	2.32	2.28	2.26
2.13	2.09	2.02	1.98	1.94	1.89	1.86	1.82	1.80	1.76	1.74	1.73
2.93	2.85	2.74	2.66	2.58	2.49	2.44	2.36	2.33	2.27	2.23	2.21
2.11	2.06	2.00	1.96	1.92	1.87	1.84	1.80	1.77	1.74	1.72	1.71
2.89	2.81	2.70	2.62	2.54	2.45	2.40	2.32	2.29	2.23	2.19	2.17
2.10	2.05	1.99	1.95	1.90	1.85	1.82	1.78	1.76	1.72	1.70	1.69
2.86	2.77	2.66	2.58	2.50	2.41	2.36	2.28	2.25	2.19	2.15	2.13
2.08	2.03	1.97	1.93	1.88	1.84	1.80	1.76	1.74	1.71	1.68	1.67
2.83	2.74	2.63	2.55	2.47	2.38	2.33	2.25	2.21	2.16	2.12	2.10
2.06	2.02	1.96	1.91	1.87	1.81	1.78	1.75	1.72	1.69	1.67	1.65
2.80	2.71	2.60	2.52	2.44	2.35	2.30	2.22	2.18	2.13	2.09	2.06
2.05	2.00	1.94	1.90	1.85	1.80	1.77	1.73	1.71	1.68	1.65	1.64
2.77	2.68	2.57	2.49	2.41	2.32	2.27	2.19	2.15	2.10	2.06	2.03
2.04	1.99	1.93	1.89	1.84	1.79	1.76	1.72	1.69	1.66	1.64	1.62
2.74	2.66	2.55	2.47	2.38	2.29	2.24	2.16	2.13	2.07	2.03	2.01
2.02	1.97	1.91	1.86	1.82	1.76	1.74	1.69	1.67	1.64	1.61	1.59
2.70	2.62	2.51	2.42	2.34	2.25	2.20	2.12	2.08	2.02	1.98	1.96
2.00	1.95	1.89	1.84	1.80	1.74	1.71	1.67	1.64	1.61	1.59	1.57
2.66	2.58	2.47	2.38	2.30	2.21	2.15	2.08	2.04	1.98	1.94	1.91
1.98	1.93	1.87	1.82	1.78	1.72	1.69	1.65	1.62	1.59	1.56	1.55
2.26	2.54	2.43	2.35	2.26	2.17	2.12	2.04	2.00	1.94	1.90	1.87
1.96	1.92	1.85	1.80	1.76	1.71	1.67	1.63	1.60	1.57	1.54	1.53
2.59	2.51	2.40	2.32	2.22	2.14	2.08	2.00	1.97	1.90	1.86	1.84
1.95	1.90	1.84	1.79	1.74	1.69	1.66	1.61	1.59	1.55	1.53	1.51
2.56	2.49	2.37	2.29	2.20	2.11	2.05	1.97	1.94	1.88	1.84	1.81
1.94	1.89	1.82	1.78	1.73	1.68	1.64	1.60	1.57	1.54	1.51	1.49
2.54	2.46	2.35	2.26	2.17	2.08	2.02	1.94	1.91	1.85	1.80	1.78
1.92	1.88	1.81	1.76	1.72	1.66	1.63	1.58	1.56	1.52	1.50	1.48
2.52	2.44	2.32	2.24	2.15	2.06	2.00	1.92	1.88	1.82	1.78	1.75

n_1 Degrees of Freedom (For Greater Mean Square)[a]

n_2[b]	1	2	3	4	5	6	7	8	9	10	11	12
46	4.05	3.20	2.81	2.57	2.42	2.30	2.22	2.14	2.09	2.04	2.00	1.97
	7.21	**5.10**	**4.24**	**3.76**	**3.44**	**3.22**	**3.05**	**2.92**	**2.82**	**2.73**	**2.66**	**2.60**
48	4.04	3.19	2.80	2.56	2.41	2.30	2.21	2.14	2.08	2.03	1.99	1.96
	7.19	**5.08**	**4.22**	**3.74**	**3.42**	**3.20**	**3.04**	**2.90**	**2.80**	**2.71**	**2.64**	**2.58**
50	4.03	3.18	2.79	2.56	2.40	2.29	2.20	2.13	2.07	2.02	1.98	1.95
	7.17	**5.06**	**4.20**	**3.72**	**3.41**	**3.18**	**3.02**	**2.88**	**2.78**	**2.70**	**2.62**	**2.56**
55	4.02	3.17	2.78	2.54	2.38	2.27	2.18	2.11	2.05	2.00	1.97	1.93
	7.12	**5.01**	**4.16**	**3.68**	**3.37**	**3.15**	**2.98**	**2.85**	**2.75**	**2.66**	**2.59**	**2.53**
60	4.00	3.15	2.76	2.52	2.37	2.25	2.17	2.10	2.04	1.99	1.95	1.92
	7.08	**4.98**	**4.13**	**3.65**	**3.34**	**3.12**	**2.95**	**2.82**	**2.72**	**2.63**	**2.56**	**2.50**
65	3.99	3.14	2.75	2.51	2.36	2.24	2.15	2.08	2.02	1.98	1.94	1.90
	7.04	**4.95**	**4.10**	**3.62**	**3.31**	**3.09**	**2.93**	**2.79**	**2.70**	**2.61**	**2.54**	**2.47**
70	3.98	3.13	2.74	2.50	2.35	2.23	2.14	2.07	2.01	1.97	1.93	1.89
	7.01	**4.92**	**4.08**	**3.60**	**3.29**	**3.07**	**2.91**	**2.77**	**2.67**	**2.59**	**2.51**	**2.45**
80	3.96	3.11	2.72	2.48	2.33	2.21	2.12	2.05	1.99	1.95	1.91	1.88
	6.96	**4.88**	**4.04**	**3.56**	**3.25**	**3.04**	**2.87**	**2.74**	**2.64**	**2.55**	**2.48**	**2.41**
100	3.94	3.09	2.70	2.46	2.30	2.19	2.10	2.03	1.97	1.92	1.88	1.85
	6.90	**4.82**	**3.98**	**3.51**	**3.20**	**2.99**	**2.82**	**2.69**	**2.59**	**2.51**	**2.43**	**2.36**
125	3.92	3.07	2.68	2.44	2.29	2.17	2.08	2.01	1.95	1.90	1.86	1.83
	6.84	**4.78**	**3.94**	**3.47**	**3.17**	**2.95**	**2.79**	**2.65**	**2.56**	**2.47**	**2.40**	**2.33**
150	3.91	3.06	2.67	2.43	2.27	2.16	2.07	2.00	1.94	1.89	1.85	1.82
	6.81	**4.75**	**3.91**	**3.44**	**3.14**	**2.92**	**2.76**	**2.62**	**2.53**	**2.44**	**2.37**	**2.30**
200	3.89	3.04	2.65	2.41	2.26	2.14	2.05	1.98	1.92	1.87	1.83	1.80
	6.76	**4.71**	**3.88**	**3.41**	**3.11**	**2.90**	**2.73**	**2.60**	**2.50**	**2.41**	**2.34**	**2.28**
400	3.86	3.02	2.62	2.39	2.23	2.12	2.03	1.96	1.90	1.85	1.81	1.78
	6.70	**4.66**	**3.83**	**3.36**	**3.06**	**2.85**	**2.69**	**2.55**	**2.46**	**2.37**	**2.29**	**2.23**
1,000	3.85	3.00	2.61	2.38	2.22	2.10	2.02	1.95	1.89	1.84	1.80	1.76
	6.66	**4.62**	**3.80**	**3.34**	**3.04**	**2.82**	**2.66**	**2.53**	**2.43**	**2.34**	**2.26**	**2.20**
∞	3.84	2.99	2.60	2.37	2.21	2.09	2.01	1.94	1.88	1.83	1.79	1.75
	6.64	**4.60**	**3.78**	**3.32**	**3.02**	**2.80**	**2.64**	**2.51**	**2.41**	**2.32**	**2.24**	**2.18**

5% = roman type, 1% = boldface type.

[a]Numerator.

[b]Denominator.

From Snedecor, G. W. (1938). *Statistical methods*. Ames, IA: Collegiate Press. (Table 10–3, pp. 184–187).

14	16	20	24	30	40	50	75	100	200	500	∞
1.91	1.87	1.80	1.75	1.71	1.65	1.62	1.57	1.54	1.51	1.48	1.46
2.50	2.42	2.30	2.22	2.13	2.04	1.98	1.90	1.86	1.80	1.76	1.72
1.90	1.86	1.79	1.74	1.70	1.64	1.61	1.56	1.53	1.50	1.47	1.45
2.48	2.40	2.28	2.20	2.11	2.02	1.96	1.88	1.84	1.78	1.73	1.70
1.90	1.85	1.78	1.74	1.69	1.63	1.60	1.55	1.52	1.48	1.46	1.44
2.46	2.39	2.26	2.18	2.10	2.00	1.94	1.86	1.82	1.76	1.71	1.68
1.88	1.83	1.76	1.72	1.67	1.61	1.58	1.52	1.50	1.46	1.43	1.41
2.43	2.35	2.23	2.15	2.06	1.96	1.90	1.82	1.78	1.71	1.66	1.64
1.86	1.81	1.75	1.70	1.65	1.59	1.56	1.50	1.48	1.44	1.41	1.39
2.40	2.32	2.20	2.12	2.03	1.93	1.87	1.79	1.74	1.68	1.63	1.60
1.85	1.80	1.73	1.68	1.63	1.57	1.54	1.49	1.46	1.42	1.39	1.37
2.37	2.30	2.18	2.09	2.00	1.90	1.84	1.76	1.71	1.64	1.60	1.56
1.84	1.79	1.72	1.67	1.62	1.56	1.53	1.47	1.45	1.40	1.37	1.35
2.35	2.28	2.15	2.07	1.98	1.88	1.82	1.74	1.69	1.62	1.56	1.53
1.82	1.77	1.70	1.65	1.60	1.54	1.51	1.45	1.42	1.38	1.35	1.32
2.32	2.24	2.11	2.03	1.94	1.84	1.78	1.70	1.65	1.57	1.52	1.49
1.79	1.75	1.68	1.63	1.57	1.51	1.48	1.42	1.39	1.34	1.30	1.28
2.26	2.19	2.06	1.98	1.89	1.79	1.73	1.64	1.59	1.51	1.46	1.43
1.77	1.72	1.65	1.60	1.55	1.49	1.45	1.39	1.36	1.31	1.27	1.25
2.23	2.15	2.03	1.94	1.85	1.75	1.68	1.59	1.54	1.46	1.40	1.37
1.76	1.71	1.64	1.59	1.54	1.47	1.44	1.37	1.34	1.29	1.25	1.22
2.20	2.12	2.00	1.91	1.83	1.72	1.66	1.56	1.51	1.43	1.37	1.33
1.74	1.69	1.62	1.57	1.52	1.45	1.42	1.35	1.32	1.26	1.22	1.19
2.17	2.09	1.97	1.88	1.79	1.69	1.62	1.53	1.48	1.39	1.33	1.28
1.72	1.67	1.60	1.54	1.49	1.42	1.38	1.32	1.28	1.22	1.16	1.13
2.12	2.04	1.92	1.84	1.74	1.64	1.57	1.47	1.42	1.32	1.24	1.19
1.70	1.65	1.58	1.53	1.47	1.41	1.36	1.30	1.26	1.19	1.13	1.08
2.09	2.01	1.89	1.81	1.71	1.61	1.54	1.44	1.38	1.28	1.19	1.11
1.69	1.64	1.57	1.52	1.46	1.40	1.35	1.28	1.24	1.17	1.11	1.00
2.07	1.99	1.87	1.79	1.69	1.59	1.52	1.41	1.36	1.25	1.15	1.00

Critical Values of *H* for the Kruskal-Wallis ANOVA by Rank

Sample Sizes			Critical Value of the *H*-Statistic Where p (*H*) $\leq \alpha$		
n	n	n	.10	.05	.01
2	2	2	4.5714	—	—
3	2	1	4.2857	—	—
3	2	2	4.5000	4.7143	—
3	3	1	4.5714	5.1429	—
3	3	2	4.5556	5.3611	6.2500
3	3	3	4.6222	5.6000	7.2000
4	2	1	4.5000	—	—
4	2	2	4.4583	5.3333	6.0000
4	3	1	4.0556	5.2083	—
4	3	2	4.5111	5.4444	6.4444
4	3	3	4.7091	5.7273	6.7455
4	4	1	4.1667	4.9667	6.6667
4	4	2	4.5545	5.4545	7.0364
4	4	3	4.5455	5.5985	7.1439
4	4	4	4.6539	5.6923	7.6538
5	2	1	4.2000	5.0000	—
5	3	1	4.0178	4.960	6.4000
5	3	2	4.6509	5.2509	6.8218
5	3	3	4.5333	5.6485	7.0788

(Continued)

Sample Sizes			Critical Value of the *H*-Statistic Where p (*H*) ≤ α		
n	n	n	.10	.05	.01
5	4	1	3.9873	4.9855	6.9545
5	4	2	4.5409	5.2682	7.1182
5	4	3	4.5487	5.6308	7.4449
5	4	4	4.6187	5.6176	7.7604
5	5	1	4.1091	5.1273	7.3091
5	5	2	4.5077	5.3385	7.2692
5	5	3	4.5451	5.7055	7.5429
5	5	4	4.5229	5.6429	7.7914
5	5	5	4.5600	5.7800	7.9800

Adapted from Kruskal, W. H., & Wallis, W. A. (1952). Use of ranks in one-criterion variance analysis. *Journal of the American Statistical Association, 47*(260), 583–621 and corrections in Kruskal, W. H., & Wallis, W. A. (1953). Errata: Use of ranks in one-criterion variance analysis. *Journal of the American Statistical Association, 48*(264), 907–911.

Critical Values of Dunn's Q for Nonparametric Multiple Comparison Testing

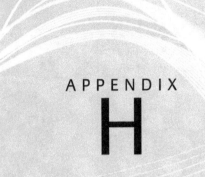

k (# Treatment Groups)	α	
	0.05	0.10
2	1.960	2.576
3	2.394	2.936
4	2.639	3.144
5	2.807	3.291
6	2.936	3.403

Adapted from Zar, J. H. (1984). *Biostatistical analysis* (2nd ed.). Englewood Cliffs, NJ: Prentice-Hall, p569. Table B. 14.

Exact Distribution of the Friedman's χ^2 for the Friedman's ANOVA by Rank Comparing Three Related Groups

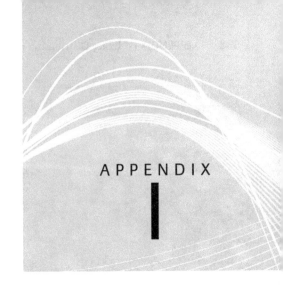

Sample Size (n)	Value of χ_r^2	Exact Probability of That Value
3	4.667	.194
3	6.0	.028
4	6.0	.069
4	6.5	.042
4	8.0	.0046
5	5.2	.093
5	6.4	.039
5	8.4	.0085
6	5.33	.072
6	6.33	.052
6	7.00	.029
6	8.33	.012
6	9.00	.0081
7	5.429	.085
7	6.0	.052
7	7.143	.027
7	8.000	.016
7	8.857	.0084
8	5.25	.079
8	6.25	.047
8	7.75	.018

(Continued)

Sample Size (n)	Value of χ^2_r	Exact Probability of That Value
8	9.0	.0099
9	4.667	.107
9	5.556	.069
9	6.000	.057
9	6.222	.048
9	8.0	.019
9	8.667	.010
9	9.556	.0060

Comparing Four Related Groups

Sample Size (n)		
2	6.0	.042
3	6.6	.075
3	7.0	.054
3	7.4	.033
3	8.2	.017
3	9.0	.0017
4	6.0	.105
4	6.3	.094
4	7.5	.052
4	7.8	.036
4	9.3	.012
4	9.6	.0069

Adapted from Friedman, M. (1937). The use of ranks to avoid the assumption of normality implicit in the analysis of variance. *Journal of the American Statistical Association, 32*(200), 675–701.

Critical Values of the Pearson Correlation Coefficient

	Level of Significance for One-Tailed Test			
	.05	.025	.01	.005
	Level of Significance for Two-Tailed Test			
df	.10	.05	.02	.01
1	.988	.997	.9995	.9999
2	.900	.950	.980	.990
3	.805	.878	.934	.959
4	.729	.811	.882	.917
5	.669	.754	.833	.874
6	.622	.707	.789	.834
7	.582	.666	.750	.798
8	.549	.632	.716	.765
9	.521	.602	.685	.735
10	.497	.576	.658	.708
11	.476	.553	.634	.684
12	.458	.532	.612	.661
13	.441	.514	.592	.641
14	.426	.497	.574	.623
15	.412	.482	.558	.606
16	.400	.468	.542	.590
17	.389	.456	.528	.575
18	.378	.444	.516	.561

(Continued)

	Level of Significance for One-Tailed Test			
	.05	.025	.01	.005
	Level of Significance for Two-Tailed Test			
df	.10	.05	.02	.01
19	.369	.433	.503	.549
20	.360	.423	.492	.537
21	.352	.413	.482	.526
22	.344	.404	.472	.515
23	.337	.396	.462	.505
24	.330	.388	.453	.496
25	.323	.381	.445	.487
26	.317	.374	.437	.479
27	.311	.367	.430	.471
28	.306	.361	.423	.463
29	.301	.355	.416	.456
30	.296	.349	.409	.449
35	.275	.325	.381	.418
40	.257	.304	.358	.393
45	.243	.288	.338	.372
50	.231	.273	.322	.354
60	.211	.250	.295	.325
70	.195	.232	.247	.303
80	.183	.217	.256	.283
90	.173	.205	.242	.267
100	.164	.195	.230	.254
125		.174		.228
150		.159		.208
200		.138		.181
300		.113		.148
400		.098		.128
500		.088		.115
1000		.062		.081

From Fisher, R. A. (1970). *Statistical methods for research workers* (14th ed.). Darien, CT: Hafner Publishing Co. (Table V. A., p. 211).

Critical Values of the Spearman Correlation Coefficient

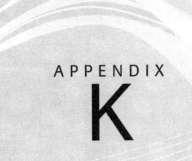

	Approximate Critical Values of the Correlation Coefficient				
	Level of Significance for the One-Tailed Test				
	.10	.05	.025	.01	.005
	Level of Significance for the Two-Tailed Test				
n	.20	.10	.05	.02	.01
4	.8000	.8000	—	—	—
5	.7000	.8000	.9000	.9000	—
6	.6000	.7714	.8286	.8857	.9429
7	.5357	.6786	.7450	.8571	.8929
8	.5000	.6190	.7143	.8095	.8571
9	.4667	.5833	.6833	.7667	.8167
10	.4424	.5515	.6364	.7333	.7818
11	.4182	.5273	.6091	.7000	.7545
12	.3986	.4965	.5084	.6713	.7273
13	.3791	.4780	.5549	.6429	.6978
14	.3626	.4593	.5341	.6220	.6747
15	.3500	.4429	.5179	.6000	.6536
16	.3382	.4265	.5000	.5824	.6324
17	.3260	.4118	.4853	.5637	.6152
18	.3148	.3994	.4716	.5480	.5975
19	.3070	.3895	.4579	.5333	.5825
20	.2977	.3789	.4451	.5203	.5684

(Continued)

Approximate Critical Values of the Correlation Coefficient

	Level of Significance for the One-Tailed Test				
	.10	.05	.025	.01	.005
	Level of Significance for the Two-Tailed Test				
n	.20	.10	.05	.02	.01
21	.2909	.3688	.4351	.5078	.5545
22	.2829	.3597	.4241	.4963	.5426
23	.2767	.3518	.4150	.4852	.5306
24	.2704	.3435	.4061	.4748	.5200
25	.2646	.3822	.3977	.4654	.5100
26	.2588	.3299	.3984	.4564	.5002
27	.2540	.3236	.3822	.4481	.4915
28	.2490	.3175	.3749	.4401	.4828
29	.2443	.3113	.3685	.4320	.4744
30	.2400	.3059	.3620	.4251	.4665

Note. The one-tailed probability is the probability that either $r \geq r$ or $r \leq -r$ (but not both).

The two-tailed probability is the sum of the probabilities that $r \geq r$ and $r \leq -r$.

Adapted from Glasser, G. J., & Winter, R. F. (1961). Critical values of the coefficient of rink correlation for testing the hypothesis of independence. *Biometrika, 48*(3/4), 444–448 (Table 3).

Distribution of χ^2 Probability

df	0.20	0.10	0.05	0.02	0.01	0.001
1	1.642	2.706	3.841	5.412	6.635	10.827
2	3.219	4.605	5.991	7.842	9.210	13.815
3	4.642	6.251	7.815	9.837	11.345	16.266
4	5.989	7.779	9.488	11.668	13.277	18.467
5	7.289	9.236	11.070	13.388	15.086	20.515
6	8.558	10.645	12.592	15.033	16.812	22.457
7	9.803	12.017	14.067	16.622	18.475	24.322
8	11.030	13.362	15.507	18.168	20.090	26.125
9	12.242	14.684	16.919	19.679	21.666	27.877
10	13.442	15.987	18.307	21.161	23.209	29.588
11	14.631	17.275	19.675	22.618	24.725	31.264
12	15.812	18.549	21.026	24.054	26.217	32.909
13	16.985	19.812	22.362	25.472	27.688	34.528
14	18.151	21.064	23.685	26.873	29.141	36.123
15	19.311	22.307	24.996	28.259	30.578	37.697
16	20.465	23.542	26.296	29.633	32.000	39.252
17	21.615	24.769	27.587	30.995	33.409	40.790
18	22.760	25.989	28.869	32.346	34.805	42.312
19	23.900	27.204	30.144	33.687	36.191	43.820
20	25.038	28.412	31.410	35.020	37.566	45.315
21	26.171	29.615	32.671	36.343	38.932	46.797

(Continued)

df	0.20	0.10	0.05	0.02	0.01	0.001
22	27.301	30.813	33.924	37.659	40.289	48.268
23	28.429	32.007	35.172	38.968	41.638	49.728
24	29.553	33.196	36.415	40.270	42.980	51.179
25	30.675	34.382	37.652	41.566	44.314	52.620
26	31.795	35.563	38.885	42.856	45.642	54.052
27	32.912	36.741	40.113	44.140	46.963	55.476
28	34.027	37.916	41.337	45.419	48.278	56.893
29	35.139	39.087	42.557	46.693	49.588	58.302
30	36.250	40.256	43.773	47.962	50.892	59.703

From Fisher, R. A. (1970). *Statistical methods for research workers* (14th ed.). Darien, CT: Hafner Publishing. (Taken from Table III, pp. 112–113).

Adachi, K., Shimada, M., & Usui, A. (2003). The relationship between the parturient's labor position and perceptions of labor pain intensity. *Nursing Research, 52*(1), 47–51.

Agresti, A., & Finlay, B. (1997). *Statistical methods for the social sciences*. Upper Saddle River, NJ: Prentice-Hall.

Ahlqvist, M., Bogren, A., Hagman, S., et al. (2006). Handline of peripheral intravenous cannulae: Effects of evidence-based clinical guidelines. *Journal of Clinical Nursing, 15*, 1354–1361.

Aiken, L., Clarke, S., Cheung, R., Sloane, D., & Silber, J. (2003). Educational levels of hospital nurses and surgical patient mortality. *Journal of the American Medical Association, 290*, 1617–1623.

Ajzen, I. (1991). Theory of planned behavior. *Organizational Behavior and Human Decision Processes, 50*, 179–211.

Akaike, H. (1987). Factor analysis and AIC. *Psychometrika, 52*(3), 317–332.

Al-Darrab, I. A., Khan, Z. A., & Ishrat, S. I. (2009). An experimental study on the effect of mobile phone conversation on drivers' reaction time in braking response. *Journal of Safety Research, 40*(3),185–189.

American Diabetes Association. (2007). Standards of medical care in diabetes. *Diabetes Care, 30*(1), S4–S41.

American Psychiatric Association. (2000). *Diagnostic and statistical manual of mental disorders* (4th ed., text revision). Washington, DC: Author.

Andersen, R. M. (1995). Revisiting the behavioral model and access to medical care: Does it matter? *Journal of Health and Social Behavior, 36*(1), 1–10.

Anderson, E., McDonald, D., Mikky, I., Brewer, T., Kosciewski, C., LaCoursiere, S., et al. (2003). Health care implications and space allocation of research published in nursing journals. *Nursing Outlook, 51*(2), 70–83.

Anderson, R. A., Isset, L. M., & McDaniel, R. R. (2003). Nursing homes as complex adaptive systems. *Nursing Research, 52*(1), 12–21.

Andrews, E. J., & Redmond, H. P. (2004). A review of clinical guidelines. *British Journal of Surgery, 91*(8), 956–964.

APA. (2010). *Publication manual of the American Psychological Association*. Washington, DC: American Psychological Association.

Armitage, C. J. (2005). Can the theory of planned behavior predict the maintenance of physical activity? *Health Psychology, 24*(3), 235–245.

Asher, A. B. (1983). Causal modeling (2nd ed.) In *Quantitative Applications in the Social Sciences Series*, 3. Newbury Park, CA: Sage.

Ashworth, C. S., DuRant, R. H., Gaillard, G., & Rountree, J. (1994). An experimental evaluation of an AIDS educational intervention for WIC mothers. *AIDS Education & B Prevention, 6*(2), 154–162.

Auerbach, D., Buerhaus, P. I., & Staiger, D. O. (2007). Trends: Better late than never: Workforce supply implications of later entry into nursing. *Health Affairs, 26*(1), 178–186.

Babbie, E. (2007). *The practice of social research*. Belmont, CA: Wadsworth.

Bachand, D. A., & Beard, M. T. (1995). Structural equation modeling. In M. T. Beard (Ed.), *Theory construction and testing* (pp. 220–230). Lisle, IL: Tucker Publishing, Inc.

Baibergenova, A., Kudyakov, R., Zdeb, M., & Carpenter, D. (2003). Low birth weight and residential proximity to PCB-contaminated waste sites. *Environmental Health Perspectives, 111*(i10), 1352–1358.

Baron, R. M., & Kenny, D. A. (1986). The moderator-mediator distinction in social psychological research: Conceptual, strategic, and statistical considerations. *Journal of Personality and Social Psychology, 51*, 1173–1182.

Beigi, A., Kabiri, M., & Zarrinkoub, F. (2003). Cervical ripening with oral misoprostol at term. *International Journal of Gynaecology and Obstetrics, 83*(3), 251–255.

Bentler, P. M. (1995). *EQS structural equations program manual*. Encino, CA: Multivariate Software.

Bentler, P. M., & Bonnett, D. G. (1980). Significance tests and goodness of fit in the analysis of covariance structures. *Psychological Bulletin, 88*(3), 588–606.

Berthiller, J., Straif, K., Boniol, M., Voirin, N., Benhaïm-Luzon, V., Ayoub, W. B., et al. (2008). Cannabis smoking and risk of lung cancer in men: a pooled analysis of three studies in Maghreb. *Journal of Thoracic Oncology, 3*(12), 1398–1403.

Bittner, F. H., Diamond, J., Myers, R., & Gill, J. M . (2008). Perception, intention, and action in adolescent obesity. D. *Journal of the American Board of Family Medicine, 21*(6), 555–561.

Block, S. (1996). The DOs and DON'Ts of poster presentation. *Biophysical Journal, 71*, 3527–3529.

Bollen, K. A. (1989). *Structural equations with latent variables*. New York, NY: John Wiley & Sons.

Bollen, K. A., & Long, J. S. (1993). Introduction. In K. A. Bollen & J. S. Long (Eds.), *Testing structural equation models* (pp. 1–9). Thousand Oaks, CA: Sage.

Boushey, C., Harris, J., Bruemmer, B., Archer, S., & Van Horn, L. (2006). Publishing nutrition research: A review of study design, statistical analyses, and other key elements of manuscript preparation, Part 1. *Journal of the American Dietetic Association, 106*(1), 89–95.

Brodeur, P. (1985). *Outrageous misconduct: The asbestos industry on trial.* New York, NY: Pantheon.

Brooks, W. (2004). The use of practice guidelines for urinary incontinence following stroke. *British Journal of Nursing, 13*(2), 1176–1179.

Brooten, D., Naylor, M., York, R., Brown, L., Roncoli, M., Hollingsworth, A., et al. (1995). Effects of nurse specialist transitional care on patient outcomes and cost: Results of five randomized trials. *American Journal of Managed Care, 1,* 35–41.

Brooten, D. (1988). Early hospital discharge and nurse specialist follow-up. Program grant, funded by the National Center for Nursing Research, PO1-NR1859.

Brostrom, A., Stromberg, A., Daahlstrom, U., & Fridlund, B. (2004). Sleep difficulties, daytime sleepiness and health-related quality of life in patients with chronic heart failure. *Journal of Cardiovascular Nursing, 19*(4), 234–242.

Brown, D. W., Dueker, N., Jamieson, D.J., Cole, J.W., Wozniak, M. A., Stern, B. J., et al. (2006). Preeclampsia and the risk of ischemic stroke among young women: results from the Stroke Prevention in Young Women Study. *Stroke, 37*(4), 1055–1059.

Browne, M. W., MacCullum, R. C., Kim, C.-T., Andersen, B. L., & Glaser, R. (2002). When fit indices and residuals are incompatible. *Psychological Methods, 7*(4), 403–421.

Brush, B. L., Sochalski, J., & Berger, A. M. (2004). Imported care: Recruiting foreign nurses to U.S. health care facilities: Importing nurses is likely to remain a viable and lucrative strategy for plugging holes in the U.S. nurse work-force. *Health Affairs, 23*(3), 78–87.

Burns, K. J. (2000). Power and effect size: Research considerations for the clinical nurse specialist. *Clinical Nurse Specialist, 14*(2), 61–68.

Burns, N., & Grove, S. K. (2001). *The practice of nursing research: Conduct, critique and utilization* (4th ed.). Philadelphia: W. B. Saunders.

Byrne, B. M. (2006). *Structural equation modeling with EQS, basic concepts, applications, and programming.* Thousand Oaks, CA: Sage.

Campbell, G., & Skillings, J. H. (1985). Nonparametric stepwise multiple comparison procedures. *Journal of the American Statistical Association, 80,* 998–998.

Can, C., Durna, Z., & Aydiner, A. (2004). Assessment of fatigue and care needs in Turkish women with breast cancer. *Cancer Nursing, 27*(2), 153–161.

Carmines, E. G., & McIver, J. P. (1983). An introduction of the analysis of models with unobserved variables. *Political Methodology, 9*(1), 51–102.

Center on an Aging Society. (2004). *Cultural competence in health care: Issue brief.* Retrieved from http://hpi.georgetown.edu/agingsociety/pdfs/cultural.pdf

Centers for Disease Control and Prevention. (2000). *Behavioral Risk Factor Surveillance System Survey data.* Atlanta, GA: Author.

Cetin, S., & Hackam, D. (2005). An approach to the writing of a scientific manuscript. *Journal of Surgical Research, 128*(2), 165–167.

Chatterjee, S., & Yilmaz, M. (1992). A review of regression diagnostics for behavioral research. *Applied Psychological Measurement, 16*(3), 209–227.

Chibnall, J. T. (2003). Statistical audit of original research articles in *International Psychogeriatrics* for the year 2003. *International Psychogeriatrics, 16*(4), 389–396.

Chou, C.-P., & Bentler, P. M. (1995). Estimates and tests in structural equation modeling. In R. H. Hoyle (Ed.), *Structural equation modeling: Concepts, issues, and applications* (pp. 37–55). Thousand Oaks, CA: Sage.

Chow, S. (Ed.). (2000). Good statistics in practice. In *Encyclopedia of biopharmaceutical statistics.* New York, NY: Marcel Dekker.

Clark, M. (2003). One-way repeated measures and corresponding multiple comparisons using SPSS and R. *RSS Matters, Benchmarks Online: Research and Statistical Support.* Retrieved from http://www.unt.edu/benchmarks/archives/2003/august03/rss.htm

Cleveland, W. (1988). *The collected works of John W. Tukey.* New York, NY: Chapman & Hall.

Cochrane Collaboration. (2010). Retrieved from http://www.cochrane.org/

Cohen, J. (1983). The cost of dichotomization. *Applied Psychological Measurement, 7,* 249–253.

Cohen, J. (1987). *Statistical power analysis for the behavioral sciences* (Rev. ed.). Hillsdale, NJ: Erlbaum.

Cohen. J. (1988). *Statistical power analysis for the behavioral sciences* (2nd ed.). Hillsdale, NJ: Erlbaum.

Cohen, J. (1992). A power primer. *Psychological Bulletin, 112*(3), 155–159.

Cohen, J., Cohen, P., West, S. G., & Aiken, L. S. (2003). *Applied multiple regression/correlation analysis for the behavioral sciences* (3rd ed.). Mahwah, NJ: Erlbaum.

Colin, P. (2011). Designing conference posters. Retrieved from http://colinpurrington.com/tips/academic/posterdesign

Cook, T. D., & Campbell, D. T. (1979). *Quasi-experimentation: Design & analysis issues for field settings.* Boston, MA: Houghton Miffin.

Curran, P. J., Bollen, K. A., Paxton, P., Kirby, J., & Chen, F. (2002). Chi-square distribution in mispecified structural equation models: Results from a Monte Carlo Simulation. *Multivariate Behavioral Research, 37*(1), 1–36.

Cuttner, J., Spiera, H., Troy, K., & Wallenstein, S. (2005). Autoimmune disease is a risk factor for the development of non-Hodgkin's lymphoma. *Journal of Rheumatology, 32*(10), 1884–1887.

Daniel, W. W. (2005). *Biostatistics: A foundation for analysis in the health sciences* (8th ed.). New York, NY: John Wiley and Sons.

Daniel, W. W. (2008). *Biostatistics: A foundation for analysis in the health sciences* (9th ed). New York, NY: John Wiley & Sons.

Davidson, F. (1996). *Principles of statistical data handling.* Thousand Oaks, CA: Sage.

DeAngelis, C. (2004). Duplicate publication, multiple problems. *Journal of the American Medical Association, 292,* 1745–1746.

Devane, D., Begley, C. M., & Clark, M. (2004). How many do I need? Basic principles of sample size estimation. *Journal of Advanced Nursing, 47*(3), 297–302.

Dinger, M. K., Heesch, K. C., & McClary, K. R. (2005). Feasibility of a minimal contact intervention to promote walking among insufficiently active women. *American Journal of Health Promotion, 20*(1), 2–6.

Dixon, J. K., Hendrickson, K. C., Ercolano, E., Quackenbush, R., & Dixon, J. P. (2009). The Environmental Health Engagement Profile: What people think and do about environmental health. *Public Health Nursing, 26,* 460–473.

Dubey, S. D. (1991). Some thoughts on the one-sided and two-sided tests. *Journal of Biopharmaceutical Statistics, 1*(1), 139–150.

Dunne, E., et al. (2007). Prevalence of HPV infection among females in the United States. *JAMA. 297*(8),813–819

Ehrenberg, A. S. C. (1977). Rudiments of numeracy. *Journal of the Royal Statistical Society A, 140*(Pt 3), 277–297.

Ertel, K. A., Koenen, K. C., Rich-Edwards, J. W., & Gillman, M. W. (2010). Maternal depressive symptoms not associated with reduced height in young children in a US prospective cohort study. *PLoS ONE, 5*(10), 1–9.

Essex-Sorlie, D. (1995). *Medical statistics & epidemiology first edition.* Norwalk, CT: Appleton & Lange.

Fan, X., Thompson, B., & Wang, L. (1999). Effects of sample size, estimation methods, and model specification on structural equation modeling fit indexes. *Structural Equation Modeling, 6*(1), 56–83.

Fan, X., & Wang, L. (1998). Effects of potential confounding factors on fit indices and parameter estimates for true and misspecified models. *Educational and Psychological Measurement, 58*(5), 701–735.

Feinstein, A. R. (1998). P-values and confidence intervals: Two sides of the same unsatisfactory coin. *Journal of Clinical Epidemiology, 51,* 355–360.

Ferketich, S., & Muller, M. (1990). Factor analysis revisited. *Nursing Research, 39,* 59–62.

Fishbein, M., & Ajzen, I. (1975). Belief, attitude, intention, and behavior: An introduction to theory and research. Reading, MA: Addison-Wesley.

Fisher, R. A. (1925). Statistical methods for research workers. London, UK: Oliver & Boyd.

Fisher, R. A. (1970). *Statistical methods for research workers* (14th ed.). Edinburgh, UK: Oliver and Boyd.

Forhan, S. E., Gottlieb, S. L., Sternberg, M. R., Xu, F., Datta, S. D., McQuillan, G. M., et al. (2009). Prevalence of sexually transmitted infections among female adolescents aged 14 to 19 in the United States. *Pediatrics, 124*(6), 1505–1512.

Fox, J. (1997). Applied regression analysis, linear models, and related methods. Thousand Oaks, CA: Sage.

Franklin, D., Senior, N., James, I., & Roberts, G. (2000). Oral health status of children in a paediatric intensive care unit. *Intensive Medical Care, 26*(3), 319–324.

Freedman, D., Pisani, R., Purves, R., & Adhikari, A. (1991). *Statistics* (2nd ed.). New York, NY: W. W. Norton.

Freedman, K. B. (2001). Sample size and statistical power of randomized, controlled trials in orthopaedics. *Journal of Bone Joint Surgery, 83B*(3), 397–402.

Freund, J. E. (1988). *Modern elementary statistics* (7th ed.). Englewood Cliffs, NJ: Prentice-Hall.

Friedman, M. (1937). The use of ranks to avoid the assumption of normality implicit in the analysis of variance. *Journal of the American Statistical Association, 32,* 675–701.

Friedman, M. (1939). A correction: The use of ranks to avoid the assumption of normality implicit in the analysis of variance. *Journal of the American Statistical Association, 34*(205), 109.

Gaddis, G. M., & Gaddis, M. L. (1990). Introduction to biostatistics. Part 4: Statistical inference techniques in hypothesis testing. *Annals of Emergency Medicine, 19*(7), 137–142.

Gardner, P. L. (1975). Scales and statistics. *Review of Educational Research, 45,* 43–57.

Garson. (2006). Statnotes: An Introduction to Multivariate Analysis. Published online by Statistics Solutions, Inc., Retrieved from http://www.statisticssolutions.com/

Gift, A., Stommel, M., Jablonski, A., & Given, W. (2003). A cluster of symptoms over time in patients with lung cancer. *Nursing Research, 52*(6), 393–400.

Gilhotra, A., & McGhee, C. (2006). Ophthalmology and vision science research. Part 4: Avoiding rejection—Structuring a research paper from introduction to references. *Journal of Refractory Surgery, 32,* 151–157.

Ginzler, E. M., & Moldovan, I. (2004). Systemic lupus erythematosus trials: Successes and issues. *Current Opinion in Rheumatology, 16*(5), 499–504.

Glantz, S. A. (1997). *Primer of biostatistics.* New York, NY: McGraw-Hill.

Glass, G. V., & Hopkins, K. D. (1996). *Statistical methods in education and psychology* (3rd ed.). Boston: Allyn and Bacon.

Gliner, J. A., Morgan, G. A., & Harmon, R. J. (2002). Basic associational designs: analysis and interpretation. *Journal of the American Academy of Child and Adolescent Psychiatry, 41*(10) 1256–1258.

Gonzalez, R., & Griffen, D. (2001). Testing parameters in structural equation modeling: Every "one" matters. *Psychological Methods, 6*(3), 258–269.

Gosset, W. S. (Student). (1908). The probable error of a mean. *Biometrika, 6,* 1–25.

Grady, P. A. (2007). *NINR Director's Page.* Retrieved from http://www.ninr.nih.gov/AboutNINR/ NINRDirectorsPage/default.htm

Greenhouse, S.W., & Geisser, S. (1959). On methods in the analysis of profile data. *Psychometrika, 24,* 95–112.

Hagen, K. B., Jamtvedt, G., Hilde, G., & Winnem, M. F. (2005). The updated Cochrane Review of bed rest for low back pain and sciatica. *Spine, 30*(5), 542–546.

Hair, J. F., Black W. C., Babin B. J., & Anderson, R. E. (2009). *Multivariate data analysis* (7th ed.). Upper Saddle River, NJ: Prentice-Hall.

Halse, R. E., Wallman, K.E., & Guelfi, K. J. (2011). Post exercise water immersion increases short-term food intake in trained men. *Medicine & Science in Sports & Exercise, 43*(4), 632–638.

Hancock, G. R., & Freeman, M. J. (2001). Power and sample size for the root mean error of approximation test of not close fit in structural equation modeling. *Educational and Psychological Measurement, 61*(5), 741–758.

Harvey, R., Roth, E., Yarnold, P., Durham, J., & Green, D. (1992). Deep vein thrombosis in stroke: The use of plasma d-dimer level as a screening test in the rehabilitation setting. *Stroke, 27*(9), 1516–1520.

Hawkins, J. W., Pearce, C. W., Kearney, M. H., Munro, B. H., Haggerty, L. A., Dwyer, J., et al. (1996). Abuse, women's self-care, and pregnancy outcomes. Funded by the National Institute for Nursing Research, National Institutes of Health AREA grant 1 R15 NRO4246-01.

Hayduk, L. A. (1987). *Structural equation modeling with LISREL: Essentials and advances.* Baltimore, MD: Johns Hopkins University Press.

Hayduk, L. A. (1996). *LISREL issues, debates, and strategies.* Baltimore, MD: Johns Hopkins University Press.

Hegyvary, S. (2005). What every author should know about redundant and duplicate publication. *Journal of Nursing Scholarship, 37*(4), 295–297.

Heise, D. R. (1969). Problems in path analysis and causal inference. In E. F. Borgatta & G. W. Bohrnstedt (Eds.), *Sociology methodology.* San Francisco: Jossey-Bass.

Henson, R. K., & Roberts, J. K. (2006). Use of exploratory factor analysis in published research: Common errors and some comment on improved practice. *Educational and Psychological Measurement, 66,* 393–416.

Heymann, A., Chodick, G., Reichman, B., Kokia, E., & Laufer, J. (2004). Influence of school closure in the incidence of viral respiratory diseases among children and on health care utilization. *Pediatric Infectious Disease Journal, 23*(7), 675–677.

Hick, W. E. (1952). A note on one-tailed and two-tailed tests. *Psychological Review, 59,* 316–318.

Hildebrand, D. K. (1986). *Statistical thinking for behavioral scientists.* Boston, MA: Duxbury Press.

Hinkle, D.E., Wiersma, W., & Jurs, S.G. (1998). *Applied statistics for the behavioral sciences* (4th ed.). Boston: Houghton Mifflin Company.

Hu, L.-T., & Bentler, P. M. (1995). Evaluating model fit. In R. H. Hoyle (Ed.), *Structural equation modeling: Concepts, issues, and applications* (pp. 76–99). Thousand Oaks, CA: Sage.

Hu, L.-T., & Bentler, P. M. (1998). Fit indices in covariance structure modeling: Sensitivity to underparameterized model misspecification. *Psychological Methods, 3*(4), 424–453.

Hu, L.-T., Bentler, P. M. (1999). Cutoff criteria for fit indexes in covariance structure analysis: Conventional criteria versus new alternatives. *Structural Equation Modeling: A Multidisciplinary Journal, 6*(1), 1–55.

Hubberty, C. J. (1993). Historical origins of statistical testing practices: The treatment of Fisher versus Neyman-Pearson views in textbooks. *Journal of Experimental Education, 61,* 317–333.

Huebner, D. M., Neilands, T. B., Rebchook, G. M., & Kegeles, S. M. (2011). Sorting through chickens and eggs: A longitudinal examination of the associations between attitudes, norms, and sexual risk behavior. *Health Psychology, 30*(1), 110–118.

Huth, M. M., & Broome, M. E. (2007). A snapshot of children's postoperative tonsillectomy outcomes at home. *Journal of Surgical and Postoperative Nursing, 12*(3), 186–195.

International Committee of Medical Journal Editors. (2005). Retrieved http://www.icmje.org/over.

Jackson, D. L. (2007). The effect of the number of observations per parameter in misspecified confirmatory factor analytic models. *Structural Equation Modeling, 14*(1), 48–76.

James-Todd, T., Tahranifar, P., Rich-Edwards, J., Titievsky, L., & Terry, M. B. (2010). The impact of socioeconomic status across early life on age at menarche among a racially diverse population of girls. *Annals of Epidemiology, 20*(11), 836–842.

Janz, N., & Becker, M. (1984). The Health Belief Model: A decade later. *Health Education Quarterly, 11*(1), 1–47.

Jöreskog, K. G., & Sörbom, D. (1988). *LISREL 7: A guide to the program and applications.* Chicago: SPSS, Inc.

Kaplan, D. (1995). Statistical power in structural equation modeling. In R. H. Hoyle (Ed.), *Structural equation modeling: Concepts, issues, and applications.* Thousand Oaks, CA: Sage.

Kaplan, D., & Wenger, R. N. (1993). Asymptomatic independence and separability in covariance structure models. *Multivariate Behavioral Research, 28*(4), 483–498.

Kenny, D. (1979). *Correlation and causality.* New York: John Wiley & Sons.

Klardie, K. A., Johnson, J., McNaughton, M. A., & Meyers, W. (2004). Integrating the principles of evidence-based practice into clinical practice. *Journal of the American Academy of Nurse-Practitioners, 16*(3), 98–105.

Kleinbaum, D. G., Klein, M. (2002). *Logistic Regression: A Self-Learning Text* (3rd ed). New York: Springer.

Klockars, A. J., & Sax, G. (1991). Multiple comparisons In *Quantitative Applications in the Social Sciences Series,* 61. Newbury Park, CA: Sage.

Knafl, K. A., & Deatrick, J. A. (2003). Further refinement of the family management style framework. *Journal of Family Nursing, 9,* 232–256.

Knafl, G., Dixon, J., O'Malley, J., Grey, M., Deatrick, J., Gallo, A., & Knafl, K. (2009). Analysis of cross-sectional univariate measurements for family dyads using linear mixed modeling. *Journal of Family Nursing, 15*(2), 130–151. PMID: 19307316.

Knapp, T. R. (1990). Treating ordinal scales as interval scales: An attempt to resolve the controversy. *Nursing Research, 39,* 121–123.

Knapp, T. R. (1993). Treating ordinal scales as ordinal scales. *Nursing Research, 42,* 184–186.

Kolmogorov, A. N. (1956). *Foundations of the theory of probability.* (2nd ed.). New York, NY: Chelsea Publishing Company.

Koppes, S. (2005). *William Kruskal, Statistician, 1919-2005.* The University of Chicago News Office. Retrieved from http://www-news.uchicago.edu/releases/05/050427.kruskal.shtml

Kraemer, H (1992). *Evaluating medical tests: Objective and quantitative guidelines.* Newbury Park, CA: Sage.

Kraemer, H. C., Morgan, G., Leech, N., Gliner, J. A., Vaske, J., & Harmon, R. J. (2003). Measures of clinical significance. *Journal of the American Academy of Child and Adolescent Psychiatry, 42*(12), 1524–1529.

Kroenke, K., Spitzer, R., & Williams, J. (2003). The Patient Health Questionnaire-2: Validity of a two-item depression screener. *Medical Care, 41*(11), 1284–1292.

Kruskal, W. H., & Wallis, W. A. (1952). Use of ranks in one-criterion analysis of variance. *Journal of the American Statistical Association, 47,* 583–621. Errata (1953) in *Journal of the American Statistical Association, 48,* 907–911.

Kurlowicz, L. (1998). Perceived self-efficacy, functional ability, and depressive symptoms in older elective surgery patients. *Nursing Research, 47*(4), 219–226.

Kurmis, A. (2003). Contributing to research: The basic elements of a scientific manuscript. *Radiography, 9,* 277–282.

Kuzma, J. W., & Bohnenblust, S. E. (2001). *Basic statistics for the health sciences.* Mountain View, CA: Mayfield.

Kuzma, J. W., & Bohnenblust, S. E. (2005). *Basic statistics for the health sciences* (5th ed.). New York: McGraw-Hill.

Laposa, J. M., Alden, L. E., & Fullerton, L. M. (2003). Work stress and post-traumatic stress disorder. *Journal of Emergency Nursing, 29*(1), 23–28.

Learman, L. A., Gerrity, M. S., Field, D. R., et al. (2003). Effects of a depression education program on residents' knowledge, attitudes and clinical skills. *Obstetrics & Gynecology, 101*(1), 167–174.

Lenoci, J. M., Telfair, J., Cecil, H., & Edwards, R. R. (2002). Self-care in adults with sickle cell disease. *Western Journal of Nursing Research, 24,* 228–245.

Lenz, E. R., Pugh, L. C., Milligan, R. A., Gift, A., & Suppe, F. (1997). The middle-range theory of unpleasant symptoms: An update. *Advances in Nursing Science, 19*(3), 14–27.

Levine, M. D., Ringham, R. M., Kalarchian, M. A., Wisniewski, L., & Marcus, M. D. (2001). Is family-based behavioral weight control appropriate for severe pediatric obesity? *International Journal of Eating Disorder, 30,* 318–328.

L'Herault, J., Petroff, L., & Jeffrey, J. (2001). The effectiveness of a thermal mattress in stabilizing and maintaining body temperature during the transport of very low–birth weight newborns. *Applied Nursing Research, 14*(4), 210–219.

Likert, R., Roslow, R., & Murphy, G. (1934). A simple and reliable method of scoring the Thurstone attitude scales. *Journal of Social Psychology, 5*(2), 228–239.

Likourezos, A., Si, M., Kim, W. O., Simmons, S., Frank, J., & Neufeld, R. (2002). Health status and functional status in relationship to nursing home subacute rehabilitation program outcomes. *American Journal of Physical Medicine & Rehabilitation, 81*(5), 373–379.

Lindbeck, A. (1992). *Nobel lectures, economics 1969–1980.* Singapore: World Scientific Publishing Co.

Liu, H. E. (2006). Fatigue and associated factors in hemodialysis patients in Taiwan. *Research in Nursing and Health, 29,* 40–50.

Lochner, H. V., Bhandari, M., & Tornetta, P., III. (2001). Type-II error rates (beta errors) of randomized trials in orthopaedic trauma. *Journal of Bone and Joint Surgery, 83-A*(11), 1650–1655.

Ludbrook, J. (2004). Detecting systematic bias between two raters. *Clinical and Experimental Pharmacology and Physiology, 31*(1–2), 113–115.

Ludwig-Beymer, P., & Gerc, S. C. (2002). An influenza prevention campaign: The employee perspective. *Journal of Nursing Care Quality, 16*(3), 1–12.

MacCallum, R. C., Browne, M. W., & Suawara, H. M. (1996). Power analysis and determination of sample size for covariance structure modeling. *Psychological Methods, 1*(2), 130–149.

Mann, H. B., & Whitney, D. R. (1947). On a test of whether one of two random variables is stochastically larger than the other. *Annals of Mathematical Statistics, 18,* 50–60.

Marsh, H. W., Balla, J. R., & Hau, K. T. (1996). An evaluation of incremental fit indices: A clarification of mathematical and empirical properties. In G. A. Marcoulides & R. E. Schumacker (Eds.), Advanced structural equation modeling: Issues and techniques. Mahwah, NJ, Erlbaum, pp. 315–353.

Maydeu-Olivares, A. (2006). Limited information estimation and testing of discretized multivariate normal structural models. *Psychometrika, 71,* 57–77.

McCormack, B. (2003). Knowing and acting: A strategic practitioner-focused approach to nursing research and practice development [Focus]. *NT Research, 8*(2), 86–100.

McGhee, C., & Gilhotra, A. (2005). Ophthalmology and vision science research. Part 3: Avoiding writer's block—Understanding the ABCs of a good research paper. *Journal of Cataract Refractive Surgery, 31,* 2413–2419.

McNaughton, M. A., Klardie, K., Meyers, W., & Johnson, J. (2004). Integrating the principals of evidence-based practice: Testing and diagnosis. *Journal of the American Academy of Nurse-Practitioners, 16*(1), 2–7.

McNemar, Q. (1969). *Psychological statistics* (4th ed.). Hoboken, NJ: Wiley & Sons.

Meyers, W. C., Johnson, J. A., Klardie, K., & McNaughton, M. A. (2004). Integrating the principles of evidence-based practice: Prognosis and the metabolic syndrome. *Journal of the American Academy of Nurse Practitioners, 16*(5), 178–184.

Mezzacappa, E. S., Arumugam, U., Chen, S. Y., Stein, T. R., Oz, M., & Buckle, J. (2010). Coconut fragrance and cardiovascular response to laboratory stress. *Holistic Nursing Practice, 24*(6), 322–332.

Miles, K., Penny, N., Power, R., & Mercey, D. (2003). Comparing doctor and nurse-led care in a sexual health clinic: Patient satisfaction questionnaire. *Journal of Advanced Nursing, 42*(1), 64–72.

Miller, P. E. (2008). The relationship between job satisfaction and intention to leave of hospice nurses in a for-profit corporation. *Journal of Hospice and Palliative Nursing, 10*(4), 56–64.

Mitchell, J. C., & Counselman, F. L. (2003). A taste comparison of three different liquid steroid preparations: Prednisone, prednisolone, and dexamethasone. *Academic Emergency Medicine, 10*(4), 400–403.

Mood, A. M., Graybill, F. A., & Boes, D. (1974). *Introduction to the theory of statistics.* New York: McGraw-Hill.

Morgan, S., Reichert, T., & Harrison, T. (2002). *From numbers to words: Reporting statistical results for the social sciences.* Boston: Allyn and Bacon.

Moye, L. A., & Tita, A. T. N. (2002). Defending the rational for the two-tailed test in clinical research. *Circulation, 105,* 3062–3065.

Muthén, B. (2001). Second-generation structural equation modeling with a combination of categorical and continuous latent variables: New opportunities for latent class–latent growth modeling. In L. M. Collins, A. G. Sayer, L. M. Collins, & A. G. Sayer (Eds.), *New methods for the analysis of change* (pp. 291–322). Washington, DC: American Psychological Association.

Norris, A. E., & Devine, P. G. (1992). Linking pregnancy concerns to pregnancy risk avoidant action: The role of construct accessibility. *Personality and Social Psychology Bulletin, 18*(2), 118–192.

Norris, A. E., & Ford, K. (1995). Condom use by African American and Hispanic youth with a well-known partner: Integrating the Health Belief Model, Theory of Reasoned Action, and Construct Accessibility Model. *Journal of Applied Social Psychology, 25,* 1801–1830.

Norusis, M. J. (2003). *SPSS 12.0: Statistical procedures companion.* Upper Saddle River, NJ: Prentice-Hall.

nQuery (2007). Retrieved from http://www.statsol.ie/html/nQuery/nQuery_home.html

Nunnally, J. C., & Bernstein, I. H. (1994). *Psychometric theory* (3rd ed.). New York, NY: McGraw-Hill.

O'Connor, J. J., & Robertson, E. F. (2003). *William Sealy Gosset.* Retrieved from http://turnbull.mcs.st-and.ac.uk.

Ogden, T. E., & Goldberg, I. A. (2002). *Research proposals: A guide to success* (3rd ed.). San Diego: Academic Press.

Okusun, I. K., Chandra, K. M. D., Boev, A., et al. (2004). Abdominal adiposity in U.S. adults: Prevalence and trends, 1960–2000. *Preventive Medicine, 39,* 197–206.

Ostir, G. V., & Uchida, T. (2000). Logistic regression a non-technical review. *American Journal of Physical Medicine and Rehabilitation, 79*(6), 565–572.

Ott, L., & Mendenhall, W. (1990). *Understanding statistics* (5th ed.). Boston: PWS-Kent Publishing.

Ottenbacher, K. J., & Maas, F. (1999). How to detect effects: Statistical power and evidence-based practice in occupational therapy research. *American Journal of Occupational Therapy, 53*(2), 181–888.

Owen, S. V., & Froman, R. D. (1998). Uses and abuses of the analysis of covariance. *Research in Nursing & Health, 21,* 557–562.

Parshall, M. B. (2002). Psychometric characteristics of dyspnea descriptor ratings in emergency department patients with exacerbated chronic obstructive pulmonary disease. *Research in Nursing and Health, 25,* 331–344.

Paton, L. M., Alexander, J. L., Nowson, C. A., et al. (2002). Pregnancy and lactation have no long-term deleterious effect on measures of bone mineral in healthy women: A twin study. *American Journal of Clinical Nursing, 77,* 707–714.

Pearson, K. (1930). *The life, letters and labours of Francis Galton.* Cambridge, UK: Cambridge University Press.

Pedhazur, E. J. (1997). *Multiple regression in behavioral research, explanation and prediction* (3rd ed.). Orlando, FL: Harcourt Brace.

Pedhazur, E. J., & Schmelkin, L. P. (1991). *Measurement, design, and analysis: An integrated approach.* Hillsdale, NJ: Erlbaum.

Pender, N. J. (1987). *Health promotion in nursing practice* (2nd ed). Norwalk, CT: Appleton & Lange.

Penney, G., & Foy, R. (2007). Do clinical guidelines enhance safe practice in obstetrics and gynaecology? *Best Practice & Research Clinical Obstetrics and Gynaecology, 21*(4), 657–673.

Pettit, N. N., DePestel, D. D., Malani, P. N., & Riddell, J. (2010). Factors associated with seroconversion after standard dose hepatitis B vaccination and high-dose revaccination among HIV-infected patients. *HIV Clin Trials, 11*(6), 9–332.

Plichta, S. B., Vandecar-Burdin, T., Odor, K., Reams, S., & Zhang, Y. (2007). The emergency department and victims of sexual violence: An assessment of preparedness to help. *Journal of Health and Human Services Administration, 29*(3), 285–308.

Plichta, S., & Garzon, L. (2010). *Statistics for Nursing and Allied Health.* Philadelphia: Lippincott Williams & Wilkins.

Polit, D. F., & Beck, C. T. (2008). *Nursing research: Generating and assessing evidence for nursing practice* (8th ed.). Philadelphia: Lippincott Williams & Wilkins.

Purrington, C. B. (2011). *Advice on designing scientific posters.* Retrieved March 2011 from http://www.swarthmore.edu/NatSci/cpurrin1/posteradvice.htm

Rabius, V., McAlister, A. L., Geiger, A., & Huang, P. (2004). Telephone counseling increases cessation rates among young adult smokers. *Health Psychology, 23*(5), 539–541.

Radloff, L. S. (1977). The CES-D scale: A self-report depression scale for research in the general population. *Applied Psychological Measurement, 1,* 385–401.

Raftery, A. E. (1993). Bayesian model selection in structural equation models. In K. A. Bollen & J. S. Long (Eds.), *Testing stuctural equation models* (pp. 163–180). Beverly Hills, CA: Sage.

Raftery, A. E. (1995). Bayesian model selection in social research. In P. V. Marsden (Ed.), *Sociological methodology* (pp. 111–163). Cambridge: Basil Blackwell.

Roberts, S., & Martin, M. A. (2006). Using supervised principal components analysis to assess multiple pollutants effects. *Environmental Health Perspectives, 114,* 1877–1882.

Robinson, J. H. (1995). Grief responses, coping processes, and social support of widows: Research with Roy's model. *Nursing Science Quarterly, 8*(4), 158–164.

Rosenfeldt, F., Dowling, J., Pepe, S., & Fullerton, M. (2000). How to write a paper for publication. *Heart, Lung, and Circulation, 9,* 82–87.

Ryser, G. R., Campbell, H. L., & Miller, B. K. (2010). Confirmatory factor analysis of the scales for diagnosing attention deficit hyperactivity disorder (SCALES). *Educational and Psychological Measurement, 70*(5), 844–857.

Sakuta, H., Suzuki, T., Katayama, Y., Yasuda, H., & Ito, T. (2005). Heavy alcohol intake, homocysteine and type 2 diabetes. *Diabetic Medicine, 22,* 1359–1363.

Salsburg, D. (2001). *The lady tasting tea: How statistics revolutionized science in the twentieth century.* New York: W.H. Freeman.

Sapnas, K. G., & Zeller, R. A. (2002). Minimizing sample size when using exploratory factor analysis for measurement. *Journal of Nursing Measurement, 10,* 135–154.

Saris, W. E., & Satorra, A. (1993). Power evaluations in structural equation models. In K. A. Bollen & J. S. Long (Eds.), *Testing structural equation models* (pp. 181–204). Thousand Oaks, CA: Sage.

Satorra, A., & Bentler, P. M. (1994). Corrections to test statistics and standard errors in covariance structure analysis. In A. von Eye & C. C. Clogg (Eds.), *Latent variable analysis: Applications for developmental research* (pp. 399–419). Thousand Oaks, CA: Sage.

Schermelleh-Engel, K., Moosbrugger, H., & Müller, H. (2003). Evaluating the fit of structural equation models: Tests of significance and descriptive goodness-of-fit measures. *Methods of Psychological Research, 8*(2), 23–74.

Schilling, L.S., Dixon, J.K., Knafl, K.A., Grey, M., Ives, B., & Lynn, M. R.(2007). Determining content validity of a self-report instrument for adolescents using a heterogeneous expert panel. *Nursing Research, 56,* 361–366.

Schilling, L.S., Dixon, J.K., Knafl, K.A., Lynn, M.R., Murphy, K., Dumser, S., & Grey, M. (2009). A new self-report measure of self-management of Type 1 diabetes for adolescents. *Nursing Research, 58,* 228–236.

Schilling, L.S., Knafl, K. A., & Grey, M. (2006). Changing patterns of self-management in youth with type 1 diabetes. *Journal of Pediatric Nursing, 21*(6), 412–424.

Schmid, C. F. (1983). *Statistical graphics: Design principles and practices.* New York, NY: John Wiley & Sons.

Schroeder, M. A. (1990). Diagnosing and dealing with multicollinearity. *Western Journal of Nursing Research, 12*(2), 175–187.

Schulberg, H. C., Saul, M., Ganguli, M., Christy, W., & Frank, R. (1985). Assessing depression in primary medical and psychiatric practices. *Archives of General Psychiatry, 42*, 1164–1170.

Schumacker, R. E., & Lomax R. G. (2004). *A beginner's guide to structural equation modeling* (2nd ed.). Mahwah, NJ: Erlbaum.

Seaborg, E. (2007). *Reference ranges and what they mean.* Retrieved from http://www.labtestsonline.org/understanding/features/ref_ranges-6.html

Spearman, C. (1904). The proof and measurement of association between two things. *American Journal of Psychology, 15*, 86–92.

SPSS, Inc. (1999a). *SPSS Base 10.0 applications guide.* Chicago, IL: Author.

SPSS, Inc. (1999b). *SPSS Base 10.0 user's guide.* Chicago, IL: Author.

SPSS, Inc. (2006). *SPSS Base 15 user's guide.* Chicago: Author.

SPSS SamplePower. (2007). Retrieved from http://www.spss.com/samplepower/web_demo.htm

Stanton, J. M. (2001). Pearson, and the peas: A brief history of linear regression for statistics instructors. *Journal of Statistics Education, 9* (3). Retrieved from http://www.amstat.org/publications/jse/v9n3/stanton.html.

Stevens, S. S. (1946). On the theory of scales of measurement. *Science, 102*, 677–680.

Stevens, S. S. (1968). Measurement, statistics, and the schemapiric view. *Science, 161*, 849–856.

Stevens, S. S. (2001). Systematic reviews: The heart of evidence-based practice. *AACN Clinical Issues, 12*(4), 529–538.

Stewart, J. C., Janicki, D. L., & Karmarck, T. W. (2006). Cardiovascular reactivity to and recovery from psychological challenge as predictors of 3-year change in blood pressure. *Health Psychology, 25*(1), 111–118.

de Szendeffy, J. (2005). *A practical guide to using computers in language teaching.* Ann Arbor, MI: University of Michigan Press.

Tabachnick, B. G., & Fidel, L. S. (2006). *Using multivariate statistics* (5th ed). New York, NY: Allyn & Bacon.

Tanguma, J. (2001). Effects of sample size on the distribution of selected fit indices: A graphical approach. *Educational and Psychological Measurement, 61*(5), 759–776.

Tarkka, M. T. (2003). Predictors of maternal competence by first-time mothers when the child is 8 months old. *Journal of Advanced Nursing, 41*(3), 233–240.

Teijlingen, E., & Hundley, V. (2002). Getting your paper to the right journal: A case study of an academic paper. *Journal of Advanced Nursing, 37*(6), 506–511.

Templin, T., & Peters, R. (2002). *Rules for calculating degrees of freedom in structural equation modeling.* Paper presented at the annual meeting of the Midwest Nursing Research Society, Chicago, March 2002.

Thorpe, L., et al. (2009). Prevalence and control of diabetes and impaired fasting glucose in New York City. *Diabetes Care, 32*,57–62.

Thurstone, L. L. (1947). Multiple factor analysis. Chicago: University of Chicago Press.

Toothaker, L. E. (1993). Multiple comparison procedures In *Quantitative Applications in the Social Sciences*, 89. Newbury Park, CA: Sage.

Truong, K. D., & Sturm, R. (2005). Weight gain trends across sociodemographic groups in the United States. *American Journal of Public Health, 95*(9), 1602–1606.

Tucker, L. A., & Maxwell, K. (1992). Effects of weight training on the emotional well-being and body image of females: Predictors of greatest benefit. *American Journal of Health Promotion, 6*(6), 338–344.

Tufte, E. R. (1983). *The visual display of quantitative information.* Cheshire, CT: Graphics Press.

Tulman, L. R., & Jacobsen, B. S. (1989). Goldilocks and variability. *Nursing Research, 38*, 377–379.

U.S. Census Bureau. (2010). *2006-2008 American Community Survey 3-year estimates. S1201. Marital status.* Retrieved from http://factfinder.census.gov/servlet/STTable?_bm=y&-geo_id=01000US&-qr_name=ACS_2008_3YR_G00_S1201&-ds_name=ACS_2008_3YR_G00_.

U.S. Preventive Services Task Force. (2007). Retrieved from http://www.ahrq.gov/clinic/uspstfix.htm.

van der Akker-Scheek, I., Stevens, M., Spriensma, A., & van Horn, J. R. (2004). Goningen Orthopaedic Social Support Scale: Validity and reliability. *Journal of Advanced Nursing, 47*(1), 57–63.

Vaughan, E. D. (1998). Statistics: Tools for understanding data in the behavioral sciences. Upper Saddle River, NJ: Prentice-Hall.

Verran, J. A., & Ferketich, S. L. (1987). Testing linear model assumptions: Residual analysis. *Nursing Research, 36*(2), 127–129.

Vogt, W. P. (2005). *Dictionary of statistics & methodology: A nontechnical guide for the social sciences.* London, England: Sage.

Wallgren, A., Wallgren, B., Persson, R., Jorner, U., & Haaland J. (1996). *Graphing statistics & data creating better charts.* Thousand Oaks, CA: Sage.

Wang, L., Fan, X., & Willson, V. L. (1996). Effects of nonnormal data on parameter estimates and fit indices for a model with latent and manifest variables: An empirical study. *Structural Equation Modeling, 3*(3), 228–247.

Wang, S., Yu, M., Wang, C., & Huang, C. (1999). Bridging the gap between the pros and cons in treating ordinal scales as interval from an analysis point of view. *Nursing Research, 48*(4), 226–229

Weisberg. (1992). Central Tendency and Variation, monograph for the Sage series on Quantitative Applications in the Social Sciences. Newbury Park, CA: Sage.

Weng, L., Dai, Y., Huang, H., & Chiang, Y. (2010). Self-efficacy, self-care behaviours and quality of life of kidney transplant recipients. *Journal of Advanced Nursing, 66*(4), 828–838.

West, S. G., Finch, J. F., & Curran, P. J. (1995). Structural equation models with non-normal variables: Problems and remedies. In R. H. Hoyle (Ed.), *Structural equation modeling: Concepts, issues, and applications* (pp. 56–75). Thousand Oaks, CA: Sage.

White, H., McConnel, E. S., Bales, C. W., & Kuchibhatla, M. (2004). A 6-month observational study of the relationship between weight loss and behavioral symptoms in institutionalized Alzheimer's disease subjects. *Journal of the American Medical Directors Association, 5*, 89–97.

Wilks, S., & Vonk, M. (2008). Private prayer among Alzheimer's caregivers: Mediating burden and resiliency. *Journal of Gerontological Social Work, 50*(3–4), 113–131.

Wills, T. A., Pokhrel, P., Morehouse, E., & Fenster, B. (2011). Behavioral and emotional regulation and adolescent substance use problems: A test of moderation effects in a dual-process model. *Psychology of Addictive Behaviors*. Advance online publication.

Winer, B. J. (1971). *Statistical principles in experimental design* (2nd ed.). New York, NY: McGraw-Hill.

Wright, S. (1934). The method of path coefficients. *Annals of Mathematical Statistics, 5*(September), 161–215.

Wood, M. J. (2006). *Basic steps in planning nursing research: From question to proposal* (6th ed.). Boston: Jones & Bartlett.

Wood, R. Y., Duffy, M. E., Morris, S. J., & Carnes. J. E. (2002). The effect of an educational intervention on promoting breast self-examination in older African American and Caucasian women. *Oncology Nursing Forum, 29*(7), 1087.

Woo, J., Hong, A., Lau, E., & Lynn, H. (2007). A randomized controlled trial of Tai Chi and resistance exercise on bone health, muscle strength and balance in community-living elderly people. *Age and Aging, 36*(3), 262–268. World Health Organization. (2000). *Obesity: Preventing and managing the global epidemic. Report of a WHO Consultation* (WHO Technical Report Series 894). Geneva: Author.

Wright, S. (1934). The method of path coefficients. *Annals of Mathematical Statistics, 5*(September), 161–215.

Yang-Wallentin, F., & Jöreskog, K. G. (2001). Robust standard errors and chi-squares for interaction models. In G. A. Marcoulides & R. E. Schumacker (Eds.), *New developments and techniques in structural equation modeling* (pp. 159–171). Mahwah, NJ: Erlbaum.

Yang, Y., & Dunson, D. (2010). Bayesian semi parametric structural equation models with latent variables. *Psychometrika, 75*(4), 675–693.

Yang, Y., & Green, S. B. (2010). A note on structural equation modeling estimates of reliability. *Structural Equation Modeling, 17*(1), 66–81.

Page numbers followed by "t" indicate table; those followed by "f" indicate figure.